D1293953

Pathology
of the
Placenta

OTHER MONOGRAPHS IN THE SERIES
MAJOR PROBLEMS IN PATHOLOGY

VIRGINIA A. LIVOLSI, M.D.
Series Editor

Published

Forthcoming

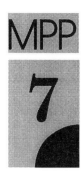

MPP

7

HAROLD FOX
M.D., F.R.C.Path., F.R.C.O.G.

Emeritus Professor of Reproductive Pathology
Department of Pathological Sciences
The University of Manchester
Manchester, England

Pathology of the Placenta

Volume 7 in the Series

MAJOR PROBLEMS IN PATHOLOGY

second edition

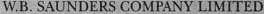

W.B. SAUNDERS COMPANY LIMITED
A Division of Harcourt Brace & Company
LONDON PHILADELPHIA TORONTO SYDNEY TOKYO

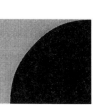

This book is printed on acid-free paper

W. B. Saunders   24–28 Oval Road
Company Ltd   London, NW1 7DX

The Curtis Center
Independence Square West
Philadelphia, PA 19106–3399, USA

Harcourt Brace & Company
55 Horner Avenue
Toronto, Ontario, M8Z 4X6, Canada

Harcourt Brace & Company, Australia
30–52 Smidmore Street
Marrickville
NSW 2204, Australia

Harcourt Brace & Company, Japan
Ichibancho Central Building, 22-1 Ichibancho
Chiyoda-ku, Tokyo 102, Japan

© 1997 W. B. Saunders Company Ltd

First edition published 1978

All rights reserved. No part of this publication may be reproduced, stored in
a retrieval system or transmitted, in any form or by any means, electronic,
mechanical, photocopying or otherwise, without the prior permission of
W. B. Saunders Company Ltd, 24–28 Oval Road, London NW1 7DX

A catalogue record for this book is available from the British Library

ISBN 0-7020-2196-2

Typeset by Saxon Graphics Ltd, Derby
Printed by The Bath Press, Bath

Preface to the First Edition

The placenta is one of the most readily available of all human organs, but it is not often routinely subjected to detailed and critical pathological scrutiny; this is largely because the view that placental pathology is difficult to interpret and can rarely be correlated with events during pregnancy is one that has gained a wide and enduring credence in many pathological laboratories. Until about twenty-five years ago there was some justification for this attitude, for a technique of placental examination had not been established and descriptions of placental pathology were characterized chiefly by their undue emphasis on gross abnormalities, their lack of accurate histopathological detail, and their use of an archaic and misleading terminology. During the last quarter of a century the placenta has, however, increasingly attracted the attention of workers from a wide range of scientific disciplines, and as a result of their labour it is now possible to give, as I have attempted to do in this volume, a logical and systematic account of placental pathology.

This book is directed principally towards pathologists, but I would hope that it conveys my belief that pathology is concerned as much with function as with morphology. I have, it is true, dwelt at some length on the morbid anatomy of the placenta, but I have also attempted to assess the functional significance and the clinical implications of the various structural changes; indeed, I have been at pains to stress that a lesion, no matter how impressive it may be in morphological terms, cannot be regarded as important unless it can be shown to impair placental function to an extent that the continuing growth and well-being of the fetus is endangered. Because of this attitude I have perhaps been guilty of introducing some repetition into the text, for before discussing the overall pattern of placental abnormalities in specific complications of gestation I have thought it necessary to consider first, as discrete entities, each of the individual abnormalities that form the components of this pattern; I do not feel unduly apologetic about this, for the degree of confusion in the past about the pathogenesis and functional significance of placental lesions has been such as to make it worthwhile sacrificing brevity for clarity.

I have tried throughout to review, in a fairly full fashion, the published work on each aspect of placental pathology, but I have not hesitated to quote my own observations and opinions. I did not feel that I was able to do this on the subject of trophoblastic neoplasia, of which I have had very little personal experience. I have therefore been extremely fortunate in obtaining the agreement of Dr C.W. Elston to contribute a chapter on this topic and I am most grateful to him.

My ultimate hope in writing this text on the placenta is that it may encourage an increasing number of pathologists to share my interest in this short-lived but multi-faceted and fascinating organ, a study of which, though by necessity usually retrospective in nature, yields so much information about the gestation from which it has been derived and the dangers to which the growing fetus has been subject.

August, 1977

H. Fox

Preface to the Second Edition

It is 19 years since the first edition of this book. During that time interval scientific interest in the placenta has greatly increased, fuelled by such events as the formation of the European Placenta Group, the resurgence of the Rochester Trophoblast Conferences and the successful foundation of the journal *Placenta*. Basic understanding of the cell biology, molecular biology, biochemistry, physiology, pharmacology and immunobiology of the placenta has increased almost exponentially and it is a matter of regret that relatively little of this accrual of knowledge is reflected in this book. This is not because of my lack of interest in such basic science (or, as perhaps some would maintain, my lack of understanding) but because very little of this information appears to be of direct relevance to the diagnostic histopathologist, for whom this volume is principally intended, when called upon to examine a placenta.

Interest in the placenta by pathologists has also increased but, regrettably, this interest has been driven almost as much by the demands of litigation as it has by concern with the role played by the placenta in fetal development and well-being. Indeed, the pendulum has swung from an almost total neglect of the placenta by pathologists to a near deistic belief that all the problems of pregnancy can be accounted for by pathological examination of the placenta. The truth, as always, lies somewhere in between these two extreme views and I have attempted to provide a balanced account of placental pathology as seen through what I hope are the realistic, though possibly slightly iconoclastic, eyes of a diagnostic histopathologist.

The text of this new edition has been thoroughly updated, indeed largely rewritten, and I have attempted, as before, to provide a fairly full review of the relevant literature. One change has been that the chapter on gestational trophoblastic disease has been written by myself rather than, as in the first edition, by Christopher Elston. This is partly because of the enormous demands placed upon Professor Elston to write on other topics and partly because my previous inexperience in this slightly esoteric field of placental pathology has now been rectified.

I hope that this volume will be of help to the diagnostic histopathologist when required, often quite unrealistically, by obstetricians to provide an explanation for an adverse fetal outcome and will be of value to pathologists in critically evaluating the placenta for medico-legal purposes.

H. Fox

Acknowledgements

Professor F. A. Langley died in 1995 but my debt of gratitude to him for originally stimulating my interest in the placenta remains undiminished. Any faults, and I have no doubt that there are many, in my scientific and pathological development have been entirely of my own making but any virtues were installed by Frederick Langley. His scientific integrity and curiosity, allied to a degree of iconoclasm, have served as a personal touchstone to me and I am proud to have followed in his footsteps.

Help has been afforded me by Linda Chawner in the preparation of new microphotographs, whilst Carolyn Jones has been unstinting in her aid, particularly in the drawing of line diagrams. Hazel Morgan and Wilma Lamb have proved assiduous in the tracing of references.

I have to thank Sean Duggan of W. B. Saunders Company for his help, encouragement and, above all, patience. This latter quality has also been displayed by my wife who has had to endure, with considerable forbearance, months of my sitting crouched morosely over a word processor and the presence of vast mounds of paper in all nooks and crannies of her house.

H. Fox

Acknowledgements for Illustrations

Chapter One
   Figures 1.1, 1.4 and 1.5. Courtesy of Dr P. Wilkin. Figure 1.17. Courtesy of the late Dr F. Bøe. Figure 1.26. Courtesy of Dr J. S. Wigglesworth and by kind permission of the Editors of *British Journal of Obstetrics and Gynaecology* and of *Nature*. Figure 1.11. By kind permission of the Editor of *Journal of Pathology*. Figures 1.12 and 1.16 are modifications of diagrams originally published by Professor P. Kaufmann and were, with his permission, redrawn by Dr C. J. P. Jones. Figures 1.9, 1.13, 1.14, 1.32, 1.33, 1.36 and 1.37. Courtesy of Dr C. J. P. Jones. Figures 1.28, 1.29, 1.30 and 1.31. By kind permission of the Editor of *European Journal of Obstetrics, Gynecology and Reproductive Biology* and of Elsevier/North Holland Biomedical Press B.V.

Chapter Two
   Figure 2.1. Courtesy of Dr R. Thau. Figure 2.2. Courtesy of Dr J. Dancis.

Chapter Three
   Figure 3.7. Courtesy of Dr J. Pryse-Davies and by kind permission of the Editor of *British Journal of Obstetrics and Gynaecology*. Figure 3.12. By kind permission of the Editor of *Obstetrical and Gynecological Survey* and Williams and Wilkins Company, Baltimore.

Chapter Four
   Figures 4.1, 4.3 and 4.5. Courtesy of Dr A. H. Cameron. Figure 4.2 Courtesy of Dr E. S. E. Hafez. Figure 4.4. Courtesy of Dr N. F. Th. Arts. Figure 4.6. Reproduced from *Haines and Taylor: Textbook of Obstetrical and Gynaecological Pathology* (H. Fox ed.), by permission of Dr A. H. Cameron and Churchill Livingstone. Figures 4.7 and 4.8. Courtesy of Dr V. J. Baldwin (Vancouver). Figure 4.9. Courtesy of Dr H. G. Kohler. Figure 4.10. Courtesy of Dr M. Shannon Allen Jr. Figure 4.13. By kind permission of Dr G. Corney, the Editor of *Annals of Human Genetics*, and the Cambridge University Press.

Chapter Five
   Figures 5.1, 5.3, 5.7, 5.9, 5.19, 5.35, 5.36, 5.44 and 5.46. By kind permission of the Editor of *British Journal of Obstetrics and Gynaecology*. Figures 5.2 and 5.6. From Fox, H. (1967). Perivillous fibrin deposition in the human placenta. *American Journal of Obstetrics and Gynecology*, volume 98, pp. 245–251. By kind permission of C. V. Mosby Company. Figure 5.4. By kind permission of the Editor of *Journal of Clinical Pathology*. Figures 5.26 and 5.27. Courtesy of Professor J. S. Scott and by kind permission of the Editor of *British Journal of Obstetrics and Gynaecology*. Figures 5.13, 5.14, 5.16 and 5.18. By kind permission of the Editor of *Biology of the Neonate* and S. Karger A. G., Basel. Figure 5.23. Courtesy of Dr J. E. Gillan (Dublin) and reproduced with the permission of the Editor of *Placenta*. Figures 5.15, 5.34, 5.39 and 5.42. Courtesy of Professor F. A. Langley and by kind permission of the Editor of *Journal of Clinical Pathology*. Figure 5.45. Courtesy of Dr J. G. B. Russell.

Chapter Six

Figures 6.2, 6.3, 6.5, 6.7, 6.11, 6.12, 6.13, 6.21 and 6.23. By kind permission of the Editor of *British Journal of Obstetrics and Gynaecology*. Figures 6.9 and 6.17. By kind permission of the Editor of *Journal of Pathology*. Figure 6.19. By kind permission of the Editor of *Obstetrics and Gynecology*. Figure 6.24. Reproduced with the permission of the Editor of *Placenta*. Figures 6.27, 6.28. Courtesy of Professor W. B. Robertson and by kind permission of the Editor of *European Journal of Obstetrics, Gynecology and Reproductive Biology* and of Elsevier/North Holland Biomedical Press B.V.

Chapter Seven

Figures 7.1, 7.2, 7.3 and 7.4. By kind permission of the Editor of *British Journal of Obstetrics and Gynaecology*. Figures 7.8 and 7.9. Courtesy of Dr C. J. P. Jones.

Chapter Eight

Figure 8.2 By kind permission of the Editor of *Journal of Clinical Pathology*. Figures 8.6 and 8.7. Courtesy of Dr C. J. P. Jones. Figures 8.10, 8.11 and 8.12. By kind permission of the Editor of *Obstetrics and Gynecology*. Figures 8.13 and 8.14. By kind permission of the Editor of *Journal of Pathology*. Figure 8.15. Courtesy of Dr H. G. Kohler. Figure 8.16. Reproduced with the permission of the Editor of *Placenta*.

Chapter Nine

Figures 9.1, 9.2, 9.3 and 9.4. By kind permission of the Editor of *British Journal of Obstetrics and Gynaecology*. Figures 9.12, 9.13, 9.14, 9.16 and 9.17. Courtesy of Dr C. J. P. Jones and with the permission of the Editor of *Placenta*.

Chapter Ten

Figure 10.2. Courtesy of Dr. D. I. Rushton. Figures 10.3, 10.7 and 10.8. Courtesy of Dr L. H. Honoré and by kind permission of the Editor of *Teratology*. Figures 10.10 and 10.11. Courtesy of Dr B. Gustavii and by kind permission of the Editor of *Acta Obstetrica et Gynecologica Scandinavica*.

Chapter Eleven

Figures 11.1, 11.9, 11.10, 11.15, 11.18, 11.21, 11.22 and 11.24 are reproduced from *Haines and Taylor Obstetrical and Gynaecological Pathology* (H. Fox, ed.) by courtesy of Professor P. Russell (Sydney) and with permission of Churchill Livingstone. Figures 11.7 and 11.16. Courtesy of Professor F. A. Langley. Figure 11.8. Courtesy of Dr H. G. Kohler. Figure 11.11 is from material supplied by Professor J. S. Wigglesworth (London). Figures 11.12 and 11.13, courtesy of Dr J. W. Keeling (Edinburgh). Figure 11.14 is from material supplied by Dr A. J. Barson (Manchester). Figures 11.19, 11.20, 11.23 and 11.25, courtesy of Dr A. G. P. Garcia (Rio de Janeiro). Figure 11.26 is from material supplied by Dr A. G. P. Garcia (Rio de Janeiro). Figures 11.28 and 11.29, courtesy of Dr V. J. Baldwin (Vancouver).

Chapter Thirteen

Figures 13.1, 13.5 and 13.6. By kind permission of the Editors of *Journal of Clinical Pathology* and of *Obstetrical and Gynecological Survey* and Williams and Wilkins Company, Baltimore. Figure 13.7. By kind permission of the Editor of *Journal of Clinical Pathology*. Figure 13.9. From material supplied by Dr E. Jauniaux (London). Figure 13.10. By kind permission of the Editor of *Journal of Pathology*. Figures 13.11A and 11.12. From material supplied by Professor P. Russell (Sydney). Figure 13.15. Courtesy of Dr I. Jurkovic and by kind permission of Avicenum (Czechoslovak Medical Press). Figure 13.17. Courtesy of Dr H. G. Kohler.

Chapter Fourteen

Figures 14.1, 14.2, 14.10, 14.11, 14.13 and 14.35 have been previously published in *Gynecologic Oncology* (Eds Shingleton, H.M., Fowler, W.C., Jordan, J.A. and Lawrence, W.D.) and are reproduced by courtesy of the publishers. Figure 14.13 was originally supplied by Professor D. O'B. Hourihane (Dublin). Figure 14.3. Reproduced by kind permission of the Editor of *British Journal of Obstetrics and Gynaecology*. Figures 14.4, 14.5, 14.21, 14.22, 14.23 and 14.34. Reproduced from *Haines and Taylor: Obstetrical and Gynaecological Pathology* (H. Fox, ed.) by courtesy of Professor C. W. Elston and with permission from Churchill Livingstone. Figures 14.6 and 14.7. Reproduced by permission of Dr F. J. Paradinas (London), the Editor of *Current Diagnostic Pathology* and Churchill Livingstone. Figures 14.14, 14.16, 14.18, 14.20, 14.26, 14.36 and 14.37. by kind permission of the Editor of *Journal of Clinical Pathology*.

Chapter Fifteen
Figure 15.1A. By kind permission of the Editor of *Journal of Pathology*. Figure 15.7. Courtesy of Dr A. J. Barson. Figures 15.5, 15.6 and 15.9. Courtesy of Dr H. G. Kohler.

Chapter Sixteen
Figures 16.3, 16.4 and 16.6. Courtesy of Dr H. G. Kohler. Figure 16.5. Courtesy of Dr E. Gregersen and by kind permission of the Editor of *Acta Obstetrica et Gynecologica Scandinavica*. Figure 16.7. Courtesy of Dr J. O. W. Beilby and by kind permission of the Editor of *British Journal of Obstetrics and Gynaecology*.

Appendices
Figures A1.1, A1.2 and A1.3. By kind permission of the Editor of *British Journal of Obstetrics and Gynaecology*.

Contents

1

THE DEVELOPMENT AND STRUCTURE OF THE PLACENTA

It is traditional for monographs devoted to the pathology of a particular organ to have an introductory chapter in which the development and structure of that organ are described. Such a chapter gives the author a satisfying feeling of completeness, though one suspects that this is often only at the cost of an undue effort which is rarely rewarded by the close attention of his or her readers, who tend not to dwell on the finer points of normal anatomy. The temptation not to observe this tradition is one that I have reluctantly been forced to resist, for a true understanding of many aspects of placental pathology demands a sound knowledge of placental structure and development. The author faced with describing the normal structure of the placenta can, however, only look with some degree of envy at the relative ease with which more fortunate colleagues, called upon to consider the anatomy of organs such as the kidney or heart, can approach their task, because these organs have a fairly static structure that changes little with the passage of time. By contrast, the placenta, though having an exceptionally short lifespan, is in an almost constant state of morphological flux, and its histological appearances alter profoundly as gestation proceeds; furthermore the placenta, unlike most other organs, varies considerably from one area to another.

This account will, however, be relatively short and will concentrate only upon those aspects of placental anatomy that are of direct relevance to the diagnostic histopathologist.

EARLY DEVELOPMENT OF THE PLACENTA (Fig. 1.1)

The ovum is fertilized in the Fallopian tube and reaches the uterine cavity as a morula, which rapidly converts into a blastocyst and loses its surrounding zona pellucida. Following attachment to the endometrium, the outer cell layer of the blastocyst, particularly that at the implantation pole, proliferates to form the trophoblastic cell mass, from which cells infiltrate between those of the endometrial epithelium; the latter degenerate and the trophoblast thus comes into direct contact with the endometrial stroma, this apparently simple but actually extremely complex process of implantation (Denker, 1990; Aplin, 1991) being completed by the 10th or 11th post-ovulatory day. In the 7-day ovum the trophoblast forms a plaque which rapidly differentiates into two layers: an inner layer of large clear mononuclear cytotrophoblastic cells and an outer layer of multinucleated syncytiotrophoblast. That the syncytiotrophoblast is derived from the cytotrophoblast, not only at this early stage but also throughout gestation, is

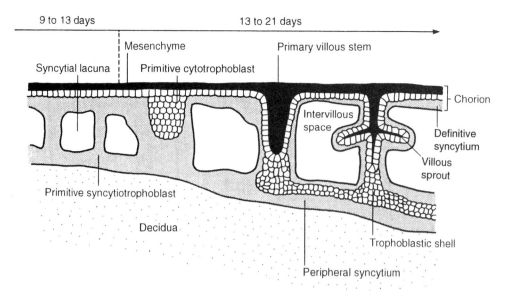

Figure 1.1. Diagrammatic representation of the early development of the placenta.

now well established, for even when the trophoblast is growing rapidly, synthesis of DNA occurs only in the nuclei of the cytotrophoblastic cells and it is only in these cells that mitotic figures are seen (Richart, 1961; Galton, 1962; Weinberg et al, 1970; Geier et al, 1975; Tedde & Tedde-Piras, 1978; Kaufmann et al, 1983; Arnholdt et al, 1991). It would appear that the syncytiotrophoblast is formed by fusion of cytotrophoblastic cells, because although no intercellular membranes can normally be seen in the syncytial layer, remnants of such membranes can occasionally be found with the aid of the electron microscope (Carter, 1964; Enders, 1965). Cells and nuclei of a type intermediate in morphology between those usually seen in the two trophoblastic layers have also been identified by electron microscopy (Terzakis, 1963; Tighe et al, 1967). It is perhaps worth noting that the syncytiotrophoblast is the only true syncytial tissue to occur in the human: this must confer a biological advantage on the trophoblast, though the nature of this is unknown. Contractor et al (1977) have suggested that in teleological terms the lack of any necessity for the syncytiotrophoblast to synthesize DNA and undergo mitotic activity allows the full metabolic activity of the tissue to be directed to its transfer function.

Between the 10th and 13th post-ovulatory days a series of intercommunicating clefts, or lacunae, appear in the rapidly enlarging trophoblastic cell mass; these clefts are possibly formed as a result of the engulfment within the syncytiotrophoblast of endometrial capillaries (Harris & Ramsey, 1966). The lacunae soon become confluent to form the precursor of the intervillous space, and it has been widely thought that as maternal vessels are progressively engulfed, or eroded, this becomes filled with maternal blood (Ramsey & Donner, 1980). It has, however, been suggested in recent years that at this stage only maternal plasma perfuses the intervillous space, a true maternal blood flow into this space not becoming established until the 12th week of gestation (Hustin et al, 1988; Schaaps & Hustin, 1988; Hustin, 1995; Jauniaux et al, 1995), a view not without its critics (Moll, 1995). The lacunae are incompletely separated from each other by trabecular columns of syncytiotrophoblast, which, between the 14th and 20th post-ovulatory days, tend to become radially orientated and come to possess a central cellular core that is produced by proliferation of the cytotrophoblastic cells at the chorionic base. These trabecular columns (Fig. 1.2A) are not true villi but serve as the framework from which villi will later develop; the placenta at this stage is a labyrinthine rather than a villous organ and the trabeculae are therefore best called 'primary villous stems' (Boyd & Hamilton, 1970). Continued growth of the cytotrophoblast leads to its distal extension into the region of decidual attachment. At the same time, a mesenchymal core appears within the villous stems; this is formed by a distal extension of the extraembryonic mesenchyme (Fig. 1.2B). Later, the villous stems become vascularized, the vessels arising within the stem and not, as previously thought, being formed as a downward extension of the chorio-allantoic arteries. Angiogenesis within the stems is almost certainly a function of the mesenchymal tissue (Dempsey, 1972; Demir et al, 1989), though it has been suggested that the vessels are formed by the cytotrophoblastic cells (Hertig, 1935; Cibils, 1968). In due course the vessels within the stems establish functional continuity with others differentiating from the body stalk and inner chorionic mesenchyme.

The distal part of the villous stem is formed almost entirely by cytotrophoblast which is not invaded by mesenchyme and not vascularized but which is anchored to the decidua of the basal plate. These cells, which form what are sometimes referred to as the 'cytotrophoblastic cell columns', proliferate and spread laterally to form a continuous cytotrophoblastic shell which splits the syncytiotrophoblast into two layers: the definitive syncytium on the fetal aspect of the shell and the peripheral syncytium between the shell and the decidua. The definitive syncytium persists as the limiting layer of the intervillous space, but the peripheral syncytium degenerates and is replaced by a layer of fibrinoid material (Nitabuch's layer). Cytotrophoblastic cells emigrate from the shell into the myometrium, where they give rise to syncytial-like giant cells which extensively colonize the placental bed (Robertson & Warner, 1974). Furthermore, cytotrophoblastic cells invade and replace the endothelium of the decidual portion of the maternal spiral arteries and disrupt the arterial wall, with the replacement of most of the muscular media by fibrinoid material (Hamilton & Boyd, 1966; Harris & Ramsey, 1966; Robertson et al, 1975). The subsequent development of the uteroplacental vasculature is discussed in a later section of this chapter.

The establishment of the trophoblastic shell is a mechanism to allow for rapid circumferential growth of the developing placenta. This leads to an expansion of the intervillous space, into which sprouts extend from the primary villous stems (Castellucci et al, 1990). These offshoots consist initially only of syncytiotrophoblast, but as they grow they pass through the stages previously seen during the development of the

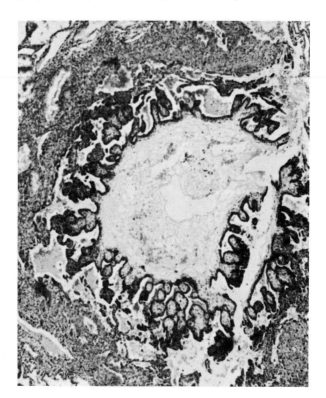

Figure 1.2A. A developing conceptus approximately 14 days after fertilization. Trabecular primary villous stems are arranged radially and divide the precursor of the intervillous space into a labyrinth (H & E ×32).

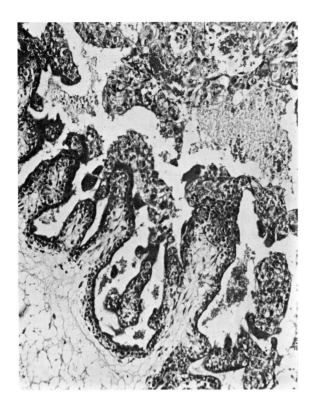

Figure 1.2B. Detail of primary villous stems in a 14-day-old conceptus. The stems have a mesenchymal core and the growing tip of each stem is formed by a mass of proliferating cytotrophoblastic cells (H & E ×90).

primary villous stems, i.e. intrusion of cytotrophoblast, formation of a mesenchymal core and eventual vascularization (Fig. 1.3). These sprouts form the primary villi and, as they are true villous structures, by the 21st day of gestation the placenta is a vascularized villous organ. Between this date and the end of the fourth month of pregnancy those villi orientated towards the uterine cavity degenerate and form the chorion laeve, whilst the thin rim of decidua covering this area gradually disappears to allow the chorion laeve to come into contact with the parietal decidua of the opposite wall of the uterus. The villi on the side of the chorion towards the decidua basalis proliferate and progressively arborize to form the chorion frondosum, which develops into the definitive placenta. During this period there is some regression of the cytotrophoblastic elements in the chorionic plate and in the trophoblastic shell, where the cytotrophoblastic cell columns degenerate and are largely replaced by fibrinoid material (Rohr's layer); however, clumps of cells remain to form the 'cytotrophoblastic cell islands'.

The placental septa appear during the third gestational month; these protrude into the intervillous space from the basal plate and divide the maternal surface of the placenta into 15 to 20 lobes. It has been much disputed in the past as to whether the septa are of maternal or fetal origin, but the available evidence now indicates that they are simply folds of the basal plate, being partly formed as a result of regional variability in placental growth and partly by the pulling up of the basal plate into the intervillous space by anchoring columns that have a poor growth rate (Boyd & Hamilton, 1966). As the basal plate is formed principally by the remnants of the trophoblastic shell embedded in fibrinoid (Kaufmann & Stark, 1971; Pisarki et al, 1975), it follows that the septa are similarly formed; some decidual cells may also be present and the relative proportions of fetal and maternal elements vary not only from septum to septum but also in different areas of individual septa (Boyd & Hamilton, 1970). The cytotrophoblastic cells, which predominate in both the basal plate and the septa, have often been referred to as 'X-cells', but their fetal origin has now been clearly confirmed both by electron microscopy (Glienke, 1974) and by studies using the quinacrine fluorescence technique to show that they always contain a Y chromosome if the fetus is male (Khudr et al, 1973;

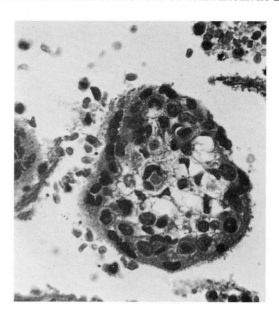

Figure 1.3. A primary stem villus in cross-section. There is a central mesenchymal core and an outer double-layered mantle of trophoblast (H & E ×180).

Maidman et al, 1973). The septa are therefore simply an incidental by-product of the architectural refashioning of the placenta and have no physiological or morphological role to play.

By the end of the fourth month of pregnancy the placenta has attained its definitive form and undergoes no further anatomical modifications. It has also achieved its full thickness, though growth in circumference continues virtually to the end of pregnancy, almost entirely as a result of progressive growth and development of the villous 'tree'.

STRUCTURE OF THE FETAL PLACENTA

The Placental Lobule

The fetal placenta is formed by several subunits, probably about 200, which have been variously titled but are now usually called 'lobules'. I use this term in preference to 'placentone', which is favoured by many German authors (Schuhmann, 1981) but which appears to me to be less descriptive. The current concept of the anatomy of the lobule is largely derived from the injection studies of Wilkin (1954, 1965), who showed it to have a structure which is comparable to that of a hollow drum (Fig. 1.4). Thus the primary stem villi break up just below the chorial plate into several secondary stem villi, which, after running for a short distance parallel to the chorionic surface, divide into a series of tertiary stem villi. The lobules are formed by these tertiary stem villi, which sweep down through the intervillous space towards the basal plate into which they insert, and then turn back upon themselves to re-enter the intervillous space; here they break up into branches which form the terminal villous network. The network is augmented by branches given off directly from the tertiary stem villi during their downward course towards the basal plate. As the tertiary stem villi run down through the intervillous space, they are arranged in a circular fashion around the periphery of an imaginary cylindrical core, this central area being relatively empty and villus-free (Fig. 1.5).

Gruenwald and his colleagues (Gruenwald, 1973, 1975a,b; Papalia-Early & Gruenwald, 1976), although agreeing in general terms with Wilkin's views, differed from him in considering that an individual lobule is not derived from a single secondary stem villus but can receive tertiary stem villi from several secondary stem villi. This is probably true, but it is a relatively minor point which does not alter significantly

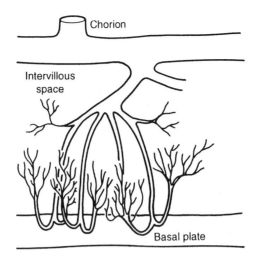

Figure 1.4. Diagram of the structure of a fetal lobule with primary stem villi dividing into secondary and tertiary stem villi.

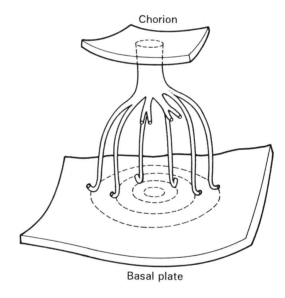

Figure 1.5. Three-dimensional concept of the fetal lobule, with the stem villi arranged in a circular fashion around a central hollow core.

the concept of the lobule. Adjacent lobules may be partially fused but are usually separated from each other by loosely textured interlobular areas that are in continuity with the subchorial lake.

It is necessary at this point to consider the meaning of the term 'cotyledon' as applied to the human placenta. This name should not be applied to the lobes seen on the maternal surface of the placenta, as these are merely the areas lying between the septa and lack any other morphological significance. The term 'cotyledon', if used at all, should be restricted to the functional unit of the fetal villous tree and this is best defined as being that part of the villous tree that has arisen from a single primary stem villus (Ramsey, 1959). According to Wilkin (1965), a single primary stem villus may give rise to a varying number of lobules, and hence there is no fixed relationship between cotyledons and lobules. Thus centrally placed cotyledons may contain as many as five lobules, whilst those more peripherally sited usually have only one or two. The situation has been made unduly confusing by the fact that some workers have described the lobule as a 'cotyledon', whilst others have referred to the same structure as a 'subcotyledon'; it is also worth noting that the structure described in this account as a 'lobule' is referred to by Gruenwald (1975a) as a 'cotyledon', and that defined here as a 'cotyledon' is considered by him as a 'lobule'. It would appear that Ramsey's (1975) suggestion that the term 'cotyledon' be abandoned when referring to the primate placenta has much to recommend it.

Basic Villous Structure

The histological appearances of the placental villi vary with gestational age and the stage of development and maturation of the villous tree. Nevertheless there is a basic villous structure that is independent of these variables.

Villous Trophoblast

The outer surface of the villi is covered by a trophoblastic mantle which consists of two easily distinguishable layers: an outer layer of syncytiotrophoblast and an inner layer of cytotrophoblastic (Langhans') cells (Fig. 1.6). The latter cells are cuboid, polyhedral or ovoid and have well-marked cell borders; their cytoplasm is clear or slightly granular whilst the nucleus is pale-staining with a finely dispersed chromatin network. These cells are prominent and form a complete layer in early pregnancy and are still present in the terminal villi of the mature placenta though they are less conspicuous than in the immature placenta. They tend to be flattened between the syncytiotrophoblast and the basement membrane and are seen best in sections stained with periodic acid-Schiff (PAS). It should be noted that although the cytotrophoblastic cells are dispersed in the mature placenta and no longer form a complete layer, their absolute number is not decreased and, indeed, continues to increase throughout pregnancy (Simpson et al, 1992). The cytotrophoblastic cells are, as noted previously, the stem cells of the trophoblast and, although largely quiescent in late pregnancy, retain their capacity to multiply and thus represent an inactive 'germinative' layer which can undergo a

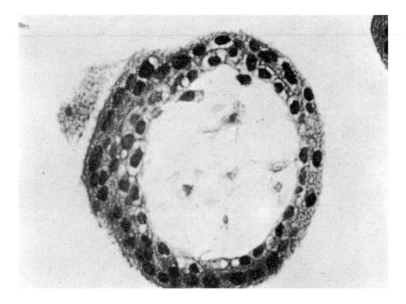

Figure 1.6. A villus from an early first-trimester placenta. The stroma is formed of loose mesenchyme in which an occasional Hofbauer cell is seen: the villus is not as yet vascularized (H & E ×200).

resurgence of proliferative activity if the need occurs to replace damaged or destroyed syncytiotrophoblast.

No cell boundaries are visible between the nuclei of the syncytiotrophoblast, which, in early pregnancy, forms a layer of uniform thickness around the periphery of the villus. Microinjection studies have shown that substances flow freely throughout this layer and the syncytiotrophoblast forms a continuous uninterrupted cytoplasmic layer that extends over the entire surface of the villous tree and completely lines the intervillous space (Gaunt & Ockleford, 1986). It is of note that the syncytiotrophoblast is in direct contact with maternal blood and thus functions as an endothelium: the structure of the syncytiotrophoblast is quite unlike that of an endothelial cell and hence its ability to act in this manner is something of a mystery. Studies with monoclonal antibodies, however, have shown that, despite their morphological dissimilarity, syncytiotrophoblast and endothelial cells share otherwise specific antigens (Voland et al, 1986) and an ability to synthesize nitric oxide (Myatt et al, 1993).

The syncytial nuclei in placentas from first trimester placentas are regularly spaced and are smaller and more darkly staining than those of the cytotrophoblast (Fig. 1.7). The syncytial cytoplasm may be homogeneous or finely granular, but is more commonly vacuolated; some of the vacuoles contain lipid. A delicate brush border may be seen, with varying degrees of ease, on the outer surface of the syncytium of young villi.

The syncytial nuclei are, in villi from term placentas, irregularly dispersed and often appear aggregated to form multinucleated protrusions from the villous surface, these being known as 'syncytial knots' (Fig. 1.8). Syncytial knots should be differentiated from 'syncytial sprouts' and 'syncytial buds'. Syncytial sprouts are present from the early stages of pregnancy and represent mainly the initial stages in the development of lateral villi. Those that do not form villi tend to become pedunculated and later break off from the villous surface to enter the intervillous space and the maternal circulation. Syncytial buds have been described as invaginations of the trophoblast into the underlying villous stroma, which may become separated from the parent tissue and appear as free multinucleated bodies within the villous stroma (Boyd & Hamilton, 1964). However, it is highly probable that these 'intrastromal buds' are, in reality, tangential sections of indenting villous surface trophoblast (Kustermann, 1981).

Some apparent syncytial knots also appear to be artefacts resulting from tangential cutting of the villous surface trophoblast (Burton, 1986a,b; Cantle et al, 1987;

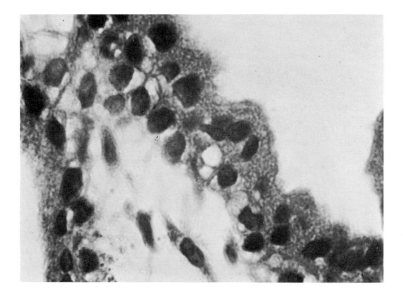

Figure 1.7. The trophoblast of an early first-trimester placental villus. There is a well-defined inner cytotrophoblastic layer and an outer layer of syncytiotrophoblast in which no cell boundaries are seen (H & E ×800).

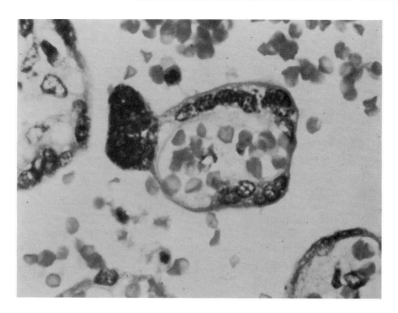

Figure 1.8. A villus bearing a syncytial knot which appears as a multinucleated protrusion from the free surface of the trophoblast (H & E ×780).

Kaufmann et al, 1987): in tangential cuts the appearances of the nuclei in the apparent knot will not differ from those in the rest of the villous syncytiotrophoblast. In true syncytial knots, however, the nuclei are small and densely staining, whilst electron microscopy shows that they have a degenerate, senescent appearance (Fig. 1.9); these appearances are in sharp contrast to those of the dispersed syncytial nuclei in a villus bearing a knot, which have a normal appearance (Jones & Fox, 1977). When considering the pathogenesis of true syncytial knots it must be borne in mind that the

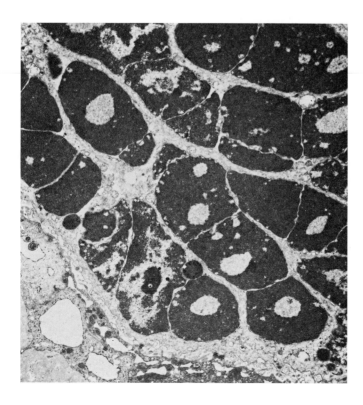

Figure 1.9. Ultra-structure of nuclei in a syncytial knot (EM ×7500).

syncytiotrophoblast is derived from the cytotrophoblast and that mitotic activity within the villous cytotrophoblast is marked in early pregnancy but continues, though to a progressively diminishing degree, into the third trimester. It follows, therefore, that the syncytial nuclei in any given villus are produced at varying stages of pregnancy and are, with respect to age, a heterogeneous population. If, as has been suggested (Martin & Spicer, 1973a), syncytiotrophoblastic nuclear senescence occurs as a programmed event, it would be expected that in the villi of the mature placenta, those formed during the earliest stages of pregnancy will show signs of ageing, whilst others, produced at a later stage of gestation, will show little or no evidence of senescence. The ultrastructural findings suggest that the oldest nuclei in the syncytium are eventually aggregated together to form knots, which may therefore be considered to represent a sequestration of unwanted aged nuclei. Teleologically there is an obvious benefit to be derived in removing senescent nuclei from areas of metabolically active syncytiotrophoblast and aggregating the effete nuclear material in one area of the villus. If it is assumed that the displaced, aged syncytial nuclei are, at least partially, replaced by fresh nuclei derived from the cytotrophoblast, it follows that villi with syncytial knots should, on average, have more syncytial nuclei than those that lack such structures. Fox (1965) and Gerl et al (1973) have shown that this is indeed the case.

It is a striking tribute to the efficiency of the placenta that it appears able to use the effete nuclear material in syncytial knots for the purpose of forming the intervillous syncytial bridges which are a not uncommon finding (Peter, 1943; Boyd & Hamilton, 1970; Burton, 1986a,b 1987; Cantle et al, 1987). These bridges contain numerous deeply staining nuclei, have a rich content of cytoplasmic fibrils, can be shown to be formed by the fusion of adjacent syncytial knots (Jones & Fox, 1977), and appear admirably suited to fulfil the mechanistic role proposed for them by Hormann (1953), namely, to act as an internal strut system which may help to protect the villous capillaries from the effects of sudden changes in intervillous space pressure during labour.

In some areas of many villi of the mature placenta the syncytiotrophoblast is focally thinned and anuclear; such areas overlie a dilated fetal capillary and may, on light microscopy, appear to fuse with the vessel wall (Fig. 1.10) to form what is now known as a 'vasculo-syncytial membrane' (Getzowa & Sadowsky, 1950). Although electron microscopy shows that there is no real fusion between trophoblast and vessel wall, it is clear that these areas differ markedly from the non-thinned areas of the syncytium and it has been claimed that they are specialized zones of the trophoblast for the facilitation of gas transfer across the placenta. The membranes appear to be formed, in part at least, by mechanical stretching of the trophoblast by ballooning capillary loops (Pisarki & Topilko, 1966; Burton & Tham, 1992).

The suggestion that these areas are important for gaseous transfer has been based principally on the fact that they represent the sites of closest approximation of maternal and fetal circulations. This would, however, only facilitate gas transfer across the placenta if membrane resistance was an important limiting factor in this process, and experimental studies suggest that this is not the case (Longo, 1972). The trophoblastic thinning is, however, only one indication of the specialized nature of the membranous areas, because not only do they differ histochemically (Amstutz, 1960) and ultrastructurally (Burgos & Rodriguez, 1966) from the non-membranous areas of the trophoblast, but scanning electron microscopy shows that there is a sharply localized loss of microvilli over their surface (Fox & Agrofojo-Blanco, 1974). It thus appears highly probable that trophoblastic gas transfer function is largely confined to the membranous areas and synthetic activity and transfer of non-gaseous substances to the non-membranous areas. This would indicate that the morphological evidence of functional regional differentiation, which can be detected at the ultrastructural level in the immature trophoblast (Dempsey & Luse, 1971; Kaufmann & Stegner, 1972), becomes sufficiently accentuated in the mature placenta to be easily visible on light microscopy. Hence, the vasculo-syncytial membranes may be considered as morphological evidence of functional topographic differentiation of the trophoblast.

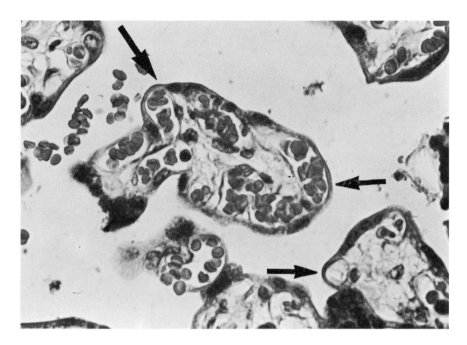

Figure 1.10. Vasculo-syncytial membranes (arrowed) in mature placenta villi (H & E ×580).

Trophoblastic Basement Membrane

The villous trophoblast is separated from the underlying stroma by the trophoblastic basement membrane which, at light microscopic level, has a fibrillary structure and measures between 20 and 50 nm thickness. The main components of the membrane are collagen IV, laminin and heparan sulphate (Duance & Bailey, 1983).

Villous Stroma

The villous stroma contains undifferentiated mesenchymal cells, mature mesenchymal (reticulum) cells, fibroblasts, myofibroblasts, pre-collagen and collagen fibres, the relative proportions of which vary with the gestational age and the stage of development of the villous tree (Kaufmann et al, 1977; Castellucci & Kaufmann, 1982a,b; Martinoli et al, 1984; Feller et al, 1985; Autio-Harmainen et al, 1991; Nanaev et al, 1991; Demir et al, 1992; Rukosuev, 1992). A sprinkling of mast cells is also present in the villous stroma (Durst-Zivkovic, 1973; Mahnke and Emmrich, 1973); their function in this site is uncertain.

Also present in the villous stroma are Hofbauer cells (Fig. 1.11); these cells may be round, ovoid or reniform, measure about 25 μm in diameter and have an eccentrically placed nucleus. Their cytoplasm is coarsely vacuolated during early pregnancy but as gestation progresses the vacuoles decrease in number and size and intracytoplasmic granules become more apparent (Castellucci et al, 1980). The nature of the Hofbauer cells has been much debated in the past but it now seems almost certain that they are simply tissue macrophages. They not only have the typical morphological, histochemical and functional characteristics of macrophages (Fox & Kharkongor, 1969; Enders & King, 1970; Castellucci & Zaccheo, 1989), but share with such cells the defining feature of possessing a surface immunoglobulin G (IgG) receptor and expressing class II major histocompatibility complex (MHC) molecules (Moskalewski et al, 1975; Wood et al, 1978; Wood, 1980; Loke et al, 1982; Bulmer & Johnson, 1984; Sutton et al, 1986, 1989; Sedmak et al, 1991; Saji et al, 1994).

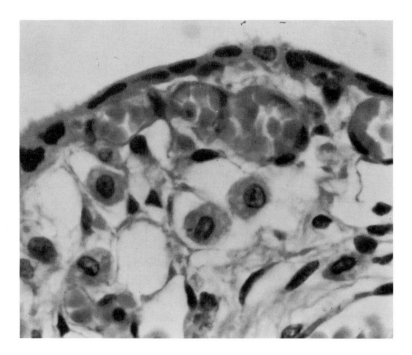

Figure 1.11. Several typical Hofbauer cells in the stroma of a first-trimester villus (H & E ×990).

Hofbauer cells are present in the villi at a very early stage of development and persist throughout pregnancy (Panigel & Anh, 1964; Fox, 1967b), though as the villous stroma becomes denser as gestation progresses, the presence of these cells tends to become masked, their presence only becoming overt if the meshes of the stroma are widened by oedema fluid. The presence of these cells in the villi before they are vascularized suggests that Hofbauer cells differentiate from mesenchymal cells in early pregnancy: at a later stage of gestation, however, this original population of Hofbauer cells may be supplemented by cells derived from fetal bone marrow-derived monocytes (Castellucci et al, 1987). The Hofbauer cells are, therefore, probably a heterogeneous population and the fact that they can show mitotic activity (Castellucci et al, 1987) suggests that a subset of these is an independent self-replicating population.

Hofbauer cells are capable of both immune and non-immune phagocytosis, can trap maternal antibodies crossing over into the placental tissues and are probably an important source of cytokines within the placenta. Other suggested functions, such as maintenance of placental water balance, involvement in transport mechanisms, a possible endocrine function and a role in the control of vasculogenesis, remain speculative.

Fetal Villous Vessels

The exact time at which villous vessels first appear is variable but by the end of the second month well-formed vessels lined by large immature endothelial cells are present. The vessels within the terminal villi of the mature placenta are of capillary size though many appear sinusoidally dilated. The endothelial cells are attached to each other by tight junctions and are supported by a delicate basal lamina which contains fibronectin, laminin and type IV collagen (Yamanada et al, 1987; Nanaev et al, 1991).

Temporal Variation in Villous Structure: Growth and Maturation of the Villous Tree

It has been usual to describe the appearances of the placental villi in terms of their changing appearance as pregnancy progresses, comparing, for instance, typical first-trimester villi with those in third-trimester placentas. It has always been recognized that this temporal variability in villous appearances was a reflection of the continuous development and branching of the villous tree but it is only relatively recently that the relationship between the growth of the villous tree and the villous appearances has been formally codified (Fig. 1.12), largely as a result of work by Kaufmann and his colleagues (Kaufmann et al, 1979; Sen et al, 1979; Castellucci & Kaufmann, 1982a,b; Kaufmann, 1982; Castellucci et al, 1984, 1990; Kosanke et al, 1993). Thus five types of villi can be identified:

1. *Mesenchymal villi.* These represent a transient stage in placental development and they can differentiate into either mature or immature intermediate villi. They comprise the first generation of newly formed villi and are derived from trophoblastic sprouts by mesenchymal invasion and vascularization. They are found mainly in the early stages of pregnancy but a few may still be found at term in the centres of the lobules. They have complete trophoblastic mantles with many cytotrophoblastic cells and regularly dispersed nuclei in the syncytiotrophoblast: their loose, immature-type stroma is abundant and contains a few Hofbauer cells together with poorly developed fetal capillaries (see Fig. 1.6).

2. *Immature intermediate villi.* These are peripheral extensions of the stem villi. They are the predominant form seen in immature placentas (Fig. 1.13) and often persist in small groups in the centres of the lobules in mature placentas, where they represent a persistent growth zone (Geier et al, 1975; Schuhmann et al, 1976; Schuhmann, 1981; Kaufmann, 1995). These villi have a well-preserved trophoblastic mantle in which cytotrophoblastic cells are numerous; the syncytial nuclei are evenly dispersed and there are no syncytial knots or vasculosyncytial membranes. They have an abundant loose

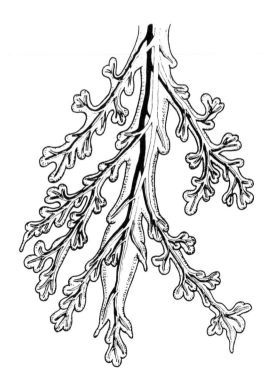

Figure 1.12. Diagrammatic representation of a peripheral villous tree. The large central stem villus runs down to terminate in a bulbous immature intermediate villus. The lateral branches from the stem villus are the mature intermediate villi from which the terminal villi protrude. (After Kaufmann, 1982, with permission.)

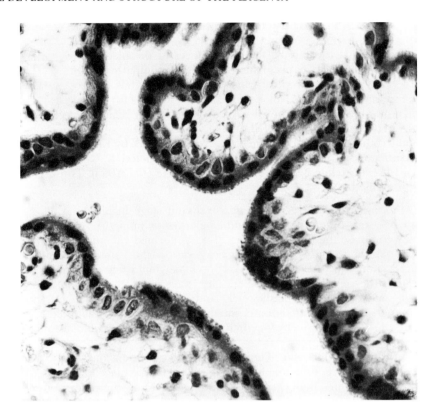

Figure 1.13. Immature intermediate villi (H & E ×450).

stroma that contains many Hofbauer cells: capillaries, arterioles and venules are present.

3. *Stem villi*. These comprise the primary stems which connect the villous tree to the chorionic plate, up to four generations of short thick branches and further generations of dichotomous branches. Their principal role is to serve as a scaffolding for the peripheral villous tree and up to one-third of the total volume of the villous tissue of the mature placenta is made up of this villous type (Kaufmann, 1995), the proportion of such villi being highest in the central subchorial portion of the villous tree. Histologically, the stem villi have a compact stroma and contain either arteries and veins or arterioles and venules whilst superficially located capillaries may also be present.

4. *Mature intermediate villi*. These are the peripheral ramifications of the villous stems from which the vast majority of terminal villi directly arise (Fig. 1.14). They are large (60–150 μm in diameter) and contain capillaries admixed with small arterioles and venules, the vessels being set in a very loose stroma which occupies more than half of the villous volume. The syncytiotrophoblast has a uniform structure, no knots or vasculo-syncytial membranes being present. Up to a quarter of the villi in a mature placenta are of this type.

5. *Terminal villi*. These are the final ramifications of the villous tree and are grape-like outgrowths from mature intermediate villi (Fig. 1.15). They contain capillaries, many of which are sinusoidally dilated to occupy most of the cross-sectional diameter of the villus. The syncytiotrophoblast is thin, the syncytial nuclei are irregularly dispersed, syncytial knots may be present and vasculosyncytial membranes are commonly seen. These terminal villi begin to appear at about the 27th week of gestation and account for 30–40% of the villous volume, 50% of the villous surface area and 60% of villi seen in

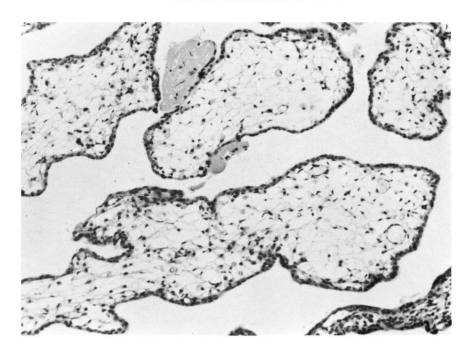

Figure 1.14. Mature intermediate villi (H & E ×150).

cross-section at term. It has been suggested that these villi are not 'outgrowths' in the true sense of the word but are formed as a result of disproportionate longitudinal growth of the capillaries within an intermediate villus compared with that of the villus as a whole: the subsequent looping of the capillaries causes them to obtrude from the villous surface (Fig. 1.16) and, with their covering of trophoblast, form the terminal villi (Kaufmann et al, 1985). The terminal villi are optimally differentiated for materno-fetal transfer and there can be no doubt that they are the site at which most transport across the placenta occurs.

The pattern of development of the villous tree envisaged by Kaufmann and his colleagues is as follows:

   i.   During the early weeks of pregnancy all the villi are of the mesenchymal type.

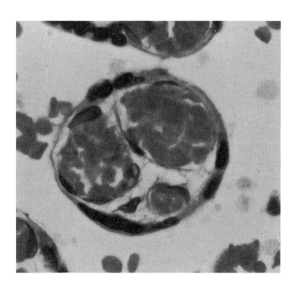

Figure 1.15. A terminal villus from a mature placenta. The stromal vessels are sinusoidally dilated and occupy most of the cross-sectional area of the villus (H & E ×780).

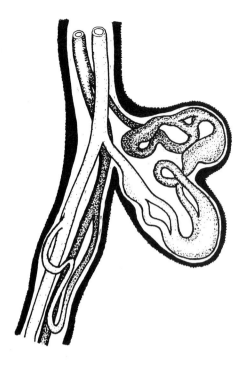

Figure 1.16. Diagrammatic representation of the formation of a terminal villus by protrusion of a capillary loop. (Adapted from Benirschke & Kaufmann, 1990, with permission.)

ii. Between the 7th and 8th weeks mesenchymal villi begin to transform into immature intermediate villi and these subsequently transform into stem villi.

iii. Development of additional immature intermediate villi from mesenchymal villi gradually ceases at the end of the second trimester but these immature intermediate villi continue to mature into stem villi and only a few persist to term as growth zones in the centres of the lobules.

iv. At the beginning of the third trimester mesenchymal villi switch from transforming into immature intermediate villi and start transforming into mature intermediate villi. These latter serve as a framework for the terminal villi which begin to appear shortly afterwards and predominate at term. The terminal villi do not result from trophoblastic proliferation but develop when longitudinal capillary growth outstrips longitudinal villous growth thus causing bulging and protrusions into the intervillous space.

Growth, Ageing and Maturation of Placental Villi

It will be clear from the description given above of the development of the villous tree that the histological appearances of the placenta vary considerably during the short life span of the organ. Thus only mesenchymal villi are seen in very early pregnancy, immature intermediate villi and stem villi form the bulk of the villous population during the second trimester whilst mature intermediate and, particularly, terminal villi predominate in the third-trimester placenta. It would not be correct, however, to describe these rather obvious changes as being an 'ageing' process; they represent a developmental and maturational process, which, in teleological terms, is designed to increase and optimize the transfer capacity of the placenta (Jackson et al, 1992; Mayhew et al, 1993). Little is known, however, of the factor (or factors) that determine placental maturation, because this is certainly not simply a reflection of fetal maturation. The condition of feto-placental asynchrony is well documented (Becker, 1975) and it is well recognized that prematurely delivered immature babies may have a placenta that is morphologically fully mature; conversely, a fully mature infant may have a morphologically immature placenta, as is sometimes the case in, for example, pregnancies complicated by maternal diabetes mellitus. It is highly probable that 'signals' are received from both the mother and the fetus but it does appear that maturation and growth within the placenta are dependent on intrinsic mechanisms. What these intrinsic mechanisms are, however, is far from clear though the placenta does contain an impressive range of growth factors and expresses an equally imposing variety of growth factor receptors (Adamson, 1987; Blay & Hollenberg, 1989; Ohlsson, 1989; Ohlsson et al, 1993; Mitchell et al, 1993).

Maturation of the villous tree is accompanied by a progressive differentiation of the trophoblast. Although these two processes are clearly intertwined they are probably independent of each other, because a placenta with fully mature terminal villi may, on occasion, show little or no evidence of trophoblastic differentiation, this latter feature being most clearly manifest by the development of vasculo-syncytial membranes.

Past claims that the placenta ages during the 9 months of gestation appear to have been largely based on a misunderstanding and a misinterpretation of the processes of villous maturation and differentiation and there is, in fact, no morphological or functional evidence to suggest that the term placenta is in any way senescent (Fox, 1979). This is not to say, however, that individual trophoblastic cells or nuclei do not become senescent, just as they do in any continuously replicating cell population. Martin and Spicer (1973a) have described ultrastructural changes of an apparently ageing nature in trophoblastic nuclei and nucleoli and thought that these were indicative of impaired protein synthesis in late pregnancy as a result of programmed senescence. Whether this interpretation of the rather subtle electron-optical abnormalities that have been observed is, however, fully justified is a question to which, at the moment, no firm answer can be given.

Regional Variation in Villous Morphology

There is a variability of villous appearances between different regions of the term placenta. Thus towards the fetal surface of the placenta, stem villi and intermediate villi are prominent whilst terminal villi form a much higher proportion of the villous population in those areas nearer the basal plate. Terminal villi in the subchorial region tend to have a more collagenous stroma, a thicker trophoblastic basement membrane, fewer vasculo-syncytial membranes and a greater number of easily visible cytotrophoblastic cells than do those nearer the basal plate (Fox, 1964; Benedetti et al, 1971). Similarly, peripherally situated terminal villi have, in general terms, a more fibrotic stroma, a thicker trophoblastic basement membrane and less vasculo-syncytial membranes than do those in the more central area of the placenta. These regional differences are probably related to variations in the flow dynamics of the maternal blood in different areas of the intervillous space, with a subsequent regional variability in villous oxygenation.

The Fetal Circulation Through the Placenta

Fetal blood passes to the placenta through the two umbilical arteries that spiral around the umbilical vein; shortly before reaching the placenta the two arteries are connected by one or two anastomotic vessels, and may even fuse into a single trunk which subsequently divides into two rami (Szpakowski, 1974). On reaching the placenta the arteries run in the chorion; the arteries are usually of equal size, and each supplies one-half of the placenta. During their chorionic course the arteries branch and at each division a proportion of the branches perforate the chorion to enter the placental substance. In addition, several perforating branches are given off directly from the undersurface of the main arteries. As these branches enter the placental substance they run in the primary stem villi and become the cotyledonary arteries. The course of the cotyledonary arteries is usually short and straight, though some workers have thought that they may sometimes run in a spiral fashion, this serving as a mechanism to control the

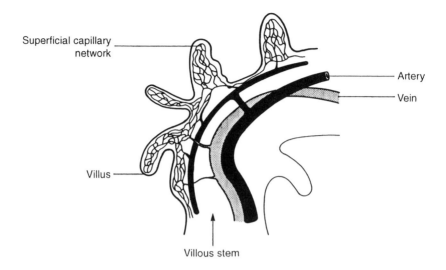

Figure 1.17. Diagram of the fetal circulation through the villi.

rate of fetal blood flow through the placenta (Romney & Reid, 1951). The cotyledonary arteries soon divide into secondary stem arteries, which in turn arborize into tertiary stem vessels. It is these latter which run through the intervillous space in the tertiary stem villi; they follow the course of these villi by inserting into the basal plate and then turning back upon themselves to re-enter the intervillous space. During their downward course, and on their re-entry into the intervillous space, they give off several villous branches which eventually break up into a capillary system that vascularizes the terminal villi. The capillary networks are found principally on the peripheral aspects of the lobules and are not seen within their interiors (Wilkin, 1965); they are most numerous towards the basal plate.

The villous capillary system was studied by Bøe (1953), who was able to inject these vessels with Indian ink. He described two separate capillary plexuses within the tertiary villous branches, each main artery being accompanied by a paravascular and a superficial capillary network (Fig. 1.17). The main artery gives off branches that in turn divide dichotomously into branches running parallel to the direction of the main artery, but with one branch running in the direction of blood flow and the other in a retrograde direction. Offshoots from these elongated branches form the superficial capillary network, which also receives a few contributory vessels from the main artery. The superficial capillary network drains directly into the main vein by a series of short stout venules. The paravascular capillary network is formed by branches arising directly from the main artery and is anatomically an arteriolar rather than a capillary system. This plexus communicates directly with the main vein and hence may be a shunt arrangement to prevent focal overloading of the terminal villous circulation.

Bøe thought that there were three patterns of terminal villous vascularization:

1. The larger villi receive a branch from the main artery plus a supply from the superficial capillary network. These villi drain directly into the main vein by a single tributary.
2. Medium-sized villi are vascularized solely from the superficial capillary network, but the venous drainage is by a separate venule directly into the main vein.
3. The small villi are vascularized only from the superficial capillary plexus and their venous drainage is solely into this plexus.

This description of the villous capillaries was largely confirmed by Crawford (1961), though he was not able to demonstrate the paravascular network: Habashi et al (1983), in a scanning electron microscopic study of corrosion casts, did define a paravascular network though only in those parts of the villous tree bathed in poorly oxygenated maternal blood. Bøe's concept has, however, been criticized by Kaufmann and his colleagues (Kaufmann et al, 1985, 1988; Leiser et al, 1985) who regard the villi described by him as mesenchymal villi arising from an immature intermediate villus: they consider that a paravascular capillary network is only present in immature intermediate villi and in young stem villi. In the mature intermediate villi the vessels are a direct continuation of the arterioles and venules in the stem villi and these progress to form capillaries which show coiling and sinusoidal dilatation, the terminal villi being vascularized only by capillary vessels which are arranged in such a way that three to five terminal villi are supplied by the same multiply-coiled capillary loop (see Fig. 1.16). This rather complex system of vascularization allows for considerable flexibility in the control of flow rate through the villi and is probably a mechanism for ensuring an optimal rate of blood flow for materno-fetal transfer.

The fetal blood flow through the placenta is about 500 ml per minute and although the main propelling force is clearly the fetal heart it is possible that there is also a peripheral villous pulse; contractile cells, now known to be myofibroblasts, are present in immature intermediate and stem villi (Krantz & Parker, 1963; Michael, 1974; Feller et al, 1985; Demir et al, 1992; Graf et al, 1994, 1995) and it has been suggested that rhythmic contraction of these cells may help to pump the venous blood back to the fetus (ten Berge, 1955).

THE MATERNAL UTEROPLACENTAL CIRCULATION

Development of Uteroplacental Arteries

The physiological changes in the spiral arteries of the placental bed which result in their conversion to uteroplacental vessels have been extensively described (Dixon & Robertson, 1958, 1961; Brosens, 1964; Brosens et al, 1967; de Wolf et al, 1973, 1980; Sheppard & Bonnar, 1974; Robertson, 1976; Pijnenborg et al, 1980, 1981, 1983; Gerretsen et al, 1983). During the early weeks of gestation, cytotrophoblastic cells stream out from the tips of the anchoring villi, penetrate the trophoblastic shell and extensively colonize the decidua and adjacent myometrium of the placental bed, these cells being the interstitial extravillous cytotrophoblastic cells (Fig. 1.18). In addition,

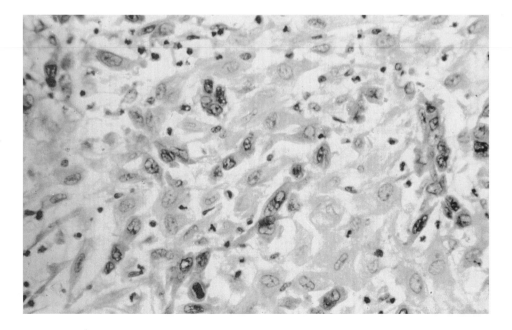

Figure 1.18. The decidua of the placental bed. The decidual cells are widely separated by interstitial extravillous cytotrophoblastic cells (H & E ×420).

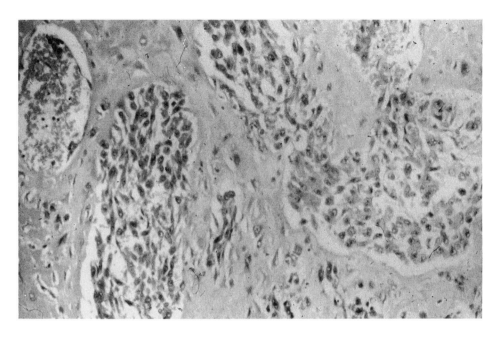

Figure 1.19. The lumens of the intradecidual portions of the spiral arteries are filled with clumps of intravascular extravillous cytotrophoblastic cells (H & E ×280).

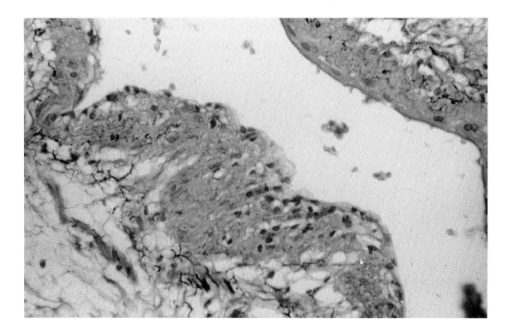

Figure 1.20. A spiral artery in the decidua of the placental bed. The endothelium has been destroyed and the media of the arterial wall is largely replaced by fibrinoid material (H & E ×470).

cytotrophoblastic cells stream into the lumens of the intradecidual portions of the spiral arteries of the placental bed where they form intraluminal plugs and constitute the intravascular extravillous cytotrophoblast (Fig. 1.19). These endovascular trophoblastic cells destroy and replace the endothelium of the maternal vessels and then invade the media where they destroy the medial elastic and muscular tissue: the arterial wall becomes replaced by fibrinoid material (Fig. 1.20) which appears to be derived partly from fibrin in the maternal blood and partly from proteins secreted by the invading trophoblastic cells. This process is complete by the end of the first trimester, at which time the physiological changes within the spiral arteries of the placental bed extend to the deciduo–myometrial junction.

After this there is a rest phase in this process but between the 14th and 16th weeks of gestation there is a resurgence of endovascular trophoblastic migration with a second wave of cells moving down into the intramyometrial segments of the spiral arteries (Fig. 1.21), these cells extending as far as the origin of these vessels from the radial arteries. Within the intramyometrial portion of the spiral arteries the same process as occurs in their intradecidual portion is repeated, i.e. replacement of the endothelium, invasion and destruction of the medial musculo-elastic tissue and fibrinoid change in the vessel wall. The end result of this trophoblastic invasion of, and attack on, the vessels of the placental bed is that the thick-walled muscular spiral arteries (Fig. 1.22) are converted into flaccid, sac-like uteroplacental vessels (Figs 1.23 and 1.24) which can passively dilate in order to accommodate the greatly augumented blood flow through this vascular system which is required as pregnancy progresses.

Although recent studies suggest that trophoblastic invasion of the placental bed vessels may not be as temporally rigidly restricted as was originally thought (Pijnenborg et al, 1991) it is nevertheless clear that the extravillous population of trophoblastic cells plays a key role in placentation. Through these cells the placenta establishes its own low-pressure, high-conductance vascular system simultaneously ensuring an adequate maternal blood flow to itself and an ample supply of oxygen and nutrients to the fetus. Several points do, however, require comment. Firstly, it is not fully settled whether the interstitial and intravascular cytotrophoblastic cells are separate populations as some believe that the intravascular cells are derived from interstitial cells which migrate

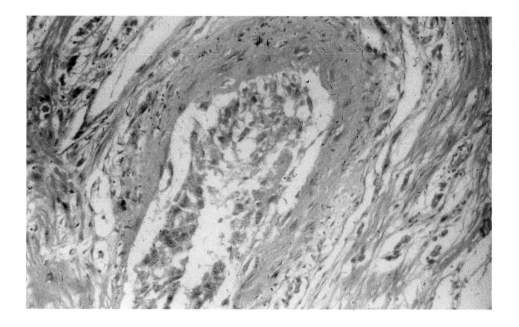

Figure 1.21. The intramyometrial portion of a spiral artery of the placental bed. The lumen contains a clump of intravascular extravillous cytotrophoblastic cells (H & E ×150).

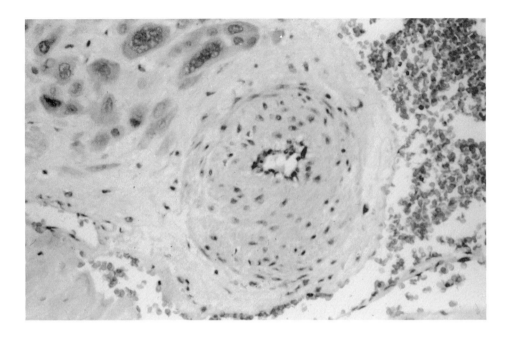

Figure 1.22. A normal thick-walled muscular spiral artery in a non-gravid uterus (H & E ×140).

through the vessel walls from their adventitial surface (Kurman et al, 1984; Fisher & Damsky, 1993). As Pijnenborg (1994) has pointed out, however, the ultimate fate of endovascular trophoblast is to be buried in the arterial wall and it seems illogical to suggest that extravascular trophoblast penetrates the full thickness of the vessel wall to lie free within the lumen only to be later incorporated within the wall of the artery. Secondly, it is far from clear why only arteries, and not veins, in the placental bed are

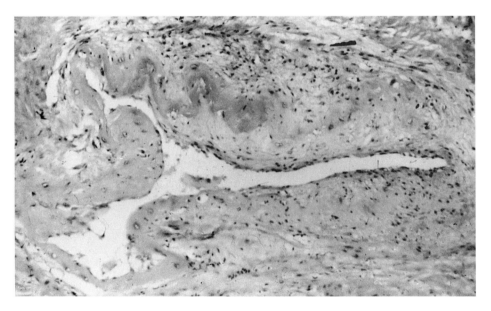

Figure 1.23. A widely dilated amuscular uteroplacental vessel in the placental bed of a gravid uterus (H & E ×120).

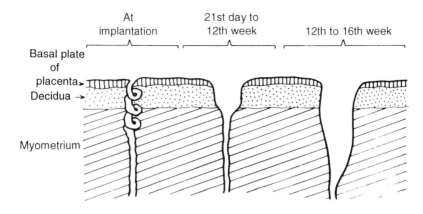

At implantation | 21st day to 12th week | 12th to 16th week

Basal plate of placenta→

Decidua →

Myometrium

Figure 1.24. Diagrammatic representation of the conversion of the spiral arteries in the placental bed into uteroplacental vessels.

invaded by trophoblast. Thirdly, the factor (or factors) controlling the well-timed waves of intravascular trophoblast movement and the limitation of interstitial trophoblastic invasion to the inner third of the myometrium are far from clear: Pijnenborg (1994) has reviewed the complex myriad of interacting factors involved in trophoblastic migration, including trophoblastic secretion of collagenases, plasminogen activator, plasminogen activator inhibitor, metalloproteinases and fibronectin, the role of cell adhesion molecules, the effects of growth factors and cytokines and the part played by immunological factors, and came to the conclusion that the control mechanisms of trophoblastic invasiveness are not understood.

The Maternal Uteroplacental Circulatory System

The studies of Ramsey and her colleagues (Ramsey, 1954, 1956, 1962, 1965; Ramsey et al, 1963; Ramsey & Donner, 1980) have shown that maternal blood enters the intervillous space from arterial inlets in the basal plate and is then driven by the head of maternal pressure towards the chorionic plate as a funnel-shaped stream (Fig. 1.25). The head of maternal pressure is gradually dissipated and is further diminished by the baffle-like action of the villi; lateral dispersion of the blood occurs and this forces the blood already present in the intervillous space out through basally placed wide venous outlets and into the endometrial venous network. In her earlier papers, Ramsey described the maternal blood as entering the intervillous space in 'spurts', whilst Borell et al (1958) described arterial 'jets'. Cineangiography has shown that these terms give an undue impression of speed and intermittency, and that the maternal blood enters the space 'much as water from an actively flowing brook penetrates a reed filled marsh' (Ramsey, 1965), producing a funnel-shaped stream that lacks both the velocity and pulsation implied by the term 'jet'.

The physiological basis for this circulatory system is believed to be a series of pressure differentials, with the pressure in the maternal arterioles being higher than the mean pressure in the intervillous space, which in turn exceeds the maternal venous pressure during myometrial diastole. It has to be emphasized, however, that the whole system is a low-pressure one, because, whereas in most organs there is a progressive decrease in the diameter of the vessels as they approach their target cells, the reverse is true for the placenta, where the spiral arteries dilate progressively as they approach their entry into the intervillous space. Therefore there is a considerable drop in pressure from the proximal non-dilated portions of the uteroplacental arterioles to the distal dilated portions, and the full arterial pressure is not transmitted to the intervillous space. The placenta itself offers very little flow resistance to maternal blood

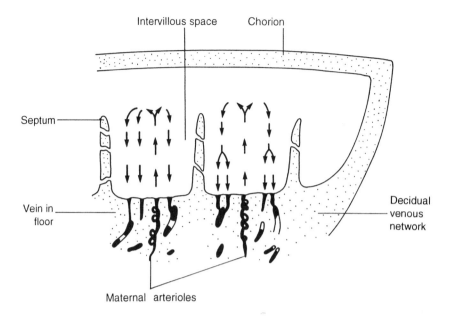

Figure 1.25. Diagrammatic representation of the circulation of maternal blood through the placenta.

and has a high vascular conductance; there is therefore very little drop in pressure across the intervillous space and the main factor governing the rate of placental blood flow is the vascular resistance of the proximal part of the uteroplacental vessels (Moll et al, 1975). Despite the fact that the pressure differences from arterial to venous sides of the intervillous space are small, they are apparently sufficient to drive arterial blood towards the chorionic plate, to stop short-cutting of the stream into adjacent venous outlets, and to prevent mixing of adjacent streams.

Cineangiography has shown that the individual spiral arterioles act independently of each other and that not all are patent and discharging blood into the intervillous space simultaneously (Ramsey et al, 1963). Furthermore, during myometrial contractions the afferent blood flow through the intervillous space may be considerably reduced or may even cease. It is not clear whether this is due to compression and obliteration of the veins draining the placenta, with a subsequent rise in intervillous space pressure, to occlusion of the afferent arterioles by a sphincter-like action, or to increased intraluminal pressure in the uterus, altering the pressure gradient between arterial and venous sides of the intervillous space (Adamsons & Myers, 1975). There is some tentative ultrasonographic evidence, however, that the intervillous space is distended during a uterine contraction (Bleker et al, 1975); this suggests that venous obstruction is the initial event and indicates that the fetus is probably not severely deprived of an oxygen supply during myometrial systole.

RELATIONSHIP OF MATERNAL CIRCULATORY SYSTEM TO FETAL LOBULE

The haemodynamic system proposed by Ramsey postulated that the arterial inflow into the intervillous space was through randomly situated arterial inlets, but it has since become clear that this is not the case and that a definite relationship exists between the maternal vessels and the fetal lobules. The nature of this relationship has not, however, been firmly established and two contrasting, and mutually incompatible, schemata have been proposed. Thus Freese (1966, 1968, 1969) and Wigglesworth (1967, 1969) believed that the arterial openings in the basal plate are so situated that the inflow from each maternal vessel is into the central villus-free space of a fetal

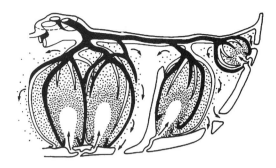

Figure 1.26. Diagrammatic representation of the relationship between the maternal circulatory system and the fetal lobule as envisaged by Wigglesworth and Freese. The density of stippling indicates the villous density.

lobule, and that the blood then flows laterally through the lobule into the interlobular areas, from which it is drained via basal venous outlets (Fig. 1.26). Others (Lemtis, 1969, 1970; Gruenwald, 1973, 1975a,b) have claimed that the maternal vessels open, not into the central space of the lobule, but into the interlobular spaces, and that the blood then circles the lobules in streams to form a shell around them, entering and leaving the lobule whilst doing this and before draining through the basal outlets (Fig. 1.27).

Which of these two theories is correct is a matter for speculation, but what is clear is that materno-fetal exchange takes place in the villi that form the lobule and that it is only here, in the shell of the lobule, that a true intervillous space, which is probably only of capillary calibre, exists. Elsewhere, in the subchorial lake, the central intra-lobular spaces and the interlobular areas, villi are either absent or sparse and these areas are functionally not part of the intervillous space.

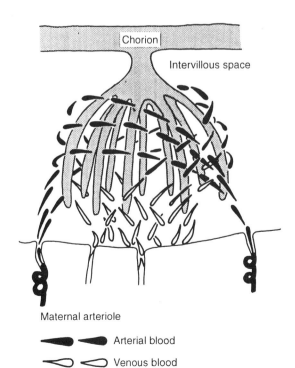

Figure 1.27. Diagrammatic representation of the relationship between the maternal circulatory system and the fetal lobule as envisaged by Gruenwald and Lemtis.

NON-VILLOUS COMPONENTS OF THE PLACENTA

Extravillous Trophoblast

Extravillous trophoblast is present in the chorion laeve, the cell columns, cell islands, basal plate and placental bed. The extravillous trophoblastic cells in the placental bed can be distinguished from decidual cells by their positive staining reaction for cytokeratins (Daya & Sabet, 1991) and they constitute the 'placental site reaction' which at term is formed by the residue of the interstitial extravillous cytotrophoblast, largely present in the decidua, and syncytiotrophoblastic-like giant cells, formed by fusion of interstitial extravillous cytotrophoblastic cells, which are largely in the adjacent myometrium. In the past it was thought that the intravascular extravillous cytotrophoblast, a prominent feature in early pregnancy, had disappeared by term but in fact it is not uncommon to encounter intravascular trophoblast in the placental bed vessels of the mature placenta (Gosseye & van der Veen, 1992).

The interstitial extravillous cytotrophoblastic cells have also been classed as 'intermediate trophoblast' (Kurman et al, 1984) though this term had been previously well established to describe those villous cytotrophoblastic cells that are beginning to differentiate into syncytiotrophoblast (Tighe et al, 1967). It had also been previously shown that many of the interstitial extravillous cytotrophoblastic cells were showing evidence of beginning syncytiotrophoblast differentiation and were also thus of the intermediate type (Wynn, 1972, 1975a; Robertson & Warner, 1974). It should be stressed, however, that intermediate cytotrophoblastic cells simply represent a transitory phase in the pathway of trophoblastic differentiation from stem cells. There is, therefore, little justification for regarding 'intermediate' cytotrophoblastic cells as a distinct sub-population of trophoblastic cells and it is preferable to retain the term 'extravillous cytotrophoblast'. Having said that there are several distinctive features of the extravillous cytotrophoblastic cells, namely their positive staining reaction for human placental lactogen (HPL) (Gosseye & Fox, 1984; Kurman et al, 1984) and their expression of an unusual type of class I MHC antigen (Sargent et al, 1993; Shorter et al, 1993).

The function of the intravascular extravillous cytotrophoblast appears clear because it plays a fundamental role in the conversion of spiral arteries into uteroplacental vessels. The function of the interstitial extravillous cytotrophoblast, however, is obscure: these cells tend to aggregate around spiral arteries and it has been suggested that they may, in some unknown fashion, prime these vessels to allow them to react to their eventual invasion by endovascular trophoblast (Pijnenborg et al, 1983).

Fibrin and Fibrinoid

Fibrin and fibrinoid material are found in every term placenta though in many accounts of placental structure and pathology these two substances have been confused. Classically, pathologists have considered fibrin to be derived from the blood as a result of thrombus formation whilst fibrinoid material is seen within tissues and is in part a result of transudation of plasma, usually in association with cell necrosis, and in part a secretory product. Within this conceptual framework, fibrin is seen in the roof and floor of the intervillous space and around some villi whilst fibrinoid material is present in the basal plate, septa, cell columns and in some villi. The position has been complicated by the recent introduction of a new terminology in which the classical terms of 'fibrin' and 'fibrinoid' are subsumed into 'fibrin-type fibrinoid' and 'matrix-type fibrinoid' (Frank et al, 1994). These two types of fibrinoid differ from each other in ultrastructural and immunocytochemical terms but fibrin-type fibrinoid roughly corresponds to fibrin and matrix-like fibrinoid roughly equates with fibrinoid, though in neither case is the correspondence exact. The scientific reasons for the introduction of this new terminology are impeccable but pathologists are, by nature, rather reactionary individuals and I suspect that many, including myself, will continue to use the terms fibrin and fibrinoid in the same sense as they are still used in general pathology.

ULTRASTRUCTURE OF THE PLACENTA

Surface Structure as Seen on Scanning Electron Microscopy

During the last few decades the surface ultrastructure of the placenta has been the subject of many scanning electron microscopic studies (Herbst & Multier, 1970; Bergstrom, 1971; Ludwig et al, 1971; Lerat et al, 1973; Fox & Agrofojo-Blanco, 1974; Ludwig, 1974; Cianci & Russo, 1975; Kawakami, 1975; King & Menton, 1975; Leibl et al, 1975; Demir, 1979; Kaufmann, 1982; Burton, 1987, 1990; Demir et al, 1994).

In the first-trimester placenta the villi, predominantly stem villi and immature intermediate villi, are seen as elongated or sausage-shaped structures (Fig. 1.28) with a furrowed, wrinkled surface. No cell boundaries are seen and there are no surface pores. Many villous sprouts can be observed emerging from the sides and apices of the villi (Fig. 1.29); these range from small mounds to long digitiform processes which may have a bulbous expansion at their top. All the villous surface, including that of the villous sprouts, is covered by a dense meshwork of microvilli (Fig. 1.30), these being present in a density estimated to be in the region of 600 million per cubic centimetre (Ludwig, 1974). Some of the microvilli are single but others have a complex branching structure; a minority are club-shaped but most have a leaf-like form and are seen as elongated ridges. The microvilli are closely apposed and appear almost to interlock, giving the surface an elevated mosaic pattern.

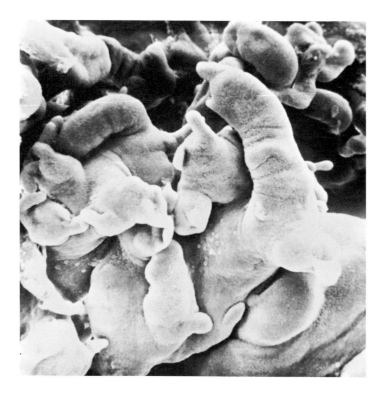

Figure 1.28. Scanning electronmicrograph of normal first-trimester villi (SEM ×210).

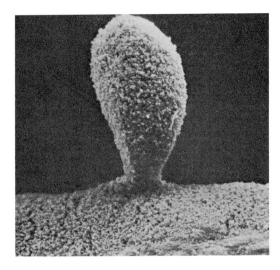

Figure 1.29. SEM of villous sprout emerging from the lateral aspect of a first-trimester placental villus (×800).

In the mature placenta the villi, predominantly terminal villi, though smaller and more digitate than during the first trimester, retain the same general form. Many are convoluted and creased with a curiously 'jowl-like' appearance which often gives them an appearance similar to that of the leg of a pachyderm. A striking feature is the presence of localized dome-shaped, blister-like swellings (Fig. 1.31) protruding from the

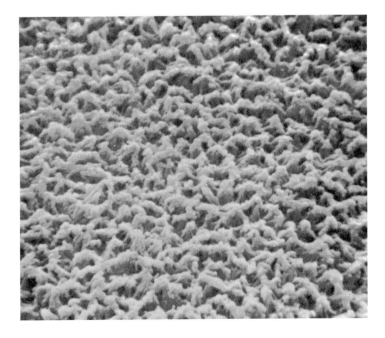

Figure 1.30. SEM of microvilli on the surface of a first-trimester villus (×5000).

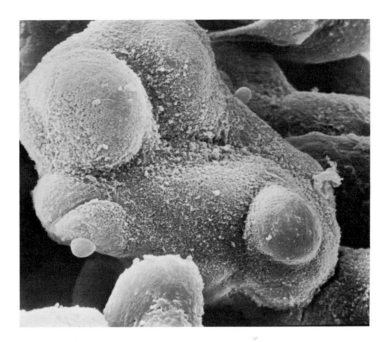

Figure 1.31. SEM of mature placental villi. Several dome-shaped swellings can be seen protruding from the villous surface; these are thought to be the vasculo-syncytial membranes (×1100).

villous surface (Fox and Agrofojo-Blanco, 1974); these are distributed in a random fashion, some being at the apex of a villus and others along its side. The finger-like syncytial sprouts are not present in the term placenta. Microvilli are present in most areas, their density at this stage being about 1200 million per cubic centimetre (Ludwig, 1974). They are now rather variable in size and, whilst a few show a leaf-like or ridge form, the majority are club-shaped or digitiform; they no longer interlock to form a mosaic. Although microvilli are present in most areas they are either absent or greatly reduced in number on the surface of the dome-shaped swellings which protrude from the villous surface; at the base of the dome there is a transition, sometimes abrupt but more often gradual, to a normal pattern.

There can be little doubt that the dome-shaped protrusions revealed by scanning electron microscopy correspond to the vasculo-syncytial membranes that are seen on light microscopy. The function of the trophoblastic microvilli is uncertain, because although King and Menton (1975) have assumed that they have an absorptive function, others have denied this role and have suggested that they are concerned either with trophoblastic excretion (Salazar & Gonzalez-Angulo, 1967) or, rather more convincingly, with receptor-mediated endocytosis (Ockleford & Whyte, 1977). If this latter assumption is correct then their localized loss from the surface of the vasculo-syncytial membranes may be considered as a mechanism for exposing the maximal possible surface of trophoblast specifically adapted for gaseous transfer to the maternal blood.

Placental Villous Ultrastructure

The first electron microscopic studies of the placenta were made over 40 years ago (Boyd & Hughes, 1954; Wislocki & Dempsey, 1955) and numerous reports since then have established the fine structure of this organ. Only a brief account of placental ultrastructure is given here, a fuller account of this topic having been published elsewhere (Jones & Fox, 1991).

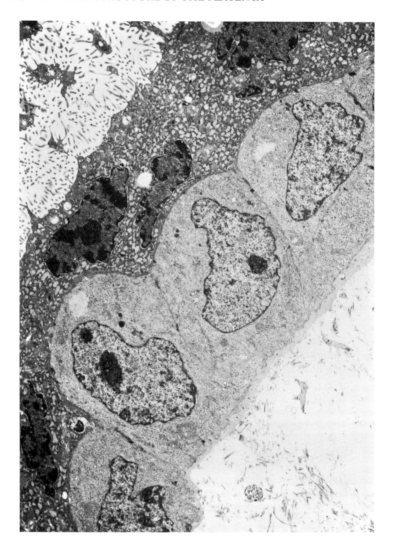

Figure 1.32. Fine structure of the trophoblast of a first-trimester placental villus. There is a continuous layer of cytotrophoblastic cells with relatively electron-lucent cytoplasm and a paucity of organelles. The overlying syncytiotrophoblast has a more complex cytoplasmic structure and is rich in organelles (×4000).

Immature Trophoblast (Fig. 1.32)

In the first-trimester placenta the syncytium is of uniform thickness; there are no plasma membranes separating the nuclei but free remnants of membranes may occasionally be seen (Enders, 1965). The free surface of the syncytiotrophoblast is covered by large microvilli that are normally about 0.5–1.2 μm in length (Fig. 1.33). Their cytoplasm is continuous with that of the syncytiotrophoblast and contains a central fibrillary core that can often be shown to be in continuity with similar fibrils in the underlying syncytium. The tips of the microvilli often show some degree of bulbous expansion and this may sometimes be so marked that a terminal vacuole is formed; these vacuoles contain flocculent material and it has been claimed that these not infrequently appear to break off from the microvilli to lie free in the intervillous space (Salazar & Gonzalez-Angulo, 1967). Between the microvilli the syncytial surface is often invaginated to form pits, which are the precursors of pinocytotic vesicles. The basal plasma membrane of the syncytiotrophoblast shows numerous complex infoldings, resulting in an

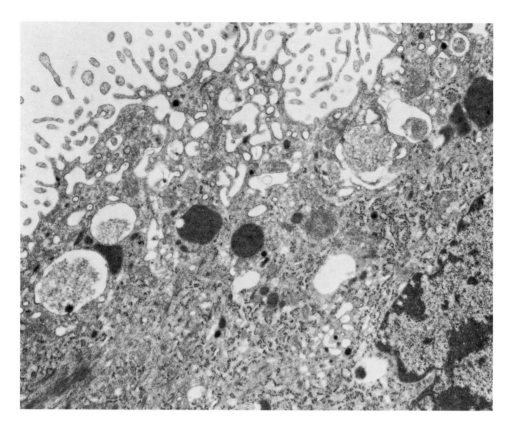

Figure 1.33. Ultrastructure of the free surface of the villous syncytiotrophoblast. There are many fine microvilli and several pinocytotic vesicles (×18,750).

interrupted extracellular space between the syncytium and the cytotrophoblast or trophoblastic basement membrane. Desmosomes are often present where the syncytium is in direct contact with a cytotrophoblastic cell.

As seen under the electron microscope, the immature syncytium is an extremely complex tissue (Fig. 1.34). It contains an abundance of rough endoplasmic reticulum, which is usually dilated to give an overall vacuolated appearance to the cytoplasm. There is some evidence that the endoplasmic reticulum forms, or contributes to, a syncytial canalicular system which passes through the full thickness of the cytoplasm and may be of considerable importance for trans-syncytial transfer (Ashley, 1965). Certainly the endoplasmic reticulum appears to communicate with the perinuclear spaces, which are often dilated to form large juxtanuclear vacuoles. The vacuolated appearance of the syncytiotrophoblast is further accentuated by the presence of pinocytotic vacuoles, which are seen most prominently in the region of the surface membrane. Free ribosomes are abundant in the syncytial cytoplasm and tend to occur in clusters or rosettes; numerous granules of glycogen are also a prominent feature. Syncytial mitochondria are moderately numerous and tend to be ovoid or rod-shaped; they have distinct lamellated cristae. There is usually a well-developed Golgi apparatus but this is often obscured by the vacuolated endoplasmic reticulum.

The complexity of the syncytiotrophoblast is compounded by the presence of a variety of granules, droplets and complex vesicles. Prominent amongst these are relatively large electron-dense lipid droplets that lack a limiting membrane and are usually quite numerous. Smaller electron-dense secretory granules, limited by a distinct double membrane, are also present and are seen most commonly in the region of the Golgi apparatus, tending to increase in size as they approach the syncytial surface. Granular

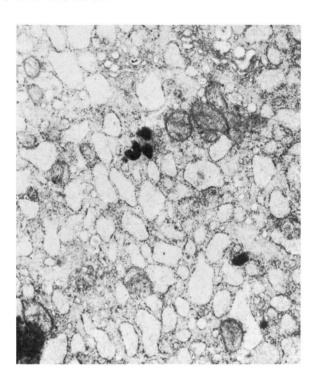

Figure 1.34. Ultrastructure of the cytoplasm of the villous syncytiotrophoblast. There are numerous profiles of rough endoplasmic reticulum, many mitochondria and a few osmiophilic granules (×12,500).

lysosomes, autophagic vacuoles, phagolysosomes, multivesicular bodies and occasional myelin bodies are also seen. The syncytial nuclei are regularly distributed and of moderate electron density, with coarsely clumped chromatin and a prominent nucleolus; the nuclear limiting membrane has a trilamellar structure and nuclear pores have been noted.

The cytotrophoblastic cells are a prominent feature of the trophoblastic layer of the immature villi (Fig. 1.35). The cytoplasm of these cells is less electron-dense than that of the syncytium and is much less richly endowed with subcellular organelles. The endoplasmic reticulum is poorly developed and does not show vacuolation. Free cytoplasmic ribosomes are, however, quite abundant, whilst mitochondria are moderately numerous and tend to be larger and less electron-dense than those of the syncytiotrophoblast. There is a well-developed Golgi complex and occasional secretory granules may be seen in the region of this organelle. Lipid droplets are rarely present in these

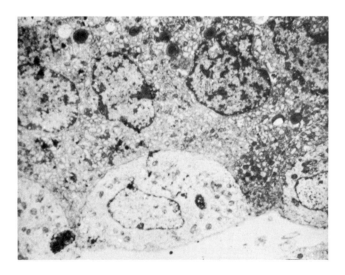

Figure 1.35. Ultrastructure of the villous trophoblast of the term placenta. A single small cytotrophoblastic cell is present in the basal portion of the trophoblast (×1250).

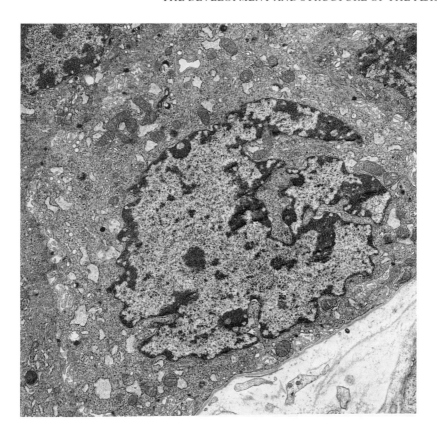

Figure 1.36. Ultrastructure of an intermediate cytotrophoblastic cell. A limiting cell membrane is still present but there is a much greater cytoplasmic complexity than is the case with a normal cytotrophoblastic cell (×7000).

cells and lysosomal structures are sparse or absent; only a little glycogen is normally recognizable but very occasional pinocytotic vesicles may be seen. The nuclei have a tri-lamellar limiting membrane and a prominent nucleolus.

Tighe et al (1967) have noted that an 'intermediate type' cell may also be found in the immature trophoblast. This cell has a more complex subcellular structure than does the normal cytotrophoblastic cell but a less complicated cytoplasmic morphology than the syncytiotrophoblast (Fig. 1.36); it is assumed that this is a cell which is in the process of being converted into a syncytiotrophoblast.

Mature Trophoblast

The ultrastructure of the mature villous trophoblast differs from that of the immature villi quantitatively rather than qualitatively, because its general morphology remains essentially unaltered. The syncytium is irregularly thinned and the nuclei are often aggregated, not infrequently with coarse clumping of their chromatin. The microvilli on the free surface of the syncytium are fewer in number and tend to be shorter and blunter than those seen in the immature placenta. The syncytial cytoplasm has a less complex structure than it does in the first trimester, as the endoplasmic reticulum is less abundant, whilst lipid droplets, secretory granules, glycogen granules, free ribosomes and mitochondria are all less frequently seen. Pinocytotic vesicles are also less numerous, but myelin bodies are more commonly seen than in the immature syncytium.

Cytotrophoblastic cells, though less numerous than in the immature placenta, are regularly present in mature villi (Fig. 1.35). Their ultrastructural characteristics are much the same as those seen in first-trimester villi, but lipid droplets, secretory granules, pinocytotic vesicles and glycogen are absent. In the mature trophoblast the syncytiotrophoblast and cytotrophoblast are linked by desmosomes and occasional tight junctions (Cavicchia, 1971).

The Villous Core

The connective tissue core of the villi contains reticulum cells, fibroblasts, myofibroblasts, Hofbauer cells and capillaries. In early gestation, undifferentiated mesenchymal cells form a loose network in the villous core with collagen fibres forming a delicate mesh around them. The mesenchymal cells differentiate into reticulum cells which have bizarre-shaped bodies and numerous elongated, thin, cytoplasmic processes: their cytoplasm contains rough endoplasmic reticulum, free ribosomes, a well-developed Golgi apparatus and a moderate number of mitochondria. The reticulum cells form a network of stromal channels that run parallel to the long axis of the villus. Fibroblasts differ from reticulum cells in that they have only a few short, thick cytoplasmic processes whilst myofibroblasts are characterized by the presence of areae densae and incomplete basal laminae. Collagen fibres are scanty in the immature villi but are moderately plentiful in the villous stroma of the mature organ.

The Hofbauer cells (Fig. 1.37) usually lie within the channels formed by reticulum cells and have a distinctive ultrastructure (Panigel & Anh, 1964). Their most characteristic feature is an abundance of cytoplasmic vacuoles, which are of variable size, have a

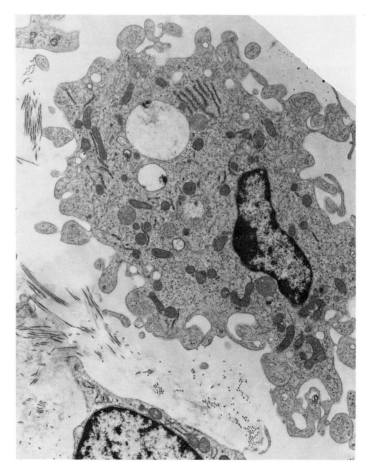

Figure 1.37. Ultrastructure of a villous Hofbauer cell (×6300).

single smooth limiting membrane, and may contain cellular debris, osmiophilic material or granular matter. The endoplasmic reticulum of the Hofbauer cells is poorly developed and there are few cytoplasmic ribosomes; their mitochondria are small.

The lumen of the fetal capillaries is lined by a single layer of endothelial cells, which are usually tapered. In immature villi the union between the cells is short and straight, but as the placenta matures the endothelial cells become thinned and elongated and their junctions become long and overlapping. Their cytoplasm is of moderate density and contains a moderate number of mitochondria, a poorly developed endoplasmic reticulum, and a well-marked Golgi complex. Pinocytotic vesicles are rarely seen in the early stages of pregnancy but are quite abundant in the endothelial cells of the mature placenta. Running through the endothelial cytoplasm are numerous fine filaments, which often form bundles that displace the cytoplasmic organelles to one side. The endothelial cells rest upon a thin, but distinct, basement membrane, which may be unilamellar or multilamellar (Martinek et al, 1975) and outside which are the pericytes, which resemble endothelial cells but have a rather dense and deeply notched nucleus.

Non-villous Trophoblast

Wynn (1972, 1975a) has drawn attention to the ultrastructure of the extravillous cytotrophoblast in the basal plate, cell islands and placental septa. In these sites the cytotrophoblastic cells have a much more complex ultrastructure than do the villous cytotrophoblastic cells; they resemble the 'intermediate type' of cytotrophoblastic cell which is sometimes seen in the villi, and indeed may have an ultrastructural complexity which approaches that of the villous syncytiotrophoblast.

Functional Significance of Ultrastructural Findings

The multiple functions and manifold metabolic activity of the syncytiotrophoblast are amply reflected in the ultrastructural complexity of this tissue. The most important activity of the trophoblast is materno-fetal transfer and it is clear that the pinocytotic vesicles are concerned in the transfer of fluid, and possibly protein, across the syncytium. These vesicles also communicate with a trans-syncytial canalicular system which probably serves as a conduit from the syncytial surface to the villous core. There is some evidence that the multivesicular bodies of the syncytiotrophoblast may also play some part in protein transfer across the syncytium (Martin & Spicer, 1973b; Jones & Fox, 1976) though this is not, as yet, fully confirmed. The function of the microvilli, and their role in syncytial absorption, is rather obscure. It is often assumed that they are a mechanism for increasing the absorptive area of the syncytial surface, and this would accord with the high concentration of alkaline phosphatase and adenosine triphosphatase on their surface (Jones & Fox, 1976). However, as Boyd & Hamilton (1970) have pointed out, the placental microvilli differ quite markedly from those seen on absorptive epithelia such as the intestine or renal tubule.

The syncytiotrophoblast contains all the organelles that one would expect to be present in both steroid-synthesizing and protein-synthesizing tissues and is clearly the major site of placental hormonal synthesis. The non-membrane limited lipid droplets seen in the syncytium are almost certainly nutritional fat *en route* from the maternal to the fetal circulation. The older view that they represent secreted hormone is unlikely, because they do not resemble secretory products as seen in other endocrine tissues. On the other hand, membrane-limited granules and droplets probably are syncytial hormones that are synthesized in the endoplasmic reticulum and 'packaged' by the Golgi apparatus.

Lysosomal structures are regularly present in the syncytium and are particularly abundant in the immature placenta. Their function in this site is uncertain but they may be of considerable significance in placentation and in the extensive restructuring of the placenta that occurs during the first three months of gestation.

Ultrastructural studies have confirmed the origin of the syncytium from the cytotrophoblast, considerable weight having been added to this concept by the demonstration of an 'intermediate' type cell and the finding of remnants of plasma membranes within the syncytium. The villous cytotrophoblastic cells have an ultrastructural simplicity which Wynn (1975b) has compared to that of neoplastic and other cells whose energies are directed principally towards growth rather than synthesis; they are unlikely, therefore, to contribute significantly to placental synthetic activities. The 'intermediate' type cells in the villi and the extravillous cytotrophoblastic cells have, however, a much more complex cytoplasmic structure and thus possess a potential for protein synthesis.

REFERENCES

Adamson, E.D. (1987) Review article: expression of proto-oncogenes in the placenta. *Placenta*, **8**, 449–466.

Adamsons, K. and Myers, R.E. (1975) Circulation in the intervillous space: obstetrical considerations in fetal deprivation. In *The Placenta and its Maternal Supply Line*, Gruenwald, P. (Ed.), pp. 158–177. Lancaster: Medical and Technical Publishing.

Amstutz, E. (1960) Beobachtungen über die Reifung der Chorionzotten in menschlichen Placenta mit besonderer Beruchsichtigung der Epithelplatten. *Acta Anatomica*, **42**, 12–30.

Aplin, J.D. (1991) Implantation, trophoblast differentiation and haemochorial placentation: mechanistic evidence in vivo and in vitro. *Journal of Cell Science*, **99**, 681–692.

Arnholdt, H., Meisel, F., Fandrey, K. and Lohrs, U. (1991) Proliferation of villous trophoblast of the human placenta in normal and abnormal pregnancies. *Virchows Archiv B Cell Pathology*, **60**, 365–372.

Ashley, D. (1965) Study of the human placenta with the electron microscope: functional implications of a canal system in the trophoblast. *Archives of Pathology*, **80**, 377–390.

Autio-Harmainen, H., Sandberg, M., Pihlajaniemi, T. and Vuorio, E. (1991) Synthesis of laminin and type IV collagen by trophoblastic cells and fibroblastic stromal cells in the early human placenta. *Laboratory Investigation*, **64**, 483–491.

Becker, V. (1975) Abnormal maturation of villi. In *The Placenta and its Maternal Supply Line*, Gruenwald, P. (Ed.), pp. 232–243. Lancaster: Medical and Technical Publishing.

Benedetti, W.L., Sala, M.A. and Alvarez, H. (1971) Zones parabasale et parachoriale du placenta humain: I. Différences d'épaisseur du trophoblaste, du nombre de cellules de Langhans et du diametre des villosites. *Gynécologie et Obstétrique*, **70**, 499–506.

Bergstrom, S. (1971) Surface ultrastructure of human amnion and chorion in early pregnancy. *Obstetrics and Gynecology*, **38**, 513–524.

Benirschke, K. and Kaufmann, P. (1990) *Pathology of the Human Placenta*, Second edn. New York: Springer-Verlag.

Blay, J. and Hollenberg, M.D. (1989) The nature and function of polypeptide growth factor receptors in the human placenta. *Journal of Developmental Physiology*, **12**, 237–248.

Bleker, O.P., Kloosterman, G.J., Mieras, D.J., Oosting, J. and Salle, H.J.A. (1975) Intervillous space during uterine contractions in human subjects: an ultrasonic study. *American Journal of Obstetrics and Gynecology*, **123**, 697–699.

Bøe, F. (1953) Studies on the vascularization of the human placenta. *Acta Obstetricia et Gynecologica Scandinavica*, **32**, Supplement 5, 1–92.

Borell, U., Fernstrom, I. and Westman, A. (1958) Eine arteriographische Studie des Plazentakreislaufs. *Geburtshilfe und Frauenheilkunde*, **18**, 1–9.

Boyd, J.D. and Hamilton, W.J. (1964) Stromal trophoblastic buds. *Journal of Obstetrics and Gynaecology of the British Commonwealth*, **71**, 1–10.

Boyd, J.D. and Hamilton, W.J. (1966) Placental septa. *Zeitschrift für Zellforschung und mikroskopische Anatomie*, **69**, 613–634.

Boyd, J.D. and Hamilton, W.J. (1970) *The Human Placenta*. Cambridge: W. Heffer and Sons.

Boyd, J.D. and Hughes, A.F.W. (1954) Observations on human chorionic villi using the electron microscope. *Journal of Anatomy*, **88**, 356–362.

Brosens, I. (1964) A study of the spiral arteries of the decidua basalis in normotensive and hypertensive pregnancies. *Journal of Obstetrics and Gynaecology of the British Commonwealth*, **71**, 222–230.

Brosens, I., Robertson, W.B. and Dixon, H.G. (1967) The physiological response of the vessels of the placental bed to normal pregnancy. *Journal of Pathology and Bacteriology*, **93**, 569–579.

Bulmer, J.N. and Johnson, P.M. (1984) Macrophage populations in the human placenta. *Clinical and Experimental Immunology*, **57**, 393–403.

Burgos, M.H. and Rodriguez, E.M. (1966) Specialized zones in the trophoblast of the human term placenta. *American Journal of Obstetrics and Gynecology*, **96**, 342–356.

Burton, D.J. (1986a) Intervillous connections in the mature human placenta: instances of syncytial fusion or section artifacts? *Journal of Anatomy*, **145**, 13–23.

Burton G.J. (1986b) Scanning electron microscopy of intervillous connections in the mature human placenta. *Journal of Anatomy*, **147**, 245–254.

Burton, G.J. (1987) The fine structure of the human placental villus as revealed by scanning electron microscopy. *Scanning Microscopy*, **1**, 1811–1828.

Burton, G.J. (1990) On the varied appearance of the human placental villous surface visualized by scanning electron microscopy. *Journal of Scanning Electron Microscopy*, **4**, 504–507.

Burton, G.J. and Tham, S.W. (1992) The formation of vasculosyncytial membranes in the human placenta. *Journal of Developmental Physiology*, **18**, 43–47.

Cantle, S.J., Kaufmann, P., Luckhardt, M. and Schweikhart, G. (1987) Interpretation of syncytial sprouts and bridges in the human placenta. *Placenta*, **8**, 221–234.

Carter, J.E. (1964) Morphologic evidence of syncytial formation from the cytotrophoblastic cells. *Obstetrics and Gynecology*, **23**, 647–656.

Castellucci, M. and Kaufmann, P. (1982a) A three dimensional study of the normal human placental villous core. *Placenta*, **3**, 269–286.

Castellucci, M. and Kaufmann, P. (1982b) Evolution of the stroma in human chorionic villi throughout pregnancy. *Biblioteca Anatomica*, **22**, 40–45.

Castellucci, M. and Zaccheo, D. (1989) The Hofbauer cells of the human placenta: morphological and immunological aspects. *Progress in Clinical Biological Research*, **269**, 443–451.

Castellucci, M., Zaccheo, D. and Pescetto, G. (1980) A three dimensional study of the normal human placental villous core. I. The Hofbauer cells. *Cell and Tissue Research*, **210**, 235–247.

Castellucci, M., Schweikhart, G., Kaufmann, P. and Zaccheo, D. (1984) The stromal architecture of the immature intermediate villus of the human placenta. *Gynecologic and Obstetric Investigation*, **18**, 95–99.

Castellucci, M., Celona, A., Bartels H. et al (1987) Mitosis of the Hofbauer cell: possible implications for a fetal macrophage. *Placenta*, **8**, 65–76.

Castellucci, M., Scheper, M., Scheffen, I., Celona, A. and Kaufmann, P. (1990) The development of the human placental villous tree. *Anatomy and Embryology*, **181**, 117–128.

Cavicchia, J.C. (1971) Junctional complexes in the trophoblast of the human full term placenta. *Journal of Anatomy* **108**, 339–346.

Cianci, S. and Russo, I. (1975) Ultrastruttura di superficie della placenta umana nel porto pretermine: studio al microscopico elettronico a scansione. *Patologia e Clinica Ostetrica e Ginecologica*, **3**, 1–7.

Cibils, L.A. (1968) Growth of the placental villi in the first trimester. *Lying-in. The Journal of Reproductive Medicine*, **1**, 377–387.

Contractor, S.F., Banks, R.W., Jones, C.J.P. and Fox, H. (1977) A possible role for placental lysosomes in the formation of villous syncytiotrophoblast. *Cell and Tissue Research*, **178**, 411–419.

Crawford, J.M. (1961) A study of the human placental capillary. *Journal of Obsetetrics and Gynaecology of the British Commonwealth*, **68**, 378–381.

Daya, D. and Sabet, L. (1991) The use of cytokeratin as a sensitive and reliable marker for trophoblastic tissue. *American Journal of Obstetrics and Gynecology*, **95**, 137–141.

Demir, R. (1979) Scanning electron microscopic observations on the surfaces of chorionic villi of young and mature placentas. *Acta Anatomica*, **105**, 226–232.

Demir, R., Kaufmann, P., Castellucci, M., Erbengi, T. and Kotowski, A. (1989) Fetal vasculogenesis and angiogenesis in human placental villi. *Acta Anatomica*, **136**, 190–203.

Demir, R., Demir, N., Kohnen, G. et al (1992) Ultrastructure and distribution of myofibroblast-like cells in human placental stem villi. *Electron Microscopy*, **3**, 509–510.

Demir, R., Demir, N., Ustunel, I. et al (1994) The fine structure of normal and ectopic (tubal) human placental villi as revealed by scanning and transmission electron microscopy. *Zentralblatt für Pathologie*, **140**, 427–442.

Dempsey, E.W. (1972) The development of capillaries in the villi of early human placentas. *American Journal of Anatomy*, **134**, 221–238.

Dempsey, E.W. and Luse, S.A. (1971) Regional specialisation in the syncytial trophoblast of early human placentas. *Journal of Anatomy*, **108**, 545–556.

Denker, H.W. (1990) Trophoblast-endometrial interactions at embryo implantation: a cell biological paradox. *Trophoblast Research*, **4**, 3–29.

de Wolf, F., de Wolf-Peeters, C. and Brosens, I. (1973) Ultrastructure of the spiral arteries in the human placental bed at the end of normal pregnancy. *American Journal of Obstetrics and Gynecology*, **117**, 833–848.

de Wolf, F., de Wolf-Peeters, C., Brosens, I. and Robertson, W.B. (1980) The human placental bed: electron microscopic study of trophoblastic invasion of spiral arteries. *American Journal of Obstetrics and Gynecology*, **137**, 58–70.

Dixon, H.G. and Robertson, W.B. (1958) A study of the vessels of the placental bed in normotensive and hypertensive women. *Journal of Obstetrics and Gynaecology of the British Empire*, **65**, 803–810.

Dixon, H.G. and Robertson, W.B. (1961) Vascular changes in the placental bed. *Pathologia et Microbiologia*, **24**, 622–630.

Duance, V.C. and Bailey, A.J. (1983) Structure of the trophoblast basement membrane. In *Biology of Trophoblast*, Loke, Y.W. and Whyte, A. (Eds), pp. 597–625. Amsterdam: Elsevier.

Durst-Zivkovic, B. (1973) Das Vorkommen der Mastzellen in der Nachgeburt. *Anatomischer Anzeiger*, **134**, 225–229.

Enders, A.C. (1965) Formation of syncytium from cytotrophoblast in the human placenta. *Obstetrics and Gynecology*, **25**, 378–386.

Enders, A.C. and King, B.F. (1970) The cytology of Hofbauer cells. *Anatomical Record*, **167**, 231–252.

Feller, A.C., Schneider, H., Schmidt, D. and Parwaresch, M.R. (1985) Myofibroblast as a major cellular constituent of villous stroma in human placenta. *Placenta*, **6**, 405–415.

Fisher, S.J. and Damsky, C.H. (1993) Human cytotrophoblast invasion. *Seminars in Cell Biology*, **4**, 183–188.

Fox, H. (1964) The pattern of villous variability in the normal placenta. *Journal of Obstetrics and Gynaecology of the British Commonwealth*, **71**, 749–758.

Fox, H. (1965) The significance of villous syncytial knots in the human placenta. *Journal of Obstetrics and Gynaecology of the British Commonwealth*, **72**, 347–355.

Fox, H. (1967a) The incidence and significance of Hofbauer cells in the mature placenta. *Journal of Pathology and Bacteriology*, **93**, 710–717.

Fox, H. (1967b) The incidence and significance of vasculo-syncytial membranes in the human placenta. *Journal of Obstetrics and Gynaecology of the British Commonwealth*, **74**, 28–33.

Fox, H. (1979) The placenta as a model of organ ageing. In *Placenta–A Neglected Experimental Animal*, Beaconsfield, P. and Villee, C. (Eds) pp. 351–378. Oxford: Pergamon.

Fox, H. and Agrofojo-Blanco, A. (1974) Scanning electron microscopy of the human placenta in normal and abnormal pregnancies. *European Journal of Obstetrics, Gynecology and Reproductive Biology*, **4**, 45–50.

Fox, H. and Kharkongor, F.N. (1969) Enzyme histochemistry of the Hofbauer cells of the human placenta. *Journal of Obstetrics and Gynaecology of the British Commonwealth*, **76**, 918–921.

Frank, H.G., Malekzadeh, F., Kertschanska, S et al. (1994) Immunohistochemistry of two different types of placental fibrinoid. *Acta Anatomica*, **150**, 55–68.

Freese, U.E. (1966) The fetal-maternal circulation of the placenta. I. Histomorphologic, plastoid injection and X-ray cinematographic studies on human placentas. *American Journal of Obstetrics and Gynecology*, **94**, 354–360.

Freese, U.E. (1968) The uteroplacental vascular relationship in the human. *American Journal of Obstetrics and Gynecology*, **101**, 8–16.

Freese, U.E. (1969) The fetal-maternal circulation: a redefinition of the utero-placental vascular relationship and the intervillous space in the human and the rhesus monkey. In *The Foeto-Placental Unit*, Pecile, A. and Finzi, C. (Eds), pp. 18–22. Amsterdam: Excerpta Medica.

Galton, M. (1962) DNA content of placental nuclei. *Journal of Cell Biology*, 13, 183–191.

Gaunt, M. and Ockleford, C.D. (1986) Microinjection of human placenta: 2. Biological application. *Placenta*, **7**, 325–332.

Geier, G., Schuhmann, R. and Kraus, H. (1975) Regional unterschiedliche Zellproliferation innerhalb der Plazentone reifer menschlicher Plazenten: autoradiographische Untersuchungen. *Archiv für Gynäkologie*, **218**, 31–37.

Gerl, D., Eichhorn, H., Eichhorn, K.-H. and Franke, H. (1973) Quantitative Messungen synzytialer Zellkernkonzentration der menschlichen Plazenta bei normalen und pathologischen Schwangerschaften. *Zentralblatt für Gynäkologie*, **95**, 263–266.

Gerretsen, G., Huisjes, H.J., Hardouk, M.J. and Elema, J.D. (1983) Trophoblast alterations in the placental bed in relation to physiological changes in spiral arteries. *British Journal of Obstetrics and Gynaecology*, **90**, 34–39.

Getzowa, S. and Sadowsky, A. (1950) On the structure of the human placenta with full term and immature foetus, living or dead. *Journal of Obstetrics and Gynaecology of the British Empire*, **57**, 388–396.

Glienke, P. (1974) Zur Ultrastruktur der Septen der menschlichen Plazenta. *Zeitschrift für mikroskopisch-anatomische Forschung*, **88**, 111–147.

Gosseye, S. and Fox, H. (1984) An immunohistological comparison of the secretory capacity of villous and extravillous trophoblast in the human placenta. *Placenta*, **5**, 329–348.

Gosseye, S. and van der Veen, F. (1992) HPL-positive infiltrating trophoblastic cells in normal and abnormal pregnancy. *European Journal of Obstetrics and Gynecology and Reproductive Biology*, **44**, 85–90.

Graf, R., Schonfelder, G., Langer, J.-U. et al (1994) Das extravasale kontraktile System der Humanplazenta: ein neuer Aspekt für die Funktion des Organs? *Zentralblatt für Gynäkologie*, **116**, 344–346.

Graf, R., Schonfelder, G., Muhlberger, M. and Gutsmann, M. (1995) The perivascular contractile sheath of human placental stem villi: its isolation and characterization. *Placenta*, **16**, 57–66.

Gruenwald, P. (1973) Lobular structure of hemochorial primate placentas, and its relation to maternal vessels. *American Journal of Anatomy*, **136**, 133–152.

Gruenwald, P. (1975a) Maternal blood supply to the conceptus. *European Journal of Obstetrics, Gynecology and Reproductive Biology*, **5**, 23–30.

Gruenwald, P. (1975b) Lobular architecture of primate placentas. In *The Placenta and its Maternal Supply Line*, Gruenwald, P. (Ed.), pp. 35–55. Lancaster: Medical and Technical Publishing.

Habashi, S., Burton, G.J. and Steven, D.H. (1983) Morphological study of of the fetal vasculature of the human placenta: scanning electron microscopy of corrosion casts. *Placenta*, **4**, 41–56.

Hamilton, W.J. and Boyd, J.D. (1966) Trophoblast in human uteroplacental arteries. *Nature*, **212**, 906–908.

Harris, J.W.S. and Ramsey, E.M. (1966) The morphology of human uteroplacental vasculature. *Contributions to Embryology. Carnegie Institution of Washington*, **38**, 43–58.

Herbst, R. and Multier, R.M. (1970) Les microvillosités à la surface des villosités chorionique du placenta humain. *Gynécologie et Obstétrique*, **69**, 609–616.

Hertig, A.T. (1935) Angiogenesis in the early human chorion and in the primary placenta of the macaque monkey. *Contributions to Embryology. Carnegie Institution of Washington*, **25**, 37–81.

Hormann, G. (1953) Ein Beiträg zur funktionellen Morphologie der menschlichen Placenta. *Archiv für Gynakologie*, **184**, 109–123.

Hustin, J. (1995) Vascular physiology and pathophysiology of early pregnancy. In *Transvaginal Colour Doppler*, Bourne, T.H., Jauniaux, E. and Jurkovic, D. (Eds), pp. 47–56. Berlin: Springer.

Hustin, J., Schaaps, J.P. and Lambotte, R. (1988) Anatomical studies of the utero-placental vascularization in the first trimester of pregnancy. *Trophoblast Research*, **3**, 49–60.

Jackson, M.R., Mayhew, T.M. and Boyd, P.A. (1992) Quantitative description of the elaboration and maturation of villi from 10 weeks of gestation to term. *Placenta*, **13**, 357–370.

Jauniaux, E., Jurkovic, D. and Campbell, S. (1995) Current topic: in vivo investigation of the placental circulation by Doppler echography. *Placenta*, **16**, 323–331.

Jones, C.J.P. and Fox, H. (1976) An ultrahistochemical study of the distribution of acid and alkaline phosphatases in placentae from normal and complicated pregnancies. *Journal of Pathology*, **118**, 143–151.

Jones, C.J.P. and Fox, H. (1977) Syncytial knots and intervillous bridges in the human placenta: an ultrastructural study. *Journal of Anatomy*, **124**, 275–286.

Jones, C.J.P. and Fox, H. (1991) Ultrastructure of the normal human placenta. *Electron Microscopy Review*, **4**, 129–178.

Kaufmann, P. (1982) Development and differentiation of the human placental villous tree. *Bibliotheca Anatomica*, **22**, 29–39.

Kaufmann, P. (1995) Development and anatomy of the placenta. In: *Haines and Taylor: Obstetrical and Gynaecological Pathology*, 4th edn, Fox, H. (Ed.), pp. 1437–1476. Edinburgh: Churchill Livingstone.

Kaufmann, P. and Stark, J. (1971) Die Basalplatte der reifen menschlichen Placenta. I. Semidunnschnitt Histologie. *Zeitschrift für Anatomie und Entwicklungsgeschichte*, **135**, 1–19.

Kaufmann, P. and Stegner, H.E. (1972) Uber die funktionelle Differenzierung des Zottensyncytiums in der menschlichen Placenta. *Zeitschrift für Zellforschung und mikroskopische Anatomie*, **135**, 361–382.

Kaufmann, P., Stark, J. and Stegner, H.E. (1977) The villous stroma of the human placenta. I. The ultrastructure of fixed connective tissue cells. *Cell and Tissue Research*, **177**, 105–121.

Kaufmann, P., Sen, D. and Schweikhart, G. (1979) Classification of human placental villi. I. Histology and scanning electron microscopy. *Cell and Tissue Research*, **200**, 409–423.

Kaufmann, P., Nagl, W. and Fuhrmann, B. (1983) Die funktionelle Bedeutung der Langhanszellen der menschlichen Placenta. *Anatomischer Anzeiger*, **77**, 435–436.

Kaufmann, P., Bruns, U., Leiser, R., Luckhardt, M. and Winterhager, E. (1985) The fetal vascularization of term human placental villi. II. Intermediate and terminal villi. *Anatomy and Embryology*, **173**, 203–214.

Kaufmann, P., Luckhardt, M., Schweikhart, G. and Cantle, S.J. (1987) Cross-sectional features and three dimensional structure of human placental villi. *Placenta*, **8**, 235–247.

Kaufmann, P., Luckhardt, M. and Leiser, R. (1988) Three dimensional representation of the fetal vessel system in the human placenta. *Trophoblast Research*, **3**, 113–137.

Kawakami, S. (1975) Scanning electron microscopic observation of human placental villi. *Acta Obstetricia et Gynaecologica Japonica*, **22**, 132–137.

Khudr, G., Soma, H. and Benirschke, K. (1973) Trophoblastic origin of the X-cells and the placental site giant cells. *American Journal of Obstetrics and Gynecology*, **115**, 530–533.

King, B.F. and Menton, D.N. (1975) Scanning electron microscopy of human placental villi from early and late in gestation. *American Journal of Obstetrics and Gynecology*, **122**, 824–828.

Kosanke, G., Castellucci, M., Kaufmann, P. and Mirinov, V.A. (1993) Branching patterns of human placental villous trees: perspectives of topological analysis. *Placenta*, **14**, 591–604.

Krantz, K.E. and Parker, J.C. (1963) Contractile properties of the smooth muscle in the human placenta. *Clinical Obstetrics and Gynecology*, **6**, 26–38.

Kurman, R.J., Main, C.S. and Chen, H.C. (1984) Intermediate trophoblast: a distinctive form of trophoblast with specific morphological, biochemical and functional features. *Placenta*, **5**, 349–369.

Kustermann, W. (1981) Uber 'Proliferationsknoten' und 'Syncytialknoten' der menschlichen Placenta. *Anatomischer Anzeiger*, **150**, 144–157.

Leibl, W., Kerjaschki, D., Rockenschaub, A. and Horandner, H. (1975) Die Oberfläche menschlicher Placentarzotten: eine rasterelektronenmikroskopische Studie. *Wiener Medizinische Wochenschrift*, **125**, 144–153.

Leiser, R., Luckhardt, M., Kaufmann, P., Winterhager, E. and Bruns, U. (1985) The fetal vascularization of term human placental villi. I. Peripheral stem villi. *Anatomy and Embryology*, **173**, 71–80.

Lemtis, H.G. (1969) New insights into the maternal circulatory system of the human placenta. In *The Foeto-Placental Unit*, Pecile, A. and Finzi, C. (Eds), pp. 25–30. Amsterdam: Excerpta Medica.

Lemtis, H.G. (1970) Physiologie der Plazenta. *Fortschritte der Geburtshilfe und Gynäkologie*, **41**, 1–52.

Lerat, M.F., Connehaye, P., Richomme, J., Magré, J. and Bonnaille, J. (1973) Etude du placenta humain au microscope electronique à balayage. *Journal de Gynécologie, Obstétrique et Biologie de la Reproduction*, **2**, 233–241.

Loke, Y.W., Eremin, O., Ashby, J. and Day, S. (1982) Characterization of the phagocytic cells isolated from the human placenta. *Journal of the Reticuloendothelial Society*, **31**, 317–324.

Longo, L.D. (1972) Disorders of placental transfer. In *Pathophysiology of Gestation*, Vol. 2, Assali, N.S. (Ed.), pp. 1–76. New York: Academic Press.

Ludwig, H. (1974) Surface structure of the human placenta. In *The Placenta: Biological and Clinical Aspects*, Moghissi, K.S. and Hafez, E.S.E. (Eds), pp. 40–64. Springfield, Illinois: Charles C. Thomas.

Ludwig, H., Junkermann, H. and Klingele, H. (1971) Oberflachen Strukturen der menschlichen Plazenta im Rasterelektonenmikroskop. *Archiv für Gynäkologie*, **210**, 1–20.

Mahnke, P.F. and Emmrich, P. (1973) Zur Mastzellhaufigkeit der menschlichen Plazentarzotte. *Zentralblatt für Gynäkologie*, **95**, 730–732.

Maidman, J.E., Thorpe, L.W., Harris, J.A. and Wynn, R.W. (1973) Fetal origin of X-cells in human placental septa and basal plate. *Obstetrics and Gynecology*, **41**, 547–552.

Martin, B.J. and Spicer, S.S. (1973a) Ultrastructural features of cellular maturation and aging in human trophoblast. *Journal of Ultrastructure Research*, **43**, 133–149.

Martin, B.J. and Spicer, S.S. (1973b) Multivesicular bodies and related structures in the syncytiotrophoblast of human term placenta. *Anatomical Record*, **175**, 15–36.

Martinek, J.J., Gallagher, M.L. and Essig, G.F. (1975) An electron microscopic study of fetal capillary basal laminas of 'normal' human term placentas. *American Journal of Obstetrics and Gynecology*, **121**, 17–24.

Martinoli, C., Castellucci, M., Zaccheo, D. and Kaufmann, P. (1984) Scanning electron microscopy of stromal cells of human placental villi throughout pregnancy. *Cell and Tissue Research*, **235**, 647–655.

Mayhew, T.M., Jackson, M.R. and Boyd, P.A. (1993) Changes in oxygen diffusive conductances of human placentae during gestation (10–41 weeks) are commensurate with the gain in fetal weight. *Placenta*, **14**, 51–61.

Michael, C. (1974) Actomyosin content of human placenta. *Journal of Obstetrics and Gynaecology of the British Commonwealth*, **81**, 307–310.

Mitchell, M.D., Trautman, M.S. and Dudley, D.J. (1993) Cytokine networking in the placenta. *Placenta*, **14**, 249–275.

Moll, W. (1995) Invited commentary: absence of intervillous blood flow in the first trimester of human pregnancy. *Placenta*, **16**, 333–334.

Moll, W., Künzel, W. and Herberger, J. (1975) Hemodynamic implications of hemochorial placentation. *European Journal of Obstetrics, Gynecology and Reproductive Biology*, **5**, 67–74.

Moskalewski, S., Ptak, W. and Czarnik, Z. (1975) Demonstration of cells with IgG receptor in human placenta. *Biology of the Neonate*, **26**, 268–273.

Myatt, L., Brockman, D.E., Eis, A.L. and Pollock, J.S. (1993) Immunohistochemical localization of nitric oxide synthase in the human placenta. *Placenta*, **14**, 487–495.

Nanaev, A.K., Rokosuev, V.S., Shirinsky, V.P. et al. (1991) Confocal and conventional immunofluorescent and immunogold electron microscopic localization of collagen types III and IV in human placenta. *Placenta*, **12**, 573–595.

Ockleford, C.D. and Whyte, A. (1977) Differentiated regions of human placental cell surface associated with exchange of materials between maternal and foetal blood: coated vessels. *Cellular Biology*, **1**, 137–146.

Ohlsson, R. (1989) Growth factors, protooncogenes and human placental development. *Cell Differentiation and Development*, **28**, 1–16.

Ohlsson, R., Glaer, A., Holmgren, L. and Franklin, G. (1993) The molecular biology of placental development. In *The Human Placenta*, Redman, C.W.G., Sargent, I.L. and Starkey, P.M. (Eds), pp. 33–81. Oxford: Blackwell.

Panigel, M. and Anh, J.N.H. (1964) Ultrastructure des cellules de Hofbauer dans le placenta humain. *Compte Rendu des Séances de l'Academie des Sciences* (Paris), **258**, 3556–3558.

Papalia-Early, A. and Gruenwald, P. (1976) The villous stems of the human placenta. *Biology of the Neonate*, **28**, 125–132.

Peter, K. (1943) Placenta-Studien. I Zotten und Zwischenzottenraume Zweier Placenta aus den Letzen Monaten der Schwangerschaft. *Zeitschrift für mikroskopische-anatomische Forschung*, **53**, 142–174.

Pijnenborg, R. (1994) Trophoblast invasion. *Reproductive Medicine Review*, **3**, 53–73.

Pijnenborg, R., Dixon, G., Robertson, W.B. and Brosens, I. (1980) Trophoblastic invasion of human decidua from 8 to 18 weeks of pregnancy. *Placenta*, **1**, 3–19.

Pijnenborg, R., Robertson, W.B., Brosens, I. and Dixon, H.G. (1981) Trophoblast invasion and the establishment of haemochorial placentation in man and laboratory animals. *Placenta*, **2**, 71–92.

Pijnenborg, R., Bland, J.M., Robertson, W.B. and Brosens, I. (1983) Uteroplacental arterial changes related to interstitial trophoblast migration in early human pregnancy. *Placenta*, **4**, 397–414.

Pijnenborg, R, Anthony, J., Davey, D.A. et al. (1991) Placental bed spiral arteries in the hypertensive disorders of pregnancy. *British Journal of Obstetrics and Gynaecology*, **98**, 648–655.

Pisarki, T. and Topilko, A. (1966) Comparative study of the vascular syncytial membranes of the human placenta in light and electron microscopy. *Polish Medical Journal*, **5**, 630–638.

Pisarki, T., Spaczynski, M. and Glyda, A. (1975) Ksztaltowanie sie plyty podstawowej lozyska. (Formation of the placentar basal plate.) *Ginekologica Polska*, **46**, 729–735.

Ramsey, E.M. (1954) Circulation in the maternal placenta of primates. *American Journal of Obstetrics and Gynecology*, **67**, 1–14.

Ramsey, E.M. (1956) Circulation in the maternal placenta of the rhesus monkey and man, with observations on the marginal lakes. *American Journal of Anatomy*, **98**, 159–190.

Ramsey, E.M. (1959) Circulation in the placenta. In *Gestation: Transactions of the 5th Conference*, Villee, C.E. (Ed.), pp. 77–107. New York: Macey Foundation.

Ramsey, E.M. (1962) Circulation in the intervillous space of the primate placenta. *American Journal of Obstetrics and Gynecology*, **84**, 1649–1663.

Ramsey, E.M. (1965) Circulation of the placenta. *Birth Defects Original Article Series*, **1**, 5–12.

Ramsey, E.M. (1975) In discussion of Gruenwald, P. *European Journal of Obstetrics, Gynecology and Reproductive Biology*, **5**, 31.

Ramsey, E.M. and Donner, M.W. (1980) *Placental Vasculature and Circulation*. Stuttgart: Georg Thieme.

Ramsey, E.M., Corner, G.W. Jr and Donner, M.W. (1963) Serial and cineangioradiographic visualization of maternal circulation in the primate (hemochorial) placenta. *American Journal of Obstetrics and Gynecology*, **26**, 213–225.

Richart, R. (1961) Studies of placental morphogenesis. I. Radioautographic studies of human placenta utilizing tritiated thymidine. *Proceedings of the Society for Experimental Biology and Medicine (New York)*, **106**, 829–831.

Robertson, W.B. (1976) Uteroplacental vasculature. *Journal of Clinical Pathology*, **29**, Supplement (Royal College of Pathologists) **10**, 9–17.

Robertson, W.B. and Warner, B. (1974) The ultrastructure of the human placental bed. *Journal of Pathology*, **112**, 203–211.

Robertson, W.B., Brosens, I. and Dixon, G. (1975) Uteroplacental vascular pathology. *European Journal of Obstetrics, Gynecology and Reproductive Biology*, **5**, 47–65.

Romney, S.L. and Reid, D.E. (1951) Observations on the fetal aspects of placental circulation. *American Journal of Obstetrics and Gynecology*, **61**, 83–97.

Rukosuev, V.S. (1992) Immunofluorescent localization of collagen types I, III, IV, V, fibronectin, laminin, entactin, and heparan sulphate proteoglycan in human immature placenta. *Experientia*, **48**, 285–287.

Saji, F., Koyama, M. and Matsuzaki, N. (1994) Current topic: human placental Fc receptors. *Placenta*, **15**, 453–466.

Salazar, H. and Gonzalez-Angulo, A. (1967) The fine structure of human chorionic villi and placental transfer of iron in late pregnancy. *American Journal of Obstetrics and Gynecology*, **87**, 851–865.

Sargent, I.L., Redman, C.W.G. and Starkey, P.M. (1993) The placenta as a graft. In *The Human Placenta*, Redman, C.W.G., Sargent, I.L. and Starkey, P.M. (Eds), pp. 334–361. Oxford: Blackwell.

Schaaps, J.P. and Hustin, J. (1988) In vivo aspects of the materno-trophoblastic border during the first trimester of gestation. *Trophoblast Research*, **3**, 39–48.

Schuhmann, R. (1981) Plazenton: Begriff, Enstehung, funktionelle Anatomie. In *Die Plazenta des Menschen*, Becker, V., Schiebler, T.H. and Kubli, H. (Eds), pp. 199–207. Stuttgart: Georg Thieme.

Schuhmann, R., Kraus, H., Borst, R. and Geier, G. (1976) Regional unterschiedliche Enzymaktivitt innerhalb der Placentone reifer menschlicher Placenten: histochemische und biochemische Untersuchungen. *Archiv für Gynäkologie*, **220**, 209–226.

Sedmak, D.D., Davis, D.H., Singh, U., van de Winkel, J.G.J. and Anderson, C.L. (1991) Expression of IgG Fc receptor antigens in placenta and on endothelial cells in humans: an immunohistochemical study. *American Journal of Pathology*, **138**, 175–181.

Sen, D.K., Kaufmann, P. and Schweikhart, G. (1979) Classification of human placental villi. II. Morphometry. *Cell and Tissue Research*, **200**, 425–434.

Sheppard, B.L. and Bonnar, J. (1974) The ultrastructure of the arterial supply of the human placenta in early and late pregnancy. *Journal of Obstetrics and Gynaecology of the British Commonwealth*, **81**, 497–511.

Shorter, S.C., Starkey, P.M., Ferry, B.L. et al. (1993) Antigenic heterogeneity of human cytotrophoblast and evidence for the transient expression of MHC class I antigens distinct from HLA-G. *Placenta*, **14**, 571–582.

Simpson, R.A., Mayhew, T.M. and Barnes, P.R. (1992) From 13 weeks to term, the trophoblast of human placenta grows by the continuous recruitment of new proliferative units: a study of nuclear number using the dissector. *Placenta*, **13**, 501–512.

Sutton, L., Gadd, M., Mason, D.Y. and Redman, C.W.G. (1986) Cells bearing class II MHC antigens in the human placenta and amniochorion. *Immunology*, **58**, 23–29.

Sutton, L., Mason, D.Y. and Redman, C.W.G. (1989) Isolation and characterization of human fetal macrophages from placenta. *Clinical and Experimental Immunology*, **78**, 437–443.

Szpakowski, M. (1974) Morphology of arterial anastomoses in the human placenta. *Folia Morphologica (Warsaw)*, **33**, 53–60.

ten Berge, B.S. (1955) Capillaraktion in der Placenta. *Archiv für Gynäkologie*, **186**, 253–256.

Tedde, G. and Tedde-Piras, A. (1978) Mitotic index of the Langhans cells in the normal human placenta from the early stages of pregnancy to term. *Acta Anatomica*, **100**, 114–119.

Terzakis, J.A. (1963) The ultrastructure of normal human first trimester placenta. *Journal of Ultrastructure Research*, **9**, 268–284.

Tighe, J.R., Garrod, P.R. and Curran, R.C. (1967) The trophoblast of the human chorionic villus. *Journal of Pathology and Bacteriology*, **93**, 559–567.

Voland, J.R., Frisman, D.M. and Baird, S.M. (1986) Presence of an endothelial antigen on the syncytiotrophoblast of human chorionic villi: detection by a monoclonal antibody. *American Journal of Reproductive Immunology and Microbiology*, **11**, 24–30.

Weinberg, P.C., Cameron, I.L., Parmley, T., Jeter, J.R. and Pauerstein, C.J. (1970) Gestational age and placental cellular replication. *Obstetrics and Gynecology*, **36**, 692–696.

Wigglesworth, J.S. (1967) Vascular organization of the human placenta. *Nature*, **216**, 1120–1121.

Wigglesworth, J.S. (1969) The vascular organization of the human placenta and its significance for placental pathology. In *The Foeto-Placental Unit*, Pecile, A. and Finzi, C. (Eds), pp. 34–40. Amsterdam: Excerpta Medica.

Wilkin, P. (1954) Contribution a l'étude de la circulation placentaire d'origine foetale. *Gynécologie et Obstétrique*, **53,** 239–263.

Wilkin, P. (1965) *Pathologie du Placenta*. Paris: Masson.

Wislocki, G.B. and Dempsey, E.W. (1955) Electron microscopy of the human placenta. *Anatomical Record*, **123,** 133–167.

Wood, G.W. (1980) Mononuclear phagocytes in the human placenta. *Placenta*, **1,** 113–123.

Wood, G.W., Reynard, J., Krishnan, E. and Racela, I. (1978) Immunobiology of the human placenta. I. IgGFc receptors in trophoblastic villi. *Cellular Immunology*, **35,** 191–204.

Wynn, R.W. (1972) Cytotrophoblastic specializations: an ultrastructural study of the human placenta. *American Journal of Obstetrics and Gynecology*, **114,** 339–353.

Wynn, R.W. (1975a) Fine structure of the placenta. In *The Placenta and its Maternal Supply Line*, Gruenwald, P. (Ed.), pp. 56–79. Lancaster: Medical and Technical Publishing.

Wynn, R.W. (1975b) Development and ultrastructural adaptations of the human placenta. *European Journal of Obstetrics, Gynecology and Reproductive Biology*, **5,** 3–21.

Yamanda, T., Isemura, M., Yamaguchi, Y. et al. (1987) Immunohistochemical localization of fibronectin in the human placenta at their different stages of maturation. *Histochemistry*, **86,** 579–584.

2

PHYSIOLOGY OF THE PLACENTA

Despite the apparent morphological simplicity of the placenta, it is, in functional terms, a many-splendoured thing. It is an endocrine organ of some magnitude and complexity, it plays a vital role in the transfer of oxygen and nutrients to the fetus, and it acts, in an as yet undetermined manner, as an immunological barrier that prevents rejection of the fetal allograft. This last function is considered in Chapter 12 but the endocrine and transfer activities of the placenta will be discussed here; however, no attempt will be made to present these in anything more than a simplified and abbreviated form, because to do more would require a dissertation of a length and complexity that would be out of place in a pathological text.

THE PLACENTA AS AN ENDOCRINE ORGAN

The placenta can synthesize both steroid and polypeptide hormones, the latter being produced largely by its own efforts and the former usually requiring a preformed substrate. The literature on this topic is vast and rather than clutter the text with long lists of references, I feel it preferable, in this chapter only, simply to refer those wishing to pursue this topic in greater depth to several excellent reviews (Diczfalusy, 1969; Diczfalusy and Mancuso, 1969; Siiteri et al, 1974; Thau & Lanman, 1975; Shearman, 1985; Chard, 1986, 1992; Jones, 1989; Conley & Mason, 1990; Ogren & Talamantes, 1994; Solomon, 1994): a few highly specific references are, however, cited in the text.

Hormones Produced by the Placenta

Steroid Hormones

Steroid hormones are synthesized from substrates reaching the placenta from either the maternal or fetal circulation. Synthesis of these hormones is enzymatic and is not dependent, as is synthesis of peptide hormones, on the presence of specific genes and mRNAs.

Oestrogens During pregnancy the maternal excretion of oestrogens rises dramatically from under 100 μg a day in non-pregnant women to over 300 mg a day at term. A considerable proportion, about 85–90% of this rise is accounted for by oestriol and its conjugates, and it is now clear that the production of this substance is largely dependent on trophoblastic utilization of substrates produced by the fetal adrenals (Fig. 2.1). The principal substrate is dehydroepiandrosterone sulfate, which is synthesized in the fetal adrenals, hydroxylated in the 16-alpha position by the fetal liver, and then

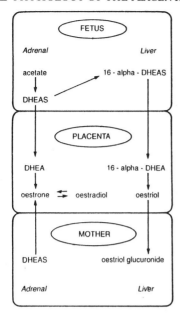

Figure 2.1. Schematic outline of oestrogen metabolism during pregnancy. DHEA, dehydroepiandrosterone; DHEAS, dehydroepiandrosterone sulfate; 16-alpha-DHEA, 16-alpha-hydroxy-dehydroepiandrosterone; 16-alpha-DHEAS, 16-alpha-hydroxy-dehydroepiandrosterone sulfate.

transferred to the placenta, where it is first hydrolysed by the enzyme sulfatase and then aromatized by the enzymes delta⁵-isomerase and delta⁵-3-beta-steroid dehydrogenase to oestriol. Unconjugated oestriol is secreted into both the maternal and fetal circulations; in the former it is conjugated largely in the liver, to be excreted subsequently in the urine as oestriol glucuronide. A little oestriol is produced by maternal hepatic conversion of oestrone and oestradiol, but this is an unimportant source of the hormone during pregnancy.

The trophoblast also synthesizes oestradiol and oestrone, but is less dependent on the fetus for the supply of a substrate for the biogenesis of these hormones than is the case with oestriol. The substrate used is dehydroepiandrosterone sulfate, which is derived, in about equal proportions, from the fetal and maternal adrenals and reaches the placenta without prior hydroxylation. The placenta also shares, in an indirect fashion, in the synthesis of oestetrol, which is excreted in considerable amounts in the maternal urine during the later months of pregnancy. This substance is produced in the fetus from oestradiol and oestrone of placental origin; these are hydroxylated in the fetal liver to form oestetrol, which is then transported unchanged into the maternal circulation.

It will be apparent that the major biosynthetic pathways of fetoplacental oestrogen synthesis are now well clarified; rather less light has been shed on the biological significance of this massive production of placental oestrogens. The role of oestrogens in the non-pregnant woman is reasonably well defined, but a consideration of this does not give an obvious indication why their levels should rise so dramatically in the gravid woman. The biological usefulness of oestriol is particularly puzzling because this substance has only a very weak oestrogenic activity. It has been suggested that the placental oestrogens account for the gestational hypertrophy of the myometrium, but such hypertrophy occurs early in pregnancy at a time when placental oestrogen output is at a relatively low level. Many other roles have been advocated, with varying degrees of plausibility, for placentally synthesized oestrogens, but the fact remains that there has been a considerable number of normal pregnancies reported in association with a placental sulfatase deficiency with consequent partial, or even complete, lack of placental oestrogen synthesis (Nakayama & Yanaihara, 1982; Taylor, 1982): the onset of labour was delayed in some of these cases but by no means all.

Progesterone The placenta is an important site of progesterone synthesis during pregnancy and at term secretes about 250 mg a day. Much of this is excreted in the maternal urine as pregnanediol, the level of which rises from about 10 mg a day at the end of the first trimester to approximately 45 mg a day at term.

Synthesis of progesterone is a function of the syncytiotrophoblast; this tissue uses maternal cholesterol as its principal substrate, as it has little or no capacity for converting acetate to progesterone. The principal intermediate along the metabolic pathway is delta^5-pregnenolone, which is converted to progesterone by delta^5-3-beta-steroid dehydrogenase and delta^5-isomerase. Very little further metabolism of progesterone occurs in the placenta; no glucocorticoids and only insignificant amounts of androgens or oestrogens are produced from the progesterone. Most progesterone passes into the fetal circulation, where it is metabolized in the fetal adrenals to a variety of corticosteroid sulfates; the remainder enters the maternal circulation, where it is conjugated in the liver and excreted in the maternal urine as pregnanediol glucuronide.

The principal function of placental progesterone is usually thought to be the maintenance of a quiescent non-contractile uterus. It is thought to act directly on the myometrium to inhibit the spread of a contractile wave, thus preventing forceful and coordinated uterine contractions. This action has, however, been questioned because the onset of labour contractions is not preceded by any fall in progesterone levels and administration of progesterone does not prevent premature onset of labour. Nevertheless, the use of a progesterone inhibitor does provoke labour and in an attempt to explain these paradoxical findings it has been suggested that myometrial contractions occur when the hormonal milieu alters from one of progesterone dominance to one of oestrogen dominance.

Despite the apparently important role of progesterone during gestation, successful pregnancies have been reported in women with homozygous familial hypobetalipoproteinaemia, a condition in which there is a grossly impaired capacity for progesterone synthesis. The fully normal gestations in these women were associated with urinary and plasma progesterone levels that were only one-third of those normally encountered in the pregnant woman (Parker et al, 1986).

Peptide Hormones

Human chorionic gonadotrophin Human chorionic gonadotrophin (hCG) was first found in the urine of pregnant women in 1927. It was later shown to be secreted by the trophoblast, which was, for many years, thought to be the only tissue capable of synthesizing this hormone. The validity of this concept has been undermined by the demonstration that a wide range of non-trophoblast-containing neoplasms also appear to produce small amounts of hCG.

hCG is a glycoprotein and is formed of two non-covalently linked subunits: the alpha-subunit is common also to luteinizing hormone (LH) and several other polypeptide hormones, whilst the beta-subunit is specific to hCG, though there is considerable homology with the beta-subunit of pituitary LH. The two subunits of hCG are translated by separate mRNAs, that for the alpha-subunit being coded by only a single gene and that for the beta-subunit by seven genes.

The villous syncytiotrophoblast is the only significant site of hCG synthesis but there is some evidence that the villous cytotrophoblastic cells can also participate in the synthesis of this hormone. The mRNA for the beta-subunit of hCG is almost entirely confined to the syncytial layer of the villous trophoblast but the mRNA for the alpha-subunit is present in both syncytiotrophoblast and cytotrophoblast. Immunofluorescence studies have shown that the cytotrophoblastic cells also have a limited capacity to synthesize the alpha-subunit and can, under exceptional circumstances, synthesize the entire molecule of hCG.

hCG is secreted almost entirely into the maternal circulation and is detectable in maternal plasma 7–10 days after implantation of the fertilized ovum. The levels of hCG then rise very rapidly, nearly doubling every 48 hours, to reach a peak at about the 8th and 10th weeks of gestation, the levels at this time being 1000 times greater than they were 6 weeks earlier. Thereafter maternal hCG levels fall markedly, by about 90%, to remain at a low level throughout the remainder of pregnancy.

hCG is luteotrophic and its best-understood function is to prolong the functional life of the ovarian corpus luteum in the cycle during which the woman conceives, this resulting in the maintenance of progesterone and oestrogen levels that are adequate to sustain the pregnancy until placental steroidogenesis attains a satisfactory level. All other proposed functions of hCG are based on *in vitro* studies and are largely speculative. A stimulatory effect on fetoplacental steroid synthesis has been suggested by the *in vitro* capacity of hCG to increase the conversion of pregnenolone to cholesterol, to stimulate the synthesis of oestrogen substrates by the fetal adrenal and to accelerate the aromatization of placental steroid precursor substances to oestrogens. This proposed role for hCG in fetoplacental steroid synthesis has to be evaluated with the knowledge that placental oestrogen synthesis continues to increase, in an unabated fashion, at a time when hCG levels undergo a steep decline. The hypothesis that hCG stimulates testosterone synthesis by the fetal testes is unproven, as is the suggestion that the hormone exerts an important immunomodulatory effect in the fetomaternal relationship. The weak thyrotrophic action of hCG is unlikely to be of any true importance in pregnancy, its activity in this respect being only 1/4000th that of pituitary thyroid-stimulating hormone (TSH). It is of interest, however, that hCG receptors are expressed in the villous syncytiotrophoblast and in both the villous and extravillous cytotrophoblast, this raising the possibility that hCG may be an autocrine regulator of trophoblastic hormonal secretion, of trophoblastic differentiation and of the invasive capacity of extravillous trophoblast (Rodway & Rao, 1995).

Human placental lactogen Human placental lactogen (hPL), also known as human chorionic somatomammotrophin (hCS), is a single chain polypeptide that has a close chemical similarity to pituitary growth hormone, 163 of the 191 amino acids that form hPL having the same sequence as human growth hormone: hPL also shares many structural features with prolactin. The hormone is coded for by three genes, of which only two are expressed in the term placenta; the mRNA products of these genes are heterogenous though translation is identical for all.

hPL is synthesized in the villous syncytiotrophoblast and the mRNA for this hormone is restricted to the syncytial layer of the trophoblast. It is of note, however, that the extravillous cytotrophoblastic cells of the placental bed stain positively for hPL, even at the earliest stages of gestation.

hPL is first detectable in maternal plasma at about the end of the first month of gestation; its level then rises progressively to reach a plateau at approximately the 37th week of pregnancy.

A clear functional role for hPL has not been defined. The hormone has weak growth-stimulating activity but its principal effect is to act as an insulin antagonist, mobilizing fatty acids from the maternal depots and thus allowing the mother to spare glucose to meet the increasing needs of the fetus for this substance. hPL has a lactogenic action in animals and competes with prolactin for mammary gland receptors. Since, during pregnancy, the plasma levels of hPL are much higher than are those of prolactin, it is possible that hPL provokes breast development during gestation and that in the puerperium withdrawal of hPL allows pituitary prolactin to stimulate milk secretion. Whatever the true functional significance of hPL may be, its presence does not appear to be mandatory for a successful pregnancy, several fully normal gestations having been recorded in patients in whom placental hPL secretion was, presumably because of a gene deficiency, either very low or totally absent (Di Renzo et al, 1982; Hubert et al, 1983).

Human chorionic prolactin Serum prolactin levels rise considerably during pregnancy but this is probably a result of increased pituitary secretion. More interestingly, the concentration of prolactin in amniotic fluid is extremely high; levels are attained that may be as much as 100 times those reached in the plasma. There is considerable evidence that this prolactin is predominantly of decidual origin, the half-life of amniotic fluid prolactin being quite different from that of plasma prolactin. It is thought that prolactin in the amniotic fluid may be involved in the genesis and removal of amniotic fluid and that it may regulate amniotic fluid osmolarity and volume.

Human chorionic thyrotrophin   The evidence that the placenta can secrete a chorionic thyrotrophin (hCT) is now fairly convincing. This substance is immunologically distinct from human pituitary TSH and from hCG. The site of synthesis of hCT within the placenta is probably the syncytiotrophoblast but the biological function, if any, of this hormone has not, as yet, been identified.

Human chorionic adrenocorticotrophic hormone (ACTH)   There is reasonably good evidence for a chorionic ACTH but the function, if any, of a placental corticotrophin is enigmatic.

Other peptide hormones   The placenta probably produces a growth hormone that closely resembles pituitary growth hormone and also appears capable of synthesizing peptides that are either identical to, or closely resemble, all the hypothalamic releasing hormones.

Overall View of Functional Significance of Placental Hormones

It is apparent that many, indeed most, of the proposed functions of placental hormones are of a largely speculative nature and attempts to define clear-cut endocrine, metabolic or immunological roles for this galaxy of substances have, with the possible exception of hCG, failed. This, together with the fact that a normal pregnancy can be achieved in the absence of hPL, in conditions associated with a diminished capacity to synthesize progesterone and in enzyme deficiencies that can lead to a lack of placental oestrogens, has led to the view that placental hormones may have no function whatsoever as far as the mother and fetus are concerned (Chard, 1986). More recently, however, it has been proposed that the various hormones released from the placenta may act as 'scouts' rather than 'messengers', their role in this 'placental radar' system being to maintain coherent function of the syncytiotrophoblast throughout the placenta and thus achieve a constant level of materno-fetal exchange (Chard, 1993).

Control of Placental Hormone Synthesis and Release

Control mechanisms for placental endocrine activity are poorly understood and it has not proved possible to demonstrate that any feedback mechanisms of the classical type exist for this organ. It has indeed been suggested that there are no control mechanisms of any kind (Chard, 1986), and some have argued that the capacity for hormone synthesis is a direct function of trophoblastic mass and that the rate of secretion of a substance, and thus of synthesis, is determined by the concentration of that substance in the maternal blood perfusing the intervillous space, this in turn depending on the rate of maternal blood flow through the intervillous space. This is an attractive hypothesis and appears to be at least partially true insofar as placental mass is the only factor that is known to correlate with maternal hPL levels. Nevertheless this cannot be the whole story because this suggested 'control' mechanism would not account for the fact that hCG levels begin to fall steeply at a time when placental mass is increasing and hPL levels are rising. The only reasonably persuasive explanation for this switch in trophoblastic secretory activity is that the inactivation of the gene for hCG synthesis and the activation of that for hPL synthesis is a reflection of progressive trophoblastic maturation (Hoshina et al, 1985).

In vitro studies have suggested that placental hCG production may be subject to endogenous controls, prolactin having an inhibitory and placental gonadotropin-releasing hormone having a stimulatory effect on hCG synthesis. It is debatable, however, if these studies have any true *in vivo* significance.

As far as placental steroid hormone synthesis is concerned, it could be argued that substrate supply is a control factor. Substrates for progesterone synthesis are, with the rare exception of cases of hypobetalipoproteinaemia, abundantly supplied from the maternal circulation, the fetus playing no role in the synthesis of this hormone, production of which continues after fetal death. Defective fetal adrenal function, as occurs in anencephalic fetuses, is associated with low maternal levels of oestriol but in all other circumstances there is an abundant supply of substrates for oestrogen synthesis, the placenta appearing to have a virtually unrestricted capacity to produce such hormones. Maternal oestriol levels do not relate to the fetal levels of dehydroepiandrosterone and the only factor related to the placental ability to convert precursor substances to oestradiol appears to be maternal uteroplacental blood flow.

Under *in vitro* conditions both hCG and ACTH appear to influence placental steroidogenesis but it is doubtful if intrinsic regulatory mechanisms are of any real significance, the main factors controlling steroid hormone synthesis being placental size, uteroplacental blood flow and, in occasional circumstances, fetal supply of substrates.

MATERNO-FETAL TRANSFER

The role of the placenta as a transfer organ (Fig. 2.2) is, of course, of critical importance, and it is therefore not surprising that this topic has been the subject of a multitude of studies. Hence the only citations that I will make here are to several review articles, to which those with a particular interest in placental transfer mechanisms can turn for a fuller discussion (Dancis & Schneider, 1975; Reynolds, 1979; Young, 1981; Faber & Thornburg, 1983; Shennan & Boyd, 1987, 1988; Sibley & Boyd, 1988; Carter, 1989; Coleman, 1989; Page, 1993; Morriss et al, 1994). The account given here is a simple, not to say simplistic, version of a complex subject but one that nevertheless details as much information about placental transfer mechanisms as pathologists are likely to require.

General Principles

In the past the placenta was thought to be simply an inert and passive filter; it is now clear, however, that it is able to use a wide range of mechanisms for the transfer of substances from the maternal blood in the intervillous space to the fetal blood in the villous capillaries. The relative importance of each mechanism varies for each substance being transferred across the placenta, whilst more than one mechanism may be used in the exchange of any particular substance. The mechanisms involved in transplacental exchange include:

1. *Simple diffusion.* This is a process in which substances move across a membrane from an area of high concentration to one of low concentration by a process of random thermal motion. Simple diffusion occurs down a chemical or electrochemical gradient, is a passive process, and does not require energy expenditure.

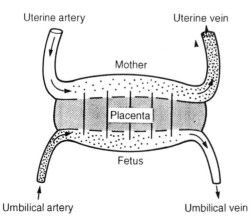

Figure 2.2. Schematic representation of the placenta as an exchange organ.

2. *Facilitated diffusion.* In this process a substance moves from an area of high concentration to one of low concentration at a rate faster than that which would be predicted on a physicochemical basis. This process requires the presence of a carrier molecule in the membrane which shuttles back and forth, accepting a molecule on one side of the membrane and releasing it at the other; the carrier increases the rate of transfer without the expenditure of energy.

3. *Active transport.* In this, the substance to be transported forms a complex with a carrier within the membrane; this complex is then linked with an energy source. Active transport occurs against a chemical gradient, requires expenditure of metabolic energy, and can often be blocked by competitive inhibition.

4. *Bulk transport.* This term is applied to the transfer of water molecules in response to an osmotic or hydrostatic pressure gradient; by a process known inelegantly as 'solvent drag', the water carries with it dissolved molecules that cross the membrane more rapidly than if they were transferred by simple diffusion.

5. *Organellar transport.* This occurs principally by the process of endocytosis, in which the surface-limiting membrane of the trophoblast invaginates to surround a small droplet, thus forming a vesicle which traverses the trophoblast to discharge its contents on the fetal side. Substances may also be transported across the placenta by coated vesicles, multivesicular bodies, or lysosomes, though it must be admitted that little is known about the possible role of these organelles in the human placenta.

6. *Breaks in placental villi.* This can hardly be classed as a physiological transfer mechanism in the placenta but, nevertheless, such breaks do occur and allow for a leak of fetal blood into the maternal circulation.

It should be noted that all the above are proposed mechanisms for transfer across a membrane and that they are all presumed to be via a transcellular route, this being in accord with the traditional view that the villous syncytiotrophoblast forms a complete, uninterrupted barrier. There is, however, increasingly convincing evidence that paracellular transfer routes are present in the villous syncytiotrophoblast and that these can be traversed by water and hydrophilic substances of up to 1.5 nm diameter (Stulc, 1989). The actual nature of these 'pores' or 'channels' in the syncytiotrophoblast has been much debated but there is now quite good proof that there is a system of membrane-lined, winding, branching, trans-syncytial channels; these channels cannot be seen on ordinary electron microscopy but can be visualized, albeit in incomplete form, with the aid of a marker such as lanthanum hydroxide (Kertschanska et al, 1994). The functional significance and importance of this paracellular transport system remains to be determined.

Transfer of Specific Substances

Gas Exchange

Oxygen The transfer of oxygen from the maternal blood to the fetus is, of course, a supremely important function of the placenta, and it is believed that this process occurs largely, probably entirely, by simple diffusion. There is some fragmentary and ill-supported evidence that a mechanism exists for the facilitated diffusion of oxygen across the placenta, but currently available information indicates clearly that simple diffusion is certainly the dominant method of transplacental oxygen transfer. This being so, the rate of oxygen transfer will be determined by physiochemical factors as expressed in Fick's law:

$$\frac{dQ}{dT} = \frac{D \times A \times \alpha \times \Delta P}{X}$$

In this equation:

dQ/dT = amount transferred per unit time
D = diffusion coefficient (or permeability) of the membrane
A = area available for exchange
α = solubility coefficient of the gas
ΔP = partial pressure gradient across the membrane
X = membrane thickness.

The principal force promoting oxygen transfer across the placenta is the difference in partial pressures of oxygen between maternal blood in the intervillous space and fetal blood in the villous capillaries. Unfortunately these values are not accurately known and reliance has had to be placed principally on uterine and umbilical arterial and venous partial pressures. Using these values it has been estimated that the partial pressure of oxygen in the intervillous space is about 90 mm of mercury, whilst that in uterine venous blood is about 40–50 mm of mercury. The partial pressure of oxygen in the fetal blood is thought to vary from about 15 to 30 mm of mercury whilst traversing the placenta, and hence the pressure gradient of oxygen across the placenta is in the region of 35–40 mm of mercury. This is a high pressure difference and would tend to suggest that the oxygen supply to the fetus is limited by a low diffusion capacity (or a high diffusion resistance) of the placenta. The situation as regards transplacental oxygen transfer is, however, complicated by two factors that are disregarded by Fick's law. The first of these is the presence of 'shunts' in the intervillous space, because it seems certain that some of the maternal blood passes through the space without coming into direct contact with the trophoblast; this will clearly diminish the significance of the high pressure gradient across the placenta. The second unconsidered factor is the oxygen consumption of the placenta itself, as it is estimated that between 10 and 30% of the oxygen delivered to the placenta is used by the placenta rather than transferred. If these two factors are taken into consideration it will be apparent that the diffusion coefficient of the placenta for oxygen is not as low as the considerable pressure gradient across the placenta would suggest, and, indeed, experimental studies have indicated that the diffusion resistance of the placenta is not a limiting factor in materno-fetal oxygen transfer.

When considering transplacental oxygen exchange the diffusing capacity of the maternal and fetal blood has also to be borne in mind, for oxygen must dissociate from maternal haemoglobin and combine with fetal haemoglobin. In this respect there are two mechanisms that, quite apart from the higher haemoglobin concentration in fetal blood, allow for fetal blood to be up to 13% more saturated with oxygen than maternal blood at any given partial pressure. Firstly, there is the Bohr effect, which is due to concurrent carbon dioxide transfer; by causing a rise in fetal blood pH and a fall in maternal blood pH, oxygen uptake by the fetal haemoglobin is favoured. Secondly, 2,3-diphosphoglycerate is more effective in releasing oxygen from maternal than from fetal haemoglobin.

Overall, it must be concluded that transfer of oxygen across the placenta is accomplished with great efficiency and that the single most important factor limiting this process is the maternal supply of oxygen to the placenta.

Carbon dioxide Carbon dioxide passes across the placenta from fetus to mother almost entirely in the form of physically dissolved gas, there being little or no transfer of carbonic acid or bicarbonate ions. There is a carbon dioxide partial pressure gradient, variously estimated as being between 4 and 30 mm of mercury, between fetal and maternal blood in the placenta, and carbon dioxide is exchanged by simple diffusion. The factors governing carbon dioxide transfer are similar to those that control oxygen transfer because the placental diffusion resistance to carbon dioxide is very low and cannot be considered as a limiting factor. Sufficient carbonic anhydrase is present in fetal erythrocytes to maintain adequate carbon dioxide transfer, and the release of carbon dioxide from fetal haemoglobin in the placenta is facilitated by the simultaneous uptake of oxygen (the Haldane effect). The partial pressure gradient across the placenta is thought to be due partly to vascular shunts and partly to placental production of carbon dioxide.

Transfer of Nutrients

Carbohydrates   Glucose is the principal metabolic fuel of the fetus. Because maternal blood glucose levels always exceed those in the fetal blood by about 20 mg/100 ml, it was originally thought that carbohydrates crossed the placenta by simple diffusion. Changes in maternal blood glucose levels are, however, very rapidly reflected in the fetal blood, and the rate of transfer is faster than that which would be predicted from the molecular weight and high polarity of the glucose molecule. Furthermore, carbohydrate transfer is stereo-specific, D-glucose being transferred more rapidly than L-glucose, and glucose being transferred more rapidly than fructose, whilst competitive inhibition amongst hexoses has also been noted. The evidence suggests, therefore, that carbohydrates cross the placenta principally by facilitated diffusion, though the possibility of active transport cannot be fully excluded. Much of the difference between maternal and fetal blood glucose levels is probably attributable to placental metabolism of glucose.

Amino acids, polypeptides and proteins   Amino acids are transferred across the placenta by an active transport mechanism. Thus, free amino acid levels are higher in the fetus than in the mother, the transfer mechanism is stereo-specific, competitive inhibition of transport has been demonstrated, the transport mechanism can be saturated by high maternal concentrations, and the process is diminished by energy uncoupling inhibitors.

The placenta is relatively impermeable to polypeptides. This is shown, for instance, by the failure of maternal ACTH to prevent adrenal hypoplasia in anencephalic fetuses and by the low fetal levels of hCG and hCS. The reason for this marked limitation of polypeptide transfer is unknown.

Maternal plasma proteins are, despite their large molecular size, transferred to the fetus, though at a slower rate than amino acids and probably by a process of receptor-mediated endocytosis. There is a considerable variation in transfer rates between different proteins which is not explicable on the basis of differences in molecular weight, e.g. IgG is transferred more rapidly than the much smaller albumin molecule. This selectivity appears to depend on specific surface receptors on the placenta.

Lipids   Fetal fat is derived, in the main, either from free fatty acids transferred across the placenta or from the fetal synthesis of lipid from carbohydrate and acetate. Free fatty acids appear to traverse the placenta by simple diffusion and maternal and fetal blood levels show a moderately good correlation. Cholesterol passes rather slowly through the placenta, whilst phospholipids are hydrolysed and then resynthesized in the placenta during their passage across it. Steroids cross the placenta with ease, as is shown by the masculinization of female fetuses following the administration of exogenous steroids to the mother; steroids passing through the placenta may undergo enzymatic alteration.

Vitamins   The fetal levels of the lipid-soluble vitamins (A, D, E and K) are, in general, slightly lower than those found in the maternal blood, and it is thought that these substances are transferred across the placenta by simple diffusion. The carotene (pro-vitamin A) levels in the fetus are considerably lower than those in the mother, whilst fetal levels for retinol (vitamin A) appear to vary in a manner that is quite independent of maternal levels. This suggests that maternal carotene is transferred across the placenta and then converted into retinol by the fetal liver, and that retinol itself is probably poorly transferred by the placenta.

The water-soluble vitamins (B and C) are generally presumed to be actively transported across the placenta because fetal levels of these substances exceed the maternal values. The possibility of placental synthesis must, however, be taken into account, and it has not yet been proved that these vitamins require an energy-dependent transfer system. Vitamin C is found in the blood both as the reduced L-ascorbic acid and as the oxidized dehydroascorbic acid. The levels of dehydroascorbic acid in maternal and fetal blood approximate to each other, but fetal values for L-ascorbic acid exceed those found in the mother. This, together with the fact that dehydroascorbic acid is transferred across the placenta more rapidly than L-ascorbic acid, suggests that the oxidized form is preferentially transferred across the placenta and then converted to L-ascorbic acid either in the placental tissue or in fetal liver. The fetal levels of riboflavin (vitamin B_2) are twice the maternal values, but flavine adenosine dinucleotide is present in higher concentration in the maternal than in the fetal blood. It is postulated that the placenta is relatively impermeable to both these substances, but binds flavine adenosine dinucleotide and converts it to riboflavin, which is subsequently released into the fetal circulation.

Electrolytes   Sodium is transported rapidly across the placenta; its transfer rate reaches a peak at about the 35th week of gestation and then declines somewhat towards term. Transplacental passage of sodium is thought to be largely due to simple diffusion, but solvent drag may also play a minor role. In general, the transfer of sodium is thought to be both flow and membrane limited, though the way in which the placenta limits sodium exchange is not known.

Potassium is also thought to traverse the placenta by a combination of simple diffusion and solvent drag, and an increase in maternal potassium level is rapidly followed by an elevation of the fetal potassium values. Nevertheless, experimental studies have shown that the fetus retains its potassium in the face of maternal depletion of this electrolyte, and this raises the possibility that an active transport system is involved in potassium exchange.

Most other ionic substances, such as calcium, iodine, iron and phosphate, are found in higher concentration in the fetus than in the mother and would therefore appear to be transferred by an active transport system. The placental handling of iron is of particular interest because the placenta is able to release iron from transferrin by an energy-dependent mechanism and it continues in experimental conditions to concentrate iron in itself even after removal of the fetus.

Water   Water probably passes from mother to fetus by a bulk flow mechanism which is responsive to minor differences in hydrostatic or osmotic pressure.

Transfer of Pharmacological Agents

A knowledge of the ability of the placenta to transfer pharmacological substances from the maternal to fetal circulations is of considerable importance to teratologists, physicians, pharmacologists and anaesthetists, but is of only secondary interest to the pathologist. It is, however, of value to be aware that anaesthetic gases cross the placenta readily, as do sodium thiopentone, barbiturates, salicylates, phenacetin, pethidine and morphine. Most sulfonamides and antibiotics also traverse the placenta with ease, though erythromycin is relatively poorly transferred.

It should not be thought that the placenta is necessarily a passive bystander to a pharmacological attack on the fetus because there is good evidence that drug-metabolizing enzymes may be induced in placental tissue and that drug substrates may undergo biotransformation within the trophoblast.

REFERENCES

Carter, A.M. (1989) Factors affecting gas transfer across the placenta and the oxygen supply to the fetus. *Journal of Developmental Physiology*, **12**, 305–322.

Chard, T. (1986) Placental synthesis. *Clinics in Obstetrics and Gynaecology*, **13**, 447–467.

Chard, T. (1992) Placental hormones and metabolism. In *Medicine of the Fetus and Mother*, Reece, E.A., Hobbins, J.C., Mahoney, M.J. and Petrie, R.H. (Eds), pp. 88–96. Philadelphia: Lippincott.

Chard, T. (1993) Placental radar. *Journal of Endocrinology*, **138**, 177–179.

Coleman, R.A. (1989) The role of the placenta in lipid metabolism and transport. *Seminars in Perinatology*, **51**, 94–101.

Conley, E.D. and Mason, J.I. (1990) Placental steroid hormones. *Ballière's Clinical Endocrinology and Metabolism*, **4**, 249–272.

Dancis, J. and Schneider, H. (1975). Physiology: transfer and barrier function. In *The Placenta and its Maternal Supply Line*, Gruenwald, P. (Ed.), pp. 98–124. Lancaster: Medical and Technical Publishing.

Diczfalusy, E. (1969). Steroid metabolism in the foeto-placental unit. In *The Foeto-Placental Unit*, Pecile, A. and Finzi, C. (Eds), pp. 65–109. Amsterdam: Excerpta Medica.

Diczfalusy, E. and Mancuso, S. (1969) Oestrogen metabolism in pregnancy. In *Foetus and Placenta*, Klopper, A. and Diczfalusy, E. (Eds), pp. 191–248. Oxford and Edinburgh: Blackwell Scientific.

Di Renzo, G.C., Angeschia, M.M. and Volpe, E. (1982). Deficiency of human placental lactogen in an otherwise normal pregnancy. *Journal of Obstetrics and Gynaecology*, **2**, 153–154.

Faber, J.J. and Thornburg, K.L. (1983). *Placental Physiology*. New York: Raven Press.

Hoshina, M., Boothby, M., Hussa, R. et al (1985). Linkage of human chorionic gonadotrophin and placental lactogen biosynthesis to trophoblast differentiation and tumorigenesis. *Placental*, **4**, 163–172.

Hubert, C., Descombey, D., Mondon, F. and Daffos, F. (1983). Plasma human chorionic somatomammotropin deficiency in a normal pregnancy is the consequence of low concentration of messenger RNA coding for human chorionic somatomammotropin. *American Journal of Obstetrics and Gynecology*, **147**, 676–678.

Jones, C.T. (1989) Endocrine function of the placenta. *Ballière's Clinical Endocrinology and Metabolism*, **3**, 755–780.

Kertschanska, S., Kosanke, G. and Kaufmann, P. (1994) Is there morphological evidence for the existence of transtrophoblastic channels in human placental villi? *Trophoblast Research*, **8**, 591–596.

Morriss, F.H., Boyd, R.D.H. and Mahendran, D. (1994). Placental transport. In *The Physiology of Reproduction*, 2nd edn, Knobil, E. and Neill, J.D. (Eds), pp. 813–861. New York: Raven Press.

Nakayama, T. and Yanaihara, T. (1982). Placental sulphatase deficiency. *Contributions to Gynecology and Obstetrics*, **9**, 145–156.

Ogren, L. and Talamantes, F. (1994). The placenta as an endocrine organ: polypeptides. In *The Physiology of Reproduction*, 2nd edn, Knobil, E. and Neill, J.D. (Eds), pp. 875–945. New York: Raven Press.

Page, K. (1993) *The Physiology of the Human Placenta*. London: UCL Press.

Parker, R.C., Illingworth, D.R., Bissonnette, J. and Carr, B.R. (1986) Endocrine changes during pregnancy in a patient with familial hypobetalipoproteinemia. *New England Journal of Medicine*, **314**, 557–560.

Reynolds, F. (1979) Transfer of drugs. In *Placental Transfer*, Chamberlain, G. and Wilkinson, A. (Eds), pp. 166–181. Tunbridge Wells: Pitman Medical.

Rodway, M.R. and Rao, Ch.V. (1995) A novel perspective on the role of human chorionic gonadotropin during pregnancy and in gestational trophoblastic disease. *Early Pregnancy: Biology and Medicine*, **1**, 176–187.

Shearman, R.P. (1985). *Clinical Reproductive Endocrinology*. Edinburgh: Churchill Livingstone.

Shennan, D.B. and Boyd, C.A.R. (1987) Ion transport by the placenta: a review of membrane transport systems. *Acta Biochemica et Biophysica*, **906**, 437–457.

Shennan, D.B. and Boyd, C.A.R. (1988) Placental handling of trace elements. *Placenta*, **9**, 333–343.

Sibley, C.P. and Boyd, R.D.H. (1988) Control of transfer across the mature placenta. *Oxford Reviews of Reproductive Biology*, **10**, 382–435.

Siiteri, P.K., Gant, N.F. and MacDonald, P.C. (1974) Synthesis of steroid hormones by the placenta. In *The Placenta, Biological and Clinical Aspects*, Moghissi, K.S. and Hafez, E.S.E. (Eds), pp. 238–257. Springfield, Illinois: Charles C. Thomas.

Solomon, S. (1994) The primate placenta as an endocrine organ: steroids. In *The Physiology of Reproduction*, 2nd edn, Knobil, E. and Neill, J.D. (Eds), pp. 863–873. New York: Raven Press.

Stulc, J. (1989). Extracellular transport pathways in the haemochorial placenta. *Placenta*, **10**, 113–119.

Taylor, N.F. (1982) Review: placental sulphatase deficiency. *Journal of Inherited Metabolic Disorders*, **5**, 164–176.

Thau, R.B. and Lanman, J.T. (1975) Endocrinological aspects of placental function. In *The Placenta and its Maternal Supply Line*, Gruenwald, P. (Ed.), pp. 125–144. Lancaster: Medical and Technical Publishing.

Young, M. (1981) Placental amino acid transfer and metabolism. In *Placental Transfer Methods and Interpretations*, Young, M., Boyd, R.D.H., Longo, L.D. and Telegdy G. (Eds), pp. 177–184. London: Saunders.

ABNORMALITIES
OF PLACENTATION

3

In this chapter several anomalous forms of placentation will be considered, most of which fall rather conveniently into the broad group of 'abnormalities of placental shape'. Placenta accreta will, however, also be discussed, though the purist may well remark that this condition is possibly better considered as an endometrial abnormality rather than as an aberration of placentation.

ABNORMALITIES OF PLACENTAL SHAPE

The placenta is normally a round discoid organ: whether this is necessarily the optimal shape for efficient function is a moot point, because in pregnancy at high altitudes the placenta, which is presumably unduly stressed under such circumstances, is more commonly ovoid in outline (Chabes et al, 1968). In most cases in which the placenta is unusually shaped, there is good, though not conclusive, evidence that the abnormality develops at a very early stage of pregnancy, either during implantation of the fertilized ovum or during the first stages of placental development.

Placenta Extrachorialis

In this anomaly the chorionic plate of the placenta, from which the villi arise, is smaller than the basal plate: hence the transition from membranous to villous chorion takes place, not at the edge of the placenta, but at some distance within the circumference of the fetal surface of the placenta, thus leaving a ridge of villous tissue projecting beyond the limits of the chorionic plate (Fig. 3.1).

If the transition from villous to membranous chorion is marked by a flat ring of membrane the placenta is classed as 'circummarginate', whilst if this marginal ring is plicated with a raised, often rolled, edge the placenta is of the 'circumvallate' type (Figs. 3.2–3.4). Sometimes the placenta is marginate or vallate in one area whilst elsewhere the villous chorion extends to the placental periphery (Fig. 3.5); these partial forms of the anomaly are common and it is by no means exceptional to encounter a placenta that is marginate in one area and vallate in another. Scott (1960) considers that the distinction between these two forms of extrachorial placenta is unwarranted, but this is a view I cannot share, partly because the two varieties are clearly distinctive on macroscopic examination and partly because they are of differing clinical importance.

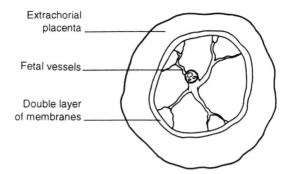

Extrachorial placenta

Fetal vessels

Double layer of membranes

Figure 3.1. Diagrammatic representation of a placenta extrachorialis as viewed from the fetal aspect.

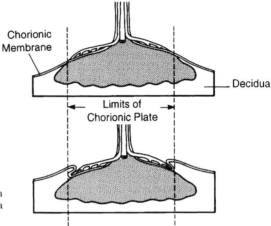

Chorionic Membrane

Decidua

Limits of Chorionic Plate

Figure 3.2. Diagrammatic representation of a circummarginate placenta (above) and a circumvallate placenta (below).

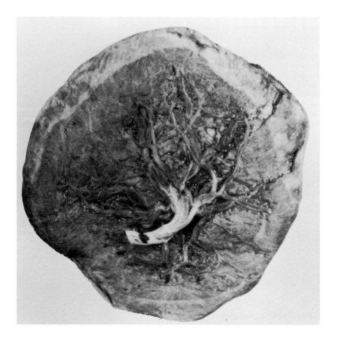

Figure 3.3. A circumarginate placenta viewed from the fetal aspect.

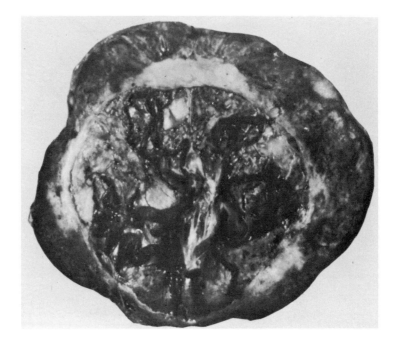

Figure 3.4. A circumvallate placenta viewed from the fetal aspect.

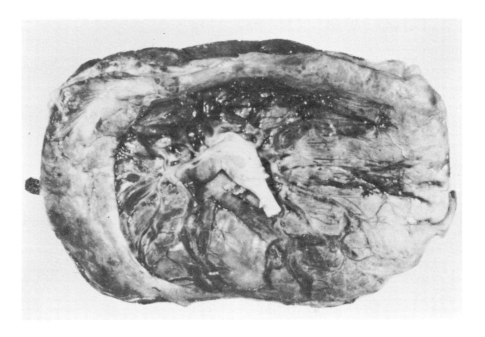

Figure 3.5. A partially circumvallate placenta. On the left side the placenta is vallate but on the right side it is normal.

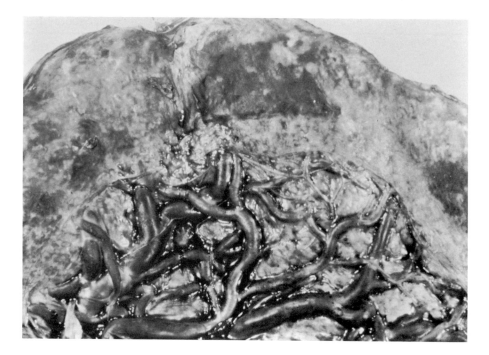

Figure 3.6. The chorionic plate of a placenta extrachorialis. The fetal vessels appear to terminate at the marginal membranous fold.

The fetal vessels in the chorionic plate of an extrachorial placenta appear to terminate at the marginal membranous fold (Fig. 3.6) and the membranes overlying the villous tissue that protrudes beyond this fold are avascular and can be easily stripped off without causing any tearing. Scott (1960) has shown that the vessels do in fact continue their course beyond the limiting fold but run at a deeper plane, beneath the membranes. Histological examination of the ring in a circummarginate placenta will reveal only amnion and chorion, often with some fibrin. The raised fold of a circumvallate placenta may be equally bereft of other components but more commonly also contains decidual tissue, 'ghost-like' placental villi, blood clots or, rarely, apparently normal functioning villi. Extrachorial placentas are otherwise usually unremarkable and their villi do not show any abnormal features.

Incidence (Table 3.1)

One of the few aspects of this topic about which some measure of agreement has been reached is that between 18 and 30% (averaging about 25%) of placentas are of the extrachorial variety. Less unanimity has been attained regarding the incidence of circumvallate placentas, a high proportion of students of this anomaly finding it in about 1% of deliveries and a smaller group noting an incidence of between 3.6 and 6.9%. My own inclination is towards those quoting the higher incidence (not unnaturally, as the highest cited incidence was that noted in our own material) and it is worth remarking that the authors quoting a low incidence often do not state whether or not they have included the partial form of this anomaly; one suspects that they have not, because those workers finding a high incidence have usually made it clear that they were including both partial and complete forms of the circumvallate placenta within their totals.

There is general agreement that circumvallate placentas are found more commonly in multigravidae, but maternal age does not appear to influence the incidence. Benson and Fujikura (1969), working in the USA, noted a significantly higher

Table 3.1. Reported incidence of placenta extrachorialis and placenta circumvallata

Author	Incidence of Placenta Extrachorialis (%)	Incidence of Placenta Circumvallata (%)
Hobbs and Rollins (1934)	—	0.5
Hobbs and Price (1940)	—	0.8
Hunt et al (1947)	—	0.5
Paalman and Vander Veer (1953)	—	0.5
Pavoni (1954)	24	1.6
Pinkerton (1956)	25	2.5
Aguero (1957)	28	1.8
Sauramo (1960)	—	1.7
Scott (1960)	18	—
Ziel (1963)	—	0.6
Wilson and Paalman (1967)	—	1.0
Maqueo-Topete et al (1968)	6	1.0
Wentworth (1968)	32	6.5
Benson and Fujikura (1969)[a]	30	3.6
Malkani and Bhasin (1970)	19	—
Foss and Vogel (1972)[b]	—	1.0
Fox and Sen (1972)	24	6.9
Glinski (1973)	—	1.0
Lal (1975)	19	2.2
Benirschke and Kaufmann (1990)	—	5.2

[a] White women only.
[b] Placentas from 'high-risk' cases.

incidence of extrachorial placentas in white than in black women, but we did not find an unusually low incidence in non-Caucasians in our own population in Manchester (Fox & Sen, 1972).

Aetiology and Pathogenesis

The causation of placenta extrachorialis has proved a fertile field for speculative theories. Some, such as the belief that the abnormality is due to an endometritis or to cornual implantation, are demonstrably incorrect and have been discarded. The others, the earlier of which have been reviewed and critically evaluated by Scott (1960), include:

1. A popular theory in the last century was that excessive proliferation of decidua around the young placenta might restrict the area of the chorionic plate: if this was so, one would expect always to find decidual tissue in the limiting fold and this, whilst frequently present, is often absent.
2. Liepmann (1906) considered that the folds were due to variations in amniotic pressure relative to the growth of the uterine wall, but he did not explain why, under these circumstances, the fold should often contain tissue other than membranes.
3. Sfameni (1908) postulated that circumvallation was the result of an incoordination between placental and uterine growth, but he did not enter into any discussion as to why this should produce this anomaly rather than marginal placental separation.
4. Goodall (1934) thought that the abnormal shape of a circumvallate placenta was due to compensatory lateral growth, this being a response to placental infarction; this theory is untenable if only for the reason that most circumvallate placentas show no evidence of infarction.

5. Williams (1927) believed that the chorionic plate was unduly small from the onset because of poor development of the chorion frondosum. He argued that as pregnancy progressed the peripheral villi would have to grow laterally, and he incorporated a previous suggestion of von Herff (1896) by proposing that such growth could only be attained by lateral splitting of the decidua. This concept has won several adherents (Hobbs & Rollins, 1934; Morgan, 1955) but has been criticized by Scott (1960) on the grounds that, when excessive placental growth does occur, as in severe rhesus incompatibility, a circumvallate placenta does not develop.

6. Nesbitt (1957) also thought that circumvallation was the result of an unduly small chorionic plate and maintained that this was due to unusually shallow implantation of the ovum. Although Hertig (1960) tended to accept this hypothesis, it is purely speculative.

7. Torpin (1953, 1955a,b, 1958, 1966) has for many years enthusiastically espoused his view that placenta extrachorialis is due to an excessively deep implantation of the ovum. His argument, which is rather complex, is that under such circumstances the original placenta forms more than half of the ovular sac and this will lead to the formation of a ring at the placental margin, through which the membranes will herniate to give a circumvallate placenta. His theory is similar in concept to an earlier one of Lahm (1924), who suggested that deep implantation is followed by rupture of the decidua capsularis with herniation of the membranes and their contents. Scott (1960) has examined Torpin's theory in a rather oblique fashion by arguing that deep implantation should develop in women with an unduly thick decidua, that the depth of the decidua should be related to endometrial thickness at the end of a non-fertile period, and that a thick endometrium should lead to an excessive menstrual flow. He was unable to find any correlation between a history of heavy menstrual flow and subsequent development of a circumvallate placenta and thus concluded that the available evidence did not lend support to Torpin's theory. Scott himself points out the indirect nature of this evidence and indicates the not necessarily correct assumptions that he had made; to me, the views of Torpin are moderately persuasive, especially as they can be extended to give a unitary concept of other placental abnormalities such as bilobate placenta or placenta membranacea.

8. Pinkerton (1956) attributed circumvallation to haemorrhage around the placental edge during the early stages of pregnancy. This theory has been supported partially by Benirschke and Driscoll (1967), and fully by Naftolin et al (1973) and Lal (1976), but Scott (1960), whilst agreeing that such haemorrhage does occur and that it can influence the shape of the placenta, maintained that in many extrachorial placentas there was no evidence of any marginate bleeding, either recent or old, a finding with which I am in agreement.

9. Benirschke and Driscoll (1967) think that fresh reconsideration should be given to Grosser's (1927) suggestion that a reduction in intra-amniotic pressure is an important aetiological factor in placenta extrachorialis, and point to the high incidence of this type of placenta in women in whom there has been prolonged leakage of fluid (Bain et al, 1964) and to the association, noted by some workers, of hydrorrhoea and circumvallate placentas. In retrospect it is clear that many of the cases reported by Bain and his colleagues were examples of extramembranous pregnancy and, indeed, a circumvallate placenta is always found in a gestation of this type (Kohler et al, 1970). This would, at first sight, appear to lend support to Benirschke and Driscoll's view, but there is no clear correlation between oligohydramnios, caused, for example, by fetal renal agenesis, and circumvallate placentation, and it is at least equally possible that a circumvallate placenta limits the growth of the membranes and thus predisposes to extramembranous pregnancy and hydrorrhoea.

10. Deacon et al (1974) and Lademacher et al (1981) have suggested that at least some cases of circumvallate placentation may be of genetic origin, though they

do not elaborate on how this abnormal gene exerts its effect: their evidence for this hypothesis is, to say the least, scanty in the extreme.

Which, if any, of this plethora of theories is correct is, at the moment, a matter for speculation, but some are mutually contradictory, few are wholly satisfactory, and none appears to be of universal application to all examples of this anomaly.

Clinical Significance

Opinion has been sharply divided between those who consider placenta extrachorialis to be simply an anatomical variant of little or no clinical importance (Williams, 1927; Pavoni, 1954; Pinkerton, 1956; Wentworth, 1968) and others who maintain that it is causally related to a very high incidence of abortion, antepartum haemorrhage, premature onset of labour and perinatal death (Hobbs & Price, 1940; Hunt et al, 1947; Morgan, 1955; Ziel, 1963; Ayala et al, 1965; Martin, 1967; Wilson & Paalman, 1967; Maqueo-Topete et al, 1968; Lal, 1975). In his extensive survey, Scott (1960) found the extrachorial placenta to be accompanied unduly frequently by antepartum bleeding but to be otherwise of no significance.

Some of the responsibility for this state of confusion rests on those who have indiscriminately included both the circummarginate and the circumvallate placenta under the single heading of placenta extrachorialis, because it has emerged clearly from several studies that the circummarginate form is totally devoid of any clinical importance (Benson & Fujikura, 1969; Fox & Sen, 1972). Even if consideration is limited to the circumvallate placenta it is also necessary to distinguish between the complete and the partial forms of the anomaly, because Benson and Fujikura (1969), who found that the totally circumvallate placenta was associated with increased rates of antepartum bleeding, premature labour and perinatal mortality, noted that the inclusion of the partial form in their study would have diminished, and probably almost negated, these positive findings. My experience has been somewhat similar, as I found that the totally, but not the partially, circumvallate placenta is accompanied by a relatively high rate of threatened abortion and premature onset of labour (Fox & Sen, 1972). I could not, however, confirm that any form of circumvallate placenta was associated with an excess of antepartum bleeding or perinatal death. Lademacher et al (1981) did, by contrast, find circumvallate placentation to be associated with an increased perinatal mortality and also with an excess of congenital fetal malformations; this latter finding, unique to their series, has received little further attention and has been neither confirmed nor refuted.

An interesting finding in our survey was that infants with either type of circumvallate placenta tended unduly frequently to be of low birth weight for the length of their gestational period, a finding also noted by Benson and Fujikura (1969), Glinski (1973), Rolschau (1978), Sandstedt (1979), Suska et al (1989) and Liu (1990). This may indicate that the circumvallate placenta is relatively inefficient, but it could also be argued that both the tendency towards fetal undernutrition and circumvallate placentation are due to a common, and as yet unidentified, maternal factor. It is of note that the deficit of fetal growth associated with circumvallate placentation is usually relatively slight with most neonates only just falling into the defined category of small for gestational age.

A circumvallate placenta can be diagnosed antenatally by ultrasound (Jauniaux et al, 1989; Sherer et al, 1991; McCarthy et al, 1995), though the practical value of this diagnostic achievement would appear to be very limited.

Placenta Membranaces (Synonym: Placenta Diffusa)

Classically, this term denotes a thin membranous placenta enveloping the entire or greater part of the gestational sac. The condition is sometimes described as 'partial' if less than the entire surface of the gestational sac is involved and this term is certainly justified if, for instance, only two-thirds of the membranes are covered by villous tissue;

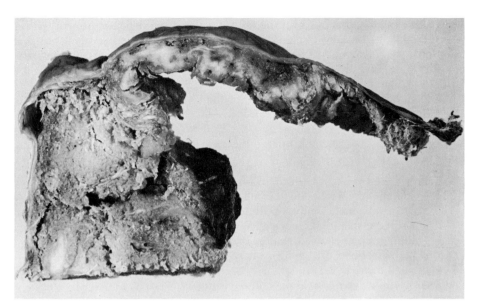

Figure 3.7. A placenta membranacea. The membranes are covered by villous tissue which extends to the gestation sac opening. The edge of a thicker placental disc is also shown.

however, it is probably not warranted if this concept is extended, as it has been (Wilkins et al, 1991), to the finding of a 2–3 cm rim of thin villous tissue around the placental disc. The expression 'membranacea' is, in itself, somewhat inaccurate and misleading, as this form of placenta is not necessarily either thin or membranous. The essential, and only, defining feature of the anomaly is that all, or most, of the membranes are covered on their outer aspect by chorionic villi. Exceptionally there may be a focal thickening to form a placental disc (Fig. 3.7), but more commonly the gestational sac is diffusely covered by villous tissue, albeit of varying thickness. During the early weeks of gestation the placenta is, of course, normally of this type and remains so until those villi which are orientated towards the uterine cavity, and which are covered by the decidua capsularis, atrophy to form the chorion laeve. It is also worthy of note that this form of placenta is the norm, throughout gestation, in the pig, donkey and elephant.

Placenta membranacea is rare and only a few cases have been described, the more recent reports and reviews being those of Finn (1954), Aguero (1957), Janovski and Granowitz (1961), Culp et al (1973), Pryse-Davies et al (1973), Mathews (1974), Wladimiroff et al (1976), Las Heras et al (1982), Molloy et al (1983), Hurley and Beischer (1987), Greenberg et al (1991), Wilkins et al (1991), Dinh et al (1992) and Ekoukou et al (1995). It has been suggested by Aguero (1957) that the anomaly occurs once in every 3300 deliveries, but this is contrary to all other workers' experiences and is an unacceptably high figure. The estimate by Hurley and Beischer (1987) that placenta membranacea occurs only once in 25,500 pregnancies would appear to be nearer the correct mark.

In nearly all cases there is recurrent antepartum bleeding, often starting quite early in pregnancy; the bleeding is probably due to the fact that a placenta membranacea must also of necessity be a placenta praevia. An antepartum diagnosis of placenta membranacea can, under these circumstances, sometimes be made by ultrasonography (Molloy et al, 1983; Dinh et al, 1992) but this technique is not invariably successful (Las Heras et al, 1982).

Most cases end either in abortion or premature onset of labour and the outlook for fetal survival has, in the past, been poor, largely because of prematurity; survival rates have, however, improved considerably over the last 20 years. Janovski and Granowitz (1961) maintained that the fetus is often very underweight for the length of the gestational period, and suggested that, in humans, a placenta membranacea was a relatively inefficient mode of placentation. This belief has, however, not been substantiated in more recent case reports in which the fetus has shown no deficit of growth (Hurley & Beischer, 1987; Greenberg et al, 1991). Following delivery there is often postpartum haemorrhage and a morbid adherence of the placenta, which necessitates manual removal or, in extreme cases, hysterectomy. It is extremely rare for there to be a fully normal pregnancy, labour and delivery (Aguero, 1957).

The pathogenesis of this condition is quite clear, as it is obviously due to a complete failure of the normal process of atrophy of those villi away from the chorion frondosum during the early stages of gestation. The aetiology is, however, less overt, though there has been no shortage of proffered theories; these have been reviewed by Janovski & Granowitz (1961) and include:

1. Previous endometritis, which, by producing excessive endometrial vascularization, encourages the development of villi over the entire surface of the gestational sac.
2. Poor development of the decidual blood supply, which necessitates the persistence of the villi on the chorion laeve.
3. Unduly deep implantation of the ovum.
4. A faulty trophoblastic anlage, whereby the placenta reverts to a more primitive atavistic form.
5. Atrophy or hypoplasia of the endometrium.

None of these theories (or, to be more exact, hypotheses) is particularly persuasive, though the possible importance of endometrial insufficiency is suggested by the tendency of this type of placenta to be unduly adherent. On the other hand, the vast majority of examples of placenta accreta are clearly not of the membranacea variety.

Ring-shaped Placenta

This rare anomaly (which is also known variously as a 'girdle', 'collar' or 'annular' placenta) was the subject of a surprisingly large number of reports and reviews in the German literature between 1928 and 1937 (Klaften, 1928; Antoine, 1930; Philipp, 1930, 1932; Abraham, 1932; Grahbner, 1932; Siedentopf, 1932; Rüder, 1933; Fauvet, 1935; Fraenkel & Granzow, 1936; Kiefer, 1937), but it has since received little notice apart from the reports of Kleine (1956), Walsen (1958), Cavalli (1961), Vahlenkamp (1961), and Keefer and Cope (1963).

The incidence of this abnormality is usually quoted as being about 1 per 5500 deliveries, but this figure is not based on any firm data and is, in my opinion, far too high, as I doubt if many obstetricians or pathologists will see more than one example (usually not even that) in a lifetime of clinical practice. As its name implies, the placenta in this condition is annular in shape and resembles a segment of a hollow cylinder. Sometimes a complete ring of placental tissue is seen, but more commonly a portion of the ring undergoes atrophy, which results in a placenta that is approximately horseshoe shaped. In these latter circumstances, fetal placental vessels will be found running across the gap left by the process of villous atrophy.

It will come as no surprise to the reader of this chapter to learn that amongst the explanations offered for the development of this aberrant form of placenta are endometrial insufficiency, excessively deep implantation of the fertilized ovum, unduly superficial implantation of the ovum, and an atavistic regression towards a more primitive form of placentation. None of these hypotheses withstands even the most superficial critical scrutiny, whilst the suggestion that the ring-shaped placenta is actually a central placenta praevia in which the central area has undergone atrophy and degeneration has been disposed of by Kleine's (1956) demonstration of a placenta of this type within the upper uterine segment. I would regard the ring-shaped placenta as a variant of a placenta membranacea and it almost certainly results from a distortion of the normal process of orderly villous atrophy during the early months of gestation.

The clinical significance of this aberration is uncertain but it does appear to be associated with a high incidence of both ante- and postpartum bleeding, whilst the fetus is often of low birth weight for the length of the gestational period.

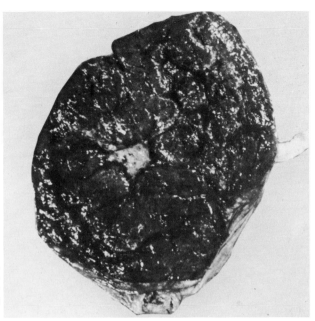

Figure 3.8. A fenestrate placenta seen from the maternal aspect. There is a focal deficiency of villous tissue in the centre of the placenta but the chorionic plate is present.

Fenestrate Placenta

This is an exceptionally rare abnormality of unknown pathogenesis in which the central portion of a discoidal placenta is missing (Kleine, 1956); sometimes there is an actual hole in the centre of the placenta, but more commonly the defect is one of villous tissue only and the chorionic plate is present (Fig. 3.8). The only clinical significance of this abnormality is that it may be mistakenly thought that the missing portion is still retained in the uterus and the mother thus be subjected to an unnecessary uterine exploration.

Accessory Lobe

Adjacent to the main placenta may be found one or more accessory lobes of variable size (Fig. 3.9). These are often called 'succenturiate lobes' but this is a somewhat inappropriate term as the Latin verb 'succinere' means 'to accompany' in a choral or musical rather than in a physical sense. The accessory lobe may be linked to the main placental mass by a narrow isthmus of chorionic tissue, but it is not infrequently entirely separate and connected only by the membranes. The umbilical cord is usually inserted into the main placenta and the vascular supply of the lobe is from an artery on the fetal surface of the main placenta; the artery to the lobe may, therefore, run an intramembranous course.

Accessory lobes are usually relatively small, but are thought by some to represent one extreme of a continuous spectrum, at the other end of which is the bilobate placenta (Torpin & Hart, 1941). I would, however, regard the accessory lobe as an entity distinct from a bilobate placenta, partly because I have not been convinced that such a spectrum exists, partly because the two conditions are possibly of different pathogenesis, and partly because in bilobate placentation the cord is usually, though admittedly not invariably, inserted between the two lobes, a situation encountered only rarely with an accessory lobe.

Torpin and Hart (1941) found accessory lobes in 6.6% of their series of 4098 placentas, but Earn (1951) estimated that they occurred only once in 600 deliveries, whilst Sauramo (1960) noted an incidence of 0.7% in his study of 5000 placentas. Sirivongs

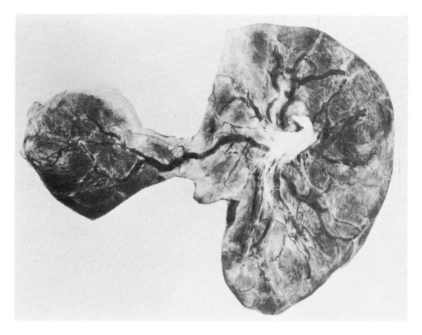

Figure 3.9. An accessory lobe: this is joined to the main placental mass only by a bridge of membranes. The cord is inserted into the main placenta and a vessel is running intramembranously to the lobe.

(1974) encountered accessory lobes in 3% of a very large series of placentas, and this is approximately the frequency with which I have found them in my own material.

Most accessory lobes are, fortunately, devoid of clinical importance, but occasionally the lobe is retained *in utero* after delivery of the main placenta and this can lead to sub-involution and delayed postpartum bleeding. Rarely, the lobe may lie over the internal os and thus present as a placenta praevia, whilst very exceptionally there may be fetal haemorrhage as a result of trauma to vessels running intramembranously to the lobe. A forewarning of such complications can be achieved by antenatal ultrasound recognition of an accessory lobe (Hata et al, 1988).

Most of the early concepts of the pathogenesis of this anomaly were largely, or entirely, speculative; these included double nidation, regional variation in the nutrient capacity of the endometrium, and irregular endometrial insufficiency. More modern views, though more persuasive, are perhaps equally devoid of a factual basis. Torpin and Hart (1941) suggested that the anomaly is due to the development of the placenta on both the anterior and posterior walls of the uterus, the main lobe thus being on one wall and the accessory lobe on the other. They attribute this to either unduly superficial implantation of the fertilized ovum (which is thus able to adhere to both walls) or a fortuitous implantation of the ovum into the lateral or apical sulcus. Boyd and Hamilton (1970) regard the accessory lobe as a remnant of the previously complete shell of villous tissue, the lobe thus representing a focal failure of the normal process of villous atrophy in the chorion laeve. I have no personal evidence or bias for or against of these two hypotheses.

Bilobate Placenta

A bilobate placenta (also known as a 'bipartite' placenta or as a 'placenta duplex') is one consisting of two nearly equally-sized lobes (Fig. 3.10), which may be connected to each other by a bridge of chorionic tissue or which may be quite separate and discrete. The umbilical cord is usually inserted between the two lobes, sometimes into the connecting bridge but often velamentously.

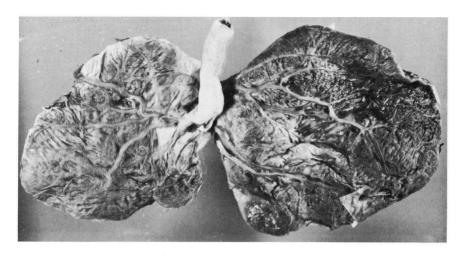

Figure 3.10. A bilobate placenta. The cord is inserted between the two placental masses.

Despite the ease with which this anomaly can be identified, there have been widely varying estimates of its frequency. Torpin and Hart (1941) found that 2.2% of placentas were of this type, whilst Fujikura et al (1970) reported an incidence of 4.2% in placentas from white women in Boston. On the other hand, Sauramo (1960) encountered only two bilobate placentas in 5000 deliveries, whilst Sirivongs (1974) found only 25 such placentas of this type in 12,120 deliveries. Earn (1951) considered that a bilobate placenta was found once in 350 deliveries, and this figure approximates more closely to my own experience than do those cited in the other studies of this anomaly.

Fujikura et al (1970) have been the only workers who have attempted to define the clinical significance of this placental maldevelopment. They noted that bilobate placentation occurred with undue frequency in women of high gravidity, in older women and in patients with a previous history of infertility. The only pregnancy complications to occur unduly frequently in association with a bilobate placenta were first-trimester bleeding and adherent placenta, there being no tendency towards premature labour and no effect on fetal development or well-being.

The pathogenesis of this condition is not fully understood, but Torpin and his colleagues (Torpin & Hart, 1941; Torpin, 1953, 1958; Torpin & Barfield, 1968) have presented quite persuasive evidence that the two lobes are on opposing walls of the uterine cavity and have suggested that this results from unusually superficial implantation of the fertilized ovum, which is thus able to attach itself to both anterior and posterior walls. The process postulated is thus very similar to that known to occur in several subhuman primates in which bilobate placentation is the norm. Benirschke and Driscoll (1967) suggest that abnormal lateral growth of the placenta produces the bilobate form, but do not present this concept with any firm conviction.

Multilobate Placenta

Placentas consisting of three or more lobes are extremely rare. Torpin and Hart (1941) noted that 10 of their series of 4098 placentas were trilobate, but this seems an unusually high incidence. Little is known about the clinical significance of this anomaly, but one would expect that the complications described as a possible consequence of an accessory lobe would also occur with a trilobate placenta. Sudha et al (1973) have reported an example of fetal haemorrhage from rupture of an interlobar vessel in a case of trilobate placentation.

Placentas consisting of four or five lobes occur with great rarity; Earn (1951) cites a report of a placenta that was formed of seven lobes. It must be assumed that these multilobate placentas develop as a result of irregular atrophy of the villous shell and that they thus represent a perversion of the normal differentiation of the chorion into chorion laeve and chorion frondosum.

PLACENTA ACCRETA

This condition was defined by Irving and Hertig (1937) as 'the abnormal adherence, either in whole or in part, of the afterbirth to the underlying uterine wall'. They considered that the pathological basis for this undue tenacity was a complete or partial absence of the decidua basalis, and a placenta accreta is now regarded as being one in which the placental villi adhere to, invade into, or penetrate through the myometrium.

It is usual to delineate several subdivisions of this condition. Thus, if the placental villi are attached to the myometrium but do not invade the muscle it is classed as placenta accreta vera, if the villi invade the myometrium it is known as placenta increta, whilst if the villi penetrate through the full thickness of the myometrium the stage of 'placenta percreta' (Fig. 3.11) has been reached. Luke et al (1966) criticized this classification on the grounds that the degree of villous penetration of the myometrium is rarely uniform and suggested that the name 'the adherent or invasive placenta' be used to cover all these various contingencies. This phrase, though correct in a pedantic sense, is unduly cumbersome for routine usage and I prefer to use the term 'placenta accreta' to include all degrees of the adhesive placenta.

It is also the rule to further subdivide cases of placenta accreta into 'total' (involving the whole placenta), 'partial' (involving one or more lobes) and 'focal' (involving isolated areas in a lobe). This additional classification has also been argued against by Luke et al (1966) on the basis that histological examination of the placenta is rarely complete and that, very frequently, attempts at manual removal so distort uteroplacental relationships that a pathological judgement as to whether adhesion was total or partial is virtually impossible.

Incidence

The true frequency of placenta accreta is almost impossible to determine. The reported incidence in any given institution or area varies widely from a maximum of one case of placenta accreta per 436 deliveries (Barss & Misch, 1990) to a minimum of one per 93,000 deliveries (Althabe & Althabe, 1963). Between these two extremes there is a very variable range of quoted incidences, from which it is impossible to select any one figure as being representative. The highest incidences have been in series reported from Papua New Guinea (Barss & Misch, 1990), Thailand (Sumawong et al, 1966) and Chile (Thonet, 1949); it is by no means the case, however, that placenta accreta occurs unduly commonly in the relatively 'underdeveloped' countries and no demonstrable pattern of geographic variation has emerged from the reported studies.

Information about ethnic incidence is also scanty. In Israel, placenta accreta appears to occur equally commonly in Jews of occidental and oriental origin (Goldman, 1963), whilst in series reported from the USA there is no obvious predilection for either black or white patients. Only a very few cases have been reported from Africa (Bourrel et al, 1964), and information about ethnic variation in Asia is virtually non-existent.

The difficulties encountered in attempting to determine the true incidence of placenta accreta reflect, to a considerable extent, problems in definition of this condition. In some series the diagnosis has only been made after pathological examination of a hysterectomy specimen whilst in others the diagnosis has rested entirely upon clinical grounds. The situation is further complicated by the fact that a diagnosis of partial placenta accreta, based solely on examination of a delivered placenta, may be made in cases in which a clinical diagnosis of placenta accreta had not been entertained (Jaques et al, 1996). Furthermore, some have considered that manual removal of the placenta

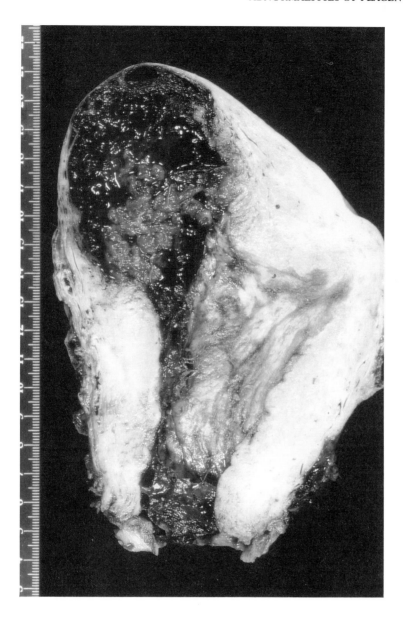

Figure 3.11. A placenta percreta.

can, in itself, be considered as a surrogate for at least a partial degree of placenta accreta (Khong et al, 1991): this belief may, in fact, have some validity though it is difficult to believe that there are not other causes of a failure of normal placental separation.

Quite irrespective of an inability to define a true incidence of placenta accreta there is a well-marked impression in individual centres in the USA that the incidence of clinically diagnosed cases is increasing (Read et al, 1980; Clark et al, 1985; Weckstein et al, 1987).

Pathology

The pathological basis of placenta accreta has been reviewed by Meyer (1955). The characteristic histological feature is a total or partial absence of the decidua basalis (Fig. 3.12); not uncommonly the decidua is replaced by loose connective tissue, throughout which are scattered occasional groups of decidual cells. The decidua parietalis may be normal but is more commonly partially or completely deficient.

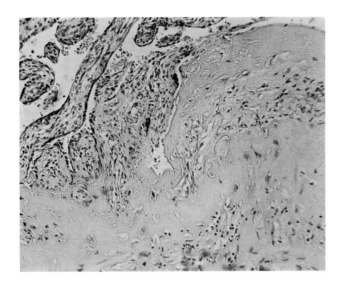

Figure 3.12. Photomicrograph of the implantation of the villi in a placenta accreta. The decidua is represented only by hyaline connective tissue in which there a few scattered decidual cells (H & E × 80).

Where the decidua basalis is lacking, the placental villi are separated from the myometrium by Nitabuch's fibrinoid layer: this latter may appear normal but is frequently thinned or irregular and sometimes completely absent. If the villi penetrate into the myometrium, the muscle may be locally thinned; the myometrial fibres are often hyalinized and can show degenerative changes. There is commonly a local increase in myometrial fibrous tissue and the uterine wall may show a moderate infiltration by acute or chronic inflammatory cells.

The placental villi are usually normal and do not, as a general rule, show any evidence of trophoblastic abnormality or hyperplasia.

The appearances described above are those that are seen in a hysterectomy specimen with the placenta still partially or totally *in situ*. Hutton et al (1983) showed, however, that a clinical diagnosis of placenta accreta could be confirmed by examination of the delivered placenta by the finding, on the maternal surface, of myometrial tissue with either immediately adjacent placental villi or myometrial tissue separated from the villi only by a layer of fibrin: myometrial tissue was invariably absent from the maternal surface of placentas from women in whom there were no clinical features to suggest placenta accreta. Jaques et al (1996) and Salafia et al (submitted) also used this technique but some of the cases they thus diagnosed as 'mild' placenta accreta did not appear to have any clinical features suggestive of a truly adherent placenta. This does therefore raise a question about the validity of a purely pathological diagnosis made in this fashion.

Aetiology

In 1972 I reviewed the 622 cases of placenta accreta that had been reported during the 25-year period from 1945 to 1969 (Fox, 1972). It was noticeable that there was a particular tendency for women with a placenta of this type to be either unusually elderly (this term being used within an obstetrical rather than a social context) or of high gravidity or, not uncommonly, both. Only a small proportion of the women were primigravidas and only rarely was there a previous history of menstrual disturbance or involuntary infertility.

The predisposing causes of a placenta accreta that were suggested by the various authors included:

1. *Placenta praevia.* This was present in 213 cases (34.3%); in some examples of partial placenta praevia it was noted that only the portion of the placenta implanted in the lower uterine segment was abnormally adherent (e.g. Kistner et al, 1952; Foster, 1960; Bruce, 1966; Dreishpoon, 1967; Torbet & Tsoutsopliades, 1968).

2. *Previous uterine curettage*. A history of this was given by 188 patients (30.2%); the operation was usually performed after a previous delivery or abortion. Of particular interest amongst this group were a small number of women in whom curettage had been followed by prolonged amenorrhoea and the formation of intrauterine synechiae, the breaking down of which was followed by a pregnancy complicated by placenta accreta (Musset et al, 1960; Beard, 1966; Dmowski & Greenblatt, 1969). Several further examples of this particular sequence of events have since been reported by Georgakopoulos (1974).

3. *Previous Caesarean section*. One hundred and fifty-four (24.8%) of the women had been subjected to a previous section; only rarely, however, was it known that the placenta was implanted over the scar. In a few exceptional cases it was demonstrated that the placenta was unduly adherent only in that part directly overlying the scar (Segur-Ferrer et al, 1964; Botha, 1969).

4. *Previous manual removal of the placenta*. This had been necessary in 64 patients (10.3%) and had invariably occurred in the pregnancy immediately prior to that complicated by a placenta accreta.

5. *Cornual implantation*. This was noted in 25 patients (4%), most of whom were, however, reported by just two groups of workers (Thonet, 1949; Sumawong et al, 1966).

6. *Previous uterine sepsis*. Twenty-four women (3.8%) had a history of uterine sepsis; this nearly always occurred as a complication of manual removal in the immediately prior pregnancy.

7. *Uterine fibroids*. A placenta accreta was associated with fibroids in 18 cases (2.9%); in only three of these, however, was the placenta shown to be implanted directly over a submucous tumour (Monti & Guglielmone, 1958; Lordy & Machado, 1961; Tovena & Someda de Marco, 1963).

8. *Previous uterine surgery (apart from Caesarean section)*. This was thought to be an aetiological factor in nine patients (1.5%); the operative procedures to which these women had been subjected included cornual resection, myomectomy, resection of a rudimentary horn and removal of an interstitial pregnancy.

9. *Uterine malformation*. Malformed uteri were noted in eight cases, these being mainly of the bicornuate type.

In many patients there was a combination of possible aetiological factors, whilst in only 7% was there no obvious predisposing cause.

There have, since my review in 1972, been several subsequent reports and series which have, in general, tended to confirm the aetiological factors discussed above (Breen et al, 1977; Morison, 1978; Hutton et al, 1983; Mahmood & Kok, 1990; Sfar et al, 1994) though the proportion of cases in which previous Caesarean section appears to be an aetiological factor is increasing (Clark et al, 1985). Additional aetiological factors that have been recently identified include planned partial endometrial resection (Wood & Rogers, 1993) and myotonic dystrophy (Freeman, 1991).

Pathogenesis

The common end-point of all the various factors that appear to predispose to the development of a placenta accreta is a deficiency of the decidua. The pathogenesis appears fairly clear-cut when a placenta accreta complicates implantation on a uterine scar, on a submucous fibroid, in the lower uterine segment, in a rudimentary horn, or in the uterine cornua, in all of which circumstances the underlying decidua is often deficient or poorly developed.

There is no doubt that over-enthusiastic curettage can cause an endometrial and decidual deficiency; this is exemplified by those cases in which the operation is followed by the development of uterine synechiae. In most cases of placenta accreta, however, any previous curettage has usually been performed after either a normal delivery or an abortion and has not led to any disturbance of menstruation. It is quite possible that in such patients the operation had been necessitated by the retention of chorionic tissue because of a partial placental adherence. This argument can also be applied to a history of a previous manual removal, because this manoeuvre is unlikely to be a true aetiological factor in the development of a placenta accreta, and the necessity for its use is more probably an indication of a minor degree of abnormal placental adherence in the previous pregnancy.

Uterine sepsis can obviously lead to endometrial fibrosis and decidual deficiency but it is nowadays an uncommon cause of placenta accreta. It has been suggested that uterine adenomyosis is of some importance in the development of an adherent placenta (Roman, 1960) but there is scant evidence to support this contention.

If, in many patients, a history of previous curettage or manual removal is indicative of a recurring, or progressive, tendency to form an unduly adherent placenta, it becomes clear that in about one-third of women with a placenta accreta there are no obvious aetiological or predisposing factors to account for the decidual deficiency. It has been suggested that in such cases there is a primary hormonal deficiency and endometrial hypoplasia (Millar, 1959), but it is difficult to reconcile this theory with the very low incidence of placenta accreta in primigravidas, with the paucity of previous menstrual disturbances, and with the infrequency of previous involuntary infertility.

It has been maintained that a placenta accreta may be due, not to an inadequacy of the decidua, but to an undue invasiveness of the placenta (Tovena & Someda de Marco, 1963; da Fonseca & da Luz Roris, 1965; Teppa et al, 1968). This view is supported to some extent by Khong and Robertson (1987) who showed that the intravascular extravillous trophoblast of the placental bed extended unusually deeply in cases of placenta accreta, reaching as far as the large arteries of the radial/arcuate system. Khong and Robertson also noted a failure to form multinucleated giant cells in the placental bed and a decreased density of interstitial trophoblast in the deeper parts of the myometrium and concluded that placenta accreta resulted from an abnormal interaction between the maternal tissues and migratory trophoblast in the early stages of placentation. This theory is at variance with the usual histological findings in placenta accreta and Benirschke and Kaufmann (1995) believe that the changes noted in the placental bed are a result of the absence of decidua and not a primary causal factor for undue adherence of the placenta. Salafia et al (submitted) have, up to a point, supported the concept of undue trophoblastic invasiveness as the primary pathogenetic mechanism in placenta accreta though their findings differ from those of Khong and Robertson insofar as they found presumed evidence of deep invasion in association with lack of trophoblastic invasion of placental bed vessels. They suggested that local hypoxia acts as a spur to increased depth of trophoblastic invasion, basing this view on the experimental, and highly unphysiological, study of Zhou et al (1993). The concept that uteroplacental ischaemia is responsible for increased trophoblastic invasiveness appears untenable if only for the reason that most trophoblastic invasion of the placental bed occurs at a time when there is probably no perfusion of the intervillous space by maternal blood. The suggestion that the unduly deep invasion of the villi is due to the deficiency of a hypothetical immunological mechanism that normally limits the depth of penetration (Schaupe et al, 1974) is also not in accord with the histological findings. Nevertheless, in a recent, and as yet not fully documented, study it was shown that there is an absence of detectable beta-hCG in the syncytiotrophoblast of the penetrating villi in placenta percreta, this, because of the presence of beta-hCG mRNA, being apparently due to a post-transcriptional defect in hCG synthesis. It was therefore suggested that the absence of beta-hCG at the site of advancing trophoblast may result in inappropriate maternofetal immunological recognition (Coppola et al, 1995). This is an intriguing observation which requires confirmation; it is, however, possible that the failure to synthesize hCG may be due to the lack of a decidual 'signal' and thus is a secondary, rather than a primary, phenomenon. It should be noted that the extravillous trophoblast population in cases of placenta accreta is immunohistologically fully normal (Earl et al, 1987).

It will be apparent that the long, and perhaps complacently, held view that a deficiency of decidua is the primary factor in the pathogenesis of a placenta accreta is currently under attack by those proposing a more dynamic view of the relationship between trophoblast and maternal tissues. Nevertheless the newer hypotheses do not adequately explain either the histological findings or the known and proven aetiological factors for this condition.

van Thiel et al (1972) have noted an increased incidence of placenta accreta amongst women becoming pregnant after successful treatment for gestational trophoblastic disease, and they have postulated that the mechanism responsible for the control of placental invasion may be altered in such women, this leading, in some circumstances, to trophoblastic disease and, in others, to a placenta accreta. This is an interesting speculation for which, however, there is little factual evidence and against which there are strong histologically based arguments: Breen et al (1977) have commented on the absence of any instances of placenta accreta in a large series of patients who had received chemotherapy for a trophoblastic disease.

Clinical Effects

Antepartum bleeding is common in any series of women with placenta accreta; this is due almost entirely to the high proportion of cases of placenta praevia. The haemorrhage may be copious and is sometimes intensified by the development of afibrinogenaemia (Ochshorn et al, 1969).

Uterine rupture occurs in about 14% of patients, the placenta in such cases being of the 'percreta' type and penetrating through the myometrium. This catastrophe can occur before, during or after labour, but most commonly complicates the antepartum period, frequently during the second trimester and sometimes as early as the first trimester (Katzman, 1960; Shram & Askari, 1965; Botha, 1969; Camlibel, 1981). Occasionally the placental tissue invades the bladder (Taefi et al, 1970; Grabert et al, 1970; Silber et al, 1973; Mathews, 1983; Trenton, 1984; Aho et al, 1985; Melchor et al, 1987; Litwin et al, 1989; Altintas et al, 1991; Price et al, 1991; Roux et al, 1992; Bakri et al, 1993; Lymperopoulou et al, 1993) commonly with resulting severe haematuria or, very occasionally, the formation of a vesico-uterine fistula (Krysiewicz et al, 1988).

Cases have been reported in which placenta accreta presented as profuse haemorrhage during or immediately after curettage in early pregnancy for elective or incomplete abortion (Begneard et al, 1965; Veridiano et al, 1986; Woolcott et al, 1987; Harden et al, 1990; Ecker et al, 1992; Rashbaum et al, 1995). These are unusual, however, and the outstanding clinical characteristic of placenta accreta is a failure of placental separation during the third stage of labour. If the placenta is totally adherent there will be no separation at all and no postpartum bleeding, but if the adherence is less than total there will be partial separation and postpartum haemorrhage; the bleeding is often very heavy and it has been suggested that this is due to the decidual deficiency being accompanied by a lack of local thromboplastic substance (Kistner et al, 1952).

A rare, but serious, complication of placenta accreta is uterine inversion; this may occur spontaneously but usually follows an attempted manual removal of the placenta.

The net effect of these various misfortunes that may befall a woman with a placenta accreta led, in the past, to a maternal mortality rate in the order of 10% (Fox, 1972): this is now almost certainly very much lower. It should be noted that a placenta accreta may be associated with a raised maternal serum alpha-fetoprotein level (Ginsberg et al, 1992; Zelop et al, 1992; McCool et al, 1992; Kupferminc et al, 1993) and that the condition can be diagnosed antenatally by ultrasonography or by magnetic resonance imaging (Kerr de Mendonca, 1988; Hoffman-Tretin et al, 1992; Rosemond & Kepple, 1992; Thorp et al, 1992; Fejgin et al, 1993). Until relatively recently, the optimal treatment for a placenta accreta was hysterectomy and this is still generally the case when the condition is complicated by severe bleeding. In the absence of haemorrhage there is, however, an increasing tendency to leave the placenta *in situ* and administer a course of methotrexate (Arulkumaran et al, 1986; Legro et al, 1994).

REFERENCES

Abraham, E.G. (1932) Placenta zonaria humana incompleta. *Zentralblatt für Gynäkologie*, **56**, 221–228.
Aguero, O. (1957) *Anomolias Morfologicas de la Placenta y su Significado Clínico*. Caracas, Venezuela: Artegrafia.

Aho, A.J., Pulkkinen, M.O. and Vaha-Eskeli, K. (1985) Acute urinary tamponade with hypovolemic shock due to placenta percreta with bladder invasion. *Scandinavian Journal of Urology and Nephrology*, **19**, 157–159.

Althabe, O. and Althabe, O. (1963) Placenta accreta. *Semana Médica* (Buenos Aires), **123**, 118.

Altintas, A., Ozgunen, F.T., Doran, S. and Doran, F. (1991) Placenta percreta invading the urinary bladder. *Australian and New Zealand Journal of Obstetrics and Gynaecology*, **31**, 371–372.

Antoine, T. (1930) Placenta pseudozonaria und fenestrata. *Zentralblatt für Gynäkologie*, **54**, 749–751.

Arulkumaran, S., Ng, C.S., Ingemarsson, I. and Ratnam, S.S. (1986) Medical treatment of placenta accreta with methotrexate. *Acta Obstetricia et Gynecologica Scandinavica*, **65**, 285–286.

Ayala, L.C., Topete, M.M., Mondragon, H.L. and Pinsker, V.S. (1965) Placenta extracorial: valoracion anatomoclinica de 86 casos. *Ginecologia y Obstetricia de México*, **20**, 593–598.

Bain, A.D., Smith, I.I. and Gauld, I.K. (1964) Newborn after prolonged leakage of liquor amnii. *British Medical Journal*, **ii**, 598–599.

Bakri, Y.N., Sundin, T., Mansi, M. and Jaroudi, K. (1993) Placenta percreta with bladder invasion: report of three cases. *American Journal of Perinatology*, **10**, 468–470.

Barss, P. and Misch, K.A. (1990) Endemic placenta accreta in a population of remote villagers in Papua New Guinea. *British Journal of Obstetrics and Gynaecology*, **97**, 167–174.

Beard, R.M. (1966) Placenta accreta in a patient with Asherman's syndrome. *Australian and New Zealand Journal of Obstetrics and Gynaecology*, **6**, 316–320.

Begneard, W., Dougherty, C.M. and Mickal, A. (1965) Placenta accreta in early gestation: report of two cases. *American Journal of Obstetrics and Gynecology*, **95**, 267–268.

Benirschke, K. and Driscoll, S.G. (1967) *The Pathology of the Human Placenta*. Berlin, Heidelberg, New York: Springer-Verlag.

Benirschke, K. and Kaufmann, P. (1990) *Pathology of the Human Placenta*, 2nd edn. New York: Springer-Verlag.

Benirschke, K. and Kaufmann, P. (1995) *Pathology of the Human Placenta*, 3rd edn. New York: Springer-Verlag.

Benson, R.C. and Fujikura, T. (1969) Circumvallate and circummarginate placenta: unimportant clinical entities. *Obstetrics and Gynecology*, **34**, 799–804.

Botha, M.C. (1969) Spontaneous rupture of the uterus due to placenta percreta: a case report. *South African Medical Journal*, **43**, 39–41.

Bourrel, P., Tournier-Lasser, C. and Gerome, M. (1964) Placenta accreta chez l'Africaine; trois observations. *Medicine Tropicale (Marseilles)*, **24**, 185–191.

Boyd, J.D. and Hamilton, W.J. (1970) *The Human Placenta*. Cambridge: W. Heffer & Sons.

Breen, J.L., Neubecker, R., Gregori, C.A. and Franklin, J.E. Jr (1977) Placenta accreta, increta and percreta: a survey of 40 cases. *Obstetrics and Gynecology*, **49**, 43–47.

Bruce, D.F. (1966) Placenta praevia accreta. *Scottish Medical Journal*, **5**, 155–157.

Camlibel, F.T. (1981) Spontaneous rupture of uterus caused by placenta percreta. *New York State Journal of Medicine*, **81**, 1373–1376.

Cavalli, D. (1961) Le anomalie morfologiche della placenta (si du un caso di rara anomalia) *Rivista di Ostetricia e Ginecologia Pratica*, **43**, 388–401.

Chabes, E., Pereda, J., Hyams, L. et al (1968) Comparative morphometry of the human placenta at high altitude and at sea level. I. The shape of the placenta. *Obstetrics and Gynecology*, **31**, 178–185.

Clark, S.L., Koonings, P.P. and Phelan, J.P. (1985) Placenta previa/accreta and prior cesarean section. *Obstetrics and Gynecology*, **66**, 89–92.

Coppola, D., Putong, P.B., Finkelstein, S. and Cooper, H. (1995) Defective synthesis of beta-human chorionic gonadotropin (beta-HCG) in placenta percreta. *Abstract. United States and Canadian Academy of Pathology Annual Meeting, Toronto.*

Culp, W.C., Bryan, R.N. and Morettin, L.B. (1973) Placenta membranacea: a case report with arteriographic findings. *Radiology*, **108**, 309–310.

da Fonseca, M.A.A. and da Luz Roris, M. (1965) Um caso de placenta acreta. *Revista Clínica do Instituto Maternal de Lisboa*, **15**, 71–81.

Deacon, J.S.R., Gilbert, E.F., Viseskul, C., Herrmann, J. and Opitz, J.M. (1974) Polyhydramnios and neonatal haemorrhage in three sisters: a circumvallate placenta syndrome. *Birth Defects Original Article Series*, **10**, 41–49.

Dinh, T.V., Bedi, D.G. and Salinas, J. (1992) Placenta membranacea, previa and accreta: a case report. *Journal of Reproductive Medicine*, **37**, 97–99.

Dmowski, W.P. and Greenblatt, R.B. (1969) Asherman's syndrome and the risk of placenta accreta. *Obstetrics and Gynecology*, **34**, 288–299.

Dreishpoon, I.H. (1967) Placenta accreta: a presentation of four interesting cases. *International Surgeon*, **47**, 541–547.

Earl, U., Bulmer, J.N. and Briones, A. (1987) Placenta accreta: an immunohistological study of trophoblast populations. *Placenta*, **8**, 273–282.

Earn, A.A. (1951) Placental anomalies. *Canadian Medical Association Journal*, **64**, 118–120.

Ecker, J.L., Sorem, K.A., Soodak, K., Robets, D.J., Safon, L.E. and Osathanondh, R. (1992) Placenta increta complicating a first-trimester abortion: a case report. *Journal of Reproductive Medicine*, **37**, 893–895.

Ekoukou, D., Ng Wing Tin, L., Nere, M.B. et al (1995) Placenta membranacea: revue de la litterature, à propos d'un cas. *Journal de Gynécologie d'Obstétrique et de la Biologie de la Reproduction*, **24**, 189–193.

Fauvet, E. (1935) Zur Frage der menschlichen 'Gürtelplacenta'. *Zentralblatt für Gynäkologie*, **59**, 1164–1169.

Fejgin, M.D., Rosen, D.J., Ben-Nun, I., Goldberger, S.B. and Beyth, Y. (1993) Ultrasonic and magnetic resonance imaging diagnosis of placenta accreta managed conservatively. *Journal of Perinatal Medicine*, **21**, 165–168.

Finn, J.L. (1954) Placenta membranacea. *Obstetrics and Gynecology*, **3**, 438–440.

Foss, I. and Vogel, M. (1972) Über Beziehungen zwischen Implantationsschaden der Plazenta und Plazentationsstorungen. *Zeitschrift für Geburtshilfe und Perinatologie*, **176**, 36–44.

Foster, G.S. (1960) Placenta praevia accreta: report of 2 cases and discussion of management. *Obstetrics and Gynecology*, **15**, 322–328.

Fox, H. (1972) Placenta accreta, 1945–1969. *Obstetrical and Gynecological Survey*, **27**, 475–490.

Fox, H. and Sen, D.K. (1972) Placenta extrachorialis: a clinicopathological study. *Journal of Obstetrics and Gynecology of the British Commonwealth*, **79**, 32–35.

Fraenkel, L. and Granzow, J. (1936) Gürtelplacenta. *Archiv für Gynäkologie*, **128**, 422–451.

Freeman, R.M. (1991) Placenta accreta and myotonic dystrophy: two cases. *British Journal of Obstetrics and Gynaecology*, **98**, 594–595.

Fujikura, T., Benson, R.C. and Driscoll, S.G. (1970) The bipartite placenta and its clinical features. *American Journal of Obstetrics and Gynecology*, **107**, 1013–1017.

Georgakopoulos, P. (1974) Placenta accreta following lysis of uterine synechiae (Asherman's syndrome). *Journal of Obstetrics and Gynaecology of the British Commonwealth*, **81**, 730–733.

Ginsberg, N.A., Fausone, M.E., Gerbie, M., Applebaum, M. and Verlinsky, Y. (1992) Elevated maternal serum alpha-fetoprotein associated with placenta accreta. *Journal of Assisted Reproduction and Genetics*, **9**, 497–500.

Glinski, S. (1973) Ocena wplywu lozyska obalowanego no stan noworodka. (Evaluation of the effect of circumvallate placenta upon the state of the fetus.) *Ginekologia Polska*, **44**, 123–125.

Goldman, J.A. (1963) Placenta praevia and increta: with special reference to the problem of conservative versus radical treatment. *Israel Medical Journal*, **22**, 232–241.

Goodall, J.R. (1934) Circumcrescent and circumvallate placenta. *American Journal of Obstetrics and Gynecology*, **28**, 707–722.

Grabert, H., Mossa, A., Oliveira, S.F., Hutzler, I., Fainzielber, S. and Rodriguez De Lima, C. (1970) Placenta percreta with penetration of the bladder. *Journal of Obstetrics and Gynaecology of the British Commonwealth*, **77**, 1142–1143.

Grahbner, F. (1932) Eine Gürtelplacenta. *Zentralblatt für Gynäkologie*, **56**, 1945–1948.

Greenberg, J.A., Sorem, K.A., Shifren, J.L. and Riley, L.E. (1991) Placenta membranacea with placenta increta: a case report and literature review. *Obstetrics and Gynecology*, **78**, 512–514.

Grosser, O. (1927) *Frühentwicklung, Eihautbildung und Placentation des Menschen und der Saugetiere*. Munich: J. F. Bergmann.

Harden, M.A., Walters, M.D. and Valente, P.T. (1990) Postabortal hemorrhage due to placenta increta: a case report. *Obstetrics and Gynecology*, **75**, 523–526.

Hata, K., Hata, T., Aoki, S., Takamori, H., Takamiya, D. and Kitao, M. (1988) Succenteriate placenta diagnosed by ultrasound. *Obstetric and Gynecologic Investigation*, **25**, 273–276.

Hertig, A.T. (1960) Pathological aspects. In *The Placenta and Fetal Membranes*, Villee, C.A. (Ed.), pp. 109–124. Baltimore: Williams and Wilkins.

Hobbs, J.E. and Price, C.N. (1940) Placenta circumvallata. *American Journal of Obstetrics and Gynecology*, **39**, 39–44.

Hobbs, J.E. and Rollins, P.R. (1934) Fetal death from placenta circumvallata. *American Journal of Obstetrics and Gynecology*, **28**, 78–83.

Hoffman-Tretin, J.C., Koenigsberg, M., Rabin, A. and Anyaegbunam, A. (1992) Placenta accreta: additional sonographic observations. *Journal of Ultrasound in Medicine*, **11**, 29–34.

Hunt, A.B., Mussey, R.D. and Faber, J.E. (1947) Circumvallate placenta. *New Orleans Medical and Surgical Journal*, **100**, 203–207.

Hurley, V.A. and Beischer, N.A. (1987) Placenta membranacea: case reports. *British Journal of Obstetrics and Gynaecology*, **94**, 798–802.

Hutton, L., Yang, S.S. and Bernstein, J. (1983) Placenta accreta: a 26-year clinicopathologic review (1956–1981) *New York State Journal of Medicine*, **83**, 857–866.

Irving, C. and Hertig, A.T. (1937) A study of placenta accreta. *Surgery, Gynecology and Obstetrics*, **64**, 178–200.

Janovski, N.A. and Granowitz, E.T. (1961) Placenta membranacea: report of a case. *Obstetrics and Gynecology*, **18**, 206–212.

Jaques, S.M., Qureshi, F., Trent, V.S. and Ramirez, N.C. (1996) Placenta accreta: mild cases diagnosed by placental examination. *International Journal of Gynecological Pathology*, **15**, 28–33.

Jauniaux, E., Avni, F.E., Donner, C., Rodesch, F. and Wilkin, P. (1989) Ultrasonographic diagnosis and morphological study of placenta circumvallate. *Journal of Clinical Ultrasound*, **17**, 126–131.

Katzman, H.L. (1960) Spontaneous rupture of the uterus resulting from placenta percreta: case report and review of the literature. *Harper Hospital Bulletin*, **18**, 232–238.

Keefer, F.J. and Cope, P.H. (1963) Placenta of unusual shape: report of a case. *Obstetrics and Gynecology*, **22**, 679.

Ker de Mendonca, L. (1988) Sonographic diagnosis of placenta accreta. *Journal of Ultrasound Medicine*, **7**, 211–215.

Khong, T.Y. and Robertson, W.B. (1987) Placenta creta and placenta praevia. *Placenta*, **8**, 399–409.

Khong, T.Y., Healy, D.L. and McCloud, P.I. (1991) Pregnancies complicated by abnormally adherent placenta and sex ratio at birth. *British Medical Journal*, **302**, 625–626.

Kiefer, K.H. (1937) Placenta zonaria humana completa. *Zentralblatt für Gynäkologie*, **61**, 1426–1428.

Kistner, R.W., Hertig, A.T. and Reid, D.E. (1952) Simultaneously occurring placenta praevia and placenta accreta. *Surgery, Gynecology and Obstetrics*, **94**, 141–151.

Klaften, E. (1928) Zur Klinik und Genese der Placenta pseudozonaria humana. *Zentralblatt für Gynäkologie*, **52**, 2074–2082.

Kleine, H.O. (1956) Uber seltene Plazentaformen: Gürtelplazenta, Placenta bipartita und Placenta fenestrata. *Zentralblatt für Gynäkologie*, **78**, 2029–2032.

Kohler, H.G., Peel, K.R. and Hoar, R.A. (1970) Extramembranous pregnancy and amenorrhoea. *Journal of Obstetrics and Gynaecology of the British Commonwealth*, **70**, 809–812.

Krysiewicz, S., Auh, Y.H. and Kazam, E. (1988) Vesicouterine fistula associated with placenta percreta. *Urological Radiology*, **10**, 213–215.

Kupferminc, M.J., Tamura, R.K., Wigton, T.R., Glassenberg, R. and Socol, M.L. (1993) Placenta accreta is associated with elevated maternal serum alpha-fetoprotein. *Obstetrics and Gynecology*, **82**, 266–269.

Lademacher, D.S., Vermeulen, R.C.W., van der Harten J.J. and Arts, N.F. (1981) Circumvallate placenta and congenital anomalies. *Lancet*, **i**, 732.

Lahm, W. (1924) Eine neue Erklrung der Placenta circumvallata. *Archiv für Gynäkologie*, **121**, 306–313.

Lal, K. (1975) Placenta extrachorialis: a clinico-pathological study. *Journal of Obstetrics and Gynaecology of India*, **25**, 181–185.

Lal, K. (1976) Circumvallate placenta. *Journal of Obstetrics and Gynaecology of India*, **26**, 151–152.

Las Heras, J., Harding, P.G. and Haust, M.D. (1982) Recurrent bleeding associated with placenta membranacea partialis: report of a case. *American Journal of Obstetrics and Gynecology*, **144**, 480–482.

Legro, R.S., Price, F.V., Hill, L.M. and Caritis, S.N. (1994) Non-surgical management of placenta percreta: a case report. *Obstetrics and Gynecology*, **83**, 847–849.

Liepmann, W. (1906) Beiträg zur Aetiologie der Placenta circumvallata. *Archiv für Gynäkologie*, **80**, 439–454.

Litwin, M.S., Loughlin, K.R., Benson, C.B., Droege, G.F. and Richie, J.P. (1989) Placenta percreta invading the urinary bladder. *British Journal of Urology*, **64**, 283–286.

Liu, Q.X. (1990) Pathology of the placenta from small for gestational age infants. *Chinese Journal of Obstetrics and Gynecology*, **25**, 331–334.

Lordy, C. and Machado, W. (1961) Placenta accreta. *Anais Paulistas de Medicina e Cirurgia*, **81**, 251–254.

Luke, R.K., Sharpe, J.W. and Greene, R.R. (1966) The adherent or invasive placenta. *American Journal of Obstetrics and Gynecology*, **95**, 160–168.

Lymperopoulou, A., Hainaut, F. and Crimail, P. (1993) Placenta percreta sur cicatrice de cesarienne avec envahissement vesical: revue general à propos deux cas. *Revue Francaise de Gynécologie et de l'Obstétrique*, **88**, 379–384.

McCarthy, J., Thurmond, A.S., Jones, M.K. et al (1995) Circumvallate placenta: sonographic diagnosis. *Journal of Ultrasound in Medicine*, **14**, 21-26.

McCool, R.A., Bombard, A.T., Bartholomew, D.A. and Calhoun, B.C. (1992) Unexplained positive/elevated serum alpha-fetoprotein associated with placenta increta: a case report. *Journal of Reproductive Medicine*, **37**, 826-828.

Mahmood, T.A. and Kok, K.P. (1990) A review of placenta accreta at Aberdeen Maternity Hospital, Scotland. *Australian and New Zealand Journal of Obstetrics and Gynaecology*, **30**, 108–110.

Malkani, P.K. and Bhasin, K. (1970) Clinical significance of placenta extrachorialis. *Journal of Obstetrics and Gynaecology of India*, **20**, 346–348.

Maqueo–Topete, M., Chavez–Azuela, J., Valenzuela-Lopez, S. and Espinosa-Hernandez, J. (1968) Placenta accreta and circumvallata (extrachorialis) *Obstetrics and Gynecology*, **32**, 397–401.

Martin, T.R. (1967) Circumvallate placenta. *Nova Scotia Medical Bulletin*, **46**, 29–31.

Mathews, J. (1974) Placenta membranacea. *Australian and New Zealand Journal of Obstetrics and Gynaecology*, **14**, 45–47.

Mathews, J. (1983) Placenta praevia percreta with bladder penetration. *Medical Journal of Australia*, **1**, 173–174.

Melchor, J.C., Alegre, A., Arteche, J.M., Corcostegui, B. and Rodriguez-Escudero, F.J. (1987) Placenta percreta with bladder involvement: case report and review of the literature. *International Journal of Gynaecology and Obstetrics*, **25**, 417–418.

Meyer, B. (1955) Placenta accreta: an analysis based on an unusual case. *Acta Obstetricia et Gynecologica Scandinavica*, **34**, 189–201.

Millar, W.G. (1959) A clinical and pathological study of placenta accreta. *Journal of Obstetrics and Gynaecology of the British Empire*, **66**, 353–364.

Molloy, C.E., McDowell, W., Armour, T., Crawford, W. and Bernstein, R. (1983) Ultrasound diagnosis of placenta membranacea in utero. *Journal of Ultrasound in Medicine*, **2**, 377–379.

Monti, R.L. and Guglielmone, P.L. (1958) Adherencia anormal de placenta en utero miomatosa. *Obstetricia y Ginecologia Latino–Americanas*, **16**, 352–354.

Morgan, J. (1955) Circumvallate placenta. *Journal of Obstetrics and Gynaecology of the British Empire*, **62**, 899–900.

Morison, J.E. (1978) Placenta accreta: a clinicopathologic review of 67 cases. *Obstetrics and Gynecology Annual*, **7**, 107–123.

Musset, R., Netter, A., Ravina, J. and Depoorter, L. (1960) Synechies utérines traumatiques et placenta accreta: une association fréquente et grave. *Gynécologie et Obstétrique*, **59**, 450–456.

Naftolin, F., Khudr, G., Benirschke, K. and Hutchinson, D.L. (1973) The syndrome of chronic abruptio placentae, hydrorrhea, and circumvallate placenta. *American Journal of Obstetrics and Gynecology*, **116**, 347–350.

Nesbitt, R.E.L. (1957) *Perinatal Loss in Modern Obstetrics*. Philadelphia: F. A. Davis.

Ochshorn, A., David, M.P. and Soferman, N. (1969) Placenta previa accreta: a report of 9 cases. *Obstetrics and Gynecology*, **33**, 677–679.

Paalman, R.J. and Vander Veer, C.G. (1953) Circumvallate placenta. *American Journal of Obstetrics and Gynecology*, **65**, 491–497.

Pavoni, A. (1954) Rilievi clinici ad anatomo-patologici sulla placenta marginata e circumvallata. *Rivista Italiana di Ginecologia*, **37**, 124–137.

Philipp, E. (1930) Die menschliche Gürtelplacenta und ihre Entstehung. *Zentralblatt für Gynäkologie*, **54**, 1032–1041.

Philipp, E. (1932) Die verschiedenen Formen der menschlichen Gürtelplacenta. *Zentralblatt für Gynäkologie*, **56**, 2256–2259.

Pinkerton, J.H.M. (1956) Placenta circumvallate, its aetiology and clinical significance. *Journal of Obstetrics and Gynaecology of the British Empire*, **63**, 743–747.

Price, F.V., Resnik, E., Heller, K.A. and Christopherson, W.A. (1991) Placenta previa percreta involving the urinary bladder: a report of two cases and review of the literature. *Obstetrics and Gynecology*, **78**, 508–511.

Pryse-Davies, J., Dewhurst, C.J. and Campbell, S. (1973) Placenta membranacea. *Journal of Obstetrics and Gynaecology of the British Commonwealth*, **80**, 1106–1110.

Rashbaum, W.K., Gates, E.J., Jones, J., Goldman, B., Morouls, A. and Lyman, W.D. (1995) Placenta accreta encountered during dilatation and evacuation in the second trimester. *Obstetrics and Gynecology*, **85**, 701–703.

Read, J.A., Cotton, D.B. and Miller, F.C. (1980) Placenta accreta: changing clinical aspects and outcome. *Obstetrics and Gynecology*, **56**, 31–34.

Rolschau, J. (1978) Circumvallate placenta and intrauterine growth retardation. *Acta Obstetricia et Gynecologica Scandinavica* (supplement) **72**, 11–14.

Roman, C. (1960) Placenta accreta, synechies utérines et adenomyomatoses. *Bulletin de la Fédération des Sociétés de Gynécologie et d'Obstétrique de Langue Francaise*, **12**, 279.

Rosemond, R.L. and Kepple, D.M. (1992) Transvaginal color Dopler sonography in the prenatal diagnosis of placenta accreta. *Obstetrics and Gynecology*, **80**, 508–510.

Roux, D., Horovitz, J., Pariente, J.L., Lajus, C., Le-Guillou, M. and Dubecq, J.P. (1992) Placenta praevia percreta avec envahissement vesical: un cas. *Journal de Gynécologie, Obstétrique et Biologie de la Reproduction*, **21**, 579–580.

Ruder, F.B. (1933) Die Genese und Nomenklatur der Gürtelplazenta. (Ein weiterer Fall einer Placenta zonaria humana completa.) *Zeitschrift für Geburtshilfe und Gynäkologie*, **105**, 437–444.

Salafia, C.M., Sherer, D.M., Minior, V.K. Sanders, M., Ernst, L. and Vintzileos, A.M. (1996) Histologic evidence of abnormally deep trophoblast invasion: clinical correlations. Submitted for publication.

Sandstedt, B. (1979) The placenta and low birth weight. *Current Topics in Pathology*, **66**, 2–55.

Sauramo, H. (1960) Obstetric complications due to secundines. *Annales Chirurgiae et Gynaecologiae Fenniae*, **49**, 291–297.

Schaupe, von H., Grumbrecht, C., Squarr, H.U. and Vogel, M. (1974) Placenta praevia percreta. *Zentralblatt für Gynäkologie*, **96**, 1239–1245.

Scott, J.S. (1960) Placenta extrachorialis (placenta marginata and placenta circumvallata): a factor in antepartum haemorrhage. *Journal of Obstetrics and Gynaecology of the British Empire*, **67**, 904–918.

Segur-Ferrer, J., Pascual-Moreno, A. and Quehalt-Ballestre, J.A. (1964) Placenta accreta. *Toko-Ginecologia Practica*, **23**, 287–294.

Sfameni, P. (1908) Ueber die Enstehung der Placenta marginata und circumvallata im Hinblick auf die Arbeiten von Liepmann und Kroemer. *Zentralblatt für Gynäkologie*, **32**, 234–247.

Sfar, E., Zine, S., Chaar, N. et al (1994) Analyse des facteurs de risque du placenta accreta: a propos de 8 observations. *Revue Francaise de Gynécologie et d'Obstétrique*, **89**, 202–206.

Sherer, D.M., Smith, S.S., Metlay, L.A. and Woods, J.R. Jr (1991) Sonographic and pathologic features of a circumvallate placenta associated with early amnion rupture. *Journal of Clinical Ultrasound*, **19**, 241–243.

Shram, M. and Askari, M. (1965) Spontaneous rupture of uterus caused by placenta accreta at 17 weeks of gestation. *Obstetrics and Gynecology*, **25**, 624–628.

Siedentopf, H. (1932) Placenta praevia fenestrata, eine Form der 'Gürtelplacenta'. *Zentralblatt für Gynäkologie*, **56**, 268–273.

Silber, S.J., Breakey, B., Campbell, D., Williams, H. and Fellamn, S. (1973) Placenta percreta invading bladder. *Journal of Urology*, **109**, 615–618.

Sirivongs, B. (1974) Vasa previa: report of 3 cases. *Journal of the Medical Association of Thailand*, **57**, 261–268.

Sudha, C., Schifrin, B. and Suziki, K. (1973) Trilobate placenta and an abnormal fetal heart rate pattern. *American Journal of Obstetrics and Gynecology*, **116**, 878–880.

Sumawong, V., Nondasuta, A., Thanapath, S. and Budthimedhee, V. (1966) Placenta accreta: a review of the literature and a survey of 10 cases. *Obstetrics and Gynecology*, **27**, 511–516.

Suska, P., Vierik, J., Handzo, I. and Krizko, M. (1989) Vyskyt makroskopickych zmien placent u intrauterinne rastovo retardovanych novorodencov. (Incidence of macroscopic changes in the placenta in intrauterine growth retardation in infants.) *Bratislaske Lekarske Listy*, **90**, 604–607.

Taefi, P., Kaiser, T.F., Sheffer, J.B., Courey, N.G. and Hodson, J.M. (1970) Placenta percreta with bladder invasion: report of a case. *Obstetrics and Gynecology*, **36**, 686–687.

Teppa, T.P.A., de Teppa, D.G., Dominguez, I.C. and Szczedrin, W. (1968) Placenta acreta. *Revista de Obstetricia y Ginecologia de Venezuela*, **28**, 147–167.

Thonet, C. (1949) Placenta accreta. *Boletin de la Sociedad Chilena de Obstetricia y Ginecologia*, **14**, 72–80.

Thorp, J.M. Jr, Councell, R.B., Sandridge, D.A. and Wiest, H.H. (1992) Antepartum diagnosis of placenta previa percreta by magnetic resonance imaging. *Obstetrics and Gynecology*, **80**, 506–508.

Torbet, T.E. and Tsoutsopliades, G.C. (1968) Placenta praevia accreta: conservative management. *Journal of Obstetrics and Gynaecology of the British Commonwealth*, **75**, 737–740.

Torpin, R. (1953) Classification of human pregnancy based on depth of intrauterine implantation of the ovum. *American Journal of Obstetrics and Gynecology*, **66**, 791–798.

Torpin, R. (1955a) Placenta circumvallata and placenta marginata. *Obstetrics and Gynecology*, **6**, 277–282.

Torpin, R. (1955b) Correlation of placental anomalies with spontaneous abortion or premature separation. *Journal of Obstetrics and Gynaecology of the British Empire*, **62**, 385–389.

Torpin, R. (1958) Human placental anomalies: etiology, evolution and historical background. *Missouri Medicine*, **55**, 353–357.

Torpin, R. (1966) Evolution of a placenta circumvallata. *Obstetrics and Gynecology*, **27**, 99–101.

Torpin, R. and Barfield, W.E. (1968) Placenta duplex: report of a case studied by reconstruction of the fetal sac. *Journal of the Medical Association of Georgia*, **57**, 78–80.

Torpin, R. and Hart, B.F. (1941) Placenta bilobata. *American Journal of Obstetrics and Gynecology*, **42**, 38–49.

Tovena, A. and Someda de Marco, I. (1963) Considerazioni su quattro casi di placenta previa accreta diffus. *Attualita di Ostetricia e Ginecologia*, **9**, 1249–1267.

Trenton, W.D. (1984) Placenta praevia percreta with invasion of the bladder: report of a case. *Journal of the American Osteopathic Association*, **84**, 373–375.

Vahlenkamp, H. (1961) Zum Thema Gürtelplazenta. *Geburtshilfe und Frauenheilkunde*, **21**, 980–983.

van Thiel, D.H., Grodin, J.M., Ross, G.T. and Lipsett, M.B. (1972) Partial placenta accreta in pregnancy following chemotherapy for gestational trophoblastic neoplasm. *American Journal of Obstetrics and Gynecology*, **112**, 54–58.

Veridiano, N.P., Lopes, J., Ohm, H.K. and Tancer, M.L. (1986) Placenta percreta as a cause of uterine perforation during abortion. *Journal of Reproductive Medicine*, **31**, 1049–1050.

von Herff, O. (1896) Beitrage zur Lehre von der Placenta und von den mütterlichen Eihüllen. I. Wachsthumsrichtung der Placenta, insbesondere die der Placenta circumvallate. *Zeitschrift für Geburtshilfe und Gynäkologie*, **35**, 268–325.

Walsen, O. (1958) Die menschliche Gürtelplazenta. *Zentralblatt für Gynäkologie*, **80**, 221–225.

Weckstein, N.L., Masserman, J.S.H. and Garite, T.J. (1987) Placenta accreta: a problem of increasing clinical significance. *Obstetrics and Gynecology*, **69**, 480–482.

Wentworth, P. (1968) Circumvallate and circummarginate placentas. *American Journal of Obstetrics and Gynecology*, **102**, 44–47.

Wilkins, B.S., Batcup, G. and Vinall, P.S. (1991) Partial placenata membranacea. *British Journal of Obstetrics and Gynaecology*, **98**, 675–679.

Williams, J.W. (1927) Placenta circumvallata. *American Journal of Obstetrics and Gynecology*, **13**, 1–16.

Wilson, D. and Paalman, R.J. (1967) Clinical significance of circumvallate placenta. *Obstetrics and Gynecology*, **29**, 774–778.

Wladimiroff, J.W., Wallenburg, H.C.S., Putten, P.V.D. and Drogendijk, A.C. (1976) Ultrasonic diagnosis of placenta membranacea. *Archiv für Gynäkologie*, **221**, 167–174.

Wood, C., and Rogers, P. (1993) A pregnancy after planned partial endometrial resection. *Australian and New Zealand Journal of Obstetrics and Gynaecology*, **33**, 316–318.

Woolcott, R., Nichol, M. and Gibson, J.A. (1987) A case of placenta percreta presenting in the first trimester of pregnancy. *Australian and New Zealand Journal of Obstetrics and Gynaecology*, **27**, 258–260.

Zelop, C., Nadel, A., Frigoletto, F.D. Jr, Pauker, S., MacMillan, M. and Benacerraf, B.R. (1992) Placenta accreta/increta/percreta: a cause of elevated maternal serum alpha-fetoprotein. *Obstetrics and Gynecology*, **80**, 693–694.

Zhou, Y., Chiu, K., Brescia, R.J. et al (1993) Increased depth of trophoblast invasion after chronic constriction of the lower aorta in rhesus monkeys. *American Journal of Obstetrics and Gynecology*, **169**, 224–229.

Ziel, H.A. (1963) Circumvallate placenta, a cause of antepartum bleeding, premature delivery and perinatal mortality. *Obstetrics and Gynecology*, **22**, 798–802.

4

THE PLACENTA IN
MULTIPLE PREGNANCY

The phenomenon of multiple pregnancy has attracted the attention not only of obstetricians, anthropologists, geneticists and reproductive physiologists but also of mystics, moralists, soothsayers and collectors of *curiosa* and *exotica*. It is therefore perhaps not surprising that, until relatively recently, the placentation of multiple pregnancies was a subject shrouded in disagreement, dispute and acrimony. Now, however, the dust of these old arguments has settled, the more bizarre and fanciful of the early concepts have been discarded and the anatomical features of the placenta in multiple pregnancy are reasonably well established. In this chapter only a brief and simplified outline of this topic will be given; those seeking more detailed information are referred to the excellent monograph on twin placentation by Strong and Corney (1967) and to the writings of Benirschke and his colleagues (Benirschke, 1961a,b 1972a,b; Benirschke & Kim, 1973a,b; Benirschke & Kaufmann, 1995). The entire subject of the pathology of multiple pregnancy is covered in detail in an outstanding monograph by Baldwin (1994).

TWIN PLACENTATION

Incidence of Twinning

The incidence of twin conception is very much higher than the incidence of twin births because ultrasound studies have suggested that about 12% of all conceptions are twins, as many as 70% of these being converted to singleton pregnancies by early asymptomatic loss of one of the conceptuses, the so-called vanishing twin syndrome (Robinson & Caines, 1977; Varma, 1979; Brown, 1982; Landy et al, 1982, 1986; Boklage, 1990; Landy & Nies, 1995).

Amongst white Caucasians the incidence of twinning is usually said to be in the region of one in 80 births (Strong & Corney, 1967; Benirschke & Kim, 1973a); in both Europe and the USA this rate appeared to be decreasing during the first half of the 20th century (Elwood, 1973) but is now, for reasons that are far from fully clear, once again on the increase (Bryan, 1994; Derom et al, 1995; Jewell & Yip; 1995; Taffel, 1995). The rate of twinning is higher amongst individuals of African origin, being approximately one in 70 amongst black Americans and reaching an apogee in Nigeria where, amongst the Yoruba, the incidence is one in 20 births (Nylander, 1969, 1973). By contrast, the twinning rate is low in Orientals (Baldwin, 1994), though the incidence in India and Pakistan is similar to that in Europe (Bulmer, 1970; Nylander, 1975b).

Types of Twins

Twins may be either monozygotic or dizygotic. The former are produced from a single fertilized ovum which replicates during the very early stages of development, whilst the latter are due to the independent release, and subsequent fertilization, of two separate ova. Monozygotic twins are of the same sex and are genetically identical, but dizygotic twins are no more genetically similar than any other pair of siblings and may or may not be of the same sex; it is even possible, if coitus occurs with two men in a short period of time, for apparently dizygotic twins to have separate fathers (Gedda, 1961; Hafez, 1974; Terasaki et al, 1978; Majsky & Kout, 1982; Wenk et al, 1992), though superfecundation, as this phenomenon is known, is very rare. It has been suggested that superfetation, in which a second fertilized ovum is implanted in a uterus containing a month-old pregnancy, can occur (Scrimgeour & Baker, 1974; Walter et al, 1975), but there is no conclusive proof that this actually happens (Corney & Robson, 1975; Baldwin, 1994).

The possibility of a third type of twinning in which a single ovum is fertilized by two separate spermatozoa (monovular dispermic twinning) has long been entertained (Bulmer, 1970): the resulting twins would be neither dizygotic nor monozygotic but a combination of the two. There is now evidence, derived from DNA analysis, that twinning of this type does occur, probably as a result of fertilization of a polar body as well as an oocyte from the same ovum (Baldwin, 1994), though the frequency of such twinning is unknown.

Amongst white Caucasians about a third of twins are monozygotic (Potter, 1963; Cameron, 1968; Fujikura & Froehlich, 1971; Corney et al, 1972; Cameron et al, 1983), but where the twinning rate is very high, as amongst the Yoruba of Nigeria, monozygotic twins constitute only about 8% of the total (Nylander, 1971a, 1973); conversely, where the twinning rate is low, as in the Far East, monozygotic twins tend to predominate (Chun, 1970; Dawood et al, 1975). These findings are in accord with the view that the incidence of monozygotic twinning is roughly uniform in all parts of the world, the very marked national and ethnic variations in twinning rate being due entirely to differences in the incidence of dizygotic twins (Bulmer, 1970).

The cause of twinning is uncertain, but there is a strong hereditary element, predominantly but not entirely confined to the maternal side, in dizygotic twinning, and there is a good deal of circumstantial evidence to suggest that this form of twinning may be related to a high follicle-stimulating hormone (FSH) level with resulting polyovulation (Benirschke & Kim, 1973a; Nylander, 1975a; Bomsel-Helmreich & Al Mufti, 1995). There is no evidence that hereditary factors play any role in monozygotic twinning. It has been suggested that such twinning is a form of abnormal development similar in aetiology to congenital malformation, particularly in regard to its being a response to deleterious environmental agents (Benirschke & Kim, 1973a,b; Nylander, 1975a).

Dizygotic Twin Placentation

If the two ova of dizygotic twins are implanted at some distance from each other, there will be two separate and discrete placentas, each having its own amniotic sac; the placentation is therefore clearly of the dichorionic–diamniotic type. If the two ova implant in close proximity to each other there will be two amniotic sacs but the two placentas may show varying degrees of fusion to form what appears to be a single chorionic mass (Fig. 4.1). More detailed examination reveals, however, that this is formed by two placentas and hence the form of placentation is still dichorionic and diamniotic. The theoretical possibility exists that the two placentas of dizygotic twins may show true complete fusion to form a monochorionic placenta, but nearly all the claimed examples of twins of opposite sex having a monochorionic form of placentation have been based more upon anecdotal maternal reminiscences than on any scientific evidence (Strong & Corney, 1967). The only exceptions to this rule have been the reports of Nylander and Osunkoya (1970) and Perlman et al (1990) who each described a quite convincing

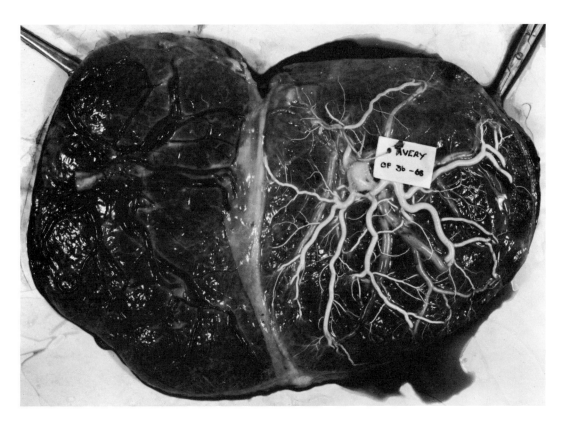

Figure 4.1. A fused dichorionic placenta. The amnion has been stripped from the fetal surface but a ridge of chorionic tissue remains at the site of the base of the septum between the two amniotic cavities. The vessels of the placenta on the right have been injected with barium solution and those of the placenta on the left with Indian ink; there is no evidence of any communication between the two vascular systems.

example of twins of opposite sex with a monochorionic placenta; however, it is quite possible that these were examples of dispermic monovular twinning rather than true dizygotic twins. It nevertheless remains true that, for all practical purposes, the finding of a monochorionic placenta excludes any possibility of the twins being dizygotic, a view occasionally disputed (Mortimer, 1987), but confirmed by genetic studies (Husby et al, 1991).

Monozygotic Twin Placentation

The form of placentation of monozygotic twins depends on the stage at which duplication occurs (Fig. 4.2). It is believed (Corner, 1955) that if the single fertilized ovum separates into two during the first 3 days after fertilization, i.e. before the differentiation of the trophoblast, two separate embryos will develop, each having its own placenta and amniotic sac, and the subsequent placentation of these will be identical to that seen in dizygotic twins. Thus if the two embryos implant at some distance from each other, there will be two separate placentas and amniotic sacs, and placentation will obviously be of the dichorionic–diamniotic variety. If the two developing embryos implant in close proximity to each other, there may be fusion of the two placentas but two amniotic sacs; as with dizygotic twins, the fusion is not absolute and placentation is still of the dichorionic–diamniotic type.

If splitting occurs during the blastocyst stage, i.e. between the third and eigth days after fertilization, when the trophoblast, but not the amniotic cavity, has differentiated,

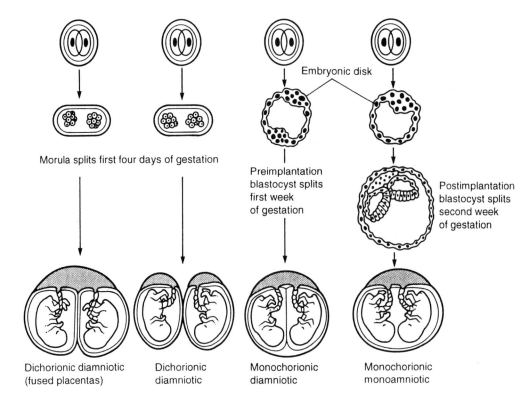

Morula splits first four days of gestation

Preimplantation blastocyst splits first week of gestation

Postimplantation blastocyst splits second week of gestation

Embryonic disk

Dichorionic diamniotic (fused placentas)

Dichorionic diamniotic

Monochorionic diamniotic

Monochorionic monoamniotic

Figure 4.2. Diagrammatic representation of the development and placentation of monozygotic twins.

the twins will develop a single placenta (Fig. 4.3) with two amniotic sacs. The placentation is then categorized as monochorionic–diamniotic.

The amniotic cavity differentiates between the 8th and 13th days after fertilization and it is thought that if splitting occurs during this period there will be only one placenta and one amniotic sac, the placentation being of the monochorionic–monoamniotic form. Not all workers are persuaded that monoamniotic placentation is produced in this fashion; some claim that in all, or most, of such cases there were originally two amniotic cavities which were converted into one by the breaking down and disappearance of the dividing membranes between the two cavities. There is good evidence that, on occasion, there may be a spontaneous or traumatic disruption of the dividing septum, the remnants of which appear as a plica on the surface of the monochorionic placenta (Foglmann, 1974; Megory et al, 1991). Benirschke and Kaufmann (1995) suggest, however, that a plica of this type is due, not to the almost total disintegration of a previously present septum, but to the splitting of the blastomere at the very moment when the amnion was forming but was as yet incomplete. This is a rather recondite dispute to which no firm answer is as yet available, and which is of theoretical rather than practical importance.

If splitting occurs at or after the 13th day of development this will result in conjoined twins, the earliest and simplest stage of which is monoamniotic twins whose umbilical cords fuse before inserting into the placenta (Larson et al, 1969).

Incidence of Various Forms of Placentation and Relationship to Zygosity

The various studies on this topic from Britain and the USA (Potter, 1963; Strong & Corney, 1967; Cameron, 1968; Fujikura & Froehlich, 1971; Corney et al, 1972) and from Nigeria (Nylander & Corney, 1969; Nylander, 1970a,b, 1971a) have been collated by Corney (1975).

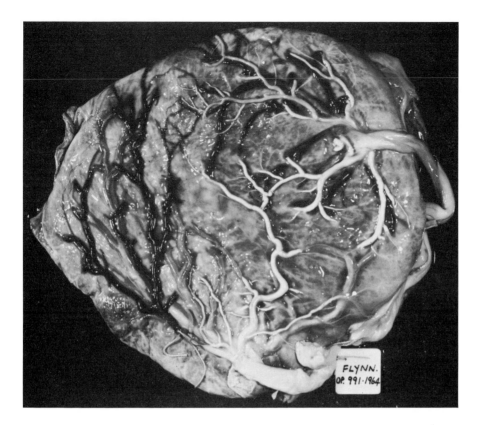

Figure 4.3. A monochorionic twin placenta. The amnion has been stripped off from the fetal aspect to leave a smooth continuous surface. The arteries of cord 1 (no label) have been injected with barium solution and this shows a direct communication with an artery from cord 2. A major artery of cord 2 has been injected with Indian ink and this substance is seen to have passed to the veins of placenta 1, indicating the presence of a deep vascular communication.

For all practical purposes all twins having a monochorionic placenta are monozygotic; twins with dichorionic placentation may, however, be either monozygotic or dizygotic. Hence the proportion of twins with dichorionic placentation will be higher than the proportion of monozygotic twins. In white Caucasian populations about 80% of twins have a dichorionic form of placentation; in Nigeria, where the proportion of monozygotic twins is low, 95% of twin placentas are dichorionic. The proportions of dichorionic placentas that are separate or fused are very roughly equal; between 10 and 15% of dichorionic placentas will be from monozygotic twins, there being in most, but not all, studies a greater tendency for monozygotic dichorionic placentas to be fused rather than separate.

Looking at the situation in the reverse fashion, the proportion of monozygotic twins having a dichorionic form of placentation is between 20 and 40%.

Vascular Anastomoses in Twin Placentas

Monochorionic Placentas

It was well established in the 19th century that vascular communications between the two territories of monozygotic twins are often found in monochorionic placentas (Hyrtle, 1870; Schatz, 1900); indeed, so complete were these early descriptions that relatively little new information on this topic has since emerged. It is agreed that such anastomoses are present in nearly all monochorionic placentas, their reported

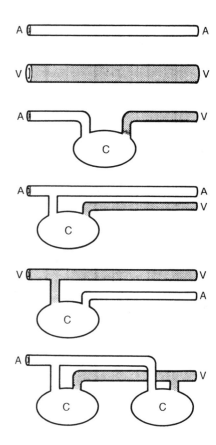

Figure 4.4. Diagrammatic representation of the various forms of vascular communication that can occur in monochorionic twin placentas. A, artery; V, vein; C, shared lobule with capillary anastomoses.

incidence varying from 76 to 100% (Benirschke, 1961a; Bleisch, 1965; Strong & Corney, 1967; Cameron, 1968; Arts & Lohman, 1971; Galea et al, 1982, Robertson & Neer, 1983; Ramos-Arroyo et al, 1988), and that these communications may be either superficial or deep. The superficial anastomoses are between relatively large vessels on the fetal surface of the placenta (Fig. 4.3) and the vast majority are direct arterio-arterial communications between a chorionic artery of one fetus and a chorionic artery of the other; a minority are of the veno-venous type, and in a few placentas both varieties of superficial communication may be present. Of perhaps greater pathological significance are arterio-venous anastomoses between the two circulatory systems; these are deep, i.e. within the placental substance, and form what Schatz (1900) referred to as the 'third circulation' (the other two being those of the two fetuses). These arterio-venous anastomoses occur in shared lobules (Fig. 4.4), which are supplied by an artery from one twin and drain into a vein from the other twin; the anastomosis is via the capillary system of the villi and there are no direct pre-capillary arterio-venous communications. Such shared lobules are often multiple and are situated along the equator separating the individual territories of the two twins. In some placentas in which there are multiple shared lobules, the arterio-venous communications may be all in the same direction, but in others some of the shared lobules may be supplied by an artery from the first twin and drain into a vein of the second twin, whilst others may be supplied by an artery from the second twin and drain into a vein from the first twin.

In many, probably most, monochorionic twin placentas both deep and superficial anastomoses are present; indeed, the arterial supply to a shared lobule is not uncommonly from a branch which arises from a superficial arterio-arterial communication (Arts & Lohman, 1971). Occasionally, venous drainage from a shared lobule is into a superficial veno-venous anastomosis.

Dichorionic Placentas

Vascular communications between dichorionic placentas that are totally separate from each other have never been described (Fig. 4.1): one placenta that macroscopically appeared to be dichorionic with superficial vascular anastomoses between the two placental masses was actually considered to be a bilobate monochorionic placenta (Kim & Lage, 1991) and a similar bilobate monochorionic placenta has been described by Altshuler and Hyde (1993). There is, however, some dispute as to whether anastomoses between the two circulatory systems ever occur in fused dichorionic placentas. Occasional claims in the earlier literature to have demonstrated such communications (Scipiades & Burg, 1930; Szendi, 1938; Perez et al, 1947; Gedda, 1961) were regarded with some scepticism by Strong and Corney (1967), who did not find any anastomoses in dichorionic placentas, an experience they shared with Benirschke (1961a), Bleisch (1964), and Arts and Lohman (1971). However, Cameron (1968) was able to prove the presence of vascular communications in two of the 500 dichorionic placentas that he studied; in each case the twins appeared to be monozygotic, and both arterio-arterial and veno-venous anastomoses were present on the placental surface. Bhargava and Chakravarty (1975) have reported finding vascular communications in seven out of 143 dichorionic placentas; even more surprisingly they claimed that in six of these the anastomoses were of the deep arterio-venous type. It is difficult to evaluate this report, because a corrosion technique, which is probably less reliable than an injection method, was used and all the illustrations of vascular communications were of such structures in monochorial placentas. Robertson and Neer (1983) described anastomoses in one of 68 fused dichorionic placentas whilst Lage et al (1989) also reported an example of both deep and superficial anastomoses across fused dichorionic placentas. A fully convincing report of proven anastomoses with substantial functional interfetal transfusion between dichorionic placentas with fusion only of the membranes has been reported by King et al (1995). There is, therefore, evidence that anastomoses between the two circulatory systems may sometimes occur in fused dichorionic placentas, a conclusion bolstered by the occasional finding of blood group chimerism in dizygotic twins of opposite sex, a finding that suggests, albeit indirectly, some degree of vascular mixing during fetal life.

Associated Pathological Features of Twin Placentas

Strong and Corney (1967) noted a very high incidence of single umbilical artery in twins; however, as discussed in Chapter 15, this has not been everyone's experience and several workers have specifically denied that any association exists between the two conditions. Velamentous insertion of the cord appears to be unduly common in twin placentas (Robinson et al, 1983; Bardawil et al, 1988; Ramos-Arroyo et al, 1988; Fries et al, 1993; Baldwin, 1994; Benirschke & Kaufmann, 1995); this high incidence has been attributed, very unconvincingly in my view, to intrauterine crowding and a secondary distortion of placental growth.

Several twin pregnancies have been reported in which one of the twins was a normal fetus and the other a complete hydatidiform mole (Sauerbrei et al, 1980; Block & Merrill, 1982; Fisher et al, 1982; Ohama et al, 1985; Khoo et al, 1986; Vejerslev et al, 1986; Monnier et al, 1987; Berrebi et al, 1988; Feinberg et al, 1988; Jauniaux et al, 1990; Adachi et al, 1992; Altaras et al, 1992; Garcia-Aguayo & Menargues Irles, 1992; van de Geijn et al, 1992; Baldwin, 1993; Miller et al, 1993; Changchien et al, 1994; Steller et al, 1994a,b; Osada et al, 1995; van de Kaa et al, 1995). In some of these cases, one of a pair of fused dichorionic twin placentas was converted into a complete hydatidiform mole whilst in others one of two separated dichorionic placentas was molar. Complete molar change in one of a fused pair of dichorionic twin placentas should not be, but has been, confused with and described as a partial hydatidiform mole: a true example of a twin gestation in which one fetus and placenta were normal whilst the other was a triploid fetus with a partial hydatidiform mole has been reported (Steller et al, 1994b). A remarkable, indeed bizarre, twin pregnancy in which one conceptus was a complete mole and the other a partial mole (with a fetus) has also been described (Ozumba & Ofodile, 1994).

Specific Features of the Various Forms of Twin Placentation

Monochorionic–Diamniotic Twin Placentation

Twins with this form of placentation have a much higher perinatal mortality than do those with dichorionic placentas; the perinatal mortality rate has, however, varied considerably in different series, ranging from just over 7% (Gruenwald, 1970) to 22–25% (Benirschke & Driscoll, 1967; Myrianthopoulos, 1970). Perhaps the most important factor contributing to this high death rate is premature onset of labour, an event often attributed to polyhydramnios. There must be some doubt, however, as to whether polyhydramnios is particularly prone to complicate monochorionic placentation in the absence of the twin-transfusion syndrome, because Nylander and MacGillivray (1975), although not noting the form of placentation, found that excessive accumulation of liquor occurred with equal frequency in monozygotic and dizygotic twin pregnancies. Nevertheless, polyhydramnios does develop unduly often as an accompaniment, or complication, of the 'twin–twin transfusion syndrome', which is an important cause of perinatal mortality in monochorionic twins.

The twin–twin transfusion (or 'feto-fetal transfusion') syndrome was defined and largely elucidated by Schatz (1900) and has been reviewed by, amongst others, Conway (1964), Corney and Aherne (1965), Rausen et al (1965), Anger and Ring (1972), Hollander and Backmann (1974), Sekiya and Hafez (1977), Tan et al (1979), Galea et al (1982), Brown et al (1989), Blickstein (1990), Giles et al (1990), Urig et al (1990), Bruner and Rosemond (1993), and Machin and Still (1995). The frequency with which this complicates monochorionic–diamniotic placentation has been estimated at about 15% (Rausen et al, 1965; Arts & Lohman, 1971), though Strong and Corney (1967) consider that its true incidence is probably over 30%. The inter-twin transfusion may be acute or chronic. In an acute twin-to-twin transfusion, which is uncommon and usually occurs during birth, the fetuses are of roughly equal size but the donor twin is pale and the recipient twin plethoric. The haemoglobin levels and red cell counts of the twins are normal at birth but within a few hours anaemia becomes apparent in the donor and polycythaemia in the recipient. A chronic twin-to-twin transfusion, by contrast, occurs as a result of a long-standing haemodynamic imbalance and a slow net transfusion from one fetus to the other. The classically described clinical features of the chronic transfusion syndrome are an excessive amount of fluid in the amniotic sac of the recipient twin and a paucity of fluid in that of the donor (the 'oligohydramnios–polyhydramnios sequence') with one twin (the donor) being pale and anaemic whilst the other (the recipient) is plethoric and polycythaemic (Fig. 4.5). There is a substantial difference in haemoglobin levels between the two twins, and increased numbers of normoblasts are seen in the peripheral blood of the anaemic infant. The anaemic twin is smaller and lighter than the plethoric one and there may be a marked difference in organ weights between the two; cardiomegaly is often present in the polycythaemic infant (Naeye, 1965). The placenta also shows marked changes (Fig. 4.6), the maternal surface of the placental territory of the anaemic, or donor, twin being pale and bulky and thus contrasting markedly with the placental substance of the plethoric, or recipient, twin. Histological examination shows that the villi in the placenta of the recipient twin have large, engorged fetal vessels but are otherwise normal, whilst those of the donor twin's placenta are oedematous and bulky with small inconspicuous vessels (Aherne et al, 1968). More recent fetal studies have, however, pointed out that haemoglobin and birth weight discrepancies are by no means common in the twin–twin transfusion syndrome and that polyhydramnios,

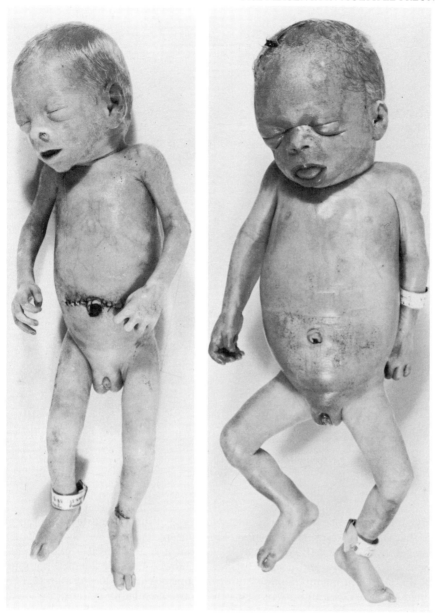

Figure 4.5. Twin–twin transfusion syndrome. The infant on the left is the donor twin and that on the right is the recipient. The placenta was monochorionic and deep vascular communications were demonstrated.

oedema and cardiac hypertrophy in the recipient twin and oligohydramnios in the donor twin are the defining, and cardinal, clinical features of the syndrome (Bajoria et al, 1995). Furthermore, there may be little difference, either grossly or histologically, between donor and recipient placentas in prenatally diagnosed cases (Wigglesworth, 1995).

Schatz (1900) proposed that the twin–twin transfusion syndrome was due to 'a dynamic asymmetry of the third circulation', i.e. that there was a shunt of arterial blood from the donor twin through arterio-venous anastomoses in shared lobules into the venous circulation of the recipient twin. This state of affairs can be compensated for if superficial large-vessel anastomoses are present to correct a unidirectional

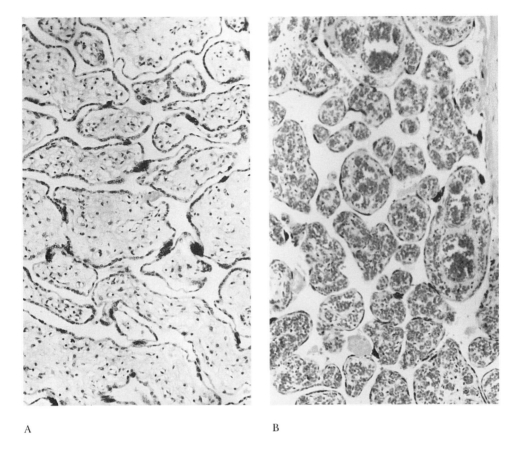

A   B

Figure 4.6. Twin–twin transfusion syndrome. The villi of the donor's placenta (A) are large and have small inconspicuous vessels whilst those of the recipient's placenta (B) have large engorged vessels.

haemodynamic imbalance in the deep anastomoses or if there are arterio-venous anastomoses that run in the reverse direction. This concept has been widely accepted, and indeed recently confirmed (Bajoria et al, 1995), but it is doubtful if it explains all the features of the syndrome, and it must further be allowed that the detailed pathophysiology of the proposed haemodynamic shunt remains obscure. Kloosterman (1963) has maintained that the communications between the two circulatory systems are too small to allow for the transfer of any appreciable amount of blood and has suggested that many of the features of the syndrome are due to hyperproteinaemia in the heavier twin. It is true that IgG levels are usually higher in the recipient than in the donor twin (Bryan & Slavin, 1974; Bryan et al, 1976), but it is not clear how this difference arises or how it could be responsible for the observed clinical and pathological features. It is nevertheless the case that the oligohydramnios–polyhydramnios sequence can occur in the absence of intertwin transfusion (Bruner & Rosemond, 1993) and that, conversely, substantial intertwin transfusion can occur without any evidence of the twin-to-twin transfusion syndrome (King et al, 1995).

A twin-transfusion syndrome, albeit of an unusual type, appears also to be responsible for the development of acardiac monsters; certainly, this malformation only occurs in monozygotic multiple pregnancies with monochorionic placentation (Moore et al, 1990; Kunz & Arnaboldi, 1991; Pinet et al, 1994). Acardiac monsters occur in about 1% of monozygotic twin gestations (Gillim & Hendricks, 1953; Napolitani & Schreiber, 1960; Amatuzio & Gorlin, 1981) and vary considerably in gross appearance and in their degree of organogenesis, ranging from a large but grossly deformed fetus to an amorphous mass (Fig. 4.7). This latter feature has been

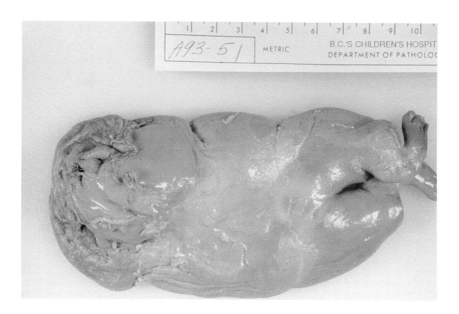

Figure 4.7. A fetus acardius (chorangiopagus parasiticus twin).

the basis of many complicated classifications (Lachman et al, 1980; Sato et al, 1984) which Baldwin (1994) has described as more confusing than helpful and are, as Benirschke and Kim (1973a) have commented, all virtually meaningless in view of their common pathogenesis. In the past the aetiology of acardia was uncertain with two contrasting theories holding sway, one maintaining that the defect was a primary one, the fetus never having had a heart, and the other proposing that the fetus did have a heart, which became atrophied as a result of an imbalance in the placental vascular communications (Keith et al, 1967; Wilson, 1972; Alderman, 1973; Severn & Holyoke, 1973). Currently it is believed that a placental vascular malfunction lies at the root of this anomaly, the abnormal twin having no placental parenchymal circulation of its own but having an arterial system that anastomoses with branches of the umbilical artery of the normal twin and a venous drainage into the umbilical veins of the normal twin. The fetal circulation is thus the reverse of normal, the abnormal twin receiving unoxygenated blood that has already perfused the normal twin, a situation known as 'twin reversed arterial perfusion' (van Allen, 1981; van Allen et al, 1983; Stephens, 1984; Shalev et al, 1992) and which leads to altered cardiovascular development with secondary abnormalities in the other tissues. Acardiac monsters can therefore be regarded as a form of conjoined twin in which the conjunction is of the chorionic circulation (Baldwin, 1994), hence the resurrection of the term 'chorangiopagus parasiticus twin' to describe this anomaly. It should be noted, in passing, that the normal, or 'pump', twin has also to circulate its blood through the abnormal twin and that this may lead to cardiomegaly and high output cardiac failure.

A further consequence of the vascular anastomoses in monochorionic placentas is that the death of one fetus may be associated with, and possibly cause, abnormalities in the surviving co-twin. Death of one twin in the third trimester of pregnancy may be associated with visceral, and especially cerebral, lesions in the survivor (Benirschke, 1961b; Yoshioka et al, 1979; Enbom, 1985; Szymoncwicz et al, 1986; Yoshida & Soma, 1986; Bulla et al, 1987; Anderson et al, 1990; Fusi et al, 1991). These have been attributed to the release of thromboplastic material from the dead fetus which passes into the circulation of the living twin and there triggers off disseminated intravascular coagulation (Moore et al, 1969; Enbom, 1985; Yoshida & Soma, 1986). An alternative, and currently more widely held, view is that the damage to the surviving twin is due to

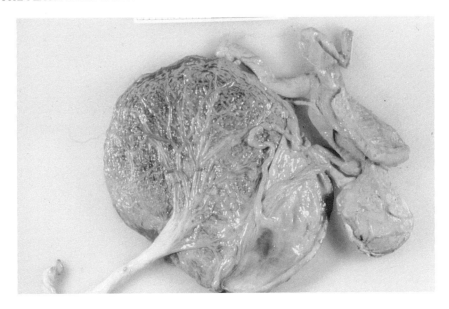

Figure 4.8. A fetus papyraceous.

hypovolaemic shock as a consequence of the dead fetus acting as a 'vascular sink', the live fetus effectively haemorrhaging into its co-twin's resistance-free blood vessels (Liu et al, 1992; Benirschke, 1993; Baldwin, 1994). This latter explanation is unlikely to be the case when fetal death at an earlier stage of gestation, with conversion of the fetus into a flattened, 'mummified' fetus papyraceous (Fig. 4.8), is associated with anatomical defects, such as intestinal atresia, in the surviving co-twin. Under these circumstances transfer of thromboplastic material or emboli through vascular anatomoses appears the more plausible mechanism (Jauniaux et al, 1988a; Wagner et al, 1990).

Monochorionic–Monoamniotic Twin Placentas

This is the least common form of twin pregnancy but despite, or perhaps because of, its relative rarity it has been the subject of a considerable number of studies, outstanding amongst which have been those of Quigley (1935), Raphael (1961), Timmons and de Alvarez (1963), Wharton et al (1968), and Pauls (1969): more recent, but less comprehensive, reviews include those of Hollingsworth (1973), Israelstam (1973), Tagawa (1974), Lumme and Saarikoski (1986), Sutter et al, (1986), Rodis et al (1987), Dorum and Nesheim (1991), Tessen and Zlatnik (1991), Olsen (1992) and Drack et al (1993).

The incidence of monoamniotic twins is a matter of some dispute, their reported frequency in multiple pregnancies having ranged from one in 65 (Librach & Terrin, 1957) to one in 666 (Acosta-Sison et al, 1946). Wenner (1956) claimed, however, that four of the 100 twins in his series had a monoamniotic placentation, and, although this figure has often been considered as grossly atypical, it has not markedly conflicted with those noted in careful prospective studies, which have shown an incidence of between 1 and 3% (Strong & Corney, 1967). Particularly striking in this respect was the finding of 18 monoamniotic twins in a series of 581 twin pregnancies investigated in Birmingham by Wharton et al (1968).

Monoamniotic placentation is associated with a high fetal mortality. Quigley (1935) found that nearly 70% of fetuses died, but more recent figures are somewhat more reassuring and suggest that between 50 and 70% of monoamniotic twins now survive (Raphael, 1961; Wensinger & Daly, 1962; Wharton et al, 1968; Baldwin, 1994;

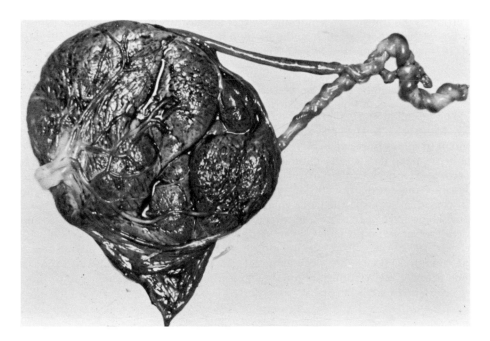

Figure 4.9. A twin placenta (presumed to have been monoamniotic) with entanglement and knotting of the two umbilical cords.

Benirschke & Kaufmann, 1995). The reasons for what is still an alarmingly high fetal death rate are not fully clear, but there is no doubt that an important contributory factor is the tendency for the two umbilical cords to become twisted and entangled with each other (Fig 4.9), with the formation of true knots, these latter being found in about 40–70% of cases (Salerno, 1959; Zuckerman & Brzezinski, 1960; Krussel et al, 1994): although cord entanglement is a potent cause of fetal death in monoamniotic pregnancies a few twins do survive this complication (Annan & Hutson, 1990). A rare event, but one that can cause considerable obstetrical embarrassment, is for the neck of the first delivered twin to be tightly encircled by the cord of the other twin; division of the cord may then lead to exsanguination of the undelivered twin (Hagood & Stokes, 1953; Goplerud, 1964; Tagawa, 1974; Ong et al, 1976; McLeod & McCoy, 1981). There is also an increased risk of obstructed labour because of interlocking of the twins.

Perhaps rather unexpectedly the transfusion syndrome is not a significant cause of fetal mortality or morbidity in monoamniotic twins and, indeed, there is some doubt as to the frequency with which placental vascular anastomoses between the two twins occur in this form of placentation. At first sight it would appear logical to expect that such anastomoses occur with at least the same frequency as in monochorionic–diamniotic placentas, but Wenner (1956) maintained that conjoined twins (which are always monoamniotic) may not have placental vascular communications, whilst Benirschke (1965) has suggested that such anastomoses occur less commonly in monoamniotic than in diamniotic placentas. This view appears to be supported by the fact that both Benirschke and Driscoll (1967) and Strong and Corney (1967) have each studied monoamniotic placentas in which no vascular anastomoses were present. On the other hand, Wharton et al (1968) found such anastomoses in 16 of their 18 monoamniotic placentas, whilst Bhargava et al (1971) demonstrated communications in all six monoamniotic placentas in their study. Currently, therefore, it appears probable that there is a high incidence of vascular communications in monoamniotic placentas, but that these are absent in a minority, which is, as yet, of ill-defined proportions.

Nevertheless the transfusion syndrome is exceptionally rare in monoamniotic twins, the only acceptable reports of such a complication being those of Hollander (1969), Meyer et al (1970) and Lumme and Saarikoski (1986).

Dichorionic–Diamniotic Twin Placentation

The perinatal mortality rate of dichorionic twins is in the region of 7–10% (Potter, 1963; Benirschke & Driscoll, 1967; Myrianthopoulos, 1970), but, in contrast to the situation in monochorionic twins, placental factors are rarely, if ever, of importance in fetal or neonatal death. The pathology of separate dichorionic placentas can be considered as identical to that of placentas from singleton pregnancies, but in fused dichorionic placentas a transfusion syndrome may occur in exceptional cases, because, as discussed previously, such placentas may very occasionally have vascular anastomoses. There have been several reports of dichorionic twins in which there was clinical evidence to suggest a possible twin-transfusion syndrome (Walker and Turnbull, 1955; Michaels, 1967; Allen, 1972). In none of these cases, however, was it proved that vascular communications were present in the placentas or that a twin-transfusion syndrome actually was responsible for the clinical features, all of which could, indeed, have been due to other factors.

Pathological Examination of the Twin Placenta

It is intended to discuss here only those aspects of placental examination that are specifically concerned with twin placentation. It is worth noting, however, that particular attention should be paid to the position of insertion of the cords and to the number of arteries in each cord; in this respect the pathologist should insist that the cords are correctly and separately labelled in the delivery room, it being made quite clear which cord is from the first and which from the second delivered twin.

From the discussion in the earlier part of this chapter it will be apparent that the pathologist is required to examine a twin placenta for one, or both, of the following two specific reasons:

1. To establish the form of placentation and hence, in some cases, the zygosity of the twins.
2. To determine whether placental vascular anastomoses are present between the two fetal circulatory systems.

Identification of Type of Placentation and Zygosity

If the two placentas are quite separate from each other they are clearly dichorionic, and if the infants are of opposite sex they are dizygotic; if the infants are of the same sex they may be either dizygotic or monozygotic, and placental examination will be of no help in determining which. If the placenta is monoamniotic then it is also monochorionic and the twins are monozygotic. The principal task of the pathologist is, therefore, to distinguish between a monochorionic–diamniotic placenta and a fused dichorionic–diamniotic placenta. It is often suggested that the first step in this investigation is to try and separate the two placental masses from each other by gentle traction: no separation will occur in monochorionic placentas, but a proportion of fused dichorionic placentas can be cleaved from each other. It should be stressed that this is the crudest possible technique of examining twin placentas; it gives no information if separation is not obtained, may make eventual identification of the nature of the septum between the two amniotic sacs more difficult, and can obviate subsequent attempts to inject the placental vasculature. One should, and indeed does, decry this form of examination, but in this imperfect world it is probable that most pathologists who require a rapid and easy answer, and who do not intend to inject the placental vessels, will find it difficult to resist giving at least a gentle tug to the chorionic mass.

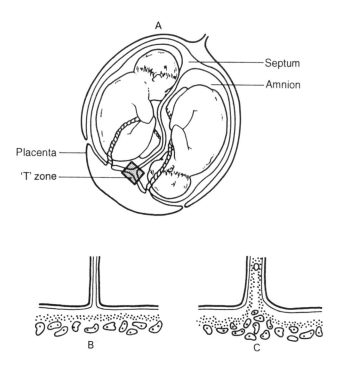

Figure 4.10. (A) Diagrammatic representation of the site of the 'T'zone in diamniotic twin placentas. (B) Diagrammatic representation of the histology of the 'T'zone in a monochorionic–diamniotic twin placenta; the septum consists solely of two layers of amnion. (C) Diagrammatic representation of the histology of the 'T'zone in a dichorionic–diamniotic twin placenta. Chorionic tissue is present in the septum between the two layers of amnion.

The real crux of the differentiation between monochorionic and fused dichorionic placentas is the presence in the latter, but not in the former, of chorionic tissue in the septum between the two amniotic cavities, and attention should first be directed to the septum itself. If the placenta is monochorionic the septum will be translucent, but in dichorionic placentas the presence of chorionic tissue makes the septum appear relatively opaque. A piece of septum should be taken for histological examination, and Benirschke and Driscoll's (1967) technique of taking a longitudinal strip of the septum which is then rolled and sectioned has much to recommend it. Next, the base of the septum should be examined; in dichorionic placentas an elevated ridge, which is at the base of the chorionic tissue in the septum, will invariably be present (Fig. 4.1), whilst in monochorionic placentas this ridge will be absent. Some workers recommend that a block for histological examination also be taken from the 'T'zone (Fig. 4.10), i.e. from the point at which the septum joins the surface of the placenta (Allen & Turner, 1971). The amnion should then be stripped off from the fetal surface of the placenta; in monochorionic placentas the amnion peels off easily, leaving a smooth continuous surface (Fig. 4.3), but in dichorionic placentas there will be tearing of the placental substance at the base of the septum, at the site of the ridge.

Subsequent histological examination of the membrane roll from the septum should give a good indication of the type of placentation, because in monochorionic placentas it will consist solely of two layers of amnion (Fig. 4.11), whilst in dichorionic placentas the two layers of amnion will be separated by two layers of chorionic tissue (Fig. 4.12). In practice, unfortunately, a clear-cut answer will not always be obtained because by the time the placenta is received in the laboratory the septal membranes may be distorted and their relationships disturbed (Bleisch, 1964). Under such circumstances the histology of the 'T'zone' may be more rewarding, as this will show more clearly the extension of the chorion into the septum.

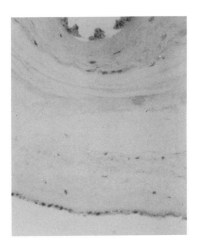

Figure 4.11. Histological appearances of the septum separating the two amniotic cavities of a monochorionic–diamniotic twin placenta: this consists solely of two layers of amnion (H & E ×150).

Demonstration of Vascular Anastomoses

Theoretically an attempt should be made to demonstrate the possible presence of vascular communications in all monochorionic or fused dichorionic placentas. In practice, most pathologists will simply content themselves with noting whether or not there are any superficial anastomoses between large vessels which are easily visible to the naked eye, and only those with a special interest in the topic will routinely proceed to injection studies. Nevertheless any pathologist who is prepared to examine twin placentas must also be prepared to study their vascular systems under certain specific circumstances. These are:

1. If, after gross and microscopic examination, the type of placentation still remains in doubt.
2. If there is any suspicion of the twin-transfusion syndrome.
3. If there is any abnormality in the surviving twin following death of one infant *in utero*.
4. In any case in which intrauterine or neonatal death of a twin has occurred for no obvious reason.

Large superficial anastomoses may be relatively easy to detect because they are often visible on the fetal surface of the placenta; however, the nature of such communications is not always obvious because in the placenta it may be quite difficult to distinguish between veins and arteries. Some workers inject air bubbles into the superficial vessels and show that they can be pushed from the vessels of one twin to those of the other; unfortunately the inherent vagaries of this technique, which are largely due to the surface tension properties of air bubbles, restrict considerably its value. Several

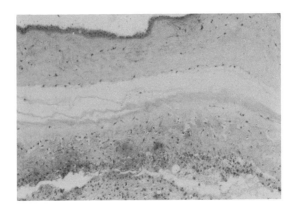

Figure 4.12. Histological appearances of the septum separating the two amniotic cavities of a dichorionic–diamniotic twin placenta. The two layers of amnion are separated from each other by chorionic tissue (H & E ×120).

other substances have been suggested for the demonstration of large superficial anastomoses, these including milk and red wine. The former has been used by some workers
(Coen & Sutherland, 1970) and can give a quite clear demonstration of the vascular
communications (50 ml being injected into a superficial vessel); one feels, however, that
a vintage burgundy can be put to better use than for the demonstration of placental
vascular anastomoses. Perhaps the simplest and best substance to use routinely is
coloured saline (Benirschke, 1961a).

The identification of the deep arterio-venous anastomoses is, of course, of more
importance in investigating a case of possible twin–twin transfusion syndrome, in
which superficial anastomoses are frequently absent. For this purpose two methods are
available: the first is to inject a radio-opaque dye and then trace the vascular communications by radiological study, and the other is to inject a coloured plastic substance and then prepare a corrosion specimen. It cannot be claimed that accurate
results are achieved by either technique without a considerable amount of experience,
and if one is content simply to show that communications exist, is not concerned with
their actual physical demonstration, and is satisfied by showing that fluid injected into
one twin's vascular territory will appear in that of the other twin, it is probable that
injection of coloured saline will suffice.

THE VANISHING TWIN SYNDROME

A pathologist may be required to examine a placenta from a singleton birth following a pregnancy in which there was, during its early stages, ultrasound evidence of a
twin gestation – the so-called 'vanishing twin phenomenon'. It should be noted that this
term is only applied to very early death of a twin and does not refer to the presence of
an obvious second fetus that takes the form of a fetus papyraceus, death in such cases
probably having occurred during the early second trimester.

A twin may indeed vanish completely leaving no morphological residue though
genetic evidence of an absorbed twin is occasionally detectable in the form of a restricted placental chimerism, i.e the presence of both 46,XX and 46,XY cell lines in a
singleton placenta (Callen et al, 1991; Reddy et al, 1991; Falik-Borenstein et al, 1994);
this differs from a restricted placental mosaicism for which there is no conceptual
necessity to invoke the prior presence of a second fetus.

Morphological remnants of a second gestation may, however, be found, albeit
often with some difficulty, in placentas from pregnancies complicated by a vanishing
twin. Sulak and Dodson (1986) noted a collapsed gestational sac within the membranes of a placenta from such a case, this appearing macroscopically as a plaque-like
thickening within the membranes. Jauniaux et al (1988b) examined 10 placentas from
pregnancies complicated by the vanishing twin phenomenon and found in one case
remnants of an embryonic vertebral column immediately adjacent to a peripheral
plaque of perivillous fibrin. They noted peripherally situated and well-delineated
plaques of perivillous fibrin deposition in four other cases and implied, but did not
clearly state, that they considered these plaques to be the remains of the placental
tissue of the vanished fetus. Others have detected fetal tissue remnants, degenerate
placental villi or empty gestational sacs either at the placental margin, within the membranes or on the fetal surface of the surviving twin's placenta in a high proportion of
placentas from pregnancies in which a twin had apparently vanished (Yoshida &
Soma, 1986; Huter et al, 1990; Rudnicki et al, 1991; Nerlich et al, 1992; Baldwin,
1994), these usually being visible, on careful examination, as small nodules or foci of
thickening (Yoshida, 1995).

TRIPLET PLACENTATION

In white Caucasians and in a Japanese population, triplets occur in about one in
10,000 deliveries, but in Ibadan, Nigeria, their frequency is one in 563 deliveries
(Nylander, 1971b, 1975b; Shanklin & Perrin, 1984; Imaizumi, 1990). Triplets may be

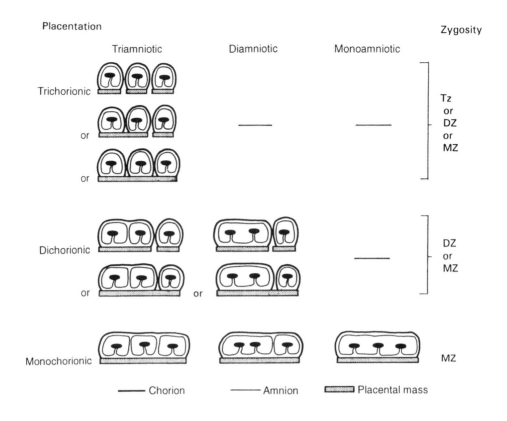

Figure 4.13. Diagrammatic representation of triplet placentation.

trizygotic, dizygotic or monozygotic. Trizygotic triplets are due to the fertilization of three ova, whilst dizygotic triplets are produced by the fertilization of two ova, one of which subsequently replicates; monozygotic triplets result from the fertilization of a single ovum which then undergoes replication, a further replication then occurs in one of the already replicated zygotes.

The placentation of triplets (Fig. 4.13) has been discussed by Boyd and Hamilton (1970), Nylander and Corney (1971), Corney (1975) and Baldwin (1994), and follows the same principles as those already described for dizygotic and monozygotic twin placentation. Thus trizygotic triplets have a trichorionic–triamniotic placentation, but there may be three separate placentas, two fused placentas and one separate placenta, or fusion of the three placentas to form a single mass. Dizygotic triplets may have a placentation identical to that of trizygotic triplets, or may be dichorionic; if dichorionic, the two placentas may be separate or fused and there may be two or three amniotic sacs. Monozygotic triplets may show any of the forms of placentation seen in dizygotic or trizygotic triplet placentation, or may be monochorionic, in which case they may be monoamniotic, diamniotic or triamniotic.

In practice, in white Caucasian populations, about 16% of triplets are monochorionic, 42% dichorionic and 42% trichorionic; in Nigeria, however, 72.5% of triplets are trichorionic and only 2.5% are monochorionic (Nylander & Corney, 1971).

HIGHER MULTIPLE BIRTHS

It would be merely repetitious to detail here the possible permutations of forms of placentation found in higher multiple births. Suffice it to say that the principles of monozygotic and dizygotic placentation apply to these with equal cogency, that quadruplet placentation is discussed in some detail by Boyd and Hamilton (1970) and Hafez

(1974), and that case reports of placentation in still higher multiple pregnancies include those of Hamblen et al (1937), Gibbs et al (1960), Neubecker et al (1962), Berbos et al (1964), Turksoy et al (1967), Cameron et al (1969), Lachelin et al (1972), Bender and Brandt (1974), Metler et al (1974), Garrett et al (1976), Giovannucci-Uzielli et al (1981), Serreyn et al (1984) and Egwuato et al (1992).

REFERENCES

Acosta-Sison, H., Aragon, G.T. and de la Paz, A. (1946) Monoamniotic twins: danger to the life of at least one twin (First case report in Philippines) *Journal of the Philippine Medical Association*, **22**, 43–46.

Adachi, N., Ihara, Y. and Ito, H. (1992) Two cases of twin pregnancy with complete hydatidiform mole. *Acta Obstetricia et Gynaecologica Japonica*, **44**, 1463–1466.

Aherne, W., Strong, S.J. and Corney, G. (1968) The structure of the placenta in the twin transfusion syndrome. *Biologia Neonatorum*, **12**, 121–135.

Alderman, B.A. (1973) Foetus acardius amorphus. *Postgraduate Medical Journal*, **49**, 102–105.

Allen, J.P. (1972) Twin transfusion syndrome. *Northwest Medicine*, **71**, 296–298.

Allen, M.S. and Turner, U.G. (1971) Twin birth – identical or fraternal twins? *Obstetrics and Gynecology*, **37**, 538–542.

Altaras, M.M., Rosen, D.J., Ben-Nun, I., Aviram, R., Bernheim, J. and Beyth, Y. (1992) Hydatidiform mole coexisting with a fetus in twin gestation following gonadotrophin induction of ovulation. *Human Reproduction*, **7**, 429–431.

Altshuler, G. and Hyde, S. (1993) Placental pathology casebook: a bidiscoid monochorionic placenta. *Journal of Perinatology*, **13**, 492–493.

Amatuzio, J.C. and Gorlin, R.J. (1981) Conjoined acardiac monsters. *Archives of Pathology and Laboratory Medicine*, **105**, 253–255.

Anderson, R.L., Golbus, M.S., Curry, C.J.R., Callen, P.W. and Hastrup, W.H. (1990) Central nervous system damage and other anomalies in surviving fetus following second trimester antenatal death of co-twin: report of four cases and literature review. *Prenatal Diagnosis*, **10**, 513–518.

Anger, H. and Ring, A. (1972) Die fetofetale Transfusion bei Zwillingen. *Zeitschrift für Geburtshilfe und Perinatologie*, **176**, 164–167.

Annan, B. and Hutson, R.C. (1990) Double survival despite cord entwinement in monoamniotic twins: case report. *British Journal of Obstetrics and Gynaecology*, **97**, 950–951.

Arts, N.F.Th. and Lohman, A.H.M. (1971) The vascular anatomy of monochorionic diamniotic twin placentas and the transfusion syndrome. *European Journal of Obstetrics and Gynecology*, **3**, 85–93.

Bajoria, R., Wigglesworth, J. and Fisk, N.M. (1995) Angioarchitecture of monochorionic placentas in relation to the twin–twin transfusion syndrome. *American Journal of Obstetrics and Gynecology*, **172**, 856–863.

Baldwin, V.J. (1994) *Pathology of Multiple Pregnancy*. New York: Springer-Verlag.

Bardawil, W.A., Reddy, R.L. and Bardawil, L.W. (1988) Placental considerations in multiple pregnancy. *Clinics in Perinatology*, **15**, 13–40.

Bender, H.G. and Brandt, G. (1974) Morphologie und Morphometrie der Fünflings-Placenta. *Archiv für Gynäkologie*, **216**, 61–72.

Benirschke, K. (1961a) Accurate recording of twin placentation – a plea to the obstetrician. *Obstetrics and Gynecology*, **18**, 334–347.

Benirschke, K. (1961b) Twin placenta in perinatal mortality. *New York State Journal of Medicine*, **61**, 1499–1508.

Benirschke, K. (1965) Major pathologic features of the placenta, cord and membranes. *Birth Defects Original Articles Series*, **1**, 52–56.

Benirschke, K. (1972a) Multiple births. In *Pediatrics*, 15th edn, Barnett, H.L. and Einhorn, A.H. (Eds), pp. 117–125. New York: Appleton-Century-Crofts.

Benirschke, K. (1972b) Origin and clinical significance of twinning. *Clinical Obstetrics and Gynecology*, **15**, 220–235.

Benirschke, K. (1993) Intrauterine death of a twin: mechanisms, implications for surviving twin, and placental pathology. *Seminars in Diagnostic Pathology*, **10**, 222–231.

Benirschke, K. and Driscoll, S.G. (1967) *The Pathology of the Human Placenta*. Berlin, Heidelberg, New York: Springer-Verlag.

Benirschke, K. and Kaufmann, P. (1995) *Pathology of the Human Placenta*, 3rd edn. New York: Springer-Verlag.

Benirschke, K. and Kim, C.K. (1973a) Medical progress: multiple pregnancy. *New England Journal of Medicine*, **288**, 1276–1284.

Benirschke, K. and Kim, C.K. (1973b) Medical progress: multiple pregnancy. *New England Journal of Medicine*, **288**, 1329–1336.

Berbos, J.D., King, B.F. and Janusz, A. (1964) Quintuple pregnancy. *Journal of the American Medical Association*, **188**, 813–816.

Berrebi, A., Mercier, N., Sarramon, M.F. et al (1988) Un nouveau cas de mole hydatiforme survenant dans l'un des oeufs d'une grossesse gemellaire. *Revue Francaise de Gynécologie et d'Obstétrique*, **83**, 429–441.

Bhargava, I. and Chakravarty, A. (1975) Vascular anastomoses in twin placentae and their recognition. *Acta Anatomica*, **93**, 471–480.

Bhargava, J., Chakravarty, A. and Raja, P.T.K. (1971) An anatomical study of the foetal blood vessels on the chorial surface of the human placenta. III. Multiple pregnancies. *Acta Anatomica*, **80**, 465–479.

Bleisch, V.R. (1964) Diagnosis of monochorionic twin placentation. *American Journal of Clinical Pathology*, **42**, 277–284.

Bleisch, V.R. (1965) Placental circulation of human twins: constant arterial anastomoses in monochorionic placentas. *American Journal of Obstetrics and Gynecology*, **91**, 862–869.

Blickstein, I. (1990) The twin–twin transfusion syndrome. *Obstetrics and Gynecology*, **76**, 714–722.

Block, M.F. and Merrill, J.A. (1982) Hydatidiform mole with coexisting fetus. *Obstetrics and Gynecology*, **60**, 129–134.

Boklage, C.E. (1990) Survival probability of human conceptus from fertilization to term. *International Journal of Fertility*, **35**, 75–94.

Bomsel-Helmreich, O. and Al Mufti, W. (1995) The mechanism of monozygosity and double-ovulation. In *Multiple Pregnancy: Epidemiology, Gestation and Perinatal Outcome*, Keith, L.G., Papiernik, E., Keith, D.M. and Luke, B. (Eds), pp. 25–40. New York: Parthenon.

Boyd, J.D. and Hamilton, W.J. (1970) *The Human Placenta*. Cambridge: W. Heffer and Sons.

Brown, B.St.J. (1982) Disappearances of one gestational sac in the first trimester of multiple pregnancies – ultrasonographic findings. *Journal of the Canadian Association of Radiologists*, **33**, 273–275.

Brown, D.L., Benson, C.B., Driscoll, S.G. and Doubilet, P.M. (1989) Twin transfusion syndrome: sonographic findings. *Radiology*, **170**, 61–63.

Bruner, J.P. and Rosemond, R.L. (1993) Twin-to-twin transfusion syndrome: a subset of the twin oligohydramnios–polyhydramnios sequence. *American Journal of Obstetrics and Gynecology*, **169**, 925–930.

Bryan, E. (1994) Trends in twinning rates. *Lancet*, **343**, 1151–1152.

Bryan, E.M. and Slavin, B. (1974) Serum IgG levels in feto-fetal transfusion syndrome. *Archives of Disease in Childhood*, **49**, 908–910.

Bryan, E.M., Slavin, B. and Nicholson, E. (1976) Serum immunoglobulins in multiple pregnancy. *Archives of Disease in Childhood*, **51**, 354–359.

Bulla, M., von Lilien, T., Goecke, H., Roth, B., Ortmann, M. and Heising, J. (1987) Renal and cerebral necrosis in survivors after in utero death of co-twin. *Archives of Gynecology*, **240**, 119–124.

Bulmer, M.G. (1970) *The Biology of Twinning in Man*. Oxford: Clarendon Press.

Callen, D.F., Fernandez, H., Hull, Y.J., Svigos, J.M., Chambers, H.M. and Sutherland, G.R. (1991) A normal 46,XX infant with a 46,XX/69,XXY placenta: a major contribution to the placenta is from a resorbed twin. *Prenatal Diagnosis*, **11**, 437–442.

Cameron, A.H. (1968) The Birmingham twin survey. *Proceedings of the Royal Society of Medicine*, **61**, 229–234.

Cameron, A.H., Robson, E.B., Wade-Evans, J. and Wingham, J. (1969) Septuplet conception: placental zygosity studies. *Journal of Obstetrics and Gynaecology of the British Commonwealth*, **76**, 692–698.

Cameron, A.H., Edwards, J.H., Derom, R., Thiery, M. and Bolaert, R. (1983) The value of twin surveys in the study of malformations. *European Journal of Obstetrics, Gynecology and Reproductive Biology*, **14**: 347–356.

Changchien, C.C., Eng, H.L. and Chen, W.J. (1994) Twin pregnancy with hydatidiform mole (46,XX) and a coexistent fetus (46,XY) *Journal of the Formosa Medical Association*, **93**, 337–339.

Chun, F.Y. (1970) Some data on twinning in Singapore. *Journal of the Singapore Paediatric Society*, **12**, 44–58.

Coen, R.W. and Sutherland, J.M. (1970) Placental vascular communications between twin fetuses: a simplified technique for demonstration. *American Journal of Diseases of Children*, **120**, 332.

Conway, C.F. (1964) Transfusion syndrome in multiple pregnancy. *Obstetrics and Gynecology*, **23**, 745–751.

Corner, G.W. (1955) The observed embryology of human single-ovum twins and other multiple births. *American Journal of Obstetrics and Gynecology*, **70**, 933–951.

Corney, G. (1975) Placentation. In *Human Multiple Reproduction*, MacGillivray, I., Nylander, P.P.S. and Corney, G. (Eds), pp. 40–76. London: W. B. Saunders.

Corney, G. and Aherne, W. (1965) The placental transfusion syndrome in monozygous twins. *Archives of Disease in Childhood*, **40**, 264.

Corney, G. and Robson, E.B. (1975) Types of twinning and determination of zygosity. In *Human Multiple Reproduction*, MacGillivray, I., Nylander, P.P.S. and Corney, G. (Eds), pp. 16–39. London: W. B. Saunders.

Corney, G., Robson, E.B. and Strong, S.J. (1972) The effect of zygosity on the birth weight of twins. *Annals of Human Genetics*, **36**, 45–59.

Dawood, M.Y., Ratnam, S.S. and Lim, Y.C. (1975) Twin pregnancy in Singapore. *Australian and New Zealand Journal of Obstetrics and Gynaecology*, **15**, 93–98.

Derom, R., Orlebeke, J., Eriksson, A. and Thiery, M. (1995) The epidemiology of multiple births in Europe. In *Multiple Pregnancy: Epidemiology, Gestation and Perinatal Outcome*, Keith, L.G., Papiernik, E., Keith, D.M. and Luke, B. (Eds), pp. 145–162. New York: Parthenon.

Dorum, A. and Nesheim, B.I. (1991) Monochorionic monoamniotic twins – the most precarious of twin pregnancies. *Acta Obstetricia et Gynecologica Scandinavica*, **70**, 381–383.

Drack, G., Kind, C. and Lorenz, U. (1993) Management monoamnioter Zwillingsschwangerschaften. *Gebürtshilfe und Frauenheilkunde*, **53**, 100–104.

Egwuato, V.E., Iloabachie, G.C., Okezie, O. and Ibe, B.C. (1992) Quintuplet pregnancy: case report. *West African Journal of Medicine*, **11**, 154–157.

Elwood, J.M. (1973) Decline in dizygotic twinning. *New England Journal of Medicine*, **289**, 486.

Enbom, J.A. (1985) Twin pregnancy with intrauterine death of one twin. *American Journal of Obstetrics and Gynecology*, **152**, 424–429.

Falik-Borenstein, T.C., Korenberg, J R. and Schreck, R.R. (1994) Confined placental chimerism: prenatal and postnatal cytogenetic and molecular analysis, and pregnancy outcome. *American Journal of Medical Genetics*, **50**, 51–56.

Feinberg, R.F., Lockwood, C.J., Salafia, C. and Hobbins, J.C. (1988) Sonographic diagnosis of a pregnancy with a diffuse hydatidiform mole and coexistent 46,XX fetus: a case report. *Obstetrics and Gynecology*, **72**, 485–488.

Fisher, R.A., Sheppard, D.M. and Lawler, S.D. (1982) Twin pregnancy with complete hydatidiform mole (46,XX) and fetus (46,XY); genetic origin proved by analysis of chromosome polymorphisms. *British Medical Journal*, **284**, 1218–1220.

Foglmann, R. (1974) Monoamniotic twins. *Acta Geneticae Medicae et Gemellologiae*, **23,** Supplement 17.

Fries, M.H., Goldstein, R.B., Kilpatrick, S.J., Golbus, M.S., Callen, P.W. and Filly, R.A. (1993) The role of velamentous cord insertion in the etiology of twin–twin transfusion. *Obstetrics and Gynecology*, **81,** 569–574.

Fujikura, T. and Froehlich, L.A. (1971) Twin placentation and zygosity. *Obstetrics and Gynecology*, **37**, 34–43.

Fusi, L., McParland, P., Fisk, N., Nicolini, U. and Wigglesworth, J. (1991) Acute twin–twin transfusion: a possible mechanism for brain damaged survivors after intrauterine death of a monochorionic twin. *Obstetrics and Gynecology*, **78**, 517–520.

Galea, P., Scott, J.M. and Goel, K.M. (1982) Feto-fetal transfusion syndrome. *Archives of Disease in Childhood*, **57**, 781–794.

Garcia-Aguayo, F.J. and Menargues Irles, M.A. (1992) Evolution of diamniotic–dichorionic pregnancy into complete hydatidiform mole and normal fetus. *Journal of Clinical Ultrasound*, **20**, 604–607.

Garrett, W.J., Carey, H.M., Stevens, L.H., Climie, C.R. and Osborn, R.A. (1976) A case of nonuplet pregnancy. *Australian and New Zealand Journal of Obstetrics and Gynaecology*, **16**, 193–202.

Gedda, L. (1961) *Twins in History and Science*. Springfield, Illinois: Charles C. Thomas.

Gibbs, C.E., Boldt, J.W., Daly, J.W. and Morgan, H.C. (1960) A quintuplet gestation. *Obstetrics and Gynecology*, **16**, 464–468.

Giles, W.B., Trudinger, B.J., Cook, C.M. and Connelly, A.J. (1990) Doppler umbilical studies in the twin–twin transfusion syndrome. *Obstetrics and Gynecology*, **76**, 1097–1099.

Gillim, D.M. and Hendricks, C.H. (1953) Holocardius: a review of the literature and case report. *Obstetrics and Gynecology*, **2**, 647.

Giovannucci-Uzielli, M.L., Vecchi, G., Donzelli, G.P., D'Ancona, V.L. and Lapi, E. (1981) The history of the Florence sextuplets: obstetric and genetic considerations. *Progress in Clinical Biology Research*, **69**, 217–220.

Goplerud, C.P. (1964) Monoamniotic twins with double survival: report of a case. *Obstetrics and Gynecology*, **23**, 289–290.

Gruenwald, P. (1970) Environmental influence on twins apparent at birth: a preliminary study. *Biology of the Neonate*, **15**, 79–93.

Hafez, E.S.E. (1974) Physiology of multiple pregnancy. *Journal of Reproductive Medicine*, **12**, 88–98.

Hagood, M. and Stokes, R.H. (1953) Double survival of monoamniotic twins. *American Journal of Obstetrics and Gynecology*, **65**, 1152–1154.

Hamblen, D.C., Baker, R.D. and Derieux, G.D. (1937) Roentgenographic diagnosis and anatomic studies of quintuple pregnancy. *Journal of the American Medical Association*, **109**, 10–12.

Hollander, H.-J. (1969) Monoamniotische Zwillinge. *Zeitschrift für Gebürtshilfe und Gynäkologie*, **171**, 292–300.

Hollander, H.-J. and Backmann, R. (1974) Das Transfusionssyndrom bei Zwillingen. *Gebürtshilfe und Frauenheilkunde*, **34**, 931–936.

Hollingsworth, W.C. (1973) Monoamniotic twin pregnancy: a case report. *North Carolina Medical Journal*, **34**, 443–444.

Husby, H., Holm, N.V., Gernow, A., Thomsen, S.G., Kock, K. and Gurtler, H. (1991) Zygosity, placental membranes and Weinberg's rule in a Danish consecutive twin series. *Acta Geneticae Medicae et Gemellologiae*, **40**, 147–152.

Huter, O., Brezinka, C., Busch, G. and Pfaller, C. (1990) Zur Frage der 'Vanishing Twin'. *Gebürtshilfe und Frauenheilkunde*, **50**, 989–992.

Hyrtle, J. (1870) *Die Blutgefässe der menschlichen Nachgeburt*. Vienna: Braumüler.

Imaizumi, Y. (1990) Triplets and higher order births in Japan. *Acta Geneticae Medicae et Gemellologiae*, **37**, 295–306.

Israelstam, D.M. (1973) Mono-amniotic twin pregnancy: a case report. *South African Medical Journal*, **47**, 2026–2027.

Jauniaux, E., Elkhazen, N., Vanrysselberge, M. and Leroy, F. (1988a) Aspects anatomo-cliniques du syndrome du foetus papyrace. *Journal de la Gynécologie, Obstétrique et Biologie de la Reproduction*, **17**, 653–659.

Jauniaux, E., Elkhazen, N., Leroy, F., Wilkin, P., Rodesch, F. and Hustin, J. (1988b) Clinical and morphologic aspects of the vanishing twin phenomenon. *Obstetrics and Gynecology*, **72**, 577–581.

Jauniaux, E., de Lannoy, E., Moscoso, G. and Campbell, S. (1990) Diagnose prenatal des pathologies molaires associees a un fetus: revue de la litterature recente a propos d'un cas. *Journal de la Gynécologie, Obstétrique et Biologie de la Reproduction*, **19**, 941–946.Jewell, S.E. and Yip, R. (1995) Increasing trends in plural births in the United States. *Obstetrics and Gynecology*, **85**, 229–232.

Keith, L., Cestaro, A. and Elias, I. (1967) Fetus holoacardius: a complication of monochorial twinning. *Chicago Medical School Quarterly*, **27**, 30–35.

Khoo, S.K., Monks, P.L. and Davies, N.T. (1986) Hydatidiform mole coexisting with a live fetus: a dilemma of management. *Australian and New Zealand Journal of Obstetrics and Gynaecology*, **26**, 129–135.

Kim, K. and Lage, J.M. (1991) Bipartite diamnionic monochorionic twin placenta with superficial anastomoses: report of a case. *Human Pathology*, **22**, 501–503.

King, A.D., Soothill, P.W., Montemagno, R., Young, M.P., Sams, V. and Rodeck, C.H. (1995) Twin-to-twin blood transfusion in a dichorionic pregnancy without the oligohydramnios–polyhydramnios sequence. *British Journal of Obstetrics and Gynaecology*, **102**, 334–335.

Klebe, J.G. and Ingomar, C.J. (1972) The fetoplacental circulation during parturition illustrated by the interfetal transfusion syndrome. *Pediatrics*, **49**, 112–116.

Kloosterman, G.J. (1963) The 'third circulation' in identical twins. *Nederlands Tijdschrift voor Verloskunde en Gynaecologie*, **63**, 395–412.

Krussel, J.S., von Eckardstein, S. and Schwenzer, T. (1994) Doppelter Nabelschnurknoten bei monoamniotischer Geminigraviditat als Ursache des intrauterinen Fruchttods beider Zwillinge. *Zentralblatt für Gynäkologie*, **116**, 497–499.

Kunz, J. and Arnaboldi, M. (1991) Acardiacus bei Zwillingsschwangerschaft. *Zeitschrift für Geburtshilfe und Perinatologie*, **195**, 275–279.

Lachelin, G.C.L., Brant, H.A., Swyer, G.I.M., Little, V. and Reynolds, E.O.R. (1972) Sextuplet pregnancy. *British Medical Journal*, **i**, 787–790.

Lachman, R., McNabb, M., Furmanski, M. and Karp, L. (1980) The acardiac monster. *European Journal of Pediatrics*, **134**, 195–200.

Lage, J.M., Vanmarter, L.J. and Mikhael, E. (1989) Vascular anastomoses in fused, dichorionic twin placenta resulting in twin transfusion syndrome. *Placenta*, **10**, 55–59.

Landy, H.J. and Nies, B.M. (1995) The vanishing twin. In *Multiple Pregnancy: Epidemiology, Gestation and Perinatal Outcome*, Keith, L.G., Papiernik, E., Keith, D.M. and Luke, B. (Eds), pp. 59–72. New York: Parthenon.

Landy, H.J., Keith, L. and Keith, D. (1982) The vanishing twin. *Acta Geneticae Medicae et Gemellologiae*, **31**, 179–194.

Landy, H.J., Weiner, S., Corson, S.L., Batzer, F.R. and Bolognese, R.J. (1986) The 'vanishing twin'; ultrasonographic assessment of fetal disappearance in the first trimester. *American Journal of Obstetrics and Gynecology*, **155**, 14–19.

Larson, S.L., Kempers, R.D. and Titus, J.L. (1969) Monoamniotic twins with a common umbilical cord. *American Journal of Obstetrics and Gynecology*, **105**, 635–636.

Librach, S. and Terrin, A.J. (1957) Monoamniotic twin pregnancy. *American Journal of Obstetrics and Gynecology*, **74**, 440–443.

Liu, S., Benirschke, K., Scioscia, A.L. and Mannino, F.L. (1992) Intrauterine death in multiple gestation. *Acta Geneticae Medicae et Gemellologiae*, **41**, 5–26.

Lumme, R.H. and Saarikoski, S.V. (1986) Monoamniotic twin pregnancy. *Acta Geneticae Medicae et Gemellologiae*, **35**, 99–105.

Machin, G.A. and Still, K. (1995) The twin–twin transfusion syndrome: vascular anatomy of monochorionic placentas and their clinical outcome. In *Multiple Pregnancy: Epidemiology, Gestation and Perinatal Outcome*, Keith, L.G., Papiernik, E., Keith, D.M. and Luke, B. (Eds), pp. 367–394. New York: Parthenon.

McLeod, F. and McCoy, D.R. (1981) Monoamniotic twins with an unusual cord complication: case report. *British Journal of Obstetrics and Gynaecology*, **88**, 774–775.

Majsky, A. and Kout, M. (1982) Another case of occurrence of two different fathers of twins by HLA typing. *Tissue Antigens*, **20**, 305.

Megory, E., Weiner, E., Shalev, E. and Ohel, G. (1991) Pseudoamniotic twins with cord entanglement following genetic funipuncture. *Obstetrics and Gynecology*, **78**, 915–918.

Metler, S., Meyer, J. and Rudzinski, L. (1974) Morphology of the afterbirth of the Danzig quintuplets. *Acta Geneticae Medicae et Gemellologiae*, **22**, 164–167.

Meyer, W.C., Keith, L. and Webster, A. (1970) Monoamniotic twin pregnancy with the transfusion syndrome: a case report. *Chicago Medical School Quarterly*, **29**, 42–51.

Michaels, L. (1967) Unilateral ischemia of the fused twin placenta: a manifestation of the twin transfusion syndrome. *Canadian Medical Association Journal*, **96**, 402–405.

Miller, D., Jackson, R., Ehlen, T. and McMurtrie, E. (1993) Complete hydatidiform mole with a twin live fetus: clinical course of 4 cases with complete cytogenetic analysis. *Gynecologic Oncology*, **50**, 119–123.

Monnier, J.C., Nihouarn, G., Vinatier, D., Lanciaux, B., Savary, B. and LecomtHoucke, M. (1987) Grossesse gemellaire associant une mole hydatidiforme et un oeuf normal. *Journal de Gynécologie, d'Obstétrique et Biologie de la Reproduction*, **16**, 213–218.

Moore, C.M., McAdams, A.J. and Sutherland, J.M. (1969) Intrauterine disseminated intravascular coagulation: a syndrome of multiple pregnancy with a dead twin fetus. *Journal of Pediatrics*, **74**, 523–528.

Moore, T.R., Gate, S.A. and Benirschke, K. (1990) Perinatal outcome of forty-nine pregnancies complicated by acardiac twinning. *American Journal of Obstetrics and Gynecology*, **163**, 907–912.

Mortimer, G. (1987) Zygosity and placental structure in monochorionic twins. *Acta Geneticae Medicae et Gemellologiae*, **36**, 417–420.

Myrianthopoulos, N.C. (1970) An epidemiologic survey of twins in a large prospectively studied population. *American Journal of Human Genetics*, **22**, 611–629.

Naeye, R.L. (1965) Organ abnormalities in a human parabiotic syndrome. *American Journal of Pathology*, **46**, 829–842.

Napolitani, F.D. and Schreiber, L. (1960) The acardiac monster: a review of the world literature and presentation of two cases. *American Journal of Obstetrics and Gynecology*, **80**, 582–589.

Nerlich, A., Wiser, J. and Krone, S. (1992) Plazentabefunde bei 'Vanishing Twins'. *Geburtshilfe und Frauenheilkunde*, **52**, 230–234.

Neubecker, R.D., Blumberg, J.M. and Townsend, F.M. (1962) A human monozygotic quintuplet placenta: report of a specimen. *Journal of Obstetrics and Gynaecology of the British Commonwealth*, **69**, 137–139.

Nylander, P.P.S. (1969) The value of the placenta in the determination of zygosity – a study of 1052 Nigerian twin maternities. *Journal of Obstetrics and Gynaecology of the British Commonwealth*, **76**, 699–704.

Nylander, P.P.S. (1970a) Placental forms and zygosity determination of twins in Ibadan, Western Nigeria. *Acta Geneticae Medicae et Gemellologiae*, **19**, 45–54.

Nylander, P.P.S. (1970b) Twinning in Nigeria. *Acta Geneticae Medicae et Gemellologiae*, **19**, 457–464.

Nylander, P.P.S. (1971a) Biosocial aspects of multiple births. *Journal of Biosocial Science*, Supplement 3, 29–38.

Nylander, P.P.S. (1971b) The incidence of triplets and higher multiple births in some rural and urban populations in Western Nigeria. *Annals of Human Genetics*, **34**, 409–415.

Nylander, P.P.S. (1973) The placenta and zygosity of twins. *Acta Geneticae Medicae et Gemellologiae*, **22**, 234–237.

Nylander, P.P.S. (1975a) The causation of twinning. In *Human Multiple Reproduction*, MacGillivray, I., Nylander, P.P.S. and Corney, G. (Eds), pp. 77–86. London: W. B. Saunders.

Nylander, P.P.S. (1975b) Frequency of multiple births. In *Human Multiple Reproduction*, MacGillivray, I., Nylander, P.P.S. and Corney, G. (Eds), pp. 87–97. London: W. B. Saunders.

Nylander, P.P.S. and Corney, G. (1969) Placentation and zygosity of twins in Ibadan, Nigeria. *Annals of Human Genetics*, **33**, 31–38.

Nylander, P.P.S. and Corney, G. (1971) Placentation and zygosity of triplets and higher multiple births in Ibadan, Nigeria. *Annals of Human Genetics*, **34**, 417–426.

Nylander, P.P.S. and MacGillivray, I. (1975) Complications of twin pregnancy. In *Human Multiple Reproduction*, MacGillivray, I., Nylander, P.P.S. and Corney, G. (Eds), pp. 137–146. London: W. B. Saunders.

Nylander, P.P.S. and Osunkoya, B.O. (1970) Unusual monochorionic placentation with heterosexual twins. *Obstetrics and Gynecology*, **36**, 621–625.

Ohama, K., Katsunori, U., Okamoto, I. and Fujiwara, A. (1985) Two cases of dizygotic twins with andro-genetic mole and normal conceptus. *Hiroshima Journal of Medical Sciences*, **34**, 371–375.

Olsen, M.E. (1992) Monoamniotic twin gestations. *Journal of the Tennessee Medical Association*, **85**, 511–512.

Ong, H.C., Puvan, I.S. and Chan, W.F. (1976) An unusual complication on a twin pregnancy – umbilical cord of twin 2 around the neck of twin 1. *Australian and New Zealand Journal of Obstetrics and Gynaecology*, **16**, 57–58.

Osada, H., Iitsuka, Y., Matsui, H. and Sekiya, S. (1995) A complete hydatidiform mole coexisting with a normal fetus was confirmed by variable number tandem repeat (VNTR) polymorphism analysis using polymerase chain reaction. *Gynecologic Oncology*, **56**, 90–93.

Ozumba, B.C. and Ofodile, A. (1994) Twin pregnancy involving complete hydatidiform mole and partial mole after five years of amenorrhoea. *European Journal of Obstetrics and Gynecology and Reproductive Biology*, **53**, 230–234.

Pauls, F. (1969) Monoamniotic twin pregnancy: a review of the world literature and a report of two new cases. *Canadian Medical Association Journal*, **100**, 254–256.

Perez, M.L., Firpo, J.R. and Baldi, E.M. (1947) Sobre las anastomosis circulatorias de las placentas dizig-oticas. *Obstetricia y Ginecologia Latino-Americanas*, **5**, 5–22.

Perlman, E.J., Stetten, G., Tuck-Muller, C.M. et al (1990) Sexual discordance in monozygotic twins. *American Journal of Medical Genetics*, **37**, 551–557.

Pinet, C., Colau, J.C., Delezoide, A.L. and Menez, F. (1944) Les jumeaux acardiaques. *Journal de Gynécologie, Obstétrique et Biologie de la Reproduction*, **23**, 85–92.

Potter, E.L. (1963) Twin zygosity and placental form in relation to the outcome of pregnancy. *American Journal of Obstetrics and Gynecology*, **87**, 566–577.

Quigley, J.K. (1935) Monoamniotic twin pregnancy: a case record with review of the literature. *American Journal of Obstetrics and Gynecology*, **29**, 354–362.

Ramos-Arroyo, M.A., Ulbright, T.M. and Christian, J.C. (1988) Twin study: relationship between birth weight, zygosity, placentation, and pathologic placental changes. *Acta Geneticae Medicae et Gemellologiae*, **37**, 229–238.

Raphael, S.I. (1961) Monoamniotic twin pregnancy: a review of the literature and a report of 5 new cases. *American Journal of Obstetrics and Gynecology*, **81**, 323–330.

Rausen, A.R., Seki, M. and Strauss, L. (1965) Twin transfusion syndrome: a review of 19 cases studied at one institution. *Journal of Pediatrics*, **66**, 613–628.

Reddy, K.S., Petersen, M.B., Antonarakis, S.E. and Blakemore K.J. (1991) The vanishing twin: an explanation for discordance between chorionic villi karotype and fetal karotype. *Prenatal Diagnosis*, **11**, 679–684.

Robertson, E.G. and Neer, K.J. (1983) Placental injection studies in twin gestation. *American Journal of Obstetrics and Gynecology*, **147**, 170–174.

Robinson, H.P. and Caines, J.S. (1977) Sonar evidence of early pregnancy failure in patients with twin conceptions. *British Journal of Obstetrics and Gynaecology*, **84**, 22–25.

Robinson, L.K., Jones, K.L. and Benirschke, K. (1983) The nature of structural defects associated with velamentous and marginal insertion of the umbilical cord. *American Journal of Obstetrics and Gynecology*, **146**, 199–204.

Rodis, J.F., Vintzileos, A.M., Campbell, W.A., Deaton, J.L., Fumia, F. and Nochimson, J. (1987) Antenatal diagnosis and management of monoamniotic twins. *American Journal of Obstetrics and Gynecology*, **157**, 1255–1257.

Rudnicki, M., Vejerslev, L.O. and Junge, J. (1991) The vanishing twin: morphologic and cytogenetic evaluation of an ultrasonographic phenomenon. *Gynecological and Obstetrical Investigation*, **31**, 141–145.

Salerno, L.J. (1959) Monoamniotic twinning: a survey of the American literature since 1935 with a report of four new cases. *Obstetrics and Gynecology*, **14**, 205–213.

Sato, T., Kaneko, K., Konuma, S., Sato, I. and Tamada, T. (1984) Acardiac anomalies: review of 88 cases in Japan. *Asia and Oceania Journal of Obstetrics and Gynaecology*, **10**, 45–52.

Sauerbrei, E.E., Salem, S. and Fayle, B. (1980) Coexistent hydatidiform mole and live fetus in the second trimester. *Radiology*, **135**, 415–417.

Schatz, F. (1900) *Klinische Beitrage zur Physiologie des Fetus*. Berlin: Hirschwald.

Scipiades, E. and Burg, E. (1930) Über die Morphologie der menschlichen Placenta mit besonderer Rücksicht auf unsere eigenen Studienen. *Archiv für Gynäkologie*, **141**, 577–619.

Scrimgeour, J.B. and Baker, T.G. (1974) A possible case of superfetation in man. *Journal of Reproduction and Fertility*, **36**, 69–73.

Sekiya, S. and Haez, E.S.E. (1977) Physiomorphology of twin transfusion syndrome: a study of 86 twin gestations. *Obstetrics and Gynecology*, **50**, 288–292.

Serreyn, R., Thiery, M. and Vandekerckhove, D. (1984) Outcome of an octuplet pregnancy. *Archives of Gynaecology*, **234**, 283–293.

Severn, C.B. and Holyoke, E.A. (1973) Human acardiac anomalies. *American Journal of Obstetrics and Gynecology*, **116**, 358–365.

Shalev, E., Zalel, Y., Ben-Ami, M. and Weiner, E. (1992) First trimester ultrasonic diagnosis of twin reversed arterial perfusion sequence. *Prenatal Diagnosis*, **12**, 219–222.

Shanklin, D.R. and Perrin, E.V.D.K. (1984) Multiple gestation. In *Pathology of the Placenta*, Perrin, E.V.D.K. (Ed.), pp. 165–182. New York: Churchill Livingstone.

Steller, M.A., Genest, D.R., Bernstein, M.R., Lage, J.M., Goldstein, D.P. and Berkowitz, R.S. (1994a) Natural history of twin pregnancy with complete hydatidiform mole and coexisting fetus. *Obstetrics and Gynecology*, **83**, 35–42.

Steller, M.A., Genest, D.R., Bernstein, M.R., Lage, J.M., Goldstein, D.P. and Berkowitz, R.S. (1994b) Clinical features of multiple conception with partial or complete molar pregnancy and coexisting fetuses. *Journal of Reproductive Medicine*, **39**, 147–154.

Stephens, T.D. (1984) Muscle abnormalities associated with the twin-reversed-arterial-perfusion (TRAP) sequence (acardia) *Teratology*, **30**, 311–318.

Strong, S.J. and Corney, G. (1967) *The Placenta in Twin Pregnancy*. Oxford: Pergamon Press.

Sulak, L.E. and Dodson, M.G. (1986) The vanishing twin: pathologic confirmation of an ultrasound phenomenon. *Obstetrics and Gynecology*, **68**, 811–815.

Sutter, J., Arab, H. and Manning, F.A. (1986) Monoamniotic twins: antenatal diagnosis and management. *American Journal of Obstetrics and Gynecology*, **155**, 836–837.

Szendi, B. (1938) Über die Bedeutung der Struktur der Eihüte und des Gefässnetzes der Placenta auf Grund von 112 Zwillingsgeburten. *Archiv für Gynäkologie*, **167**, 108–129.

Szymonowicz, W., Preston, H. and Yu, Y.Y.H. (1986) The surviving monozygotic twin. *Archives of Disease in Childhood*, **61**, 454–458.

Tafell, S.M. (1995) Demographic trends in twin births: USA. In *Multiple Pregnancy: Epidemiology, Gestation and Perinatal Outcome*, Keith, L.G., Papiernik, E., Keith, D.M. and Luke, B. (Eds), pp. 133–144. New York: Parthenon.

Tagawa, T. (1974) Monoamniotic twins with double survival: report of a case with a peculiar cord complication. *Wisconsin Medical Journal*, **73**, 131–132.

Tan, K.L., Tan, R., Tan, S.H. and Tan, A.M. (1979) The twin transfusion syndrome: clinical observations in 35 affected pairs. *Clinical Pediatrics*, **18**, 111–114.

Terasaki, P.I., Gjertson, D., Bernoco, D., Perdue, S., Mickey, M.R. and Bond, J. (1978) Twins with two different fathers identified by HLA. *New England Journal of Medicine*, **299**, 590–592.

Tessen, J.A. and Zlatnik, F.J. (1991) Monoamniotic twins: a retrospective controlled study. *Obstetrics and Gynecology*, **77**, 832–834.

Timmons, J.D. and de Alvarez, R.R. (1963) Monoamniotic twin pregnancy. *American Journal of Obstetrics and Gynecology*, **86**, 875–881.

Turksoy, R.N., Toy, B.L., Rogers, J. and Papageorge, W. (1967) Birth of septuplets following human gonadotrophin administration in Chiari–Frommel syndrome. *Obstetrics and Gynecology*, **30**, 692–698.

Urig, M.A., Clewell, W.H. and Elliott, J.P. (1990) Twin–twin transfusion syndrome. *American Journal of Obstetrics and Gynecology*, **163**, 1522–1526.

Urig, M.A., Simpson, G.F., Elliott, J.P. and Clewell, W.H. (1988) Twin–twin transfusion syndrome: the surgical removal of one twin as a treatment option. *Fetal Therapy*, **3**, 185–188.

van Allen M.I. (1981) Fetal vascular disruptions: mechanisms and some resulting birth defects. *Pediatric Annual*, **10**, 219–233.

van Allen, M.I., Smith, D.W. and Shepard, T.H. (1983) Twin reversed arterial perfusion (TRAP) sequence: a study of 14 twin pregnancies with acardius. *Seminars in Perinatology*, **7**, 285–293.

van de Geijn, E.J., Yedema, C.A., Hemrika, D.J., Schutte, M.F. and ten Velden, J.J. (1992) Hydatidiform mole with coexisting twin pregnancy after gamete intra-fallopian transfer. *Human Reproduction*, **7**, 568–572.

van de Kaa, C.A., Robben, J.C.M., Hopman, A.H.N., Hanselaar, A.G.J.M. and Vooijs, G.P. (1995) Complete hydatidiform mole in twin pregnancy: differentiation from partial mole with interphase cytogenetic and DNA cytometric analyses on paraffin embedded tissues. *Histopathology*, **26**, 123–129.

Varma, T.R. (1979) Ultrasound evidence of early pregnancy failure in patients with multiple conceptions. *British Journal of Obstetrics and Gynaecology*, **86**, 290–292.

Vejerslev, L.O., Dueholm, M. and Nielsen, F.H. (1986) Hydatidiform mole: cytogenetic marker analysis in twin gestation. *American Journal of Obstetrics and Gynecology*, **155**, 614–617.

Wagner, D.S., Klein, R.L., Robinson, H.B. and Novak, R.W. (1990) Placental emboli from a fetus papyraceous. *Journal of Pediatric Surgery*, **25**, 538–542.

Walker, J. and Turnbull, E.P.N. (1955) The environment of the foetus in human multiple pregnancy. *Etudés Néo-natales*, **3**, 123–148.

Walter, A., Hasenohr, G. and Kerin, J.F.P. (1975) Superfetation in man. *Australian and New Zealand Journal of Obstetrics and Gynaecology*, **15**, 240–246.

Wenk, R.E., Houtz, T., Brooks, M. and Chiafari, F.A. (1992) How frequent is heteroparental superfecundation? *Acta Geneticae Medicae et Gemellologiae*, **41**, 43–47.

Wenner, R. (1956) Les examens vasculaires des placentas gemellaires et le diagnostic des jumeaux homozygotes. *Bulletin de la Société Belge de Gynécologie et Obstétrique*, **26**, 773–781.

Wensinger, J.A. and Daly, R.F. (1962) Monoamniotic twins. *American Journal of Obstetrics and Gynecology*, **83**, 1254–1256.

Wharton, B., Edwards, J.H. and Cameron, A.H. (1968) Monoamniotic twins. *Journal of Obstetrics and Gynaecology of the British Commonwealth*, **75**, 158–163.

Wigglesworth, J.S. (1995) The placenta in twins. In *Multiple Pregnancy*, Ward, R.H. and Whittle, M. (Eds), pp. 48–55. London: RCOG Press.

Wilson, E.A. (1972) Holoacardius. *Obstetrics and Gynecology*, **40**, 740–748.

Yoshida, K. (1995) Documenting the vanishing twin by pathological examination. In *Multiple Pregnancy: Epidemiology, Gestation and Perinatal Outcome*, Keith, L.G., Papiernik, E., Keith, D.M. and Luke, B. (Eds), pp. 51–58. New York: Parthenon.

Yoshida, K. and Soma, H. (1986) Outcomes of the surviving co-twin of a fetus papyraceous or of a dead fetus. *Acta Geneticae Medicae et Gemellologiae*, **35**, 91–98.

Yoshioka, H., Kadomoto, Y., Mino, M., Morikawa, Y., Kasubuchi, Y. and Kusunok, T. (1979) Multicystic encephalomacia in liveborn twin with a stillborn macerated co-twin. *Journal of Pediatrics*, **95**, 798–800.

Zuckerman, H. and Brzezinski, A. (1960) Monoamniotic twin pregnancy: report of two cases with review of the literature. *Gynaecologia*, **150**, 290–298.

5

MACROSCOPIC ABNORMALITIES OF THE PLACENTA

The study of gross placental lesions has, until quite recently, been made unnecessarily complicated by the use of classifications based solely on macroscopic characteristics, by a frequent failure to apply even the most basic of pathological principles, and by the use of a ludicrous, indeed almost fatuous, system of terminology. Thus, in the past, the term 'infarct' has been used quite indiscriminately to cover all visible lesions, even, as an extreme example, being applied to thrombi, cysts or foci of calcification. Fortunately, much of this archaic terminology has now sunk into well-deserved oblivion although traces of it still remain to pollute the obstetrical literature. The terminology used here for the various gross placental lesions is a rational one that is based largely upon their pathology and which leaves relatively little room for confusion.

There is no single ideal or logical way of classifying gross placental lesions; they can, with equal validity, be grouped according to their appearance, their pathogenesis or their functional significance. I prefer to consider these lesions in pathogenetic terms, thus:

1. Lesions due to disturbances of maternal blood flow to or through the placenta.
2. Lesions due to disturbances of fetal blood flow to or through the placenta.
3. Thrombi and haematomas.
4. Non-vascular lesions.

I recognize that this is not a fully logical classification because some of the lesions classed as thrombi or haematomas may well be secondary to changes in one or other of the two placental circulatory systems. Nevertheless it serves as a useful, albeit flawed, framework for a discussion of the various gross lesions of the placenta. These lesions are not described in any particular order of significance or importance, this latter quality being related more to the space allotted to them than to their ranking in a descriptive hierarchy.

It should be noted that this chapter does not include a discussion of macroscopic abnormalities of the cord or membranes and does not consider non-trophoblastic tumours of the placenta, these aspects of the gross pathology of the placenta being discussed in Chapters 13, 15 and 16.

LESIONS DUE TO DISTURBANCES OF MATERNAL BLOOD FLOW

Massive Perivillous Fibrin Deposition

Some degree of perivillous fibrin deposition in the intervillous space occurs in nearly every full-term placenta and is indeed visible macroscopically in most placentas as a fine speckling. In a proportion, however, perivillous fibrin deposition is sufficiently extensive to form a clearly visible, and often quite large, plaque-like lesion; it is only to these latter cases that I apply the term 'massive perivillous fibrin deposition'. It should be noted that this lesion has also been referred to as 'perivillous fibrinoid deposition' (Benirschke & Kaufmann, 1995): for reasons discussed in Chapter 1 I think that most pathologists would prefer to retain the term 'fibrin' for material that is, without doubt, derived from the maternal blood in the intervillous space.

Macroscopic Features

Massive perivillous fibrin deposition is seen most frequently in the peripheral area of the placenta and often fills in the marginal angle (Fig. 5.1). However, it is not unusual for it to occur in the more central portion of the placenta, where it tends to take the form either of an irregular vertical strip running between maternal and fetal surfaces (Fig. 5.2) or of a roughly circular or ovoid plaque in the basal or intermediate zones. The lesion is hard and, although often very irregular in outline, sharply demarcated from the surrounding normal tissue. The cut surface is usually white but may have a brown or slightly yellow tinge and, although often appearing slightly granular, may be smooth and featureless.

Histology

On microscopy a plaque of this type is seen to consist of widely separated villi entrapped in fibrin which is completely obliterating the intervillous space (Fig. 5.3). In freshly formed lesions a few degenerate syncytial nuclei may be seen around the periphery of individual encased villi; the trophoblastic basement membrane is only slightly thickened and the villous stroma and vessels are normal. In older plaques the

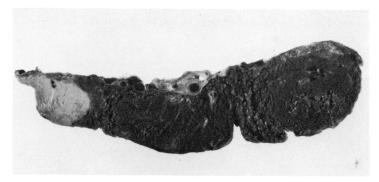

Figure 5.1. A peripherally situated plaque of perivillous fibrin which fills in the lateral angle of the placenta.

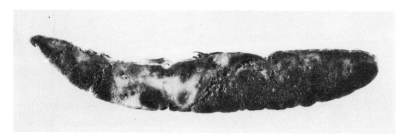

Figure 5.2. A centrally situated plaque of perivillous fibrin; this is irregular in outline and whitish-yellow in colour.

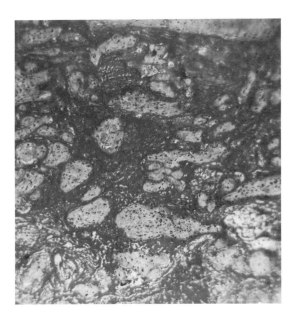

Figure 5.3. Histological appearances of a plaque of perivillous fibrin. The villi are widely separated from each other by fibrin, which is filling in and obliterating the intervillous space (H & E ×55).

syncytiotrophoblast of the involved villi has completely disappeared, the trophoblastic basement membrane is thickened, and there is a progressive fibrosis of the stroma together with sclerosis, and eventual obliteration, of the villous vessels, so that, in the well-established lesion, the villi appear as avascular fibrotic islands in a sea of fibrin (Fig. 5.4). Although the syncytiotrophoblast is lost, the villous cytotrophoblastic cells not only persist but proliferate, often forming a prominent mantle around individual villi (Fig. 5.5). Quite frequently, the cytotrophoblastic cells spread out into the surrounding fibrin and groups of such cells may become detached from their parent villus to appear as isolated cell masses in the enveloping fibrin (Fig. 5.6).

For reasons that I cannot understand, it has been remarked that the lesion which I

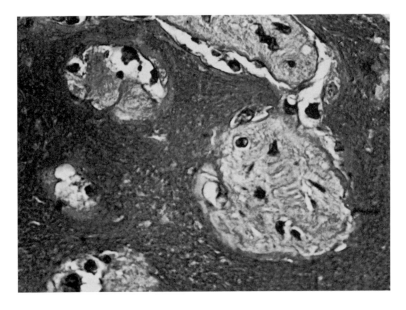

Figure 5.4. Villi entrapped in a plaque of perivillous fibrin. The villi are fibrotic, avascular and have lost their trophoblastic covering (H & E ×350).

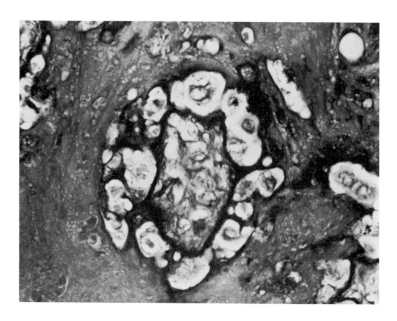

Figure 5.5. Proliferation of cytotrophoblastic cells to form a mantle around a villus embedded in a plaque of fibrin: the gross thickening of the trophoblastic basement membrane is also apparent (PAS ×450).

have described as massive perivillous fibrin deposition (Fox, 1967a) refers only to deposition of fibrin around stem villi (Nelson et al, 1990; Redline & Patterson, 1994); whether this misapprehension is due to the opaqueness of my writing, the lack of clarity of my microphotographs or a misreading of my text is a moot point. For clarification,

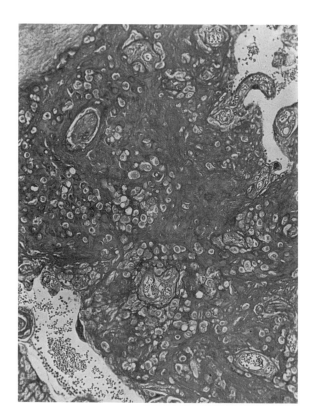

Figure 5.6. A plaque of perivillous fibrin in which there has been marked proliferation of the villous cytotrophoblastic cells: many of these have become detached from their parent villi and have spread out into the enveloping fibrin (PAS ×65).

however, I am unequivocally referring to deposition of fibrin around terminal villi; some stem villi may be included within the plaque by perchance but most of the villi entrapped in fibrin are usually terminal villi, i.e. those villi that are of greatest functional importance.

Incidence

Plaques of perivillous fibrin are found in about 22% of placentas from full-term uncomplicated pregnancies (Fox, 1967a); they are uncommon in placentas from premature deliveries (6%) but their incidence is not increased in prolonged pregnancy. Perivillous fibrin is, at all stages of pregnancy, seen relatively infrequently in placentas from women with pre-eclampsia or essential hypertension (12–13%) and in those from diabetic mothers (6%).

Aetiology and Pathogenesis

It is generally accepted that the material obliterating the intervillous space is fibrin and that the fibrin is derived from the maternal blood in the intervillous space. Eden (1897) was the first to offer an explanation for the thrombosis of maternal blood in the intervillous space around groups of villi, arguing that the villous syncytio-trophoblast is the physiological equivalent of an endothelium in the intervillous space, and that therefore any degenerative changes in this tissue would lead to thrombosis of maternal blood. His suggestion won many adherents, the syncytial degeneration being variously attributed to obliterative lesions of the fetal stem arteries, an ageing change or to toxic factors in the maternal blood (McNalley, 1924; Strachan, 1926; Hunt et al, 1940; Steigrad, 1952; Thomsen, 1954; Gregor, 1961; Kérisit & Toulouse, 1970b). Benirschke and Kaufmann (1995) also favour this hypothesis, arguing that focal syncytial degeneration allows for exposure of maternal blood to the villous tro-phoblastic basement membrane which, with its content of collagens, laminin and fibronectins, activates the coagulation system in the maternal blood. To some extent this view is based upon the study of Nelson et al (1990) who demonstrated focal fibrin deposition on areas of villous syncytial denudation: it is clear from the micro-photographs accompanying the paper that Nelson and his colleagues were referring to focal deposition of fibrin on areas of syncytial loss, a finding that I would not contest, and not to massive perivillous fibrin deposition. Further, Nelson et al (1990) do not rule out the possibility that the syncytial damage may have been secondary to stasis of maternal blood in the intervillous space. The problems with the view expressed by Benirschke and Kaufmann (1995) are two-fold: firstly they do not explain why syncytial degeneration should occur in otherwise normal pregnancies and, secondly, they do not explain why the incidence of massive perivillous fibrin deposition is lower in pregnancies complicated by pre-eclampsia (a condition in which ischaemic damage to the villous syncytiotrophoblast would be expected) than it is in uncomplicated pregnancies.

In reality, fetal vascular lesions of an obliterative nature do not cause syncytial damage, and syncytial degeneration does not appear to be the primary change that precipitates massive perivillous fibrin deposition. Moe and Jorgensen (1968) have, with the aid of the electron microscope, shown quite clearly that the initial event is the adherence of maternal platelets to normal, healthy villous syncytiotrophoblast, and there seems little doubt of the correctness of the view that fibrin deposition is due to thrombosis of maternal blood as a result of eddy currents and stasis within the inter-villous space (Siddall & Hartman, 1926; Ashworth & Stouffer, 1956; Carter et al, 1963a,b). The nature of this closed irregular space, the splitting in direction and change in velocity of the maternal blood flow as it reaches the subchorial space, and the baffling action of the villi all predispose to turbulence, eddies, stasis and throm-bosis. The villi are therefore simply bystanders in this pathological process and their inclusion within the fibrinous plaque is purely accidental. Once entrapped within the thrombotic plaque, however, the villi suffer a marked reduction in their supply of oxygen, as this is derived from the maternal blood from which they become cut off by the enveloping fibrin. The syncytiotrophoblast of the trapped villi will therefore undergo ischaemic necrosis, as this tissue is markedly sensitive to hypoxia. It will thus be apparent that the syncytial damage is a consequence rather than a cause of perivillous fibrin deposition. Enough oxygen appears to reach the villi to preserve the viability of the villous cytotrophoblast and core, these being less sensitive to oxygen lack; indeed, in response to this state of relative hypoxia, the cytotrophoblastic cells will proliferate (see Chapter 6).

Significance

In my experience the vast majority of plaques of perivillous fibrin deposition are devoid of any clinical significance. They occur infrequently in placentas from stillbirths and their incidence or size is not excessive in placentas from infants of low birth weight; furthermore, there is, in general terms, an inverse relationship between the presence of placental plaques of perivillous fibrin and fetal hypoxia, this latter complication occurring much less frequently in pregnancies in which the placenta contains lesions of this type than in those in which this placental abnormality is absent (Fox, 1967a). The banal nature of perivillous fibrin deposition is not confined to lesions in which only a few villi are involved but is equally applicable to those in which 20–30% of the villous population is included in fibrin. This is, at first sight, surprising, because although the entrapped villi are not infarcted, they serve no physiological function and are lost to the fetus for the purposes of transfer of oxygen or nutrients. Surprise will, however, only be evoked from those who believe that the placenta has, during a normal pregnancy, little or no functional reserve capacity and cannot stand a loss of more than about 10% of its functioning villi without serious consequences for the continuing welfare of the fetus. This view is wrong, because the placenta has a considerable reserve capacity and can withstand the loss of up to 30%, and probably considerably more, of its villous population without there being any discernible effect on the growth or oxygenation of the fetus, a fact to which the trivial nature of perivillous fibrinous plaques bears eloquent witness. It should be noted, however, that this functional reserve can be dissipated by a reduced maternal uteroplacental blood flow, and that perivillous fibrin deposition appears to occur usually in the setting of a good maternal blood flow through the placenta. This is suggested by the low incidence of this lesion in placentas from pregnancies complicated by a hypertensive disorder and by the notably low frequency of accompanying fetal hypoxia. It could be proposed that the greater the amount of maternal blood entering the irregular intervillous space per unit of time, the higher is the risk of turbulence and thrombosis.

Despite the generally unimportant nature of perivillous fibrin deposition, very occasionally placentas are encountered in which as much as 70–80% of the villous population is entrapped in fibrin, sometimes, but not exclusively, in association with maternal floor infarction: clearly, villous loss of this degree would dissipate the functional reserve of the placenta and all such cases I have seen were associated with intrauterine fetal death. Perivillous fibrin deposition of this extent is, however, extremely rare. Kaplan (1994) has also commented that in exceptional cases over half of the villous tissue is enveloped in perivillous fibrin and that lesions of this extent are associated with fetal growth retardation and death, whilst Fuke et al (1994) noted that two-thirds of live born infants with placentas showing massive perivillous fibrin deposition were growth retarded.

It is only fair to point out that not everyone concurs with the view that perivillous fibrin deposition is usually a banal lesion. Redline and Patterson (1994) found that perivillous fibrin deposition was associated unusually frequently with an adverse fetal outcome, particularly intrauterine growth retardation. Their definition of perivillous fibrin was, however, a rather restricted one because they limited this diagnosis to cases in which at least 20–30% of the villi in the central basal part of the placental parenchyma were entrapped in fibrin; this definition would exclude most plaques of perivillous fibrin from consideration.

Subchorionic Fibrin Plaque

A layer of subchorionic fibrin, in the roof of the intervillous space, is present in most placentas but in some there is focal excess fibrin deposition to form a hard, white, laminated plaque in the subchorionic area which, on microscopy, is seen to consist solely of fibrin.

Macroscopic Features

Subchorionic fibrin deposition is seen as a laminated white plaque that is usually roughly triangular, with the base of the triangle fused with the undersurface of the chorionic plate and the apex protruding into the placental substance (Fig. 5.7). Occasionally a plaque is roughly rectangular, with the long axis of the plaque lying in a plane parallel to that of the chorionic plate (Fig. 5.8). Rarely, the whole of the subchorionic zone is filled in by laminated fibrin. Where the plaque is in contact with the intervillous space, it is not uncommon to see fresh laminated thrombus that is being progressively transformed into fibrin and incorporated into the plaque. The fibrin plaques are very sharply demarcated from normal placental tissue.

Histology (Fig. 5.9)

Microscopy shows a plaque of this type to consist solely of laminated fibrin in which no villi are present. The fibrin is intimately attached to the undersurface of the chorionic plate, which is itself usually normal in all respects.

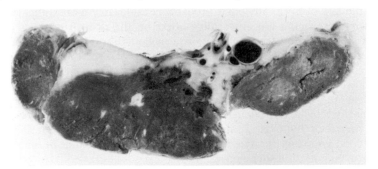

Figure 5.7. A roughly triangular plaque of subchorionic fibrin.

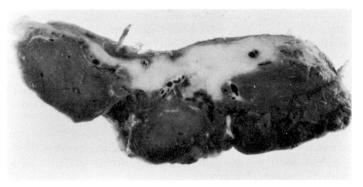

Figure 5.8. A rectangular plaque of subchorionic fibrin.

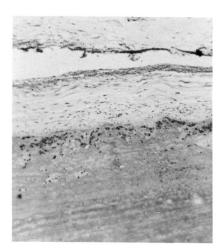

Figure 5.9. Histological appearances of a subchorionic fibrin plaque showing laminated fibrin (below) fused with a normal chorionic plate (above) (H & E ×55).

Incidence

Subchorionic fibrin plaques are found in about 20% of placentas; this incidence is almost entirely unaffected by maternal factors.

Aetiology and Pathogenesis

There is no doubt that the material in these plaques is fibrin (Moe, 1969), and little doubt that it is deposited in this site from the maternal blood in the intervillous space, a view first put forward by Langhans (1877) over a century ago. Sorba (1948) thought that the fibrin was deposited at a site of chorionic inflammation, but the very frequent absence of a chorionitis in the presence of subchorionic fibrin makes this theory untenable. It seems clear that the fibrin deposition is a result of stasis of maternal blood in the subchorionic area of the intervillous space (Geller, 1959). In the subchorionic zone there is a change in both direction and flow of the maternal blood and this, together with the mixing at the lateral margins of inflow streams which probably occurs in this area, sets an ideal stage for turbulence, stasis and thrombosis. That turbulence does indeed occur in sites where subchorionic plaques are forming has been demonstrated by ultasonography (Jauniaux et al, 1989). Hence the pathogenesis of subchorionic fibrin is identical to that of perivillous fibrin deposition; the two lesions differ only in the absence of included villi in the subchorionic plaques, which is probably a reflection of the comparative paucity of villi in this area of the placenta and hence of the relative ease with which they can be pushed aside by an expanding mass of fibrin.

Significance

Subchorionic fibrin plaques are of no clinical importance and their presence does not interfere with fetal development or growth. It is perhaps worth mentioning here that Naeye (1990) has stressed the significance of an *absence* of subchorionic fibrin. He found, in a very large series, a statistical association between such a deficiency and features indicative of diminished fetal movement, such as a short umbilical cord, and further correlated this finding with an unduly high incidence of neurological handicap and diminished intelligence in later life. Naeye's suggestion that subchorionic fibrin deposition occurs as a result of damage produced by fetal activity to the trophoblast in the roof of the intervillous space is unconvincing: not only does this seem inherently unlikely but this layer of trophoblast is, in reality, lost at an early stage of gestation and is replaced by fibrinoid material. Whether the association between a lack of subchorionic fibrin and an increased incidence of post-natal handicap is anything more than a statistical quirk will, no doubt, be clarified with the passage of time but it is certainly a feature that should be noted by the pathologist.

Maternal Floor Infarction

This term is applied to an excess deposition of fibrin on the basal plate of the placenta (Benirschke, 1961; Benirschke & Driscoll, 1967). This lesion is not, in any sense of the word, an infarct and a more suitable name would be 'massive basal plate fibrin deposition'. Unfortunately the label of 'maternal floor infarction' has become so deeply embedded in the literature that it would be almost impossible to uproot it: I will therefore use this term, albeit with considerable reluctance. Strictly speaking there is little justification for including this lesion under the heading of 'abnormalities of maternal blood flow' but it seems reasonable to include a discussion of this lesion with those of other patterns of excess fibrin deposition in the inter-villous space.

Macroscopic Appearances

The maternal surface of a placenta with this abnormality has an almost gyriform appearance (Figs 5.10 and 5.11) and appears greyish-yellow. In the sliced placenta the basal plate is seen to be markedly thickened by firm white material which can diminish considerably the height of the intervillous space (Fig. 5.12).

Histology

The lesion consists simply of excess fibrin deposited on the basal plate of the inter-villous space: as the fibrin increases in amount, basally situated villi are often entrapped with the enlarging fibrinous mass and these will undergo the same changes as do those enmeshed in a plaque of massive perivillous fibrin deposition. In many cases there is also extensive perivillous fibrin deposition at sites away from the basal plate.

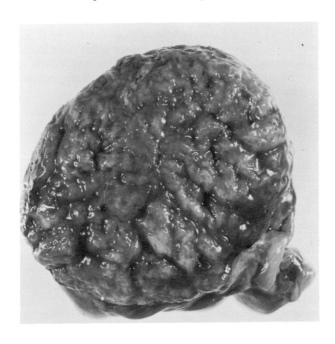

Figure 5.10. Maternal surface of a placenta showing maternal floor infarction.

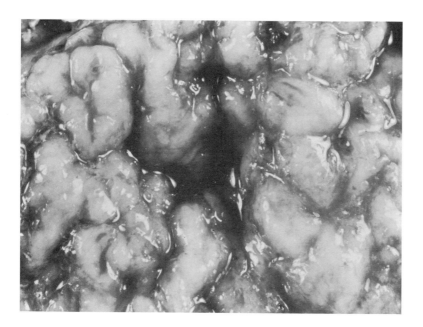

Figure 5.11. A close-up view of the maternal surface of the placenta illustrated in Fig. 5.10.

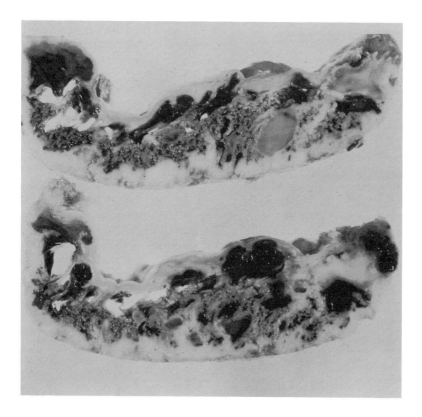

Figure 5.12. A placenta showing marked basal deposition of fibrin, this being an example of maternal floor infarction.

Incidence

Widely divergent views have been expressed about the incidence of maternal floor infarction. Naeye (1985) suggested that this lesion is found in 0.5% of placentas whilst Andres et al (1990) thought that it occurred in only 0.09% of placentas. The findings of Andres et al were based on a study that contained a significant percentage of referral material and are therefore biased: I say this because in my experience the incidence of maternal floor infarction is even less than the figure they obtained and is certainly less than that quoted by Naeye. To a very considerable extent this is a matter of definition: maternal floor infarction has never been defined in precise terms and it is a purely subjective opinion as to the point where an excess of fibrin deposition on the basal plate, which is not uncommon, reaches a sufficiency such that it can be designated as a specific lesion, i.e. maternal floor infarction. There seems to be a definite tendency for this lesion to recur in successive pregnancies (Andres et al, 1990).

Aetiology and Pathogenesis

This is completely unknown. Rushton (1987) has strongly expressed the belief that maternal floor infarction is a change that occurs only after fetal death and, indeed, this was a view to which I previously subscribed. Sufficient cases of maternal floor infarction associated with a live born infant have, however, now been described (Clewell & Manchester, 1983; Katz et al, 1987; Andres et al, 1990; Mandsager et al, 1994) for this view to be no longer tenable, though it is still perfectly possible that in some cases the lesion does develop after fetal death. Naeye (1985) thought that maternal floor infarction was a common end-point of several disorders such as acute chorioamnionitis or diminished decidual blood flow, whilst Benirschke and Kaufmann (1995) consider it to be a specific lesion caused by an abnormal host–placenta interaction, though not necessarily an immunological one. Robb et al (1986a,b) identified, by immunohistochemistry, herpes virus antigen in the basal plate of many placentas with maternal floor infarction: however, there are diagnostic pitfalls in the recognition of herpes virus infection in the gestational uterus (Yokoyama et al, 1993; Sickel & di Sant Agnese, 1994) which had not been recognized at the time of that study and any possible role for herpes virus endometritis in the pathogenesis of maternal floor infarction must remain *sub judice*.

Significance

There has been general agreement that maternal floor infarction is associated with a very high incidence of fetal death and intrauterine growth retardation (Naeye, 1985; Nickel, 1988; Andres et al, 1990; Mandsager et al, 1994) though the reasons for this are far from clear. Gersell (1993) has suggested that the fibrin interferes with the perfusion of the intervillous space by maternal blood, and this is a reasonable hypothesis.

Maternal floor infarction can be recognized ultrasonographically (Mandsager et al, 1994) and may be associated with an elevated level of alpha-fetoprotein (Katz et al, 1987).

Infarct

A placental infarct is a localized area of ischaemic villous necrosis.

Nomenclature

An astonishing number of names have been applied to placental infarcts in the past, their number being a reflection of the irrational attitude that, until relatively recently, was taken to placental pathology. It would be considered extraordinary if an infarct in any other organ, such as the heart or kidney, were encumbered with a similar plethora of largely meaningless synonyms, and it is little wonder that workers in other branches of pathology have looked askance at this sort of nonsense. It cannot be stated too strongly that there is only one type of infarct in the placenta; that this is, as are all other infarcts, an area of ischaemic tissue necrosis; that all other lesions considered to be infarcts have been wrongly classified; and that no other term but 'infarct' is required to describe this lesion.

Macroscopic Features

Infarcts occur in any part of the placental substance but are seen more commonly in the peripheral areas than in the central part. They vary considerably in size, from those measuring only 4 or 5 mm in diameter to others that involve most of the villous tissue. Infarcts are also of variable shape but most are roughly triangular, with the base of the triangle abutting onto the basal plate; less commonly they are ovoid or spherical. It is relatively unusual to see an infarct that is entirely within the placental substance and lacking contact with the basal plate; from the basal plate the infarct may extend to involve the full thickness of the placenta. A fresh infarct is dark red (Fig. 5.13) and often difficult to distinguish on naked-eye examination of the unfixed organ: indeed, if dealing with an unfixed placenta it is usually easier to feel an early infarct, because even the freshest lesion is notably firmer than healthy villous tissue. After formalin fixation it is usually quite easy to visualize a fresh infarct, which is seen to be well demarcated from the surrounding viable tissue and to have a slightly shiny cut surface.

As an infarct ages it becomes progressively firmer and its colour changes successively to brown, yellow and white. Thus the infarct that is about 10 to 14 days old has a firm, brown, slightly waxy, smooth cut surface, whilst one of long-standing appears as a hard, white plaque with a smooth or slightly granular surface (Fig. 5.14).

Histology

An early infarct is characterized by a crowding together, or aggregation, of the villi in the affected area, with an extreme narrowing or even obliteration of the intervillous space (Fig. 5.15). The villous vessels are dilated and congested (Fig. 5.16) and the

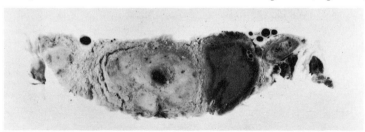

Figure 5.13. A moderately fresh placental infarct. This is dark red, firm and well delineated.

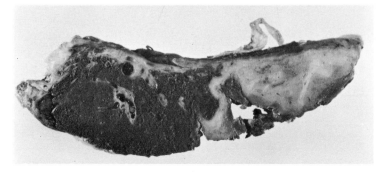

Figure 5.14. An old placental infarct. This is seen as a whitish plaque.

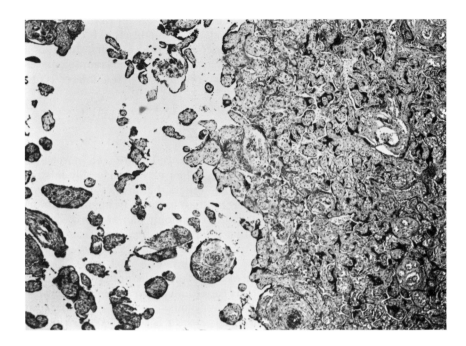

Figure 5.15. Low-power view of the histological appearances of a fresh placental infarct (on the right). The villi are aggregated together and the intervillous space is obliterated (H & E ×50).

syncytial nuclei show varying degrees of pyknosis or karyorrhexis. As the infarct ages the syncytial nuclei fragment and eventually disappear (Fig. 5.17) until the trophoblast is represented only by a thin rim of acidophilic hyaline material around the perimeter of each villus. The fetal erythrocytes trapped in the vessels of the necrotic villi undergo haemolysis and the endothelium of these vessels degenerates. The villous stroma is also degenerate and poorly staining but shows no fibrosis, whilst there is no thickening of the trophoblastic basement membrane and no proliferation of villous cytotrophoblastic cells. This process of coagulative villous necrosis continues until eventually the old

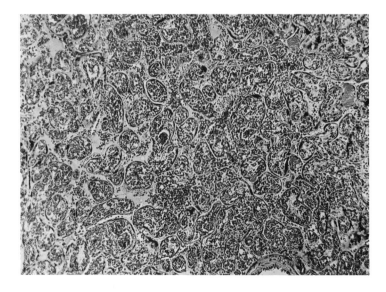

Figure 5.16. Villi in a fresh placental infarct. The villous vessels are congested and widely dilated but there is only minimal evidence of syncytial necrosis (H & E ×125).

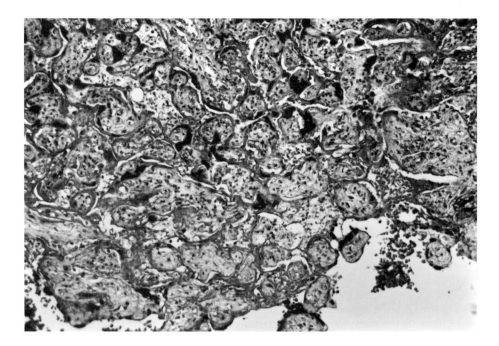

Figure 5.17. Villi in an infarct which is slightly older than that shown in Fig. 5.16. Villous congestion is less obvious and many of the erythrocytes in the fetal vessels have undergone haemolysis. Much of the villous trophoblast is showing necrotic change (H & E ×155).

infarct consists of crowded 'ghost' villi (Fig. 5.18): there is no evidence of any circulation of maternal blood through the narrowed intervillous space but quite often what little is left of this space is obliterated by a thin layer of fibrin, which is probably derived from plasma that has leaked out from the necrotic fetal vessels. There is often some deposition of fibrin around the periphery of the infarct, this being formed from the maternal

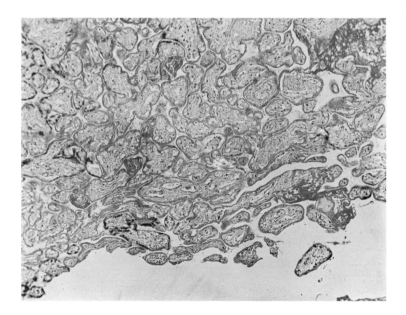

Figure 5.18. Villi in an old placental infarct. These have a 'ghost-like' appearance, whilst the villous trophoblast has undergone complete necrosis and is represented only by a perivillous rim of acidophilic material (H & E ×125).

blood, and there may be a well-marked infiltration with polymorphonuclear leucocytes, which are also derived from maternal blood in the normal areas of the intervillous space; not infrequently, however, this cellular infiltrate is surprisingly scanty or even absent. The fetal stem arteries supplying an area of freshly infarcted villi are usually normal but undergo a progressive sclerosis as the infarct ages.

The basal plate directly underlying an area of infarction may be fully normal but is more commonly necrotic.

Incidence

I have reviewed in the past the various reported studies of the incidence of placental infarction (Fox, 1967b) and there would be little point in repeating this exercise here, because the figures presented a discouraging and chaotic picture, no consensus having been reached on the frequency of infarction either in placentas from normal pregnancies or in those from pregnancies complicated by pre-eclampsia. There has been little or nothing to add since that review.

In my own experience infarcts occur in about a quarter of placentas from full-term uncomplicated pregnancies, and, whilst they are uncommon in placentas from cases of premature onset of labour, they are not found unduly frequently in those from prolonged pregnancies. There is no excess of infarcts in placentas of diabetic women nor in those of patients with materno-fetal rhesus incompatibility, but the incidence of placental infarction is significantly increased in pregnancies in which the mother has suffered from pre-eclampsia or essential hypertension. In these latter circumstances the incidence of infarction is related to the severity of the hypertensive complication, rising from 34% in placentas from women with mild pre-eclampsia to 60% in those from patients with the severe form of the disease, and from 27% in cases of mild essential hypertension to nearly 70% in placentas from severely hypertensive patients (Fox, 1967b).

Of rather more importance than the simple overall incidence is the extent of the infarction. In most placentas that are infarcted less than 5% of the villous tissue is involved in the lesion, or lesions; this is certainly the case in those from uncomplicated pregnancies, in which it is extremely unusual to find infarction involving more than this proportion of the villous parenchyma. Only in placentas from pregnancies complicated by pre-eclampsia or essential hypertension is extensive infarction, i.e. involving more than 5% of the placental tissue, found with any frequency. Infarction of this degree occurs in 30% of placentas from women with severe pre-eclampsia and in two-thirds of placentas from patients with severe essential hypertension; however, in mild pre-eclampsia, extensive placental infarction is found in only 2% of cases, whilst in women with mild essential hypertension this degree of placental infarction occurs in 20%. Extensive infarction has also been described in placentas from patients with anticardiolipin antibodies, but this is a controversial subject, which is discussed in Chapter 8.

Aetiology and Pathogenesis

The villi have a dual blood supply and for many years controversy raged between those who thought that infarction was due to obstruction of the fetal blood flow to the villi and others who maintained that the obstruction was within the maternal utero-placental vessels. The most persistent advocate of the pathogenetic importance of a fetal vascular lesion was Bartholomew, who, with his colleagues, upheld this viewpoint in a series of papers extending over a period of 30 years (Bartholomew and Kracke, 1932; Bartholomew, 1938, 1947; Bartholomew et al, 1957, 1961). He proposed a series of hypothetical aetiological factors, such as thrombosis secondary to trauma inflicted by fetal movements, or acute atherosis of the fetal vessels secondary to maternal hypercholesterolaemia, all of which were based on the assumption that the villi are oxygenated by fetal blood, a view that has become progressively more untenable as evidence has accumulated that the villi receive their oxygen supply from the maternal blood in the intervillous space. Bartholomew was eventually forced to concede that obstruction of a fetal artery could not cause villous infarction, though he was still unable to accept that infarction could result from obstruction to a maternal uteroplacental vessel, pointing out that numerous such vessels open into the lake-like intervillous space and that therefore infarction was most unlikely unless *all* the maternal vessels were occluded. He therefore postulated that infarction is due to an obstruction, caused either by a thrombus or by spasm of a sphincter, in a fetal stem vein, arguing that the resultant congestion and swelling of the villi would result in obliteration of the intervillous space with consequent infarction. This concept won a not inconsiderable degree of support (Hunt et al, 1940; Falkiner, 1942; Dieckmann, 1952; Steigrad, 1952; Thomsen, 1954; Gregor, 1961; Becker, 1963), whilst Roig (1963) went so far as to claim that the venous obstruction occurred not in the placental fetal vessels but in the umbilical veins as a result of knotting of the cord.

This theory of fetal venous obstruction later fell into disrepute, partly because venous lesions, if occurring in association with an infarct, appear clearly to be a secondary phenomenon, and partly because the view that the villi are immersed in a pool of blood into which numerous arterial inlets flow is now known to be functionally incorrect. There are, it is true, no preformed vascular pathways in the intervillous space, but nevertheless the haemodynamics of the maternal uteroplacental circulation are such that there is little or no mixing of the separate inflow streams from the individual arterioles (Ramsey, 1965). These vessels can therefore be considered as 'end arteries' and there is no theoretical reason why occlusion of such an arteriole should not result in villous infarction. Indeed, during the last 30 years it has become generally accepted that most placental infarcts are due to thrombotic occlusion of a maternal uteroplacental vessel (Fig. 5.19), a minority being secondary to a retroplacental haematoma which strips the placenta away from its supplying maternal arterioles (Zeek & Assali, 1952; Shanklin, 1959; Little, 1960; Huber et al, 1961; Fox, 1963, 1967b; Wilkin, 1965; Philippe, 1966; Littmann, 1968; Wallenburg, 1968; Wigglesworth, 1969; Kérisit & Toulouse, 1970a; Brosens & Renaer, 1972; Wallenburg et al, 1973; Nessman-Emmanuelli, 1974). Recently, however, McDermott and Gillan (1995a) have suggested that there may be a disturbance in both fetal and maternal blood flow in placental infarction. They argue that vasoconstriction of a maternal vessel will lead to slowing, and eventual thrombosis, in the villi supplied by that maternal vessel and that later thrombosis of the maternal vessel will cause infarction in the villi that have been devitalized by loss of their fetal circulation. An obvious objection to this argument is that the uteroplacental vesssels are incapable of constricting whilst villi that have been clearly deprived of their fetal circulation, as in a fetal artery thrombosis, show no signs of infarction. Further, one has only to look at an early infarct to recognize the marked

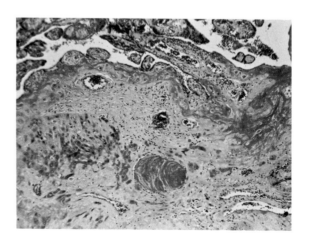

Figure 5.19. A thrombosed maternal vessel in the placental basal plate; this was immediately below an area of placental infarction (H & E ×56).

congestion and dilatation of the villous vessels. It is true that there is a secondary sclerosis of the fetal stem arteries supplying an area of infarcted villi, but I do not regard this as a primary event.

Stark and Kaufmann (1974) and Kaufmann (1975) proposed that infarction may be secondary to a primary degenerative change in the villous syncytiotrophoblast; they suggest that a block in the Embden–Meyerhof cycle leads to swelling and necrosis of the syncytium, with the formation of polypoid masses of degenerate trophoblast and secondary arrest of the maternal circulation. I have to confess to not being able to understand fully this hypothesis and it would seem difficult to accept that a metabolic disturbance should affect only a localized area of villous tissue.

Significance

There can be no doubt that the commonly occurring minor degree of placental infarction (i.e. involving less than 5% of the parenchyma) is of no clinical significance. On the other hand, extensive placental infarction is associated with a high incidence of fetal hypoxia, intrauterine growth retardation and death (Kloosterman & Huidekoper, 1952, 1954; Little, 1960; Wigglesworth, 1964; Fox, 1967b). At first sight it appears obvious that these effects on fetal well-being are a direct result of the loss of viable villous tissue and, indeed, it is this apparent influence of placental infarction that has led to the view that the placenta has little or no functional reserve capacity. It will, however, be recalled that a similar, or greater, loss of villi resulting from their entrapment in fibrin is of no consequence, and this appears to point to a paradox, villous loss due to infarction being of serious import and that due to perivillous fibrin being innocuous. The paradox is, however, a false one because, as already pointed out, the placenta has a considerable functional reserve capacity and can easily withstand the loss of 15–20% of its villous tissue as a result of ischaemic necrosis. Infarction of this degree indicates, however, that there must be extensive and widespread thrombosis of maternal vessels, an event one would not expect in a healthy vascular tree. It is, therefore, no coincidence that extensive infarction is virtually confined to pregnancies complicated by pre-eclampsia or pregnancy-induced hypertension, because it is only in these conditions that significant abnormalities of the maternal uteroplacental vasculature are found (see Chapter 6) and in which widespread thrombosis and extensive infarction occur as a consequence. Extensive placental infarction is therefore the visible hallmark of a grossly abnormal vascular tree and of a severely compromised maternal uteroplacental circulation, and it is these factors that are the true cause of the apparent effects of placental infarction on fetal growth and well-being rather than the simple destruction of villous tissue. This is not, of course, to say that the situation is not further worsened by the infarction being superimposed on a placenta, the functional reserve of which has been already dissipated by uteroplacental ischaemia, but the infarction per se is not the primary cause of the fetal abnormalities.

LESIONS DUE TO DISTURBANCES OF FETAL BLOOD FLOW

Fetal Artery Thrombosis

Thrombotic occlusion of a fetal villous stem artery produces a sharply delineated area of villous avascularity.

Macroscopic Features

The lesion appears as a roughly triangular and well-delineated area of pallor within the placental substance, with its base abutting onto the basal plate (Fig. 5.20). There is no alteration in consistence or texture and the normal 'pile' of the cut surface of the placenta is retained. An area of pallor of this type is fairly easily seen in the fixed organ but is very difficult to detect in the unfixed placenta. Localized areas of pallor

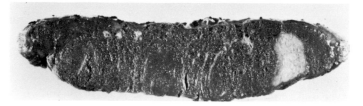

Figure 5.20. A localized area of pallor in a placenta, which is due to a fetal artery thrombosis.

may also be due to focal villous oedema, focal villous immaturity or a fixation artefact, but in such cases the pallid zone usually lacks the characteristic shape of the lesion resulting from a fetal artery thrombosis.

Histology

Microscopic examination reveals a sharply demarcated area of avascular villi (Fig. 5.21) the appearance of which is usually in stark contrast to that of the immediately adjacent vascularized villi (Fig. 5.22). The intervillous space is normally patent and contains maternal blood; there is no compression of villi or perivillous deposition of fibrin. The syncytiotrophoblast of the avascular villi is intact and usually shows a markedly excessive formation of syncytial knots; however, there is no proliferation of the cytotrophoblastic cells of the villi. The trophoblastic basement membrane is of normal thickness, whilst the villous stroma has, when stained by haematoxylin and eosin, a glazed, hyaline, pink appearance; trichrome stains show a greatly excessive amount of stromal fibrous tissue. There may be linear deposition of haemosiderin on the trophoblastic basement membrane of many of the avascular villi (Fig. 5.23) whilst some may show small specks of haemosiderin within the villous stroma (McDermott & Gillan, 1995b). Although most of the affected villi are avascular it is possible to distinguish, in a proportion, small, empty, constricted or sclerosed fetal vessels.

It has been my experience that in all instances it is possible to detect a thrombosed large fetal stem artery at the apex of the avascular area, the thrombus usually showing some degree of organization and even recanalization (Fig. 5.24). Detection of such a thrombus may require serial sectioning and hence in a single section the occluding

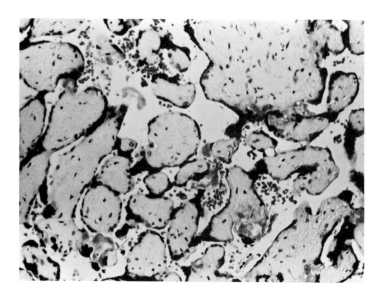

Figure 5.21. Avascular villi resulting from a fetal artery thrombosis (H & E ×125).

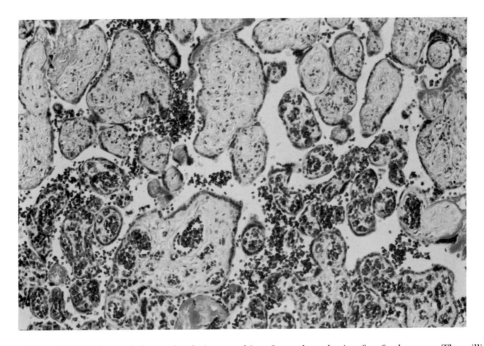

Figure 5.22. The periphery of a lesion resulting from thrombosis of a fetal artery. The villi rendered avascular as a result of the arterial occlusion (above) contrast sharply with the immediately adjacent fully vascularized villi (below) (H & E ×125).

thrombus may not be apparent (McDermott & Gillan, 1995b; Redline & Pappin, 1995). The stem vessels distal to the occlusion show a well-marked fibromuscular sclerosis: however, this is absent from fresh lesions and its severity is directly related to the age of the thrombus, its appearance being a secondary change (see Chapter 6). McDermott and Gillan (1995a) have proffered the hypothesis that the lesion described by me as a fetal artery thrombosis is actually secondary to a diminished maternal blood flow with

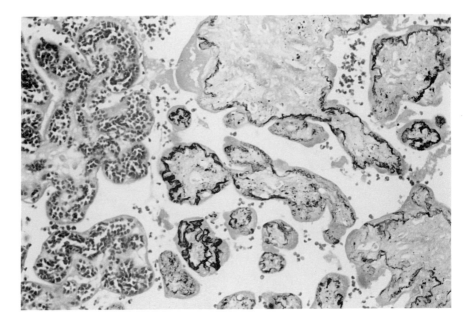

Figure 5.23. Photomicrograph of avascular villi resulting from a fetal artery thrombosis: there is mineralization of the trophoblastic basement membrane of these villi (Perls ×40).

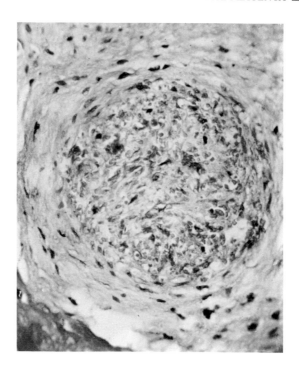

Figure 5.24. An organizing thrombus in a fetal stem artery (H & E ×200).

slowing, and eventual thrombosis, of blood in the fetal vasculature. If this was the case it would be expected that the lesion would be seen with undue frequency in placentas from women with pre-eclampsia: this is not the case.

Incidence

In my own series a single fetal artery thrombosis was present in 4.5% of placentas from full-term uncomplicated pregnancies. The only maternal factor that was associated with an increased frequency of this lesion was diabetes mellitus, because in placentas from diabetic women the incidence was approximately 10% (Fox, 1966b). There was a relatively high incidence of this lesion in placentas from stillbirths (14%) and it was notable that in all such instances the thrombi were multiple (the significance of this finding is discussed below).

Very little information is available from other sources as to the incidence of this lesion, though Driscoll (1965) has mentioned that thrombotic occlusion of fetal vessels is seen in some placentas from diabetic women. Redline and Pappin (1995) noted an incidence of between 3 and 10 per 1000 placentas.

Aetiology and Pathogenesis

The thrombi are usually found in otherwise normal fetal arteries and there are no obvious local factors that predispose to their formation. The increased incidence of this lesion in maternal diabetes mellitus is of some interest because Takeuchi and Benirschke (1961) have pointed out that renal vein thrombosis is found unduly frequently in autopsy studies of infants of diabetic mothers and have suggested that there may be a special tendency towards thrombosis in such infants. Kraus (1993) and Rayne and Kraus (1993) have noted an association between fetal artery thrombi and maternal coagulation disorders, such as positive cardiolipin antibodies, HELLP syndrome and Protein C deficiency, and have suggested that in some cases there may be a fetal coagulation disorder; a similar link with maternal coagulopathies was noted by Redline and Pappin (1995).

Significance

The villi rendered avascular by a fetal artery thrombosis are of no physiological value to the fetus and thus there is a reduction in the population of functioning villi. As has been previously discussed, the placenta can, in the presence of an unimpaired maternal circulation, withstand with ease the loss of up to 30% of its villi and it is therefore not surprising that thrombosis of a single fetal artery is of no significance in terms of placental function, as such a lesion will deprive no more than about 5% of the villi of their blood supply. Multiple thrombi are, however, more important and I have seen several placentas from fresh stillbirths in which between 40 and 50% of the villi were deprived of their fetal blood supply by thrombotic occlusion of many stem arteries. The presence of some degree of organization within the thrombi indicated that they antedated fetal death and it would not be unreasonable to assume that the functional loss of this considerable proportion of the villous population was of importance in causing fetal demise. Redline and Pappin (1995) have also noted that multiple thrombi, depriving more than 30% of the villous population of their fetal blood supply, were associated with an adverse fetal outcome. It should be stressed, however, that multiple lesions of this type occur only exceptionally.

Kraus (1993) and Rayne and Kraus (1993) have stressed that thrombosis within the placenta may be a marker for thrombosis elsewhere in the fetal vascular system and that there may be accompanying fetal brain lesions due to cerebral thrombi, a view with which Redline and Pappin (1995) concur. Nevertheless most infants whose placentas contain a fetal arterial thrombus appear to be perfectly healthy.

THROMBI AND HAEMATOMAS (Fig. 5.25)

Massive Subchorial Thrombosis

This lesion, also known as a Breus' mole, is a red thrombus that measures more than 1 cm in thickness and which separates the chorionic plate from the underlying villous tissue over much of its area.

Macroscopic Appearances

Massive subchorial thrombi are often bulbous or lobulated and tend to elevate and distort the fetal surface of the placenta by forming bulging protuberances into the amniotic cavity (Fig. 5.26). On cutting the placenta, thick nodular masses of red thrombus are seen and these appear to strip off the chorionic plate from the underlying villous tissue. The thrombus is not invariably nodular and may form a single smooth mass (Fig. 5.27). Sometimes the thrombus extends deeply into the parenchyma and may even reach the basal plate to form what is, in effect, a transplacental thrombosis.

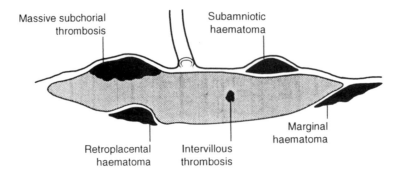

Figure 5.25. Diagram of the sites of the various haematomas and thrombi that can occur in or around the placenta.

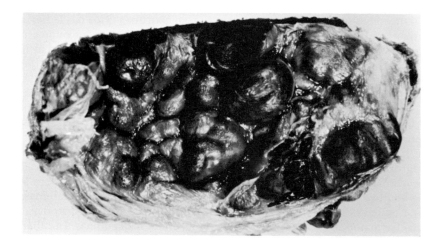

Figure 5.26. Fetal surface of a placenta in which there is a massive subchorial thrombus. The thrombus is elevating the chorionic plate to form multiple tuberous projections.

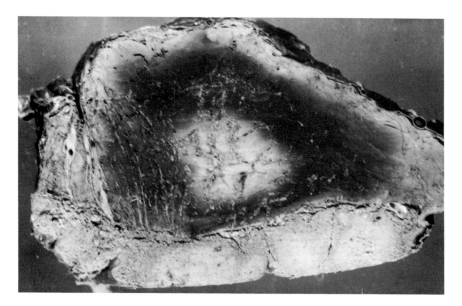

Figure 5.27. A massive subchorial thrombus. The chorionic plate is seen above and is completely stripped from the villous tissue, which is seen at the bottom of the illustration, by a massive accumulation of thrombus.

Histology

The lesion consists solely of laminated thrombus and no villi are included within it. The thrombus may be confined to the subchorionic space but not infrequently extends into and dissects the chorionic plate.

Incidence

It is extremely difficult to determine the frequency of this lesion for several reasons, prime amongst which is the assumption, either stated or implied both in Breus' (1892) original description and in many subsequent reports or studies, that a massive subchorial thrombosis is found only in placentas from abortuses. This has led to a reluctance to diagnose this entity in placentas from advanced pregnancies or live infants, and it was only relatively recently that Shanklin and Scott (1975) showed that massive subchorial thrombosis does occur in such placentas, with a frequency that they estimated as being in the region of 1 in 2000 deliveries. Furthermore, even in abortion material the true incidence of massive subchorial thrombi is difficult to define and there must be some doubt as to whether all the lesions thus designated merit this diagnosis.

The literature on this topic is further confounded by confusion as to what constitutes a subchorial haematoma or thrombus. Thus in a recent review of this topic a subchorionic haematoma was defined as 'a separation of the chorionic plate from the underlying decidua with a resultant collection of blood between the chorion and decidua' (Pearlstone & Baxi, 1993): I am far from sure what these authors were actually discussing but they certainly were not discussing massive subchorial haematomas. Some of the papers cited in this confusing review refer to retroplacental haematomas, others to marginal haematomas and yet others to true subchorial haematomas. In other ultrasonographic studies the term 'subchorionic haemorrhage' has been applied quite specifically to marginal haematomas occurring in the early stages of pregnancy (Kaufman et al, 1985; Sauerbrei & Pham, 1986; Abu-Yousef et al, 1987; Pedersen & Mantoni, 1990), a lesion that is quite different from a true subchorial thrombosis.

It has been suggested that small subchorial thrombi are more common than is generally realized and are often missed or ignored (Linthwaite, 1963). In my opinion, however, it is impossible for a *massive* subchorial thrombus to be small, and no continuous spectrum exists between the small focus of laminated subchorial thrombus, which is the precursor of a laminated plaque of subchorionic fibrin, and the massive thrombus which strips off the chorionic plate. The two conditions do not merge into each other, are readily distinguishable, and are almost certainly of differing pathogenesis.

Aetiology and Pathogenesis

These are as yet ill defined. Many have agreed with Breus that the thrombosis is a consequence of fetal death, but Shanklin and Scott (1975) disposed of this theory by their demonstration of massive subchorial thrombi in placentas from live-born infants. Other suggested aetiological factors have included an excessively deep implantation of the fertilized ovum (Torpin, 1960; Thomas, 1964), rupture of a fetal chorionic artery (Philippe, 1966; Kérisit & Toulouse, 1970b), and obstruction of the decidual veins by deposition of a thick layer of fibrinoid material (Levy, 1956). None of these is particularly convincing and I would agree with Shanklin and Scott that the blood in the thrombus is maternal in origin though Ho (1983) did describe a massive subchorial haematoma that contained a large number of nucleated red blood cells. It is probable that a massive lesion of this type is due to a sudden and marked slowing of the blood flow through the intervillous space, and the most likely cause of such a haemodynamic change is an extensive obliteration of the venous channels draining the space, a view first proposed by Hart (1902). This concept is, at the moment, entirely speculative and there are no clues available as to the factor, or factors, that might predispose to or cause a venous obstruction of this type.

Significance

This is hard to assess and whether or not a lesion of this type can lead to abortion is a moot point, though the presently available evidence suggests that it may be of some importance in this respect. Too little is known about the functional significance of a massive subchorial thrombus in placentas from advanced pregnancies for any definite conclusions to be drawn, but in Shanklin and Scott's (1975) study of 10 cases, the child was born alive in seven and survived the neonatal period in three. The thrombus is usually fresh and this suggests that the lesion predisposes to the onset of labour, often prematurely.

Retroplacental Haematoma

This is a haematoma that lies between, and separates, the basal plate of the placenta and the uterine wall (Fig. 5.25).

Macroscopic Features

A retroplacental haematoma may be large and occupy most, or even all, of the maternal surface of the placenta; lesions of this magnitude are usually readily apparent. However, it is not widely realized that many retroplacental haematomas are small, often measuring only 1 or 2 cm across; these are more easily visualized in the sliced placenta, where they are seen to be bulging up towards the chorionic plate and compressing the overlying placental parenchyma, which is often, but not always, infarcted (Figs 5.28 and 5.29). The freshly formed haematoma is soft, red and easily separated from the maternal placental surface; such detachment occurs not infrequently during delivery, under which circumstances the previous presence of a haematoma may be deduced from a crateriform depression in the maternal surface. The older haematoma is brown, hard and firmly adherent to the placental surface; it may appear to blend with, and be difficult to distinguish from, an overlying infarct and may thus be easily overlooked.

A retroplacental haematoma has to be distinguished from a simple adherent blood clot, a task that is usually not difficult, because the clot is easily stripped from the maternal surface and does not indent the placental substance.

Histology

In the early stages a retroplacental haematoma consists solely of red blood cells with only a few strands of fibrin, but as the lesion ages the erythrocytes degenerate and fibrin appears in increasing amounts. Many haematomas are infiltrated by polymorphonuclear leucocytes and macrophages, and, whilst the overlying basal plate may appear normal (Fig. 5.30), it is more often necrotic and heavily infiltrated by polymorphonuclear leucocytes (Fig. 5.31). In the later stages, haemosiderin-laden macrophages are commonly seen in the basal plate. Occasionally the basal plate ruptures and the haematoma comes into direct contact with the villous tissue. The

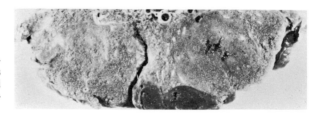

Figure 5.28. A small retroplacental haematoma which is indenting the overlying placental parenchyma: the latter is, however, not infarcted.

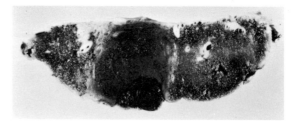

Figure 5.29. A small retroplacental haematoma which has caused infarction of the overlying placental tissue.

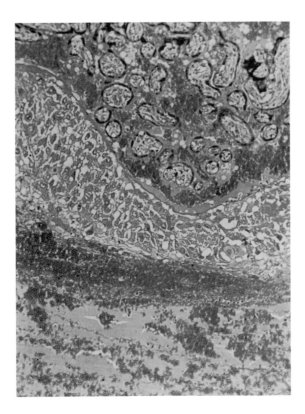

Figure 5.30. Histological appearances of a retroplacental haematoma (below). The overlying basal plate is healthy and the villi at this site are not infarcted (H & E ×100).

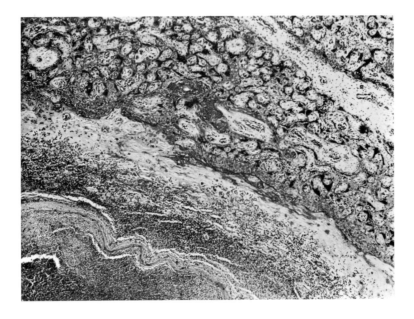

Figure 5.31. A retroplacental haematoma (below and to the left) which has caused infarction of the overlying villous tissue (above and to the right). The intervening basal plate is necrotic and infiltrated by polymorphonuclear leucocytes (H & E ×45).

directly overlying villous tissue is often infarcted, whilst Mooney et al (1994) have described diffuse haemorrhage into the stroma of villi adjacent to, or overlying the margin of, the retroplacental haematoma.

Incidence

Wilkin (1965) found retroplacental haematomas in 4.5% of all placentas and my own figure for the incidence of this lesion would be approximately the same (Fox, 1966a) as would that of Benirschke and Gille (1977). In my series the incidence was increased approximately threefold in placentas from women with pre-eclampsia, but it was not excessive in those from patients with essential hypertension. It is important to note that in women with a clinical history of abruptio placentae, it is usual to find retroplacental haematomas in no more than about 30% of their placentas, whilst, conversely, if a retroplacental haematoma is present there will be clinical evidence of abruptio placentae in only about 35% of cases.

Aetiology and Pathogenesis

The pathogenesis of retroplacental bleeding is still far from clear. It is quite certain that basal plate necrosis and villous infarction are a consequence and not a cause of the placental bleeding, but little else about this lesion allows for equal dogmatism. It would be a majority opinion that the haemorrhage is due to the rupture of a maternal decidual arteriole, it being assumed that this catastrophe occurs in a vessel the wall of which is weakened because of the changes that occur in pre-eclampsia (McKelvey, 1939; Sexton et al, 1950; van den Ende, 1959; Brosens, 1963, 1964; Marais, 1963; Renaer and Brosens, 1963). Retroplacental haematomas are, however, by no means confined to pregnancies complicated by pre-eclampsia and retroplacental bleeding may occur in patients whose decidual arterioles are perfectly normal. Egley and Cefalo (1985) suggested, as an alternative, that the process of abruption begins with uterine vasospasm, which is followed by relaxation, venous engorgement and subsequent arteriolar rupture: this is an unlikely hypothesis if only because the uteroplacental vessels, which lack a muscular wall, are incapable of undergoing vasospasm. It should be noted that only Boe (1959) has published a convincing photomicrograph of a ruptured, but otherwise normal, maternal arteriole in association with a retroplacental haematoma. Certainly, I have never been able to show that a ruptured arteriole was the cause of a retroplacental haematoma, but this is hardly surprising in view of the amount of tissue damage and distortion that is usually all too apparent in the vicinity of a haematoma.

Domisse and Tiltman (1992) performed placental bed biopsies in women who had suffered an abruption and claim to have detected abnormal, malformed vessels in the myometrium. They attributed the bleeding to rupture of such a vessel: this finding requires confirmation.

A less popular view is that obstruction of the venous outflow from the placenta is the basic pathogenetic factor in retroplacental bleeding, this hypothesis being based on experimental and clinical evidence (considered below) and lacking pathological support. Venous rupture has never been demonstrated and it has been my experience that, whilst thrombosis of a maternal draining vein is not uncommonly found in close approximation to an old retroplacental haematoma, such a lesion is never seen in association with fresh haematomas; this indicates that venous thrombosis is a secondary rather than a primary change.

A further suggestion has been that the initial event is not retroplacental haemorrhage with subsequent placental separation but rather primary placental separation with consequent retroplacental bleeding, the premature detachment being attributed to a 'faulty chorio-decidual relationship' at the time of implantation (Hibbard & Jeffcoate, 1966). This argument, based solely upon circumstantial evidence, has failed to win support.

The aetiology of retroplacental bleeding is equally uncertain and it has to be stressed that most discussions of the aetiology of this condition are actually concerned with the aetiological factors implicated in abruptio placentae. It is true that there is an overlap between the pathological syndrome of premature separation of the normally implanted placenta, of which a retroplacental haematoma is the visible hallmark, and the clinical syndrome of abruptio placentae. It is, however, equally true that abruptio placentae is a dramatic clinical event which is usually followed rapidly by delivery of the fetus and which often does not leave any pathological imprint on the placenta, whilst premature separation with retroplacental haematoma formation rarely causes clinical symptoms (Gruenwald et al, 1968) even when the haematoma is very large (Schwick et al, 1992). The only justification for considering abruptio placentae and premature separation together is the overlap already mentioned, which suggests that an episode of premature separation can occur in several bouts and that one of these may eventually result in abruption.

The aetiology of abruptio placentae, and hence, by implication, possibly also of retroplacental haematoma, is discussed fully in standard obstetrical texts and will be considered here only in outline:

1. *Maternal hypertension and pre-eclampsia.* At one time it was thought that abruptio placentae was an integral part of the pre-eclamptic process and did not occur in the absence of this condition (Bartholomew et al, 1953; Fish, 1955). This would now be regarded as an extreme view, but in most reviews of abruptio placentae a high proportion of the affected patients have been suffering from pre-eclampsia (Daro et al, 1956; Bevis, 1958; Vermelin & Braye, 1958; Hsu et al, 1960; Soferman et al, 1963; Abdella et al, 1984; Spinillo et al, 1994). On the other hand, in a few series the proportion of patients with pre-eclampsia has been low (Kimbrough, 1959; Hendelman & Fraser, 1960), and Hibbard and Jeffcoate (1966) have postulated that in many instances hypertension, oedema and albuminuria appear after the placental separation and are a result rather than a cause of the retroplacental bleeding. Pritchard et al (1970) point out, with some justification, that if this were the case, similar changes might be expected to occur after bleeding from a placenta praevia or ruptured tubal pregnancy and that this is not the case.

   Williams et al (1991b) found that although essential hypertension was associated with a high risk of abruptio placentae this was not the case for pre-eclampsia. This is in approximate accord with the findings of Abdella et al (1984) who noted that the incidence of abruption in patients with pre-eclampsia was 2.5% whilst the incidence in women with essential hypertension was 10%; in that study the highest incidence of abruption was in women with eclampsia, 23.6% of whom suffered this complication.

   This whole question has not yet been settled, but I would think it fair to say that, whilst there seems little doubt that the frequency of both abruptio placentae and retroplacental haematoma formation are increased in patients with either pre-eclampsia or essential hypertension, many examples of each condition occur in women without these diseases. An interesting point is that in one study the administration of aspirin to primigravid patients lowered the incidence of pre-eclampsia but increased that of abruptio placentae (Sibai et al, 1993).

2. *Obstruction to the venous drainage of the placental site.* Obstruction of the inferior vena cava by ligation in dogs and by manual compression in humans has been reported to cause placental separation (Howard et al, 1953; Mengert et al, 1953), and there have been isolated case reports of placental separation following antenatal examination in the supine position (Smith & Fields, 1958). Burchell and Mengert (1969) have suggested that venous obstruction may also result from natural compression of the veins by gravity when the uterus sinks low in the pelvis or by accordion-like compression of the lower uterine segment.

3. *The role of folate deficiency.* Hibbard and his colleagues (Hibbard & Hibbard, 1963; Hibbard, 1964; Hibbard & Jeffcoate, 1966; Hibbard et al, 1969) enthusiastically espoused the view that there is a causal relationship between folate deficiency and abruptio placentae. Their claims, however, have not withstood the tests of time and critical scientific scrutiny (Menon et al, 1966; Thanbu & Llewellyn-Jones, 1966; Hall, 1972) and this seductively attractive hypothesis would today have relatively little or no support.

4. *Cocaine usage.* It has been claimed that there is very strong evidence that cocaine usage during pregnancy is associated with a markedly increased incidence of abruptio placentae (Acker et al, 1983; Cohen et al, 1991; Dombrowski et al, 1991; Handler et al, 1991; Flowers et al, 1991; Slutsker, 1992; Dusick et al, 1993; Burkett et al, 1994; Miller et al, 1995). In many of these studies, however, confounding factors have not been adequately taken into account (Richardson et al, 1993). Benirschke and Kaufmann (1995) have also expressed some scepticism about this association, partly on the grounds that it is not known if the abruptio in such cases is related to chorioamnionitis or not (a valid point) and partly because the spiral arteries cannot undergo cocaine-induced vasoconstriction. It has to be borne in mind, however, that the placenta possesses specific high affinity binding sites for cocaine (Ahmed et al, 1990) and appears to be a target organ for this drug, which inhibits the placental serotonin transporter (Prasad et al, 1994): the consequences of reduced clearance of serotonin from the intervillous space are somewhat obscure but clearly potentially significant.

5. *Cigarette smoking* during pregnancy has been associated with an increased incidence of abruptio placentae in most (Naeye, 1980; Brink & Odendall, 1987; Voigt et al, 1990; Eriksen et al, 1991; Williams et al, 1991a; Raymond & Mills, 1993; Spinillo et al, 1994) but not all studies.

6. An increased incidence of abruptio placentae has been noted in women with *anticardiolipin antibodies* (De Carolis et al, 1994)

7. *Blunt trauma to the abdomen* can, perhaps not unexpectedly, cause abruptio placentae (Ribe et al, 1993; Towery et al, 1993).

8. Claims that *chorioamnionitis* is associated with an increased incidence of abruptio placentae (Darby et al, 1989) have to be set against findings of a lack of association between these two conditions (Woods et al, 1986). Placental abruption associated with chorioamnionitis has been attributed to bacterial colonization of the decidua with resultant inflammation (Darby et al, 1989).

Significance

The significance of a retroplacental haematoma is largely dependent on its size because small lesions are of no importance, whether or not they are accompanied by infarction. Large haematomas, however, may be responsible for causing an extensive area of infarction by separating a considerable proportion of the overlying villi from the maternal blood vessels, and here the functionally significant and important lesion is the infarct rather than the haematoma. The effects of placental infarction are discussed in an earlier section of this chapter, but it should be noted that if the haematoma occurs in the course of an otherwise normal pregnancy the placenta is able to suffer quite extensive infarction, involving 20–25% of the villous parenchyma, without there being any serious consequences for the fetus. Many retroplacental haematomas occur in pregnancies complicated by pre-eclampsia, however, and here the functional reserve capacity of the placenta has already been much diminished by the uteroplacental ischaemia that is an integral part of that condition. Under these circumstances a further loss of functional tissue by extensive infarction as a result of a large haematoma may compromise placental function to the extent that it fails to provide the fetus with an adequate supply of oxygen and nutrients. A huge retroplacental haematoma will cause fetal embarrassment even if it develops in an otherwise uncomplicated gestation. Such a lesion, involving more than 40% of the maternal surface, will deprive a sufficient proportion of the villi of their oxygen supply to dissipate even an uncompromised placental reserve capacity and it would be unreasonable to expect that the abrupt loss of 40–50% of the functioning villi could occur without resultant fetal hypoxia and, not uncommonly, death. Massive haematomas of this type are, however, distinctly uncommon.

Quite apart from the possible effects on fetal well-being, abruptio placentae is often complicated by a consumption coagulopathy, probably due to disseminated intravascular coagulation, in the mother; however, this is rarely seen in the much less dramatic circumstances of premature separation with retroplacental haematoma formation.

Marginal Haematoma

This is a haematoma that is formed at the lateral margin of the placenta (Fig. 5.25). In the ultrasound literature this lesion is referred to as a subchorionic haemorrhage.

Macroscopic Features

When the placenta is intact a marginal haematoma is seen as a crescentic thrombus at one placental margin; this often extends out below, and is adherent to, the maternal surface of the membranes (Fig. 5.32). The haematoma may also spread out for a little distance as a thin layer on the maternal surface of an adjacent maternal lobe. When the placenta is sliced the haematoma usually appears roughly triangular, with the base of the triangle in the plane of the basal plate of the placenta, the sides formed by the membranes and by the lateral placental margin, and the apex in the angle formed by the reflection of the membranes from the placental circumference. Any haematoma that extends onto the maternal surface of the placenta does not indent the basal plate, a feature that distinguishes this lesion from a true retroplacental haematoma.

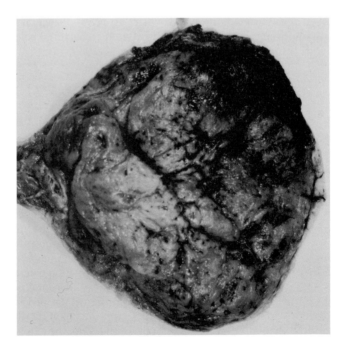

Figure 5.32. A marginal haematoma (above and to the right) which is extending onto the maternal surface of the placenta.

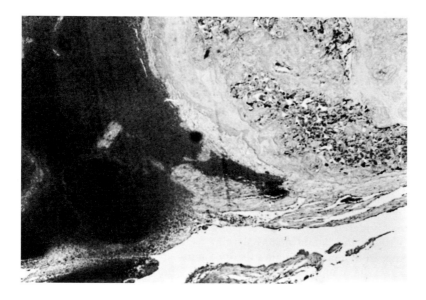

Figure 5.33. Histological appearances of a marginal haematoma. The intact lateral margin of the placenta is seen separating the haematoma from the villous tissue (H & E ×32).

Histology

Microscopy reveals a simple haematoma, usually with a moderate amount of fibrin formation and some leucocyte and macrophage infiltration: in long-standing haematomas deposits of haemosiderin may be seen in the surrounding tissue. Histological examination confirms that the coagulum lies outside the intact lateral wall of the placenta (Fig. 5.33) and thus enables one to differentiate the lesion from thrombosis of maternal blood in the lateral angle of the placenta. Microscopy also allows for the differentiation, not always easily made on naked-eye examination, between a marginal haematoma and thrombosis of a large marginal decidual venous sinus.

Incidence

Wilkin (1965) noted marginal haematomas in 0.74% of placentas. In a personal study of 715 placentas I found this lesion in 14 (1.9%): there was no association with maternal pre-eclampsia and in only three cases was there a history of antepartum haemorrhage.

Aetiology and Pathogenesis

Until relatively recently a marginal haematoma was thought to result from rupture of the placental marginal sinus. This concept grew out of Spanner's (1935) claim to have demonstrated that the sole route of venous drainage from the intervillous space was via a large marginal sinus. Rupture of this sinus was seized upon as an explanation for many cases of antepartum haemorrhage of obscure origin, and marginal sinus bleeding was rapidly elevated to the status of a clinical syndrome, the pathological stigma of which was a marginal haematoma (Fish et al, 1951; Harris, 1952; Ferguson, 1955; Fish, 1960; Schneider, 1958).

It is now realized that the marginal sinus, as described by Spanner, does not exist (Ramsey, 1956a,b; Boyd & Hamilton, 1970); there is, it is true, a peripheral area in the intervillous space in which villi are rather scanty, but there is no limited or defined venous sinus. As a non-existent sinus cannot rupture, the concept of marginal sinus bleeding has now been firmly placed in the already well-stocked repository of abandoned medical theories.

Wilkin and Picard (1961) and Wilkin (1965) produced persuasive evidence that marginal bleeding occurs in placentas that are partially implanted in the inferior segment of the uterus, the lateral margin of the placenta being, however, some distance from the internal os, i.e. in cases of lateral placenta praevia. This view was based on their finding that in cases of marginal bleeding in which the membranes were complete and the site of membrane rupture could be determined, the haematoma was always at that margin of the placenta nearest to the site of membrane rupture; furthermore, in such cases the distance between the free margin of the membranes and the lateral margin of the placenta was always less than 10 cm. These workers suggested, therefore, that the bleeding was due to rupture of uteroplacental veins at the margin of the placenta, consequent upon the partial separation of the spongy and compact layers of decidua produced by the traction of myometrial fibres during the obliteration of the inferior segment. Harris (1985, 1988) has, however, disagreed with this view because in his series of cases of marginal bleeding, lateral placenta praevia was excluded by ultrasound examination. He considered the marginal bleeding to be due to increased venous pressure in patients in whom the lateral maternal veins were unduly large, a theory that I find unconvincing. In defence of Wilkin's theory I must say that the only one of my cases in which the exact site of implantation was known was indeed a lateral placenta praevia.

Significance

A marginal haematoma may, of course, be associated with antepartum maternal haemorrhage and, in my experience, is not of any consequence for the fetus. Harris (1985, 1988) has, however, disputed this and has claimed that there is a significant relationship between marginal haematomas and premature onset of labour, arguing that extravasation of blood at the margin dissects the membranes from their decidual relationship with consequent membrane necrosis and premature rupture. The extent of membrane separation from the decidua in cases of marginal haematoma is, however, slight and, whilst accepting that Harris' findings require confirmation, I find myself unable to accept his hypothesis.

It should be noted that these remarks refer to marginal haematomas detected in placentas from third-trimester deliveries. Ultrasound studies have focused on marginal haematomas which have formed during early pregnancy and which are associated with first-trimester vaginal bleeding. There have been conflicting views about the significance of these early marginal haematomas, some finding such lesions to be associated with a high incidence of abortion and premature labour (Mantoni & Pedersen, 1981; Sauerbrei & Phan, 1986; Abu-Yousef et al, 1987) and others noting a favourable outcome in most cases (Goldstein et al, 1983; Kaufman et al, 1985; Stabile et al, 1989; Pedersen & Mantoni, 1990).

Intervillous Thrombi

These are villous-free nodular foci of coagulated blood in the intervillous space (Fig. 5.25). Some have classified these lesions as haematomas; nevertheless the lesions are entirely within the intervillous space, which can be considered as part of the vascular system, and hence can only logically be considered as thrombi. It has to be admitted, however, that they do not fulfil all the criteria usually required for the definition of a thrombus, the most notable deficiency being the absence of platelets.

Macroscopic Features

An intervillous thrombus is usually approximately round or oval and can occur in any part of the placental substance; a minority are in contact with the basal plate. There may be only a single thrombus but multiple lesions are commonly present and as many as 20 thrombi of varying size and age may be found in a single placenta. The thrombi

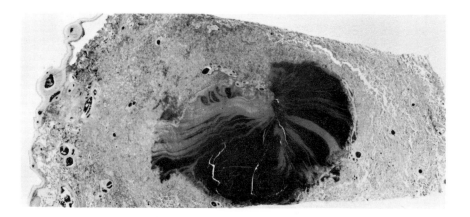

Figure 5.34. A fresh red intervillous thrombus.

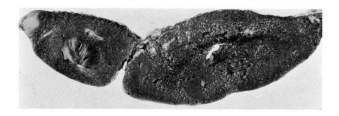

Figure 5.35. An intervillous thrombus which is older than that shown in Fig. 5.34. Linear streaks of fibrin are being laid down in the thrombus.

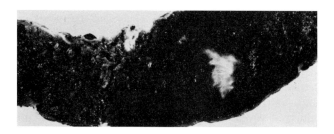

Figure 5.36. An old intervillous thrombus which is seen as a laminated white plaque.

range in size from 1 or 2 mm to 5 cm in diameter, though the majority are between 1 and 2 cm across.

A fresh intervillous thrombus is soft and dark red (Fig. 5.34), but as the thrombus ages the red cells degenerate and there is a progressive laying down of fibrin in a linear, streak-like fashion (Fig. 5.35). Hence the thrombus becomes progressively harder and its colour changes successively to brown, yellow and white. Eventually a hard, white, sharply delineated, laminated plaque is formed (Fig. 5.36).

Histology

A freshly formed thrombus consists only of red blood cells, but these gradually degenerate and fibrin is progressively laid down (Fig. 5.37), so that a lesion of some standing is formed almost entirely by laminated fibrin between the layers of which are a

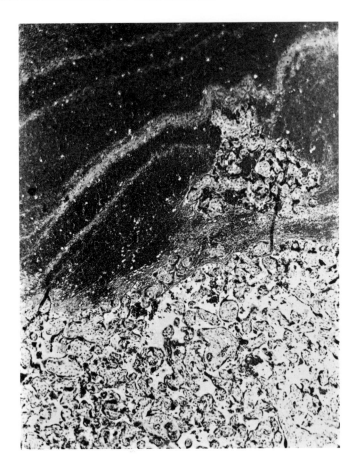

Figure 5.37. Photomicrograph of a moderately fresh intervillous thrombus (above and to the left). This consists largely of erythrocytes but a few strands of fibrin are also present (H & E ×45).

few degenerate and poorly staining erythrocytes (Fig. 5.38). A careful study of fresh intervillous thrombi will reveal the presence of nucleated red blood cells in many instances (Fig. 5.39).

Villi are absent from an intervillous thrombus, but, not uncommonly, there is a peripheral rim of compressed, and sometimes infarcted, villi around the lesion.

Incidence

Though intervillous thrombi are easily seen and readily recognized there have been striking variations in their reported incidence in placentas from full-term uncomplicated pregnancies, the figures ranging from 3 to 50%. In my own material 36% of such placentas contained intervillous thrombi (Fox, 1966a), a figure lying neatly between that reported by Wentworth (1964b) of 48% and that noted by Wilkin (1965) of 28%. There has been dispute as to whether these thrombi occur unduly commonly in placentas from women with pre-eclampsia, but in my series this was not the case; the only complication of pregnancy accompanied by an increased incidence of this lesion was materno-fetal rhesus incompatibility. This latter finding was also noted by Javert (1942), Javert and Reiss (1952) and Benirschke (1962), but not by either Wentworth (1964b) or Wilkin (1965).

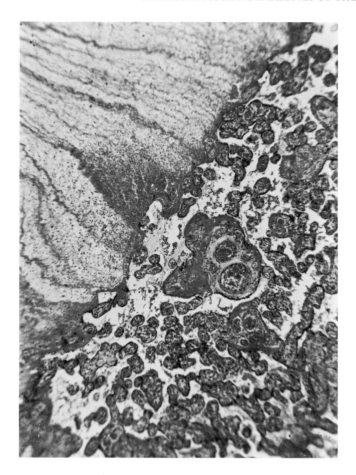

Figure 5.38. Histological appearances of an old intervillous thrombus (above and to the left); this consists almost entirely of laminated fibrin (H & E ×45).

Aetiology and Pathogenesis

Many have thought that intervillous thrombi are formed solely of maternal blood, often attributing their formation to thrombosis of a maternal decidual vein (McNalley & Dieckmann, 1923; McKay & Hertig, 1957; Huber et al, 1961). Wilkin (1965) however was not able to demonstrate venous occlusion in placentas containing intervillous thrombi. Other suggested aetiological factors have included rupture of a decidual vein (Montgomery, 1933), coagulation of the inflow from a diseased maternal arteriole (Marais, 1962), thrombosis of a spiral arteriole (Wigglesworth, 1969), and focal degeneration of villous syncytiotrophoblast with release of thromboplastic substances (Ashworth & Stouffer, 1956; Isidor & Aubry, 1957; Wilkin, 1965).

The alternative view is that the thrombi are formed of a mixture of fetal and maternal blood, and this would be in accord with the observation that nucleated erythrocytes are often seen in intervillous thrombi (Naeslund & Aren, 1947; Kline, 1948, 1949; Bichenbach & Kivel, 1950; Javert & Reiss, 1952; Rindi, 1958; Fox, 1963; Pisarki, 1964; Benirschke & Driscoll, 1967). Potter (1948) suggested that the cells classed as nucleated erythrocytes were, in fact, lymphocytes superimposed on red cells, whilst Wilkin (1965) has claimed that they are maternal red cells with overlying fragments of syncytiotrophoblast, but from my own observations I am quite sure that the cells considered both by myself and others to be nucleated red cells have been correctly characterized. Their identity as fetal cells has been conclusively confirmed by Kaplan et al (1982) who used an immunocytochemical technique to identify fetal haemoglobin.

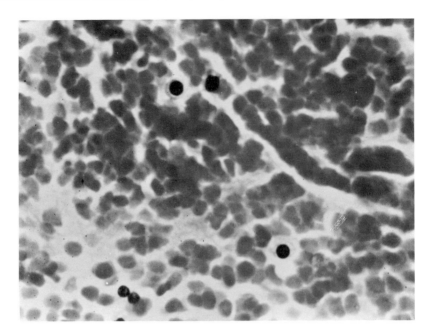

Figure 5.39. Nucleated erythrocytes in a fresh intervillous thrombus (H & E ×850).

Potter (1948) also maintained that the blood group of the cells in an intervillous thrombus is always the same as that of the mother and may differ from that of the fetus, but this view was conclusively disproved by Gille et al (1986). It is not, however, claimed that the thrombi are formed solely of fetal blood, because they are almost certainly a mixture of both maternal and fetal erythrocytes, with it being probable that, in many, the latter form only a small proportion of the total. This being so, it is perhaps not surprising that Potter, who based her results on the study of only a small number of placentas and who did not detail the techniques used, was not able to detect the fetal component.

Fetal bleeding into the intervillous space would appear to be via a rupture of thinned, attenuated syncytiotrophoblast overlying a dilated villous fetal capillary, because breaks of this nature are not uncommonly found in carefully studied placentas (Naeslund & Aren, 1947; Kline, 1948; Fox, 1964). Isolated breaks of this nature do not appear to be due to trauma during preparation, whilst the presence of a small 'blob' of fibrin at their margins indicates that they do not develop during delivery of the placenta. Leakage of fetal blood through such a break would, especially if maternal and fetal blood cells were incompatible with each other, trigger off local coagulation.

Significance

Intervillous thrombi have no effect on placental function or fetal well-being; their only significance is that they mark a site of fetal bleeding into the intervillous space and hence into the maternal circulation. It is now well established that between 15 and 30% of women have, during the third trimester, fetal red cells in their circulation in numbers that indicate a chronic low-grade leakage of such cells from the fetal circulation (Zipursky et al, 1965; Renaer et al, 1976), and it is therefore not surprising that there is a good correlation between the presence of intervillous thrombi in the placenta and the appearance of fetal erythrocytes in the maternal blood (Banti et al, 1968). This association is quantitative as well as qualitative, because the greater the number of intervillous thrombi in a placenta the greater is the leak of fetal red cells across the placenta.

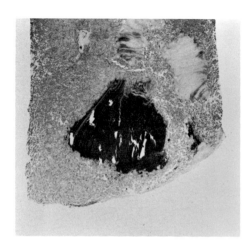

Figure 5.40. A Kline's haemorrhage.

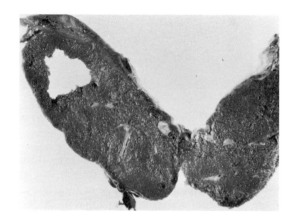

Figure 5.41. A sharply delineated cavity in the placental substance. This marks the site of a Kline's haemorrhage, from which the semi-liquid blood exuded during cutting of the placenta.

Kline's Haemorrhage

This name is applied, in a rather loose fashion, to haemorrhagic areas in the placental substance. The lesion was first noted by Kline (1948), whose description was notable chiefly for its vagueness. In essence, it consists of a nodular focus of semi-fluid or fluid blood within the placental parenchyma (Fig. 5.40); on slicing the placenta the blood may flow out from the slice to leave a sharply delineated cavity (Fig. 5.41), this being described by Wilkin (1965) as a 'caverne' and by German authors as a 'Plazentar-Hohlraum'. These collections of blood contain nucleated erythrocytes and there is a clear correlation between their presence within a placenta and the appearance of fetal red cells in the maternal blood (Wentworth, 1964a; Banti et al, 1968). I have, therefore, little doubt that the so-called 'Kline's haemorrhage' is, in reality, a very fresh intervillous thrombus (Fig. 5.42) and as such does not merit being classified as a separate entity.

Subamniotic Haematoma

This is a collection of free blood lying between amnion and chorion on the fetal surface of the placenta. The lesion is readily apparent as a plum-coloured tumefaction, which lifts the amnion away from the chorion, is usually small, and often has a roughly triangular shape. Haematomas of this type have attracted little attention, as most are clearly very fresh and are due to trauma to the surface venous tributaries of the umbilical veins during delivery, this commonly being the result of excessive traction on the

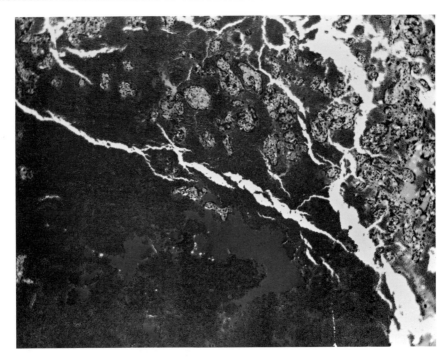

Figure 5.42. Histological appearances of the margin of a Kline's haemorrhage (H & E ×45).

umbilical cord. DeSa (1971) has, however, drawn attention to older haematomas which have clearly been formed some time before delivery of the infant and has noted an association between the presence of such lesions and a low birth weight. He found that these haematomas were accompanied by evidence of old thrombi in the chorionic veins. I have no data on this point and DeSa's findings have been neither confirmed nor refuted.

NON-VASCULAR LESIONS

Calcification

Macroscopic Features

Macroscopically visible calcification of the placenta is by no means uncommon and may be quite extensive. The calcium is often seen on the maternal surface of the placenta as small, hard, scattered flecks, whilst there may, if the placenta is heavily calcified, be a gritty feel to the knife when cutting into the organ. In placental slices the flecks of calcium occur principally in the basal plate and in the septa (Fig. 5.43); calcification of the chorionic plate is unusual. Healthy villous tissue is rarely visibly calcified but there may be considerable deposition of calcium in old infarcts and in plaques of perivillous or subchorial fibrin.

Histology

Histological examination confirms the sites of calcium deposition, the mineral being readily recognized as structureless, basophilic material that is deposited either as plaques or as coarse granules that are strongly PAS positive and give a positive reaction with von Kossa's stain (Fig. 5.44). Calcification of single or multiple villi is sometimes seen.

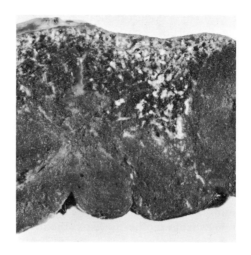

Figure 5.43. Flecks of calcium in, and adjacent to, a placental septum.

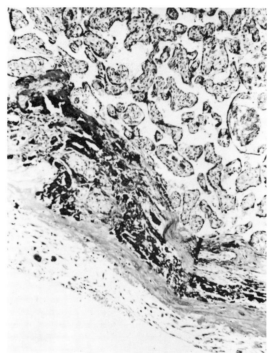

Figure 5.44. Histological appearances of calcification in the basal plate of the placenta (PAS ×65).

Incidence

The incidence of gross placental calcification, of the type detectable by a pathologist, has varied in different studies from 14 to 37% (Simon, 1951; Fujikura, 1963a; Wentworth, 1965; Wiegand, 1969; Brandt, 1973), the incidence in my own material being approximately 19% (Fox, 1964). This latter figure is very similar to that noted on antenatal radiology by Russell and Fielden (1969), but differs considerably from those obtained by postnatal radiography of the placenta, a technique that gives an incidence of calcification ranging from 75 to 90% (Masters & Clayton, 1940; Fleming, 1943; Hartley, 1954; Tindall & Scott, 1965). This disparity between the results obtained by pathological and radiological examination is not as dispiriting as may at first sight appear, because Schonig (1928) has shown that there are two forms of placental calcification: the first, 'physiological calcification', occurs during the first 6 months of pregnancy in the form of tiny granules which are not visible to the naked eye; whilst the second, 'dystrophic calcification', occurs during the later months of gestation as plaque-like deposits of easily visible calcium. This is perhaps an oversimplified view, as there is no evidence that the plaque-like deposits occur in dead or degenerate tissue, this type of calcification being metastatic in nature rather than dystrophic. Nevertheless Hassler (1969), using a sophisticated microradiographic technique, has confirmed that several different types of calcification occur in the placenta, only one of which would be likely to be macroscopically visible. It therefore appears that whilst the radiologist is able to detect both the physiological and 'dystrophic' or 'metastatic' forms of calcification (Fig. 5.45), the pathologist is able only to discern the latter type of calcium deposition. This assumption is bolstered by the fact that the incidence of 'gross' or 'heavy' calcification noted on radiological examination approximates to the overall incidence of placental calcification found in pathological studies. It should perhaps be added that chemical analyses of placental calcium content estimate not only 'dystrophic' and structural calcium in the organ but also the calcium of the intracellular fluid and transport calcium *en route* from mother to fetus (Einbrodt et al, 1962). It is therefore not too surprising that such analyses have yielded results that have often not only been mutually contradictory but that have also been difficult to reconcile with those obtained by either pathological or radiological examination.

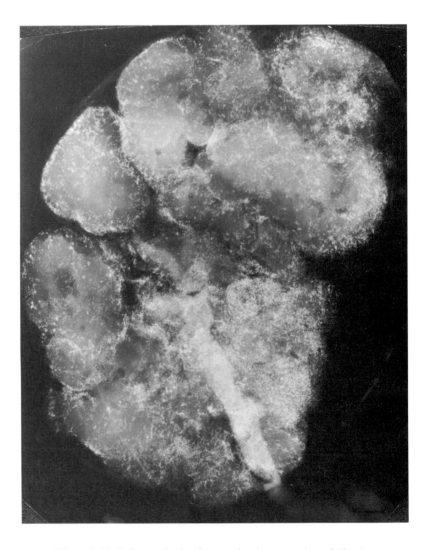

Figure 5.45. Radiograph of a placenta showing extensive calcification.

Gross calcification is distinctly uncommon in placentas from pregnancies terminating before the 36th week of gestation, but then increases rapidly in incidence as term is approached. It would appear logical to assume that prolonged pregnancy would be accompanied by a continued increase in both the incidence and degree of placental calcification, but it has been my own, and other workers', experience that this is not the case and that there is no excess of calcification in placentas from prolonged pregnancies (Masters & Clayton, 1940; Simon, 1951; Tindall & Scott, 1965; Wentworth, 1965; Russell & Fielden, 1969). Despite intermittent claims to the contrary, there is no increase in the incidence of placental calcification in maternal pre-eclampsia, essential hypertension or diabetes mellitus (Fox, 1966a; Brandt, 1973).

Aetiology and Pathogenesis

The view that calcification is a hallmark of placental senescence or degeneration is no longer tenable, despite the fact that it is still sometimes quoted in obstetrical and pathological textbooks. It has been clearly shown that there is a highly significant association between primigravidity and placental calcification (Fujikura, 1963a; Fox, 1964; Tindall & Scott, 1965; Wentworth, 1965; Brandt, 1973). Women whose placentas are calcified also tend to be younger than those whose placentas are uncalcified, though there is some dispute as to whether or not this is simply a reflection of the fact that the younger a woman is the more likely she is to be a primigravida. It is also established that calcification is more common in placentas from babies delivered during the late summer and early autumn (Fujikura, 1963b; Tindall & Scott, 1965; Russell & Fielden, 1969; Brandt, 1973), and in those from women who belong to the higher socioeconomic groups within the community (Russell & Fielden, 1969).

It may be offered as at least a partial explanation for these observations that Paupe et al (1961) noted a tendency for the serum calcium level to be higher in primigravid women at the time of delivery than in multigravid women, whilst Mull and Bill (1934) showed that in women with only a short interval between pregnancies there was a slight but definite reduction in serum calcium levels in each successive gestationary period. These latter workers also demonstrated that maternal serum calcium levels tended to be highest during the late summer and early autumn. These findings suggest that the maternal serum calcium level is a factor in the pathogenesis of placental calcium deposition, a view strengthened by the fact that placental calcification is increased in women given dietary calcium supplements during pregnancy (Fleming, 1943; Ritala, 1946; Linsman & Chalek, 1952). This is certainly not the whole story, however, because Tindall and Scott (1965) have pointed out that the degree of calcification may be notably different in each of a pair of dichorionic twin placentas. This indicates strongly that a further mechanism is involved that is independent of maternal calcium levels.

Significance

Gross placental calcification is now known to be of no pathological or clinical significance (Tindall & Scott, 1965; Wentworth, 1965; Brandt, 1973). Calcification is no more common in placentas from fresh stillbirths than in those from live-born infants and in prolonged intrauterine death there appears to be, not an accumulation, but a progressive loss of calcium from the placenta.

Septal Cyst

A septal cyst is round or oval, sharply demarcated from the surrounding tissue and usually measures 5–10 mm in diameter (Fig. 5.46). The cyst wall is formed by a smooth, thin, glistening membrane and the cyst contents are grey and gelatinous. The cysts are

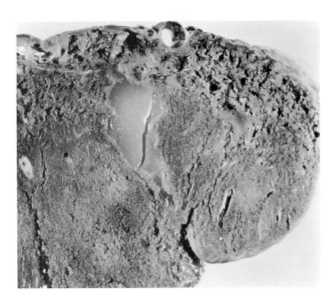

Figure 5.46. A septal cyst in the substance of a placenta.

usually in the subchorionic zone and it can often be seen that the cyst walls are in direct continuity below with a septum.

Histlogical examination confirms that the cyst is actually in the apex of a septum (Fig. 5.47), the cyst wall being formed by septal tissue (Fig. 5.48). The contents of the cyst appear quite structureless but stain weakly with PAS. Kaplan (1994) maintains that these cysts develop in masses of proliferating trophoblast associated with perivillous fibrin deposition but this view is clearly not compatible with the histological findings.

In most series, septal cysts have been present in between 11 and 20% of placentas (Paddock & Greer, 1927; Harer, 1936; Carter et al, 1963a; Wilkin, 1965) and in my own material were found in 19% of placentas from full-term uncomplicated pregnancies (Fox, 1965). The cysts occur more commonly in oedematous placentas and are

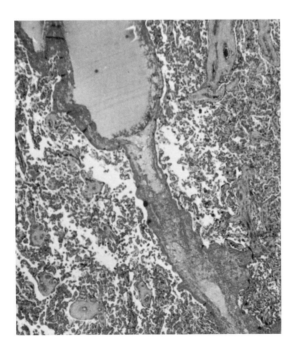

Figure 5.47. Low-power photomicrograph of a septal cyst (above): this can be clearly seen to have developed within a septum (H & E ×6).

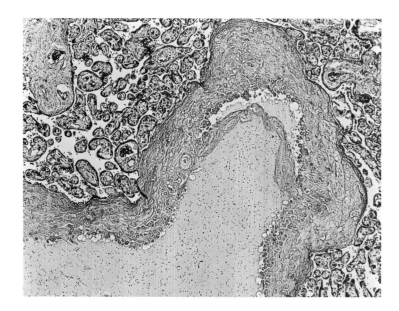

Figure 5.48. Higher power view of the wall of a septal cyst (H & E ×60).

therefore more frequently found in those from diabetic women or from cases of materno-fetal rhesus incompatibility.

The pathogenesis of these cysts is unknown but older views that they represent cystic degeneration of infarcts or intervillous thrombi (Bret et al, 1960; Barthomolew et al, 1961) are clearly invalid. The reason for their increased incidence in oedematous placentas is also obscure because the septa in which the cysts arise do not appear oedematous in such cases.

A septal cyst is of no clinical importance.

GENERAL COMMENTS ON GROSS LESIONS OF THE PLACENTA

It will be clear to the reader of this chapter that most macroscopically visible lesions of the placenta are of little or no clinical importance and that, in the past, their significance has been markedly overemphasized. This has been largely due to the ease with which such lesions can be detected and their convenience as pegs upon which to hang a facile diagnosis of placental insufficiency, a situation compounded by the incorrect assumption that the placenta has only a minimal functional reserve capacity. This is not to say, however, that gross examination of the placenta is unimportant, because some visible lesions are significant as a direct cause of fetal death, hypoxia or growth retardation, these including very extensive perivillous fibrin deposition, multiple fetal artery thrombi and large retroplacental haematomas. Infarction is very rarely of sufficient degree to be a direct cause of fetal complications but, when extensive, serves as an indicator of a markedly abnormal maternal vasculature whilst the presence of a fetal artery thrombosis may be associated with thrombi elsewhere in the fetal vasculature.

With these few exceptions, however, very few gross lesions of the placenta are of any clinical or functional significance.

REFERENCES

Abdella, T.N., Sibai, B.M., Hays, J.M. and Anderson, G.D. (1984) Relationship of hypertensive disease to abruptio placentae. *Obstetrics and Gynecology*, **63**, 365–370.

Abu-Yousef, M.M., Bleicher, J.J., Williamson, R.A. and Weiner, C.P. (1987) Subchorionic hemorrhage: sonographic diagnosis and clinical significance. *American Journal of Roentgenology*, **149**, 737–740.

Acker, D., Sachs, B.J., Tracey, K.J., Wise, W.E. (1983) Abruptio placentae associated with cocaine use. *American Journal of Obstetrics and Gynecology*, **146**, 220–221.

Ahmed, M.Z., Zhou, D.H., Maulik, D. and Eldefrawi, M.E. (1990) Characterization of a cocaine binding protein in human placenta. *Life Sciences*, **46**, 553–561.

Andres, R.L., Kuyper, W., Resnik, R., Piacquadio, K.M. and Benirschke, K. (1990) The association of maternal floor infarction of the placenta with adverse perinatal outcome. *American Journal of Obstetrics and Gynecology*, **163**, 935–938.

Ashworth, C.T. and Stouffer, J.G. (1956) A study of fibrin deposition in the placenta. *American Journal of Clinical Pathology*, **26**, 1031–1043.

Banti, D., Jennison, R.F. and Langley, F.A. (1968) Significance of placental pathology in transplacental haemorrhage. *Journal of Clinical Pathology*, **21**, 322–331.

Bartholomew, R.A. (1938) Pathology of the placenta: with special reference to infarcts and their relation to toxemia of pregnancy. *Journal of the American Medical Association*, **111**, 2276–2280.

Bartholomew, R.A. (1947) The possible etiological significance of thrombosis of a placental vein in mechanism of placental infarction and associated toxemia of pregnancy. *American Journal of Obstetrics and Gynecology*, **53**, 650–657.

Bartholomew, R.A. and Kracke, R.R. (1932) The relation of placental infarcts to eclamptic toxemia: a clinical, pathologic and experimental study. *American Journal of Obstetrics and Gynecology*, **24**, 797–819.

Bartholomew, R.A., Colvin, E.D., Grimes, W.H., Fish, J.S. and Lester, W.M. (1953) The mechanism of bleeding during pregnancy. *American Journal of Obstetrics and Gynecology*, **66**, 1042–1061.

Bartholomew, R.A., Colvin, E.D., Grimes, W.H., Fish, J.S., Lester, W.M. and Galloway, W.H. (1957) Facts pertinent to the etiology of eclamptogenic toxemia. *American Journal of Obstetrics and Gynecology*, **74**, 64–84.

Bartholomew, R.A., Colvin, E.D., Grimes, W.H., Fish, J.S., Lester, W.M. and Galloway, W.H. (1961) Criteria by which toxemia of pregnancy may be diagnosed from unlabelled formalin-fixed placentas. *American Journal of Obstetrics and Gynecology*, **82**, 277–290.

Becker, V. (1963) Funktionelle Morphologie der Plazenta. *Archiv für Gynäkologie*, **198**, 3–28.

Benirschke, K. (1961) Examination of the placenta. *Obstetrics and Gynecology*, **18**, 309–333.

Benirschke, K. (1962) A review of the pathologic anatomy of the human placenta. *American Journal of Obstetrics and Gynecology*, **84**, 1595–1622.

Benirschke, K. and Driscoll, S.G. (1967) *The Pathology of the Human Placenta*. Berlin, Heidelberg, New York: Springer-Verlag.

Benirschke, K. and Gille, J. (1977) Placental pathology and asphyxia. In *Intrauterine Asphyxia and the Developing Brain*, Gluck, L. (Ed.) Chicago: Year Book.

Benirschke, K. and Kaufmann, P. (1995) *Pathology of the Human Placenta*, 3rd edn. New York: Springer-Verlag.

Bevis, D.C.A. (1958) Accidental haemorrhage. *Journal of Obstetrics and Gynaecology of the British Empire*, **65**, 840–841.

Bichenbach, W. and Kivel, F. (1950) Mikroscopische Untersuchungen an Erythroblastose-Placenten. *Archiv für Gynäkologie*, **177**, 559–566.

Boe, F. (1959) Vascular changes in premature separation of the normally implanted placenta: a preliminary report. *Acta Obstetricia et Gynecologica Scandinavica*, **38**, 441–443.

Boyd, J.D. and Hamilton, W.J. (1970) *The Human Placenta*. Cambridge: Heffer.

Brandt, G. (1973) Ätiologie und Pathogenese der Kalkablagerung in der Plazenta. *Geburtshilfe und Frauenheilkunde*, **33**, 119–124.

Bret, A.J., Legros, R. and Toyoda, S. (1960) Les cystes placentaires. *Presse Medical*, **68**, 1552–1555.

Breus, C. (1892) *Das Tuberose Subchoriale-Hamatome der Decidua*. Leipzig and Vienna: Franz Deuticke.

Brosens, I. (1963) Les artérioles spiralées de la cadaque basale dans les complications hypertensives de la grossesse: étude anatomo-clinique. *Bulletin de la Societé Belge de Gynécologie et d'Obstétrique*, **33**, 61–70.

Brosens, I. (1964) A study of the spiral arteries of the decidua basalis in normotensive and hypertensive pregnancies. *Journal of Obstetrics and Gynaecology of the British Commonwealth*, **71**, 222–230.

Brosens, I. and Renaer, M. (1972) On the pathogenesis of placental infarcts in pre-eclampsia. *Journal of Obstetrics and Gynaecology of the British Commonwealth*, **79**, 794–799.

Burchell, R.C. and Mengert, W.F. (1969) Etiology of premature separation of the normally implanted placenta: preliminary observations. *American Journal of Obstetrics and Gynecology*, **104**, 795–797.

Burkett, G., Yasin, S.Y., Palow, D., LaVoie, L. and Martinez, M. (1994) Patterns of cocaine binding: effect on pregnancy. *American Journal of Obstetrics and Gynecology*, **171**, 372–378.

Carter, J.E., Vellios, F. and Huber, C.P. (1963a) Circulatory factors governing the viability of the human placenta, based on a morphologic study. *American Journal of Clinical Pathology*, **40**, 363–373.

Carter, J.E., Vellios, F. and Huber, C.P. (1963b) Histologic classification and incidence of circulatory lesions of the human placenta, with a review of the literature. *American Journal of Clinical Pathology*, **40**, 374–378.

Clewell, W.H. and Manchester, D.K. (1983) Recurrent maternal floor infarction: a preventable cause of fetal death. *American Journal of Obstetrics and Gynecology*, **147**, 346–347.

Cohen, H.R., Green, J.R. and Crombleholme, W.R. (1991) Peripartum cocaine use: estimating risk of adverse pregnancy outcome. *International Journal of Gynaecology and Obstetrics*, **35**, 51–54.

Darby, M.J., Caritis, S.N. and Shen-Schwartz, S. (1989) Placental abruption in the preterm gestation: an association with chorioamnionitis. *Obstetrics and Gynecology*, **74**, 88–92.

Daro, A.F., Gollin, H.A., Nora, E.G. and Primiano, N. (1956) Premature separation of the normally implanted placenta: a review of 306 cases. *American Journal of Obstetrics and Gynecology*, **72**, 599–604.

De Carolis, S., Caruso, A., Ferrazzani, S. et al (1994) Poor pregnancy outcome and anticardiolipin antibodies. *Fetal Diagnosis and Therapy*, **9**, 296–299.

DeSa, D.J. (1971) Rupture of foetal vessels on placental surface. *Archives of Disease in Childhood*, **46**, 495–501.

Dieckmann, W.J. (1952) *The Toxaemias of Pregnancy*, 2nd edn. London: Henry Kempton.

Dombrowski, M.P., Wolfe, H.M., Welch, R.A. and Evans, M.I. (1991) Cocaine abuse is associated with abruptio placentae and decreased birth weight, but not shorter labor. *Obstetrics and Gynecology*, **77**, 139–141.

Domisse, T. and Tiltman, A.J. (1992) Placental bed biopsies in placental abruption. *British Journal of Obstetrics and Gynaecology*, **99**, 651–654.

Driscoll, S. (1965) The pathology of pregnancy complicated by diabetes mellitus. *Medical Clinics of North America*, **49**, 1053–1067.

Dusick, A.M., Covert, R.F., Schreiber, M.D. et al. (1993) Risk of intracranial hemorrhage and other adverse outcomes after cocaine exposure in a cohort of 323 very low birth weight infants. *Journal of Pediatrics*, **122**, 438–445.

Eden, T.W. (1897) A study of the human placenta, physiological and pathological. *Journal of Pathology and Bacteriology*, **4**, 265–283.

Egley, C. and Cefalo, R.C. (1985) Abruptio placenta. In *Progress in Obstetrics and Gynaecology*, Vol. 5, Studd, J. (Ed.), pp. 108–120. London: Churchill Livingstone.

Einbrodt, H.J., Geller, H.F. and Born, J. (1962) Der 'dystropische' Kalkgehalt der normalen menschlichen Placenta. *Archiv für Gynäkologie*, **197**, 149–156.

Eriksen, G., Wohlert, M., Ersbak, V. et al. (1991) Placental abruption: a case control investigation. *British Journal of Obstetrics and Gynaecology*, **98**, 448–452.

Falkiner, N.M. (1942) Placental infarcts. *Irish Journal of Medical Science*, 6th Series, **195**, 81–93.

Ferguson, J.H. (1955) Rupture of the marginal sinus of the placenta. *American Journal of Obstetrics and Gynecology*, **69**, 995–1003.

Fish, J.S. (1955) *Hemorrhage of Late Pregnancy*. Springfield, IL: Charles C. Thomas.

Fish, J.S. (1960) Marginal placental rupture. *Clinical Obstetrics and Gynecology*, **3**, 599–615.

Fish, J.S., Bartholomew, R., Colvin, E. and Grimes, W.H. (1951) The role of marginal sinus rupture in antenatal hemorrhage. *American Journal of Obstetrics and Gynecology*, **61**, 20–31.

Fleming, A.M. (1943) The clinical significance of the degree of calcification of the placenta as demonstrated by X-ray photography. *Journal of Obstetrics and Gynaecology of the British Empire*, **50**, 135–139.

Flowers, D., Clark, J.F. and Westney, L.S. (1991) *Journal of the National Medical Association*, **83**, 230–232.

Fox, H. (1963) White infarcts of the placenta. *Journal of Obstetrics and Gynaecology of the British Commonwealth*, **70**, 980–991.

Fox, H. (1964) Calcification of the placenta. *Journal of Obstetrics and Gynaecology of the British Commonwealth*, **71**, 759–765.

Fox, H. (1965) Septal cysts of the placenta. *Journal of Obstetrics and Gynaecology of the British Commonwealth*, **72**, 745–747.

Fox, H. (1966a) *The Pathology of the Placenta*. MD Thesis, University of Manchester.

Fox, H. (1966b) Thrombosis of foetal arteries in the human placenta. *Journal of Obstetrics and Gynaecology of the British Commonwealth*, **73**, 961–965.

Fox, H. (1967a) Perivillous fibrin deposition in the human placenta. *American Journal of Obstetrics and Gynecology*, **98**, 245–251.

Fox, H. (1967b) The significance of placental infarction in perinatal morbidity and mortality. *Biologia Neonatorum*, **11**, 87–105.

Fujikura, T. (1963a) Placental calcification and maternal age. *American Journal of Obstetrics and Gynecology*, **87**, 41–45.

Fujikura, T. (1963b) Placental calcification and seasonal difference. *American Journal of Obstetrics and Gynecology*, **87**, 46–47.

Fuke, Y., Aono, T., Imai, S. et al. (1994) Clinical significance and treatment of massive intervillous fibrin deposition associated with recurrent fetal growth retardation. *Gynecologic and Obstetric Investigation*, 38, 5–9.

Geller, H.F. (1959) Über die Bedeutung des subchorialen Fibrinstreifens in der menschlichen Placenta. *Archiv für Gynäkologie*, **192**, 1–6.

Gersell, D.J. (1993) Chronic villitis, chronic chorioamnionitis, and maternal floor infarction. *Seminars in Diagnostic Pathology*, **10**, 251–266.

Gille, J., Schwerd, W. and von Criegern, T. (1986) Zusammemsetzung intervilloser Thromben aus maternem und fetalen Blut. *Zeitschrift fur Gebürtshilfe und Perinatologie*, **190**, 133–136.

Goldstein, S.R., Subramanyam, B.R., Raghavendra, B.N., Horii, S.C. and Hilton, S. (1983) Subchorionic bleeding in threatened abortion: sonographic findings and significance. *American Journal of Roentgenology*, **141**, 975–978.

Gregor, F. (1961) Histologische Veränderungen der Plazenta bei Spättoxikosen. *Zeitschrift für Geburtshilfe and Gynäkologie*. **157**, 325–340.

Gruenwald, P., Levin, H. and Yousem, H. (1968) Abruption and premature separation of the placenta: the clinical and pathologic entity. *American Journal of Obstetrics and Gynecology*, **102**, 604–610.

Hall, M.H. (1972) Folic acid deficiency and abruptio placentae. *Journal of Obstetrics and Gynaecology of the British Commonwealth*, **79**, 222–225.

Handler, A., Kistin, N., Davis, F. and Ferre, C. (1991) Cocaine use during pregnancy: perinatal outcomes. *American Journal of Epidemiology*, **133**, 818–825.

Harer, W.B. (1936) A study of one thousand placentas. *American Journal of Obstetrics and Gynecology*, **32**, 794–802.

Harris, B.A. (1952) Marginal placental bleeding: anatomical and pathological considerations. American *Journal of Obstetrics and Gynecology*, **64**, 53–61.

Harris, B.A. (1985) Peripheral placental separation: a possible relationship to premature labor. *Obstetrics and Gynecology*, **66**, 774–778.

Harris, B.A. (1988) Peripheral placental separation: a review. *Obstetrical and Gynecological Survey*, **43**, 577–581.

Hart, D.B. (1902) The nature of the tuberose fleshy mole. *Journal of Obstetrics and Gynaecology of the British Empire*, **1**, 479–481.

Hartley, J.B. (1954) Incidence and significance of placental calcification. *British Journal of Radiology*, **27**, 365–380.

Hassler, O. (1969) Placental calcifications: a biophysical and histologic study. *American Journal of Obstetrics and Gynecology*, **103**, 348–353.

Hendelman, M. and Fraser, W.D. (1960) A clinical analysis of abruptio placentae. *American Journal of Obstetrics and Gynecology*, **80**, 17–20.

Hibbard, B.M. (1964) The role of folic acid in pregnancy with particular reference to anaemia, abruptio and abortion. *Journal of Obstetrics and Gynaecology of the British Commonwealth*, **71**, 529–542.

Hibbard, B.M. and Hibbard, E.D. (1963) Aetiological factor in abruptio placentae. *British Medical Journal*, **ii**, 1430–1436.

Hibbard, B.M. and Jeffcoate, T.N.A. (1966) Abruptio placentae. *Obstetrics and Gynecology*, **27**, 155–167.

Hibbard, B.M., Hibbard, E.D., Tow, S.H. and Tan, P. (1969) Abruptio placentae and defective folate metabolism in Singapore women. *Journal of Obstetrics and Gynaecology of the British Commonwealth*, **76**, 1003–1007.

Ho, C.H. (1983) Massive subchorionic hematoma. *Archives of Pathology and Laboratory Medicine*, **107**, 438.

Howard, B.K., Goodson, J.H. and Mengert, W.F. (1953) Supine hypotensive syndrome in late pregnancy. *Obstetrics and Gynecology*, **1**, 371–377.

Hsu, C.T., Ma, Y.M., Wang, T.T. et al. (1960) Studies on abruptio placentae. *American Journal of Obstetrics and Gynecology*, **80**, 263–271.

Huber, C.P., Carter, J.E. and Vellios, F. (1961) Lesions of the circulatory system of the placenta: a study of 243 placentas with special reference to the development of infarcts. *American Journal of Obstetrics and Gynecology*, **81**, 560–573.

Hunt, H.F., Patterson, W.B. and Nicodemus, R.E. (1940) Placental infarction and eclampsia. *American Journal of Clinical Pathology*, **10**, 319–331.

Isidor, P. and Aubry, B. (1957) A propos d'un type particulier d'artériopathie de la portion foetale du placenta: essaie d'explication pathogénique, ses raports avec la toxemie et l'anoxie foetale. *Gynécologie et Obstétrique*, **56**, 152–166.

Jauniaux, E., Avni, F.E., Elkazen, N., Wilkin, P. and Hustin, J. (1989) Étude morphologique des anomalies placentaires echographiques de la deuxieme moitie de la gestation. *Journal de Gynécologie et de l'Obstétrique et Biologie de la Reproduction*, **18**, 601–613.

Javert, C.T. (1942) Erythroblastosis neonatorum: an obstetrical-pathological study of 47 cases. *Surgery, Gynecology and Obstetrics*, **74**, 1–19.

Javert, C.T. and Reiss, C. (1952) The origin and significance of macroscopic intervillous coagulation hematomas (red infarcts) of the human placenta. *Surgery, Gynecology and Obstetrics*, **94**, 257–269.

Kaplan, C.G. (1994) *Color Atlas of Gross Placental Pathology*. New York: Igaku-Shoin.

Kaplan, C., Blanc, W.A. and Elias, J. (1982) Identification of erythrocytes in intervillous thrombi: a study using immunoperoxidase identification of hemoglobins. *Human Pathology*, **13**, 554–556.

Katz, V.L., Bowes, W.A. and Sierkh, A.E. (1987) Maternal floor infarction of the placenta associated with elevated second trimester alpha-fetoprotein. *American Journal of Perinatology*, **4**, 225–228.

Kaufman, A.K., Fleischer, A.C., Thieme, G.A., Shah, D.M. and Jarnes, A.E. (1985) Separated chorioamnion and elevated chorion: sonographic features and clinical significance. *Journal of Ultrasound in Medicine*, **4**, 119–125.

Kaufmann, P. (1975) Experiments on infarct genesis caused by blockage of carbohydrate metabolism in guinea pig placentae. *Virchows Archiv. A. Pathologische Anatomie und Histologie*, **368**, 11–21.

Kérisit, J. and Toulouse, R. (1970a) Les pertubations de la circulation placentaire maternelle. Revue *Francaise de Gynécologie et de l'Obstétrique*, **65**, 321–327.

Kérisit, J. and Toulouse, R. (1970b) Les pertubations de la circulation foetale. *Revue Francaise de Gynécologie et d'Obstétrique*, **65**, 329–336.

Kimbrough, R.A. (1959) Antepartum hemorrhage: a review of 383 cases of abruptio placentae and 169 cases of placenta previa treated during the years 1944–1957. *American Journal of Obstetrics and Gynecology*, **78**, 1161–1168.

Kline, B.S. (1948) Microscopic observations of the placental barrier in transplacental erythrocytotoxic anemia (erythroblastosis fetalis) and in normal pregnancy. *American Journal of Obstetrics and Gynecology*, **56**, 226–237.

Kline, B.S. (1949) The pathogenesis of erythroblastosis fetalis. *Blood*, **4**, 1249–1255.

Kloosterman, G.J. and Huidekoper, B.L. (1952) Over de betenis van de placenta voor de 'obstetrische sterfte': een onderzoek van 2000 placentas. *Nederlands Tijdschrift voor Verloskunde en Gyneecologie*, **52**, 318–351.

Kloosterman, G.J. and Huidekoper, B.L. (1954) The significance of the placenta in obstetrical mortality. *Gynaecologica*, **138**, 529–550.

Kraus, F.T. (1993) Placental thrombi and related problems. *Seminars in Diagnostic Pathology*, **10**, 275–283.

Langhans, T. (1877) Untersuchungen über die menschliche Placenta. *Archiv für Anatomie und Physiologie*, 188–267.

Levy, H. (1956) Mola de Breus – revisao dos conceptos patogeneticos a propsito de nove casos proprios. *Gazeta Medica Portuguesa*, **9**, 341–363.

Linsman, J.F. and Chalek, J.I. (1952) Placental calcification in the roentgen pregnancy study. *American Journal of Roentgenology, Radium Therapy and Nuclear Medicine*, **67**, 267–272.

Linthwaite, R.F. (1963) Subchorial hematoma mole (Breus' mole) *Journal of the American Medical Association*, **186**, 867–869.

Little, W.A. (1960) Placental infarction. *Obstetrics and Gynecology*, **15**, 109–130.

Littmann, K.P. (1968) Zur Pathomorphologie der Deziduagefässe menschlicher Plazenten. *Geburtshilfe und Frauenheilkunde*, **28**, 554–562.

McDermott, M. and Gillan, J.E. (1995a) Chronic reduction in fetal blood flow is associated with placental infarction. *Placenta*, **16**, 165–170.

McDermott, M. and Gillan, J.E. (1995b) Trophoblast basement membrane haemosiderosis in the placental lesion of fetal artery thrombosis: a marker for disturbance of maternofetal transfer. *Placenta*, **16**, 171–178.

McKay, D.G. and Hertig, A.T. (1957) Placental insufficiency. *Bulletin of the Margaret Hague Maternity Hospital*, **10**, 3–14.

McKelvey, J.G. (1939) Vascular lesions in the decidua basalis. *American Journal of Obstetrics and Gynecology*, **38**, 815–821.

McNalley, F.P. (1924) A study of 1352 placentae with regard to white infarcts. *American Journal of Obstetrics and Gynecology*, **8**, 186–194.

McNalley, F.P. and Dieckmann, W.J. (1923) Hemorrhagic lesions of the placenta and their relation to white infarct formation. *American Journal of Obstetrics and Gynecology*, **5**, 55–66.

Mandsager, N.T., Bendon, R., Mostello, D. et al. (1994) Maternal floor infarction of placenta: prenatal diagnosis and clinical significance. *Obstetrics and Gynecology*, **83**, 750–754.

Mantoni, M. and Pedersen, J.F. (1981) Intrauterine haematoma: an ultrasound study of threatened abortion. *British Journal of Obstetrics and Gynaecology*, **88**, 47–51.

Marais, W.D. (1962) Human decidual spiral arterial studies. Part 2. A universal thesis on the pathogenesis of intraplacental fibrin deposits, layered thrombosis, red and white infarcts and toxic and non-toxic abruptio placenta. *Journal of Obstetrics and Gynaecology of the British Commonwealth*, **69**, 213–224.

Marais, W.D. (1963) Human decidual spiral arterial studies. Part 8. The aetiological relationship between toxaemia-hypertension of pregnancy and spiral arterial placental pathology. *South African Medical Journal*, **37**, 117–120.

Masters, M. and Clayton, S.G. (1940) Calcification of the human placenta. *Journal of Obstetrics and Gynaecology of the British Empire*, **47**, 437–443.

Mengert, W.F., Goodson, J.H., Campbell, R.G. and Haynes, D.M. (1953) Observations on the pathogenesis of premature separation of the normally implanted placenta. *American Journal of Obstetrics and Gynecology*, **66**, 1104–1112.

Menon, M.K.K., Sengupta, M. and Ramaswamy, N. (1966) Accidental haemorrhage and folic acid deficiency. *Journal of Obstetrics and Gynaecology of the British Commonwealth*, **73**, 49–52.

Miller, J.M. Jr, Boudreaux, M.C. and Regan, F.A. (1995) A case-control study of cocaine use in pregnancy. *American Journal of Obstetrics and Gynecology*, **172**, 180–185.

Moe, N. (1969) Deposits of fibrin and plasma proteins in the normal human placenta: an immunofluorescence study. *Acta Pathologica et Microbiologica Scandinavica*, **76**, 74–88.

Moe, N. and Jorgensen, L. (1968) Fibrin deposits on the syncytium of the normal human placenta: evidence of their thrombogenic origin. *Acta Pathologica et Microbiologica Scandinavica*, **72**, 519–541.

Montgomery, T.L. (1933) Lesions of the placental vessels. Their relationship to the pathology of the placenta: their effect upon fetal morbidity and mortality. *American Journal of Obstetrics and Gynecology*, **25**, 320–334.

Mooney, E.E., Al Shunnar, A., O'Regan, M. and Gillan, J.E. (1994) Chorionic villous haemorrhage is associated with retroplacental haemorrhage. *British Journal of Obstetrics and Gynaecology*, **101**, 965–969.

Mull, J.W. and Bill, A.H. (1934) Variations in serum calcium and phosphorus during pregnancy. 1. Normal variations. *American Journal of Obstetrics and Gynecology*, **27**, 510–517.

Naeslund, J. and Aren, P. (1947) Studies in changes in the placenta with particular reference to possible injuries to villi and foetal vessels. *Acta Obstetricia et Gynecologica Scandinavica*, **27**, 115–130.

Naeye, R.L. (1980) Abruptio placentae and placenta previa: frequency, perinatal mortality and cigarette smoking. *Obstetrics and Gynecology*, **55**, 701–704.

Naeye, R.L. (1985) Maternal floor infarction. *Human Pathology*, **16**, 823–828.

Naeye, R.L. (1990) The clinical significance of absent subchorionic fibrin in the placenta. *American Journal of Clinical Pathology*, **94**, 196–198.

Nelson, D.M., Crouch, E.C., Curran, E.M. and Farmer, D.R. (1990) Trophoblast interaction with fibrin matrix: epithelialization of perivillous fibrin deposits as a mechanism for villous repair in the human placenta. *American Journal of Pathology*, **136**, 855–865.

Nessmann-Emmanuelli, C. (1974) L'examen macroscopique du placenta a l'état frais. *Journal de Gynécologie, Obstétrique et Biologie de la Reproduction*, **3**, 1075–1086.

Nickel, R.E. (1988) Maternal floor infarction: an unusual cause of intrauterine growth retardation. *American Journal of Diseases of Children*, **142**, 1270–1271.

Paddock, R. and Greer, E.D. (1927) The origin of the common cystic structures of the human placenta. *American Journal of Obstetrics and Gynecology*, **13**, 164–173.

Paupe, J., Colin, J., Politis, E. and Lelong, M. (1961) Variations physiologiques de la calciemie chez la mere au moment de l'accouchement dans le cordon et chez le nouveau né. *Biologia Neonatorum*, **3**, 357–378.

Pearlstone, M. and Baxi, L. (1993) Subchorionic hematoma: a review. *Obstetrical and Gynecological Survey*, **48**, 65–68.

Pedersen, J.F. and Mantoni, M. (1990) Prevalence and significance of subchorionic hemorrhage in threatened abortion: a sonographic study. *American Journal of Roentgenology*, **154**, 535–537.

Philippe, E. (1966) La pathologie non-tumorale du placenta. *Archives d'Anatomie Pathologique*, **14**, 11–21.

Pisarki, T. (1964) Pathomorphology of afterbirth in perinatal death. *Polish Medical Journal*, **3**, 911–955.

Potter, E.L. (1948) Intervillous thrombi in the placenta and their possible relation to erythroblastosis fetalis. *American Journal of Obstetrics and Gynecology*, **56**, 959–961.

Prasad, P.D., Leibach, F.H., Mahesh, V.B. and Ganapathy, V. (1994) Human placenta as a target organ for cocaine action: interaction of cocaine with the placental serotonin transporter. *Placenta*, **15**, 267–278.

Pritchard, J.A., Mason, R., Corley, M. and Pritchard, S. (1970) Genesis of severe placental abruption. *American Journal of Obstetrics and Gynecology*, **108**, 22–27.

Ramsey, E.M. (1956a) Circulation in the maternal placenta of the rhesus monkey and man with observations on the marginal lakes. *American Journal of Anatomy*, **98**, 159–190.

Ramsey, E.M. (1956b) Distribution of arteries and veins in the mammalian placenta. In *Gestation: Transactions of the 2nd Conference*, Villee, C.A. (Ed.), pp. 229–251. New York: Josiah Macy Foundation.

Ramsey, E.M. (1965) Circulation of the placenta. *Birth Defects Original Article Series*, **1**, 5–12.

Raymond, E.G. and Mills, J.L. (1993) Placental abruption: maternal risk factors and associated fetal conditions. *Acta Obstetricia et Gynecologica*, **72**, 633–639.

Rayne, S.C. and Kraus, F.T. (1993) Placental thrombi and other vascular lesions: classification, morphology, and clinical correlations. *Pathology Research and Practice*, **189**, 2–17.

Redline, R.W. and Pappin, A. (1995) Fetal thrombotic vasculopathy: the clinical significance of extensive avascular villi. *Human Pathology*, **26**, 80–85.

Redline, R.W. and Patterson, P. (1994) Patterns of placental injury; correlations with gestational age, placental weight, and clinical diagnosis. *Archives of Pathology and Laboratory Medicine*, **118**, 698–701.

Renaer, M. and Brosens, I. (1963) De spiraalvorige arteriolen van de decidua basalis bij de hypertensieve verwikkelingen van de zwangerscuap. *Nederlands Tijdschrift voor Verloskunde en Gynaecologie*, **63**, 103–118.

Renaer, M., van de Putte, I. and Vermylen, C. (1976) Massive feto-maternal hemorrhage as a cause of perinatal mortality and morbidity. *European Journal of Obstetrics, Gynecology and Reproductive Biology*, **6**, 125–140.

Ribe, J.K., Teggatz, J.R. and Harvey, C.M. (1993) Blows to the maternal abdomen causing fetal demise: report of three cases. *Journal of Forensic Science*, **38**, 1092–1096.

Richardson, G.A., Day, N.L. and McGauhey, P.J. (1993) The impact of prenatal marijuana and cocaine use on the infant and child. *Clinical Obstetrics and Gynecology*, **36**, 302–318.

Rindi, V. (1958) Ulteriores contributo alla definizione morfologica della barriera placentare nella gravidanza normale e patologica. *Rivista Italiana di Ginecologia*, **33**, 488–503.

Ritala, A.M. (1946) Inorganic elements in the placenta. *Acta Obstetricia et Gynecologica Scandinavica*, **26**, Supplement **5**, 1–50.

Robb, J.A., Benirscke, K. and Barmeyer, R. (1986a) Intrauterine latent herpes simplex virus infection. I. Spontaneous abortion. Human Pathology, **17**, 1196–1209.

Robb, J.A., Benirschke, K., Mannino, F. and Voland, J. (1986b) Intrauterine latent herpes simplex virus infection. II. Latent neonatal infection. *Human Pathology*, **17**, 1210–1217.

Roig, P.P.Y. (1963) *Investigaciones Experimentales sobre Etiopatogenia de los Infartos y de los Hematomas Placentarios*. Barcelona: La Poligrafa, S.A.

Rushton, D.I. (1987) Pathology of abortion. In *Haines and Taylor: Obstetrical and Gynaecological Pathology*, 3rd edn, Fox, H. (Ed.), pp. 1117–1148. Edinburgh: Churchill Livingstone.

Russell, J.G.B. and Fielden, P. (1969) The antenatal diagnosis of placental calcification. *Journal of Obstetrics and Gynaecology of the British Commonwealth*, **76**, 813–816.

Sauerbrei, E.E. and Pham, D.H. (1986) Placental abruption and subchorionic hemorrhage in the first half of pregnancy: US appearance and clinical outcome. *Radiology*, **160**, 109–112.

Schneider, C.L. (1958) Rupture of the marginal sinus of the placenta: 'abscission windows'. *Obstetrics and Gynecology*, **11**, 715–721.

Schonig, A. (1928) Uber den Kalktransport von Mutter und Kind und über Kalkablagerung in der Plazenta. *Zeilschrift für Geburtshilfe und Gynäkologie*, **94**, 451–465.

Schwick, J., Kallenberg, A. and Wolff, F. (1992) Die symptomlose Ablatio placentae. *Zeitschrift für Geburtshilfe und Perinatologie*, **196**, 224–226.

Sexton, L.I., Hertig, A.T., Reid, D.E., Kellogg, F.S. and Patterson, W.S. (1950) Premature separation of the normally implanted placenta: a clinicopathological study of 476 cases. *American Journal of Obstetrics and Gynecology*, **59**, 13–24.

Shanklin, D.R. (1959) The human placenta with special reference to infarction and toxemia. *Obstetrics and Gynecology*, **13**, 325–336.

Shanklin, D.R. and Scott, J.S. (1975) Massive subchorial thrombohaematoma (Breus' mole) *British Journal of Obstetrics and Gynaecology*, **82**, 476–487.

Sibai, B.M., Caritis, S.N., Thom, E. et al (1993) Prevention of preeclampsia with low dose aspirin in healthy, nulliparous pregnant women. *New England Journal of Medicine*, **329**, 1265–1266.

Sickel, J.Z. and di Sant Agnese, A. (1994) Anomalous immunostaining of optically clear nuclei in gestational endometrium, a potential pitfall in the diagnosis of pregnancy-related herpes virus infection. *Archives of Pathology and Laboratory Medicine*, **118**, 831–833.

Siddall, R.S. and Hartman, F.W. (1926) Infarcts of the placenta: a study of seven hundred consecutive placentas. *American Journal of Obstetrics and Gynecology*, **12**, 683–699.

Simon, J. (1951) Calcifications placentaires: étude clinique, histologique et radiologique. *Bulletin de la Fédération des Sociétés de Gynécologie et d'Obstétrique de Langue Francaise*, **3**, 408–417.

Slutsker, L. (1992) Risks associated with cocaine use during pregnancy. *Obstetrics and Gynecology*, **79**, 778–789.

Smith, K. and Fields, H. (1958) The supine hypotensive syndrome: a factor in the etiology of abruptio placentae. *Obstetrics and Gynecology*, **12**, 369–372.

Soferman, N., Rosenberg, M. and Haimoff, M. (1963) Analyse de 108 cas de décollement prématuré du placenta normalement inséré. *Bulletin de la Fédération des Sociétés de Gynécologie et d'Obstétrique de Langue Francaise*, **15**, 362–365.

Sorba, M. (1948) *Etudes de Pathologie Foetale et Néonatale*. Lausanne: Rouge et Cie.

Spanner, R. (1935) Mutterlicher und kindlicher Kreislauf der menschlichen Placenta und seine Strombahnen. *Zeitschrift für Anatomie und Entwicklungsgeschichte*, **105**, 163–242.

Spinillo, A., Capuzzo, E., Colonna, L. et al (1994) Factors associated with abruptio placentae in preterm deliveries. *Acta Obstetricia et Gynecologica Scandinavica*, **73**, 307–312.

Stabile, I., Campbell, S. and Grudzinskas, J.G. (1989) Threatened miscarriage and intrauterine hematomas: sonographic and biochemical studies. *Journal of Ultrasound Medicine*, **8**, 289–292.

Stark, J. and Kaufmann, P. (1974) Infarktgenese in der Placenta. *Archiv für Gynäkologie*, **217**, 189–208.

Steigrad, K. (1952) Über die Beziehung von Plazentarinfarktion zur Schwangerschafts-Nephropathie: zugleich ein Beitrag zur Pathologie der Plazenta. *Gynaecologie*, **124**, 273–322.

Strachan, G.I. (1926) The pathology of the placenta. *Journal of Obstetrics and Gynaecology of the British Empire*, **33**, 262–284.

Takeuchi, A. and Benirschke, K. (1961) Renal vein thrombosis of the newborn and its relation to maternal diabetes. *Biologia Neonatorum*, **3**, 237–256.

Thanbu, J. and Llewellyn-Jones, D. (1966) Bone marrow studies in abruptio placentae. *Journal of Obstetrics and Gynaecology of the British Commonwealth*, **73**, 930–933.

Thomas, J.B. (1964) Breus' mole. *Obstetrics and Gynecology*, **24**, 794–797.

Thomsen, K. (1954) Zur Morphologie und Genese der sog. Placentarinfarkte. *Archiv für Gynäkologie*, **185**, 221–247.

Tindall, V.R. and Scott, J.S. (1965) Placental calcification: a study of 3025 singleton and multiple pregnancies. *Journal of Obstetrics and Gynaecology of the British Commonwealth*, **72**, 356–373.

Torpin, R. (1960) Subchorial haematoma mole: hypothetical aetiology. *Journal of Obstetrics and Gynaecology of the British Empire*, **67**, 990.

Towery, R., English, T.P. and Wisner, D. (1993) Evaluation of pregnant women after blunt injury. *Journal of Trauma*, **35**, 731–735.

van den Ende, I.E. (1959) The anatomy and pathology of premature separation of the placenta. *South African Medical Journal*, **33**, 737–740.

Vermelin, H. and Braye, M. (1958) Pathogenie de l'hémorrhagie rétro-placentaire. *Gynécologie et Obstétrique*, **57**, 1–18.

Voigt, L.F., Hollenbach, K.A., Krohn, M.A., Daling, J.R. and Hickok, D.E. (1990) The relationship of abruptio placentae with maternal smoking and small for gestational age infants. *Obstetrics and Gynecology*, **75**, 771–774.

Wallenburg, H.C.S. (1968) De gelokaliseerde placentalaesies: morfologie, klinische beteknis en mogelijke pathogenese. *Nederlands Tijdschrift voor Geneeskunde*, **112**, 2357–2363.

Wallenburg, H.C.S. (1969) Uber den Zusammenhang zwischen Spätgestose und Placentarinfarkt. *Archiv für Gynäkologie*, **208**, 80–90.

Wallenburg, H.C.S., Stolte, L.A.M. and Janssens, J. (1973) The pathogenesis of placental infarction: 1. A morphologic study on the human placenta. *American Journal of Obstetrics and Gynecology*, **116**, 835–840.

Wentworth, P. (1964a) A placental lesion to account for foetal haemorrhage into the maternal circulation. *Journal of Obstetrics and Gynaecology of the British Commonwealth*, **71**, 379–387.

Wentworth, P. (1964b) The incidence and significance of intervillous thrombi in the human placenta. *Journal of Obstetrics and Gynaecology of the British Commonwealth*, **71**, 894–898.

Wentworth, P. (1965) Macroscopic placental calcification and its clinical significance. *Journal of Obstetrics and Gynaecology of the British Commonwealth*, **72**, 215–222.

Wiegand, J. (1969) *Histologische Untersuchungen über die Lokalisation von Kalkniederschlgen in der menschlichen Plazenta*. Dissertation, Berlin.

Wigglesworth, J.S. (1964) Morphological variations in the insufficient placenta. *Journal of Obstetrics and Gynaecology of the British Commonwealth*, **71**, 871–884.

Wigglesworth, J.S. (1969) Vascular anatomy of the human placenta and its significance for placental pathology. *Journal of Obstetrics and Gynaecology of the British Commonwealth*, **76**, 979–989.

Wilkin, P. (1965) *Pathologie du Placenta*. Paris: Masson et Cie.

Wilkin, P. and Picard, C. (1961) La rupture du sinus marginal – existe-t-elle? Etude anatomo-clinique des lésions vasculaires de la région marginale du placenta humain. *Bulletin de la Fédération des Sociétés de Gynécologie et d'Obstétrique de Langue Francaise*, **13**, 507–511.

Williams, M.A., Schenk, B.E., Buller, H.R. and ten Cate, J.W. (1991a) Chronic hypertension, cigarette smoking, and abruptio placentae. *Epidemiology*, **2**, 450–453.

Williams, M.A., Lieberman, E., Mittendorf, R., Monson, R.R. and Schoenbaum, S.C. (1991b) Risk factors for abruptio placentae. *American Journal of Epidemiology*, **134**, 965–972.

Woods, D.L., Edwards, J.N. and Sinclair-Smith, C.C. (1986) Amniotic fluid infection syndrome and abruptio placentae. *Pediatric Pathology*, **6**, 81–85.

Yokoyama, S., Kashima, K. and Inoue, S. et al (1993) Biotin containing intranuclear inclusions in endometrial glands during gestation and puerperium. *American Journal of Clinical Pathology*, **99**, 13–17.

Zeek, P.M. and Assali, N.S. (1952) The formation, regression and differential diagnosis of true infarcts of the placenta. *American Journal of Obstetrics and Gynecology*, **64**, 1191–1200.

Zipursky, A., Pollock, J., Chown, B. and Israels, L.G. (1965) Transplacental isoimmunization by fetal red blood cells. *Birth Defects Original Article Series*, **1**, 84–88.

6

HISTOLOGICAL ABNORMALITIES OF THE PLACENTA

HISTOPATHOLOGY OF THE PLACENTAL VILLI

Villous lesions, or abnormalities, can be classified in a variety of ways. It is, for instance, perfectly acceptable to group them on a pathogenetic basis, some being due to uteroplacental ischaemia, others resulting from reduced fetal perfusion, and yet others having a non-vascular basis. For the purposes of simplicity and clarity I intend to describe the various villous abnormalities on an anatomical basis, grouping them thus:

1. Abnormalities of the trophoblast.
2. Abnormalities of the trophoblastic basement membrane.
3. Abnormalities of the stroma.
4. Abnormalities of the villous vessels.
5. Generalized abnormalities of the villi.

It will be recognized that this is a highly artificial manner in which to regard villous pathology and, at the end of this section, an attempt will be made to show how these various facets of villous structure are interrelated. It will perhaps be less apparent to those unused to the complexities of placental pathology that villous abnormalities are quantitative rather than qualitative, that no complication of pregnancy is accompanied by any specific villous changes, and that all villous lesions found in placentas from abnormal pregnancies can also occur in placentas from fully normal gestations.

Abnormalities of the Trophoblast

Excessive Number of Syncytial Knots

Syncytial knots are focal clumps of syncytial nuclei that protrude into the intervillous space from the surface of the villi. They are, as discussed in Chapter 1, to be distinguished from syncytial sprouts and buds, a precaution that has not always been observed in studies of trophoblastic pathology.

Incidence in placentas from uncomplicated pregnancies

Syncytial knots are not a feature of the first-trimester placenta and, although appearing in gradually increasing numbers during the later stages of pregnancy, are still quite uncommon before the 32nd week of gestation. After this they increase in number until term, at which time knots are normally present on between 11 and 30%

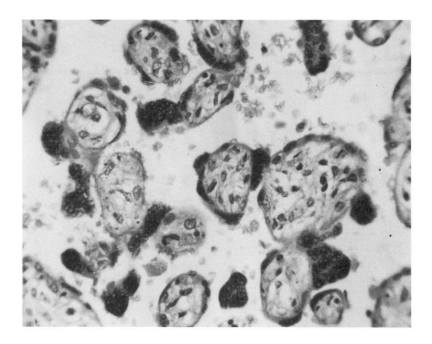

Figure 6.1. Villi in a placenta from a prolonged pregnancy; they are poorly vascularized and richly endowed with syncytial knots (H & E ×460).

of the villi; formation of knots on more than a third of the villi is considered excessive (Fox, 1965). In many, though by no means all, placentas from prolonged pregnancies (i.e. extending to, or beyond, the 42nd gestational week) there is an increase in the proportion of villi on which syncytial knots are present (Fig. 6.1).

In addition to, and distinct from, this overall increase in syncytial knot formation as pregnancy progresses, a localized, and usually very marked, excess of knots is invariably seen in the avascular villi resulting from a fetal artery thrombosis (Fig. 6.2A,B), and is often present in those villi adjacent to an infarct, which, though viable, are poorly perfused because of fibromuscular sclerosis in the fetal stem artery supplying the necrotic area (Fig. 6.3A,B). In both these circumstances the profusion of syncytial knots in the avascular or poorly vascularized villi is in sharp contrast to their relative paucity in the immediately adjacent fully vascularized villi.

Incidence in placentas from complicated pregnancies

It has often been maintained that an excessive formation of syncytial knots is a feature of placentas from pregnancies complicated by pre-eclampsia (Sauramo, 1951; Burstein et al, 1957a; Becker & Bleyl, 1961; Kubli & Budliger, 1963; Merrill, 1963; Muller et al, 1971; Holzl et al, 1974), whilst similar claims have been made for placentas from diabetic women (Kloos, 1952; Thomsen & Lieschke, 1958; Sauramo, 1961; Sani & Bottiglioni, 1964) and for those from cases of materno-fetal rhesus incompatibility (King, 1951; Thomsen & Berle, 1960; Burstein et al, 1963; Gerl et al, 1973). Others, however, have observed that these two latter conditions are associated with a normal or reduced number of knots (Benirschke, 1962; Wilkin, 1965; Wentworth, 1967; Emmrich & Godel, 1972). It should be noted that these various claims and counter-claims have largely been based more on subjective impressions than on quantitative studies and, in my own experience, which is based on actual syncytial knot counts, whilst there is a tendency, though not a very marked one, for placentas from women with pre-eclampsia, essential hypertension or diabetes mellitus to have an increased number of syncytial knots, no such trend is apparent in placentas from cases of materno-fetal rhesus incompatibility: indeed, these latter usually show a paucity of knot formation.

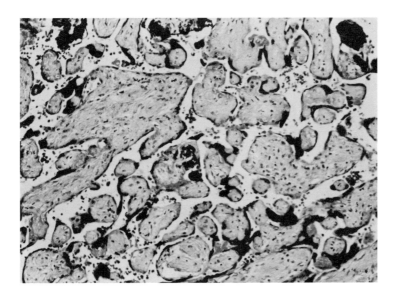

Figure 6.2A. Avascular villi resulting from a fetal artery thrombosis; many have syncytial knots (H & E ×125).

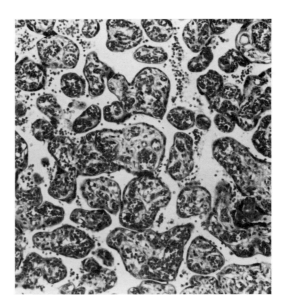

Figure 6.2B. Fully vascularized villi from a normal area of the same placenta that is shown in Fig. 6.2A; the incidence of syncytial knots is much lower than in the avascular villi (H & E ×125).

Relationship to fetal complications

I have not been able to show that there is any correlation between an excess of syncytial knots in the placenta and fetal hypoxia though their numbers are increased in a proportion of placentas from low-birth-weight infants. Knots are present in profusion in placentas from macerated stillbirths (Fig. 6.4), but are not usually unduly numerous in those from fresh stillbirths. This indicates clearly that their formation in excess is a post-mortem change.

Pathogenesis and significance

Syncytial knots have been variously considered as a degenerative phenomenon (Tenney, 1936; Tenney & Parker, 1940; Merrill, 1963), a form of syncytial hyperplasia (Riviere, 1930; Shanklin, 1958; Aladjem, 1967), a manifestation of trophoblastic amoeboid activity (Baker et al, 1944), a response to trophoblastic ischaemia or hypoxia

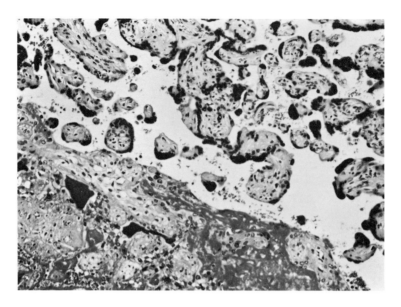

Figure 6.3A. Poorly vascularized but viable villi (above) which are immediately adjacent to an infarct (below); a very high proportion of these villi have syncytial knots (H & E ×125).

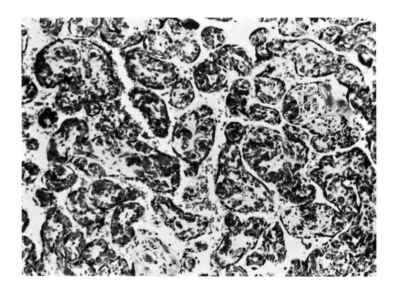

Figure 6.3B. Villi from a normal area of the same placenta as is shown in Fig. 6.3A. A much lower proportion of the villi bear syncytial knots (H & E ×125).

(Thomsen, 1955; Tominaga & Page, 1966; Schuhmann & Geier, 1972; Gerl et al, 1973; Cibils, 1974), or as an ageing change (Kubli & Budliger, 1963). Yet others have suggested that the knots are an incidental by-product of the development of vasculo-syncytial membranes in the syncytiotrophoblast, the nuclei being aggregated so as to allow for the formation of the anuclear membranous areas (Hormann, 1953; Vokaer, 1957; Alvarez, 1970). The truth of the matter is that, as discussed in Chapter 1, many, though not all, apparent syncytial knots are artefacts caused by tangential cutting of the villous syncytiotrophoblast whilst others represent a sequestration phenomena in which the oldest nuclei in the syncytiotrophoblast are aggregated together to form knots, which can therefore be regarded as collections of unwanted aged nuclei.

The view in much current writing about placental pathology is that an excessive

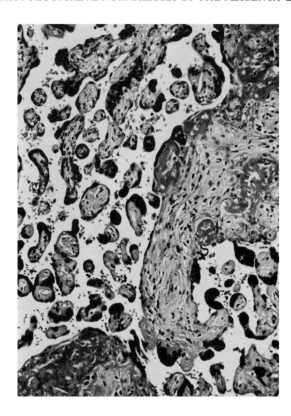

Figure 6.4. Villi in a placenta from a stillborn infant: death had occurred 6 days before delivery. There is a marked excess of villous syncytial knots (H & E ×90).

number of syncytial knots is an indication of uteroplacental ischaemia (the 'Tenney–Parker change') or fetal 'stress' (Naeye, 1989, 1992; Rayburn et al, 1989; Salafia, 1992; Altschuler, 1993; Kaplan, 1993; Benirschke & Kaufmann, 1995; Kliman et al, 1995; Salafia et al, 1995a,b). This view appears to be largely based upon the increased incidence of syncytial knots in many placentas from pregnancies complicated by pre-eclampsia and on the much cited but never confirmed experimental study of Tominaga and Page (1966) in which it was claimed that placental villi cultured under conditions of low oxygen tension showed a marked increase in syncytial knot formation. Those regarding uteroplacental ischaemia or fetal stress as the cause of an increased number of syncytial knots appear to have completely ignored the obvious correlation between reduced fetal villous perfusion and a marked increase in syncytial knots. This correlation is seen, focally and most strikingly, in the localized group of villi rendered avascular by a fetal stem artery thrombosis and is also glaringly evident in the generalized increase in syncytial knots in placentas from macerated, but not fresh, stillbirths, this reflecting the absence of a fetal circulation from villi that are still viable. It may be noted that similar changes have been observed in the experimental studies of Myers and Fujikura (1968), who showed that ligation of a fetal artery in a monkey placenta resulted in an increased formation of syncytial knots in the villi thus rendered avascular.

Once it is accepted that excess syncytial knot formation is a consequence of reduced fetal blood flow through the villi, it becomes clear that in maternal pre-eclampsia, idiopathic intrauterine growth retardation and, to a lesser extent, maternal diabetes mellitus the increased knot formation is secondary to the vasoconstriction of the fetal stem arteries, which is a characteristic feature in placentas from women with these complications of pregnancy, particularly pre-eclampsia. The fact that villous hypovascularity apparently leads to an increased formation of syncytial knots may indicate that under such circumstances the sequestration of aged nuclei is accelerated, or augmented, so as to use optimally the amount of trophoblast available for transfer purposes. Alternatively, it could be argued that diminished fetal perfusion causes an accelerated ageing of the syncytial nuclei. Either, neither or both of these hypotheses may be correct but it is also highly possible that diminished fetal perfusion of the villi leads to their collapse with increased irregularity of their contours and hence an increased incidence of artefactual tangential cutting of trophoblastic tissue. As the formation of syncytial knots appears to be an expression of nuclear ageing, it is not surprising that an excess of such structures is a feature of placentas from prolonged pregnancies. It will be recognized, however, that in prolonged pregnancy, in which fetal villous blood flow is reduced (see Chapter 7), the excess of syncytial knots is also due in part to the reduced fetal perfusion.

There is, in fact, no convincing evidence that uteroplacental ischaemia plays any direct role in the production of syncytial knots. In pre-eclampsia there is only a moderate increase in syncytial knot formation, of a degree not greater than would be expected as a result of the changes in the fetal stem arteries, whilst the localized excess of knots in villi adjacent to an infarct is clearly due principally to decreased fetal perfusion. It may be further remarked that placentas which are infarcted do not, in general, show any undue profusion of syncytial knots and that no association can be demonstrated between an increased number of syncytial knots and intrauterine fetal hypoxia or death. All these findings indicate that an excess of syncytial knots is unlikely to be a direct response to placental ischaemia, and the pathologist examining a placenta in which there is a plethora of knots can draw only the following conclusions:

1. If the villi are well vascularized the placenta is likely to be from what is at least a term pregnancy; if the duration of pregnancy is known with certainty to be less than 40 weeks it can be deduced that the villi show accelerated maturation.
2. If the villi are hypovascular then the knots are largely an expression of reduced fetal perfusion; the functional effects of this do not, in themselves, appear to be of great importance.
3. If the placenta is from a stillbirth it is probable that the excess knot formation has occurred after fetal death.

Excessive Number of Villous Cytotrophoblastic Cells

In the past it was generally believed, indeed it was almost a dogma, that the villous cytotrophoblastic cells, so prominent in the early stages of gestation, progressively disappear as pregnancy advances and are absent from the mature villi (Schroder, 1930; Hormann, 1948; Clavero-Nunez, 1962). Lone voices did occasionally remark that these cells could still be seen in the mature organ (Wislocki & Bennett, 1943; Sauramo, 1951) but these were ignored until the advent of electron microscopy, when the early studies of trophoblastic fine structure showed quite clearly that villous cytotrophoblastic cells were still present in mature placentas (Boyd & Hughes, 1954; Wislocki & Dempsey, 1955; Sawasaki et al, 1957; Ikawa, 1959). Spurred on by this knowledge, light microscopists re-studied the terminal villi of mature placentas and soon realized that they could also detect cytotrophoblastic cells (Thomsen & Blankenburg, 1956; Wigglesworth, 1962; Traub et al, 1964). It is certainly true that the villous cytotrophoblastic cells become less prominent as pregnancy proceeds and that in mature villi they tend to be flattened and inconspicuous, but they are nevertheless regularly present. Indeed, although their numbers appear to diminish, the absolute number of villous cytotrophoblastic cells actually increases progressively until term (Simpson et al, 1992), their apparent sparcity being a reflection of their wider dispersal in an increased trophoblastic volume. No special techniques of fixation or staining are necessary for the demonstration of villous cytotrophoblastic cells but they are best seen in sections stained with PAS, in which their negatively staining cytoplasm contrasts sharply with the much more positively reacting syncytial cytoplasm and their site external to the trophoblastic basement membrane is readily appreciated (Fig. 6.5).

Incidence in placentas from uncomplicated pregnancies

In the mature placenta cytotrophoblastic cells are commonly seen in about 20% of the villi, though it is by no means exceptional for them to be apparent in as many as

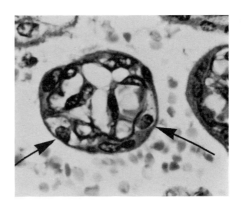

Figure 6.5. Two cytotrophoblastic cells (arrowed) are clearly visible in the trophoblastic layer of a villus in a full-term placenta (PAS ×850).

40% (Fox, 1964): these cells are, as mentioned above, inconspicuous and never form a complete mantle around the villus as they do in the immature placenta. There is a tendency, though not a very marked one, for an excessive number of cytotrophoblastic cells to be seen in placentas from prolonged pregnancies, whilst prominent cytotrophoblastic cells are a feature of the prematurely delivered placenta.

Incidence in placentas from complicated pregnancies

It has long been recognized that the presence of numerous villous cytotrophoblastic cells is a striking feature of placentas from diabetic women and from cases of materno-fetal rhesus incompatibility, but it was left to Wigglesworth (1962) to draw attention to the undue prominence and increased numbers of villous cytotrophoblastic cells frequently apparent in placentas from women whose pregnancies have been complicated by pre-eclampsia. This finding was confirmed subsequently (Fox, 1964; Maqueo et al, 1964; Kaufmann, 1972; Buckshee et al, 1974) and it may be added that in pre-eclampsia the number of villous cytotrophoblastic cells increases progressively with the severity and duration of the disease (Fig. 6.6). An excess of villous cytotrophoblastic cells is also a feature of many, though by no means all, placentas from infants with idiopathic intrauterine growth retardation.

Relationship to fetal complications

A high proportion of live-born fetuses who have suffered intrauterine hypoxia have placentas in which villous cytotrophoblastic cells are unduly numerous.

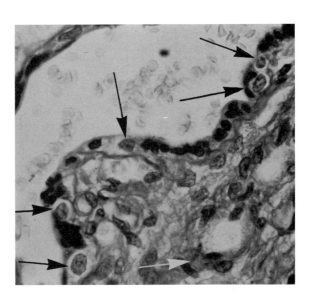

Figure 6.6. Numerous cytotrophoblastic cells (arrowed) in the villous trophoblast of a placenta from a patient with severe pre-eclampsia (H & E ×980).

Cytotrophoblastic cells tend to be obtrusively profuse in the villi of placentas from fresh stillbirths when fetal death has occurred after a prolonged period of hypoxia. This finding, however, tends to be overshadowed by the fact that after fetal demise, from any cause, the number of cytotrophoblastic cells shows a progressive increase, so that these cells are a notable feature in all placentas from macerated stillbirths.

Pathogenesis and significance

There are two mechanisms, between which a clear distinction should be drawn, that can lead to an excessive number of cytotrophoblastic cells being present in the villi. These are:

1. A failure of cytotrophoblastic regression.
2. Proliferation of cytotrophoblastic cells.

Failure of cytotrophoblastic regression is usually just one facet of a generalized failure of villous maturation, and is thus seen in those placentas in which the villi are unduly immature for the length of the gestational period. This is the principal reason for the large numbers of villous cytotrophoblastic cells in placentas from cases of diabetes mellitus or materno-fetal rhesus incompatibility.

That an excess of cytotrophoblastic cells is due to their failure to regress may usually be deduced from the general setting of villous immaturity in which this phenomenon occurs. This contrasts with the picture seen when the excess is due to hyperplasia, which usually occurs in villi that are otherwise morphologically fully mature. A further point of differentiation is that mitotic figures are seen moderately frequently in cytotrophoblastic cells undergoing hyperplasia (Fig. 6.7) but are absent from those that have failed to regress. It is, of course, possible for there to be, in a single placenta, both a failure of villous regression and some degree of cytotrophoblastic hyperplasia; evidence for this can be detected at the ultrastructural level but is not usually discernible on light microscopy. This does not detract from the fact that light microscopic recognition of the clear predominance of one or other of these processes in a placenta in which there is an excessive number of cytotrophoblastic cells does not usually present any undue difficulty.

It is largely, if not entirely, because of a hyperplasia that cytotrophoblastic cells are so numerous in placentas from women with pre-eclampsia and this also accounts for their excess in placentas from cases of intrauterine fetal hypoxia, intrauterine growth retardation and macerated stillbirths. That there is a true hyperplasia of these cells in pre-eclampsia has been confirmed by Arnholdt et al (1991) who used a monoclonal antibody to the cell proliferation marker Ki67. Wigglesworth (1962) suggested that this proliferative activity in the cytotrophoblast is a response to uteroplacental ischaemia, a view supported by the demonstration that cytotrophoblastic hyperplasia can be specifically stimulated *in vitro* (Fig. 6.8) by culturing placental villi under conditions of low oxygen tension (Fox, 1970; MacLennon et al, 1972; Amalados & Burton, 1985; Burton et al, 1989). In placentas from diabetic women and from cases of materno-fetal rhesus incompatibility in neither of which conditions is there any reason to believe that the trophoblast has been subjected to ischaemia, the failure of cytotrophoblastic regression

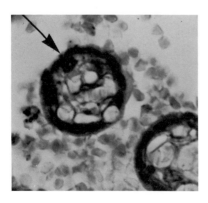

Figure 6.7. A mitotic figure (arrowed) in a villous cytotrophoblastic cell. This is from a patient with pre-eclampsia (PAS ×880).

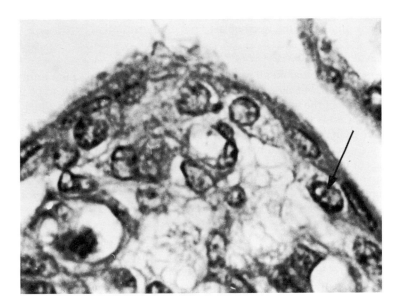

Figure 6.8. A placental villus cultured *in vitro* under conditions of low oxygen tension. The syncytiotrophoblast shows degenerative changes, and numerous prominent cytotrophoblastic cells (one of which is arrowed) are seen in the trophoblast. These features were absent from villi cultured under fully oxygenated conditions (PAS ×1170).

may be compounded by a degree of cytotrophoblastic hyperplasia that occurs in those placentas showing evidence of syncytial damage (Jones, 1976; Jones & Fox, 1976). It would appear, therefore, that cytotrophoblastic hyperplasia is a non-specific response to syncytial injury, whether this be due to ischaemia or not. This is a far from surprising conclusion, because, as discussed in Chapter 1, the cytotrophoblastic cells function as the 'stem cells' of the villous trophoblast and thus serve as a germinative zone from which the syncytiotrophoblast is derived. In the mature placenta this germinative zone is largely quiescent but it can be reactivated if the necessity arises to form fresh syncytiotrophoblast, which occurs if the syncytium is injured or destroyed. Hence cytotrophoblastic hyperplasia is essentially a repair phenomenon and is a non-specific indicator of syncytial damage or necrosis. In pre-eclampsia, in which cytotrophoblastic hyperplasia is most clearly evident, the syncytial damage is due to ischaemia, and hence the intensity of the cytotrophoblastic proliferative activity serves as a rough guide not only to the degree and extent of syncytial damage but also, by implication, to the severity and duration of the ischaemia to which the trophoblast has been subjected. Because cytotrophoblastic proliferation is a repair phenomenon which, in teleological terms, is designed to maintain placental functional efficiency, it seems almost perverse to argue, as some have done, that this process results in increased thickness of the trophoblastic villous mantle and hence impairs the oxygen transfer capacity of the placenta (Salafia et al, 1995a).

It has been suggested (Ruckhaberle & Ruckhaberle, 1976) that in addition to the two mechanisms outlined above being responsible for an excess of villous cytotrophoblastic cells, a third factor may also be operative in some cases, namely a 'maturation arrest' of the cytotrophoblastic cells which are unable to transform into syncytiotrophoblast. This is an interesting concept but such an arrest would be associated with a marked defect in syncytiotrophoblast formation, a deficiency that has not been observed.

Deficiency of Vasculo-Syncytial Membranes

Vasculo-syncytial membranes are described in Chapter 1, where it is pointed out that they are specialized areas of the syncytiotrophoblast which appear to be specifically adapted for transfer purposes and that their presence is an indication of topographic functional differentiation of the trophoblast.

Incidence in placentas from uncomplicated pregnancies

Villous vasculo-syncytial membranes are uncommon in the placenta until about the 32nd week of gestation, but thereafter they increase rapidly in number to be present, at term, on about 20% of the villi. Quantitative studies indicate that the vast majority (over 99%) of term placentas from uncomplicated pregnancies have vasculo-syncytial membranes on more than 5% of their villi (Fox, 1967a) and hence any placenta with an incidence of villous vasculo-syncytial membrane formation less than this can be considered as being deficient in these structures.

A paucity of vasculo-syncytial membranes is a feature of a proportion of placentas from prolonged, but otherwise uncomplicated, pregnancies: the reasons for, and significance of, this finding are discussed later.

Incidence in placentas from complicated pregnancies

Becker and Bleyl (1961) thought that placentas from women with pre-eclampsia tended to show a relative lack of vasculo-syncytial membranes, and this would be in accord with my own findings. I would also concur with those suggesting that the number of vasculo-syncytial membranes tends to be unduly low in placentas from cases of materno-fetal rhesus incompatibility (Hormann, 1958a,b; Becker & Bleyl, 1961) and in those from diabetic women (Hormann, 1958a,b), disagreeing in this latter respect with Horky (1964a), who claimed that the placenta of diabetic women often showed an increased incidence of these structures.

Relationship to fetal abnormalities

There is a clear-cut inverse relationship between the incidence of villous vasculo-syncytial membranes and that of fetal hypoxia (Fox, 1967a). This is not to say, of course, that every fetus whose placenta has a paucity of vasculo-syncytial membranes will show clinical evidence of hypoxia but, nevertheless, in these circumstances the incidence of hypoxia is approximately twice that occurring in fetuses whose placentas have a normal complement of these membranes. As a corollary to this there is a very low incidence of fetal hypoxia when the placenta shows a profuse formation of vasculo-syncytial membranes (i.e. on more than one-third of the villi). A relative deficiency of vasculo-syncytial membranes is also found in a significant proportion of placentas both from infants of low birth weight and from fresh stillbirths.

Pathogenesis and significance

Bremer (1916), who first described vasculo-syncytial membranes (under the name of 'epithelial plates'), likened them to renal glomeruli and suggested that they were placental excretory structures, whilst Strachan (1923) considered them as areas of syncytial degeneration. The available evidence (reviewed in Chapter 1) now indicates clearly, however, that vasculo-syncytial membranes are focally differentiated areas of the syncytiotrophoblast which are specifically concerned with materno-fetal transfer. The membranes appear at a relatively late stage of pregnancy and hence it is often assumed that their formation is a manifestation of villous maturation. Uncommonly, but significantly, placentas are encountered, however, which are in all respects morphologically mature apart from not having formed villous vasculo-syncytial membranes, and in these it is apparent that the processes of villous maturation and trophoblastic differentiation can occur independently of each other. Nevertheless the two usually proceed synchronously and, in placentas from diabetics or from cases of materno-fetal rhesus incompatibility, the relative lack of vasculo-syncytial membranes is basically a reflection of the delayed villous maturity which is frequently found in these placentas (Fig. 6.9).

A vasculo-syncytial membrane consists of attenuated anuclear syncytiotrophoblast stretched over, and in close apposition to, a sinusoidally dilated vessel. If for any reason the fetal vessels contract or collapse, the vasculo-syncytial membranes will no longer be

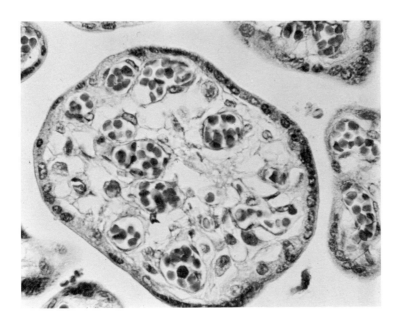

Figure 6.9. Villi in a full-term placenta from a diabetic woman. The villus is slightly immature and there is no evidence of vasculo-syncytial membrane formation (H & E ×450).

apparent even though they may have been well formed before the collapse of the fetal villous circulation. It is probably for this reason that there appears to be a lack of vasculo-syncytial membranes in placentas from prolonged pregnancies, in many of which villous hypovascularity is a typical feature (see Chapter 7). Whether this phenomenon of apparent secondary disappearance of the vasculo-syncytial membranes is accompanied by a reduction in their functional efficiency is a debatable point but there must be at least a strong suspicion that this is the case.

A paucity of villous vasculo-syncytial membranes may therefore occur under three circumstances:

1. As a component feature of a generalized retardation of villous maturation; under these circumstances there is probably a failure of both villous maturation and trophoblastic differentiation and the consequences of this are of considerable significance (see later).

2. As a secondary change following a failure of fetal villous perfusion. There is no reason in these cases to believe that there has been any primary defect of trophoblastic differentiation.

3. As an isolated phenomenon in a placenta whose villi are fully mature and adequately vascularized. This is an uncommon finding but one that is indicative of a pure failure of trophoblastic differentiation, a failure that often results in inadequate fetal oxygenation. The factors responsible for inducing trophoblastic differentiation are unknown and, in our present state of ignorance, it would be fruitless to speculate on why differentiation of this tissue should fail to occur normally in certain placentas.

Fibrinoid Necrosis of Villi

This is a lesion which, despite having a very characteristic and easily recognizable appearance, has often been confused with perivillous fibrin deposition, and which has been frequently both misinterpreted and wrongly labelled. I am, as discussed in Chapter 1, here using the term 'fibrinoid' in its traditional pathological sense as not being entirely derived from the maternal blood.

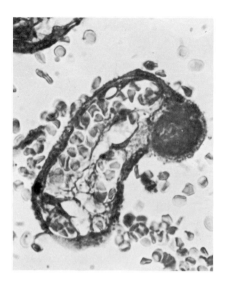

Figure 6.10. A 'blob' of homogeneous fibrinoid material in the trophoblast of a placental villus (PAS ×600).

The first step in the evolution of the abnormality is the appearance of a small 'blob' of homogeneous, acidophilic and strongly PAS-positive material in the villous trophoblast at a site beneath the syncytiotrophoblast but external to the trophoblastic basement membrane (Fig. 6.10). This abnormal substance is distinct from the trophoblastic basement membrane, which, where it lies in close contact with the fibrinoid material, shows marked, but localized, thickening.

The 'blob' of acidophilic material gradually enlarges, and hence it bulges progressively into the villous stroma (Fig. 6.11); its increase in size is apparently always due to an accretion onto its deep surface. The 'blob' does not actually invade the stromal tissue because the underlying basement membrane remains intact although becoming increasingly indented into a crescentic shape, the concavity of which is progressively deepened by the expanding mass of fibrinoid material. This process continues until eventually the whole villus is converted into a fibrinoid nodule (Fig. 6.12). The syncytiotrophoblast of the affected villi is morphologically normal in the early stages of the

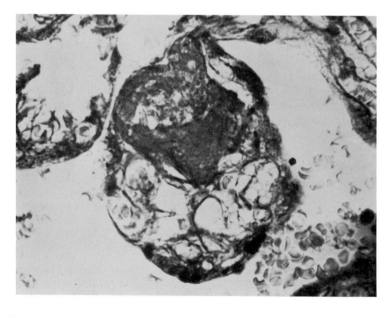

Figure 6.11. A later stage in the development of villous fibrinoid necrosis than that shown in Fig. 6.10. The mass of fibrinoid material is larger and is indenting the villous stroma (PAS ×600).

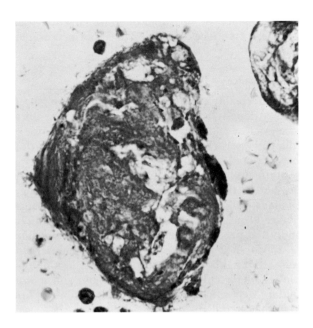

Figure 6.12. A villus that has undergone complete fibrinoid necrosis. Remnants of the syncytiotrophoblast can be seen around the perimeter of the fibrinoid mass (PAS ×600).

development of this lesion, but later shows an increasing degree of atrophy and degeneration, though even in the final stages a few remnants of this tissue still remain. Hence the eventual appearance is that of a nodular mass of homogeneous acidophilic material, around the periphery of which are a few degenerate syncytial nuclei.

Incidence in placentas from uncomplicated pregnancies

It is by no means uncommon to encounter mature placentas from uncomplicated pregnancies in which villous fibrinoid necrosis is completely absent, but in most there are occasional scattered villi that show this change. In a study of 220 placentas from term uncomplicated pregnancies I did not find any in which more than 3% of the villi had undergone complete fibrinoid necrosis (Fox, 1968a). I would therefore regard this incidence as the top limit of the 'normal range', and would consider any placenta in which more than 3% of the villi showed fibrinoid necrosis as being abnormal in this respect. The incidence of villous fibrinoid necrosis is not increased in placentas from prolonged pregnancies but tends to be rather high in those from prematurely terminating, but otherwise normal, gestations.

Incidence in placentas from complicated pregnancies

I have found the incidence of villous fibrinoid necrosis to be moderately increased in placentas from women with pre-eclampsia and to be considerably increased in those from diabetic patients and from cases of materno-fetal rhesus incompatibility; there is no excess of this villous lesion in placentas from women with essential hypertension. My findings on pre-eclampsia have been confirmed by de Ikonicoff (1970), Ehrhardt et al (1972), Sen and Langley (1974) and Sayeed et al (1976), whilst those with respect to diabetes mellitus and rhesus incompatibility have also been noted by Liebhart (1969), de Ikonicoff (1970), Ehrhardt et al (1972), Jakobovits and Traub (1972) and Mathews et al (1973).

Relationship to fetal abnormalities

I have been unable to detect any correlation between an excess of villous fibrinoid necrosis and fetal hypoxia, growth retardation or intrauterine death. On the other hand, Sen and Langley (1974) thought that placentas from stillbirths showed an abnormally high incidence of this lesion, whilst Gershon and Strauss (1961) have reported an increased frequency of villous fibrinoid necrosis in the placentas of low-birthweight infants.

Pathogenesis and significance

This villous abnormality remains something of an enigma. The suggestion that it simply represents a deposit of fibrin, derived either from the maternal blood in the intervillous space (McKay et al, 1958; Wigglesworth, 1964; Moe, 1969) or from the fetal blood in the villous vessels (Kline, 1951; Emmrich, 1966a), does not accord with the observation that fibrinoid material originates from a primary site in the villous trophoblast. This argument is also applicable to Vokaer's (1957) hypothesis that the primary abnormality lies in the villous stroma. The view that the lesion originates as a change in the villous cytotrophoblastic cells (Wilkin, 1965) is one with which I would agree; it has received considerable support from Liebhart's (1970, 1971c) electron-optical demonstration that the first discernible change in the evolution of villous fibrinoid necrosis is the appearance of masses of fibrillary material in the cytoplasm of the cytotrophoblastic cells. It has been argued that the lesion contains an admixture of fibrin and fibrinoid (Benirschke & Kaufmann, 1995) and it would not be suprising if there was secondary deposition of fibrinogen on the fibrinoid material exposed to the maternal blood in the intervillous space.

These findings merely localize the origin of the lesion and leave unanswered the question of how and why it arises. There has been, and still is, a body of support for its being the visible hallmark of an immunological reaction within trophoblastic tissue. This concept originally arose from the immunofluorescent studies of Burstein et al (1963), who showed that anti-D antibody tended to localize, in placentas from cases of materno-fetal rhesus incompatibility, in those villi showing fibrinoid necrosis; insulin showed a similar localization in diabetic women's placentas. This particular piece of work is open to considerable criticism on technical grounds and the results obtained have not been reproducible in other hands. However, other findings have emerged since which also tend to point towards an immunological basis for this lesion. First, in placentas from cases of materno-fetal rhesus incompatibility there is a direct relationship between the level of anti-D in the maternal blood and the incidence of placental villous fibrinoid necrosis (Fox, 1968a; Jakobovits & Traub, 1972). Secondly, it has been adequately demonstrated that the fibrinoid masses contain fibrinogen, fibrin, IgG, IgM and several activated components of complement (Horn & Horalek, 1961; Brzosko et al, 1965; Pisarki, 1967; McCormick et al, 1971; Oswald & Gerl, 1972; Labarrere & Faulk, 1992). Elution of the IgG shows it to be present in a bound form, which, together with the presence of complement, suggests that it is present in affected villi because of an antigen–antibody reaction (McCormick et al, 1971).

Several observations have been reported which, though of considerable interest, have tended to make the whole question of villous fibrinoid necrosis even more confused. Jakobovits and Traub (1972) have shown that injection of intra-amniotic saline appears to produce an increased number of villi showing fibrinoid necrosis, whilst Gille et al (1974a,b) have noted a similar finding after intravenous injection into the mother of a purified fragment of IgG. I must confess that I am unable fully to understand the significance of these findings and do not know whether they detract from or bolster the hypothesis of an immunological basis for villous fibrinoid necrosis.

The pathologist, noting an excess of villi showing fibrinoid necrosis in a placenta, is therefore not, at the moment, in a position to draw any valid conclusions from this finding, though the possibility that it represents an immune attack on trophoblastic tissue cannot be totally discarded and should be borne in mind.

Abnormalities of the Trophoblastic Basement Membrane

The only abnormality of the trophoblastic basement membrane recognizable on light microscopy is an increase in its thickness (Fig 6.13). It may be thought that recog-

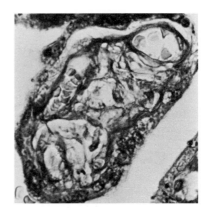

Figure 6.13. A villus in which there is a moderate degree of thickening of the trophoblastic basement membrane (PAS ×600).

nition of such a change is dependent upon highly subjective criteria, and this is indeed the case. In practice, however, this abnormality is usually easily assessed in PAS-stained sections and little difficulty is encountered in distinguishing between a normal and a thickened membrane.

Incidence in placentas from uncomplicated pregnancies

Occasional villi with a thickened trophoblastic basement membrane are found in about one-third of term placentas, but such villi rarely form more than 3% of the villous population; an incidence in excess of this is regarded as abnormal (Fox, 1968c). In many placentas from prolonged pregnancies there is a notable increase in the number of villi with abnormally thick basement membranes. It is also of note that villi entrapped in a plaque of fibrin usually have markedly thickened trophoblastic basement membranes (see Chapter 5).

Incidence in placentas from complicated pregnancies

A striking increase in the proportion of villi with unduly thick trophoblastic basement membranes is, in my experience, a common feature of placentas from women with pre-eclampsia or essential hypertension (Fox, 1968c), a finding in accord with other observations by both light and electron microscopists (Hall, 1949; Sermann & Capria, 1965; Anderson & McKay, 1966; Salvatore, 1966, 1968; Sen & Langley, 1974). A tendency towards an increased incidence of villi with thickened basement membranes is also apparent in placentas from women with diabetes mellitus and from cases of materno-fetal rhesus incompatibility.

Relationship to fetal complications

Fetuses whose placentas contain a marked excess of villi with abnormally thick trophoblastic basement membranes have a much higher incidence of clinical hypoxia than do those in whose placentas this change is absent. There is also a high incidence of this abnormality in placentas from babies of low birth weight and in those cases of fresh stillbirths caused by intrauterine hypoxia. In all placentas from macerated stillbirths, well-marked thickening of the basement membrane is found in most villi; this indicates that the lesion occurs as a post-mortem change, irrespective of whether it was also present at the time of death.

Aetiology and pathogenesis

The cause of this abnormality is unknown, but there are good grounds for suggesting that in many cases the thickening of the basement membrane is a response to utero-placental ischaemia. Such a hypothesis would accord with the striking excess of this lesion in placentas from women with the hypertensive complications of pregnancy, and would be supported by the association between this placental abnormality and fetal hypoxia. It would also be buttressed by experimental *in vitro* studies, which have shown that basement membrane thickening is seen in placental villi maintained under

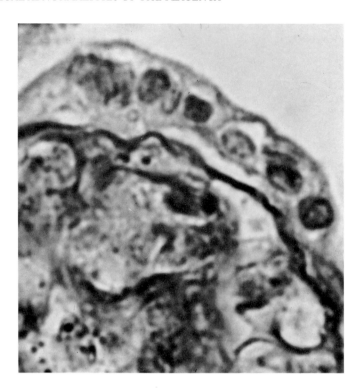

Figure 6.14. Marked thickening of the trophoblastic basement membrane of a placental villus cultured *in vitro* under hypoxic conditions. This change was not seen in fully oxygenated villi (PAS ×1170).

conditions of low oxygen tension (Fig. 6.14), but does not occur to any significant degree in those that are fully oxygenated during culture (Fox, 1970; MacLennan et al, 1972). The actual mechanism by which ischaemia induces basement changes is open to debate, but it may be related to the cytotrophoblastic hyperplasia that also occurs under ischaemic conditions and which is therefore often seen in placentas in which trophoblastic basement membrane thickening is a feature. Basement membrane material is probably secreted, in part at least, by the cytotrophoblastic cells, and the proliferative activity of these cells may be accompanied by an excessive secretion of basement membrane substance, a situation analogous to that seen in capillaries, in which thickening of the vessel basement membrane is related to an increased turnover of the endothelial cells (Vracko & Benditt, 1970). Such a view would certainly tend to explain the very gross basement membrane thickening that is often seen in villi entrapped in fibrin and which occurs in association with a degree of cytotrophoblastic proliferation beyond that encountered in non-encased villi.

If, as seems likely, basement membrane thickening is often due to uteroplacental ischaemia, this cannot be evoked as the aetiological factor in all cases, because similar basement membrane changes occur under circumstances in which there are no grounds for supposing that the villi have been subjected to ischaemia, e.g., in placentas from diabetic women or from cases of materno-fetal rhesus incompatibility. Burstein et al (1963) suggested that in these placentas the basement changes were immunologically mediated, and it is certainly easy to draw an analogy between the basement membrane changes seen in placental villi and those found in the renal glomeruli as a result of deposition of either antibodies or immune complexes. To some extent, this concept has been strengthened by Faulk et al (1974), who demonstrated that IgG can be regularly eluted from villous basement membranes, thus raising the possibility that excessive deposition of this immunoglobulin may cause an apparent increase in basement membrane width. However, a careful electron microscopic search for evidence of immune complexes in thickened villous basement membranes has proved unrewarding (Jones, 1976) and a definitive answer to this question remains to be found.

There does not seem to be, therefore, any unitary explanation for the finding of an excess of villi with thick trophoblastic basement membranes. If the pathologist encountering this change also notes that there is cytotrophoblastic proliferation, he or she can assume, with a fair degree of confidence, that there has been uteroplacental ischaemia, but if such hyperplasia is absent no definite conclusions can be drawn about the significance of this histological abnormality. It should be noted, of course, that there is no evidence that the basement membrane changes interfere with placental function; the high incidence of fetal hypoxia found in association with this abnormality is due, not to the basement membrane changes, but to the ischaemia, which is responsible both for the histological changes and the fetal complications.

Abnormalities of the Stroma

Stromal Fibrosis

The stroma of mature placental villi usually contains little collagen, but in most placentas there are occasional villi that are notably fibrotic. The decision on whether the amount of collagen in the stroma of any particular villus is excessive or not is bound to be both arbitrary and subjective, but a clear distinction can usually be drawn between normal and fibrotic villi without too much difficulty.

Incidence in placentas from uncomplicated pregnancies

A few fibrotic villi are encountered in most, but by no means all, placentas from uncomplicated pregnancies, irrespective of whether these have proceeded to term or have terminated prematurely. It is uncommon, however, for more than 3% of the villi to show a marked increase in the stromal content of fibrous tissue, and an incidence in excess of this can be considered as abnormal. In between a quarter and a third of placentas from prolonged pregnancies there is a striking increase in the number of fibrotic villi; indeed, it is in such placentas that villous fibrosis is seen most abundantly and strikingly (Fox, 1968b). It is usually notable that the villi which are fibrotic, in placentas from both term and prolonged pregnancies, are poorly vascularized (Fig. 6.15). The importance of reduced fetal perfusion is emphasized by the fact that a marked, localized excess of stromal collagen is seen in villi rendered avascular by a fetal artery thrombosis and in the poorly vascularized villi immediately adjacent to an area of infarction.

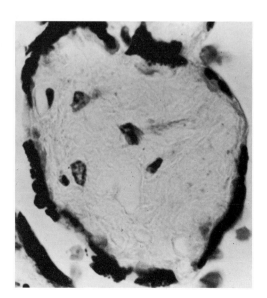

Figure 6.15. A poorly vascularized villus in a placenta from a prolonged pregnancy. There is marked fibrosis of the villous stroma (van Gieson ×780).

Incidence in placentas from complicated pregnancies

There is a tendency, though not a very striking one, for there to be an excess of fibrotic villi in placentas from women with pre-eclampsia, and a rather more marked trend towards a similar finding in placentas from diabetic women (Fox, 1968b). My observations in this latter respect are in accord with those of Sauramo (1961), Clavero-Nunez (1963), and Emmrich and Godel (1972), but are in sharp contrast to those of Liebhart (1968, 1974), who found impaired collagenization of the villous stroma in the placenta of diabetic women. No excess of stromal fibrosis is found in placentas from cases of materno-fetal rhesus incompatibility.

A scattering of fibrotic, scarred villi may result from a villitis, such as that due to rubella; this subject is discussed more fully in Chapter 11, but it may be noted here that other evidence of placental inflammation is usually also present in such circumstances.

Relationship to fetal complications

It has been claimed that stromal fibrosis is a potent cause of fetal hypoxia and death (Lawrance, 1933), but I have been unable to show an association between villous fibrosis and any fetal complication such as hypoxia or low birth weight. In placentas from macerated stillbirths most of the villi are strikingly fibrotic, but this is a post-mortem change and an excess of villous fibrosis is not a feature of placentas from fresh stillbirths.

Aetiology and pathogenesis

It is often assumed that villous fibrosis is a response to uteroplacental ischaemia, but the findings cited above, particularly the lack of any association between villous fibrosis and fetal hypoxia, the lack of any excess of fibrotic villi in placentas from fresh stillbirths, and the relatively slight tendency towards increased villous fibrosis in placentas from patients with pre-eclampsia, all argue against the acceptance of this somewhat facile hypothesis. It is much more likely that villous fibrosis is associated with, and is due to, a reduced fetal blood flow through the villi. This is specifically suggested by the fact that most fibrotic villi are poorly vascularized, by the finding of a marked degree of stromal fibrosis in the avascular villi distal to an occlusion of a fetal stem artery, and by the development of villous fibrosis after fetal death. It could, of course, be argued that the stromal collagen constricts the villous vessels and that the diminished villous vascularity is an effect rather than a cause of the excess of stromal fibrous tissue, but this argument clearly cannot be applied to the villous fibrosis that complicates a fetal artery thrombosis. The increased incidence of stromal fibrosis in both pre-eclampsia and diabetes mellitus is probably related to the 'obliterative endarteritis' of the fetal stem arteries that is found in placentas of women with these two conditions (see later in this chapter), whilst the marked excess of stromal collagen in placentas from prolonged pregnancies is seen only in those in which, very characteristically, there is a striking reduction in fetal villous vascularity.

Having said all this, it must be admitted that there is no real explanation as to how or why a reduced fetal perfusion should lead to villous fibrosis. Despite this gap in our knowledge it remains the case that the only importance of villous fibrosis to the pathologist is as a morphological hallmark of a reduced fetal villous perfusion; it is of no clinical significance.

Villous Oedema (Fig. 6.16)

Most accounts of villous oedema imply that this abnormality is easy to recognize but in practice there is no doubt that normal immature intermediate villi are often mistakenly classed as oedematous villi (Kaufman et al, 1987; Benirschke & Kaufmann, 1995). If there is true villous oedema the placenta usually appears hydropic on macroscopic examination and under these circumstances the presence of villous oedema correlates well with an increased placental water content (Barker et al, 1994). It has to be stressed, however, that in these circumstances the villous oedema is very obvious on his-

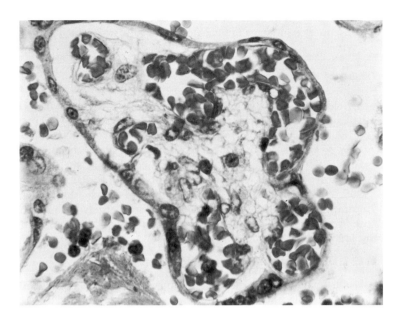

Figure 6.16. A mildly oedematous villus in a full-term placenta from a diabetic woman (H & E ×550).

tological examination and that apparently minor or moderate degrees of villous oedema are not associated with an excess of placental water. With this important codicil, villous oedema occurs in placentas from diabetic women and from cases of materno-fetal rhesus incompatibility, although only a proportion of such placentas are oedematous. Villous oedema is also occasionally seen in placentas from women with pre-eclampsia (Tarjan, 1965), whilst it should also be borne in mind that quite marked oedema of the villi is a feature of several placental infections, e.g., syphilis, toxoplasmosis and cytomegalovirus, and is often present in placentas containing a large haemangioma or metastases from a fetal neuroblastoma. It must be confessed that the cause of the fluid accumulation in the stroma is unknown, and whilst it is tempting to attribute it to a functional insufficiency of the fetal circulation, no firm evidence exists to suggest that this is the case.

The clinical significance of villous oedema has been a matter for dispute. Naeye (Naeye et al, 1983; Naeye, 1992) has maintained that villous oedema is the most important cause of stillbirth, neonatal death and neonatal morbidity in children born before the 28th week of gestation and the major cause of fetal hypoxia in infants born before the 30th week of gestation and that the finding of severe villous oedema correlates inversely with umbilical arterial blood oxygen and pH values, a view concurred with by Kovalovszki et al (1990) and Ilagan et al (1990).

Naeye considered that villous oedema is initiated by fetal stress, this being most commonly induced by acute chorioamnionitis or placental abruption, and that the oedema causes fetal hypoxia by compressing the villous vessels. It is my opinion, however, that many of the villi illustrated by Naeye as showing oedema are, in reality, normal immature intermediate villi and hence it is not altogether suprising that he found the incidence of villous oedema declined progressively after the 30th week of gestation. Further, I can see no clearly valid reason why fetal stress should result in villous oedema and I cannot visualize a haemodynamic situation in which oedema fluid could significantly reduce blood flow through the vessels from which the oedema fluid is derived; certainly, this is not a situation which is encountered in disease states elsewhere in the body. Alvarez et al (1972) have suggested that the increased size of the oedematous villi may decrease the capacity of the intervillous space and thus limit the maternal blood flow through the placenta. Haemodynamic studies to confirm this suggestion are lacking and Shen-Schwartz et al (1989) could not confirm that villous oedema was, in itself, of any consequence in terms of fetal welfare, a view with which I tend to concur.

Excessive Number of Villous Hofbauer Cells

The long-held view that the villous Hofbauer cells disappear from the placenta after the fourth month of pregnancy (Hofbauer, 1925; Stieve, 1941; Hormann, 1947, 1948) resisted the occasional claims to the contrary that were expressed by light microscopists (Rodway & Marsh, 1956; Geller, 1957) but eventually succumbed to the electron microscopists, who were able to show convincingly that such cells were indeed present in the mature placenta (Bargmann & Knoop, 1959; Panigel & Anh, 1964a,b; Nagy et al, 1965; Wynn, 1965, 1967). It remains true, of course, that the Hofbauer cells appear to diminish in number as gestation progresses, largely because they are compressed by the increasingly compact stroma, but they can still be seen in most full-term placentas and are probably present in all.

Incidence in placentas from uncomplicated pregnancies

Villous Hofbauer cells are seen in abundance in young placentas, are present in moderate numbers in placentas from pregnancies terminating during the early third trimester, and can be seen, in scattered villi, in 80% of term placentas (Fox, 1967b). In the mature organ it is unusual to find Hofbauer cells in more than 2–3% of the villi, and it is an almost invariable rule that they are never seen in fully mature, non-oedematous villi, only occurring in those that are less mature than the bulk of the villous population or in those showing some degree of oedema (Fig. 6.17).

Incidence in placentas from complicated pregnancies

An excess of villous Hofbauer cells is not a feature of placentas from women with pre-eclampsia or essential hypertension, but it is commonly, though not invariably,

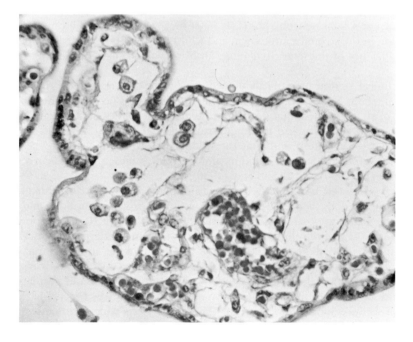

Figure 6.17. A markedly oedematous villus in a placenta from a diabetic woman. Many Hofbauer cells are seen in the widely dilated interfibrillary spaces of the oedematous villous stroma (H & E ×350).

found in placentas from cases of maternal diabetes mellitus or fetal hydrops. In these latter conditions this profusion of Hofbauer cells is only apparent if the villi are either unduly immature or oedematous, the number of such cells being directly proportional to the degree of immaturity or to the severity of the oedema.

Relationship to fetal complications

No association exists between an excess of villous Hofbauer cells and any disturbance of fetal well-being.

Aetiology and pathogenesis

Hofbauer cells are seen in villi that have a wide-meshed loose stroma, whether this is due to immaturity or oedema (Geller, 1957; Horky, 1964b; Fox, 1967b), and they are not visible on light microscopy in fully mature villi, which have a condensed stroma and narrowed or obliterated interfibrillary spaces. Nevertheless, electron microscopy often reveals compressed and distorted Hofbauer cells in the stromal core of such villi, and Bleyl (1962) has shown that Hofbauer cells become easily demonstrable in villi that are artificially rendered oedematous by saline perfusion after delivery, whilst remaining inapparent in those villi that escape perfusion. All this suggests that the apparent reduction in the number of villous Hofbauer cells as pregnancy progresses is largely, if not entirely, due to their being compressed and masked by the progressive condensation of the villous stroma during placental maturation, and that their presence is only revealed if the interfibrillary spaces become widened by oedema fluid. It is possible, however, that their abundance in oedematous villi is accentuated by a true increase in their number, if Enders and King's (1970) postulation that these cells have an unusual capacity for water uptake and help to maintain the intravillous fluid volume, is correct: certainly, the Hofbauer cells do have a proliferative capacity (Castellucci et al, 1987).

From the purely practical point of view, the finding of an excess of villous Hofbauer cells in a mature placenta is an indication of villous immaturity or oedema only and is otherwise of no significance.

Abnormalities of the Villous Vessels

The terminal villi of the mature placenta usually contain between two and six capillary vessels, which are sinusoidally dilated so as to occupy most of the cross-sectional area of the villus. Three possible deviations from this norm can be envisaged, namely villous avascularity, hypovascularity and hypervascularity.

Avascular villi were noted by Gruenwald (1961) in placentas from babies of low birth weight, and it has subsequently often been assumed that he was ascribing this abnormality to a primary failure of villous vascularization. In fact it is clear from his report that he was describing examples of villous avascularity occurring as a consequence of a fetal artery thrombosis. This lesion, which is considered fully in Chapter 5, is the only cause of villous avascularity in placentas from live-born or freshly stillborn infants. In placentas from macerated stillbirths the villi often appear avascular, but there is little doubt that under these circumstances the regression of the villous vessels is a post-mortem change.

The term 'villous hypovascularity' does not imply that there are too few vessels in a villus but indicates that the vessels present are small and non-dilated. Vessels of this type are a characteristic, indeed a defining, feature of the immature villus, and hence villous hypovascularity in the term placenta may be simply one facet of a delay in villous maturation. Diminished vascularity in mature villi is often secondary to an obstructive lesion of the fetal stem arteries, such as a thrombus, an obliterative endarteritis or a fibromuscular sclerosis, but small inconspicuous vessels may also be encountered in fully mature villi with normally patent stem arteries (see Fig. 6.15), this abnormality being seen particularly in placentas from prolonged pregnancies (Emmrich and Mülzer, 1968; Fox, 1969; Mülzer et al, 1970). The factors causing this collapse, or constriction, of the villous vasculature in prolonged pregnancy are unknown, but it may be

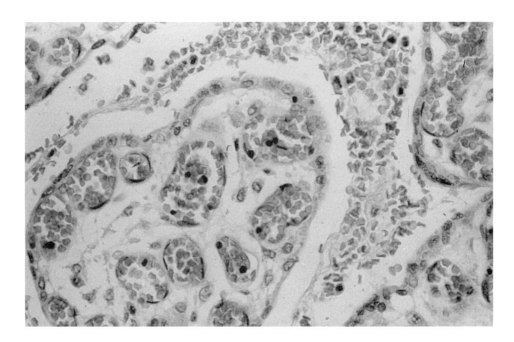

Figure 6.18. Villi showing chorangiosis (H & E ×240).

noted that the diminished villous vascularity does not, in itself, appear to have any detrimental effect on fetal well-being.

Villous hypervascularity, in which individual villi contain an excessive number of vessels, has been classed as 'chorangiosis' by Altshuler (1984) who considered that this abnormality could be diagnosed when microscopy with a ×10 objective showed 10 villi, each with 10 or more fetal vessels, in 10 or more non-infarcted areas of the placenta (Fig. 6.18). Altshuler found chorangiosis to be strongly associated with perinatal death and congenital malformations and considered that this abnormality was a response to low-grade tissue hypoxia (Altshuler, 1991). There have been remarkably few other reports of chorangiosis though Sheehan et al (1990) did describe a case of neonatal death associated with a placenta showing this abnormality to a very marked and extensive degree. Benirschke (1994) considers chorangiosis to be due to chronic fetal hypoxia and has pointed out that it is a lesion which probably takes a long time to develop. There is, however, very little evidence that chronic hypoxia does result in increased villous vascularization. It is true that placental vascular endothelial growth factor does appear to be up-regulated in hypoxic conditions (Wheeler et al, 1995) but Burton et al (1996) studied the villous vascular response to hypoxic stress in pregnancies at high altitude, in placentas from women with severe anaemia and in pregnancies complicated by pre-eclampsia and concluded that dilatation, rather than proliferation, of capillaries was the principal adaptation to hypoxia in all these circumstances. It may be further noted that chorangiosis is commonly focal rather than diffuse and it is difficult to see how chronic fetal oxygen deficiency could result in a patchy villous hypervascularization.

Chorangiosis is easily recognized and its presence should certainly be noted: I would, however, consider that both its pathogenesis and significance are unknown.

Generalized Abnormalities of the Villi

The only abnormalities that affect the whole villus are the various disorders of placental maturation.

Villous Immaturity

The placental villi may appear unduly immature for the length of the period of gestation; it has, however, been my experience that villous immaturity is difficult to recognize and assess in placentas from pregnancies of less than 36 weeks' gestation, a view recently confirmed in a study which concluded that experienced pathologists can have considerable difficulties in assessing villous maturity (Khong et al, 1995). In this section I limit my discussion of this villous abnormality to its occurrence in the placenta after the 36th week of gestation.

At and after the 36th week of gestation terminal villi are the predominant form amongst the villous population: these villi are small, have sinusoidally dilated vessels which compress and almost obliterate the stromal core, and have an irregular trophoblastic covering in which syncytial knots and vasculo-syncytial membranes are present. By contrast, villi that are, for this stage of gestation, immature, i.e. are intermediate villi, can be recognized by their relatively large diameter, small non-dilated vessels, relative abundance of stroma, and uniform trophoblast which lacks both syncytial knots and vasculo-syncytial membranes.

Immature, or intermediate, villi occur in the term placenta in two forms. The first is as small, isolated groups scattered amongst villi that are normally and fully mature (Fig. 6.19), a pattern that is seen in 97% of placentas from full-term uncomplicated pregnancies (Fox, 1968d) and thus cannot be considered as abnormal. Bleyl and Stefek (1965) suggested that these are freshly formed villi arising directly from villous stems and hence are indicative of continuing placental growth. Later studies that used the techniques of autoradiography and enzyme histochemistry confirmed this view by showing that the groups of immature villi are invariably situated in the centre of a fetal lobule and have all the characteristics of young and actively growing tissue (Schuhmann & Wehler, 1971; Geier et al, 1975; Schuhmann et al, 1976). The only significance of the finding of immature villi in this form is therefore that they represent an index of persistent villous growth.

The second, and more important, form of this abnormality is that in which all, or most, of the villi are markedly immature for the length of the pregnancy (Fig. 6.20): there is a deficiency of terminal villi and immature intermediate villi predominate. Becker (1963, 1971, 1975) has made a detailed study of this phenomenon, which he has

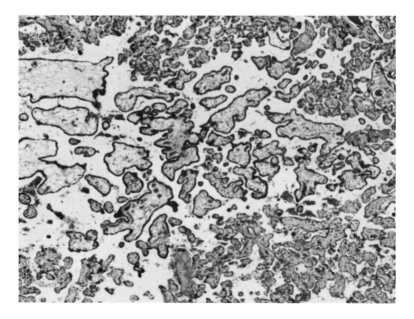

Figure 6.19. A group of extremely immature intermediate villi in an otherwise fully mature placenta: these are in the centre of a fetal lobule (H & E ×32).

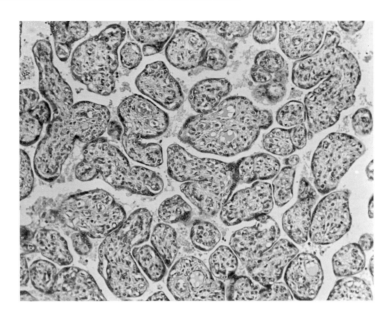

Figure 6.20. Generalized villous immaturity in a placenta from a gestation of 40 weeks: there has been a failure of terminal villus formation (H & E ×100).

described as 'maturitas retardata placentae', and ascribed it to an asynchrony between the rates of placental and fetal maturation. Kloos and Vogel (1968) have elaborated on this concept and have evolved a rather complicated classification of villous immaturity which is based on the supposed point during pregnancy at which villous maturation became retarded; their system is difficult to apply in practice and I am not fully satisfied that it is valid.

A delay in villous maturation occurs in a proportion of placentas from diabetic women and is a relatively common feature of placentas from cases of materno-fetal rhesus incompatibility. It is also seen in syphilitic infection of the placenta, in some placentas from anencephalic fetuses, in some instances of fetal Down's syndrome, and may also be found in placentas from uncomplicated pregnancies.

The process of villous maturation is, in teleological terms, designed to increase the area of trophoblast in contact with the maternal blood, to approximate to each other as closely as possible the fetal and maternal circulations, and to allow for the optimal efficiency of trophoblastic transfer mechanisms. It is therefore not surprising that a generalized failure of villous maturation is associated with a relatively high incidence of fetal hypoxia (Becker, 1975) and fetal growth retardation (Busch, 1972, 1974; Bender et al, 1976b; Altshuler, 1991). It should not be thought, however, that these complications are an inevitable accompaniment of villous immaturity because many infants whose placental villi are immature are of normal weight for the length of the gestational period.

The cause of a failure of villous maturation is unknown; it is not simply a reflection of a failure of fetal maturation, and the infrequency with which it is found in placentas from women with pre-eclampsia indicates that uteroplacental ischaemia is not a signi ficant aetiological factor. A failure of villous perfusion does not result in villous immaturity, because this change is not seen in villi rendered avascular by a fetal artery thrombosis, and there is no evidence that infection or immunological attack can be held responsible for this abnormality.

Accelerated Villous Maturation

A completely mature villous pattern, with a predominance of terminal villi, is found in a proportion of placentas from immature, prematurely delivered infants (Becker, 1975; Schweikhart et al, 1986) and this form of feto-placental asynchrony is known as 'maturitas praecox placentae'. Accelerated maturation has also been described in placentas from women with pre-eclampsia (Schuhmann & Geier, 1972; Holzl et al, 1974), though this is far from being a common finding in such placentas. The significance of this acceleration in the maturation process of the villi is uncertain, but it is possible that it is a compensatory mechanism to counter the effects of an inadequate uteroplacental blood flow (Schuhmann, 1975). It should be stressed, however, that this process of accelerated maturation is not one of accelerated ageing; ageing and maturation are two different processes and there is no evidence that the prematurely matured placenta is senescent in any way.

General Comments on Villous Histopathology

It will be appreciated that many of the abnormalities seen in the villi represent a response, often of a compensatory nature, to disturbances in blood flow. Thus a decrease in uteroplacental blood flow results in cytotrophoblastic hyperplasia and trophoblastic basement membrane thickening, whilst decreased fetal perfusion of the villi produces an increase in syncytial knots and stromal fibrosis. Other changes are of uncertain origin, e.g., villous fibrinoid necrosis, but they affect too few villi to be of any functional significance. The only two villous abnormalities that do not appear to be simply a reflection of extravillous vascular disorders, and which affect a sufficiently high proportion of villi to be of possible functional significance, are abnormalities of villous maturation, as manifested by a generalized villous immaturity, and a failure of trophoblastic differentiation, as shown by a lack of vasculo-syncytial membranes. Both these abnormalities diminish the functional efficiency of the placenta and pose a potential threat to the well-being, and even to the life, of the fetus; it is therefore particularly unfortunate that both these disorders are of unknown aetiology and pathogenesis.

HISTOPATHOLOGY OF THE FETAL STEM ARTERIES

Apart from thrombotic occlusion, which is discussed in Chapter 5, the only lesions seen in the fetal stem vessels within the placenta are fibromuscular sclerosis and obliterative endarteritis (Fox, 1967c). A haemorrhagic endovasculitis of the stem vessels has also been described but, as discussed below, there is some dispute as to whether this condition is a true pathological entity.

Fibromuscular Sclerosis

This is characterized by a marked hyperplasia of the fibrous and muscular tissue of the media, with a proliferation of intimal fibrous tissue which grows into, and eventually obliterates, the vascular lumen (Figs 6.21 and 6.22). Fibromuscular sclerosis is seen in two forms in the placental fetal vasculature: 'localized' and 'generalized'. The localized variety occurs under three circumstances:

1. In stem arteries supplying an area of villous infarction.
2. In stem arteries supplying villi which are embedded in a fibrinous plaque.
3. In stem arteries distal to an occluding thrombus.

It seems certain that, under these circumstances, the fibromuscular sclerosis is a secondary phenomenon; thus, for instance, the vessels supplying a group of freshly infarcted villi do not show any sclerosis, whilst the older an infarct the more marked is the sclerosis of the fetal vessels.

The generalized form of fibromuscular sclerosis is found only in placentas from stillbirths. It is not present in placentas from fresh stillbirths, but the longer the time interval between fetal death and delivery the more marked is the sclerosis in the fetal stem arteries (Fox, 1968e).

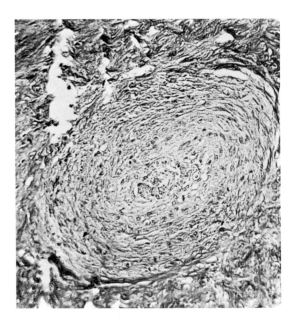

Figure 6.21. Fibromuscular sclerosis of a fetal stem artery (van Gieson ×180).

These findings point, inescapably in my view, to the conclusion that fibromuscular sclerosis is a reactive phenomenon secondary to cessation of fetal blood flow through the vessels, and that the generalized form seen in placentas from stillbirths is a post-mortem change consequent upon fetal death, a conclusion also reached by Wilkin (1965), Emmrich (1966b), Theuring (1968) and Genest (1992). The view that the vascular sclerosis is an ante-mortem lesion due either to placental inflammation (Fujikura & Benson, 1964) or to maternal infection (Becker & Dolling, 1965) is clearly indefensible, as is that maintaining it to be a manifestation of prolonged pregnancy (Dring & Kloos, 1964).

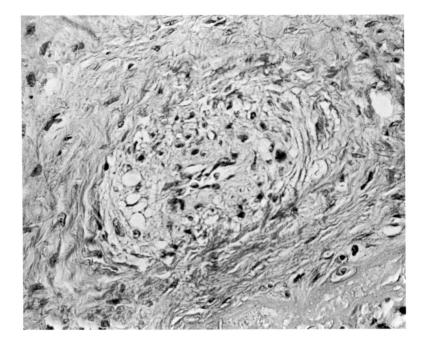

Figure 6.22. Higher power view than seen in Fig. 6.21 of a fetal stem artery in which the lumen is almost totally obliterated by a fibromuscular sclerosis (van Gieson ×620).

Obliterative Endarteritis

This abnormality is characterized by an apparent swelling and proliferation of the intimal cells of the fetal stem arteries, with thickening of the subendothelial basement membrane (Fig. 6.23). The degree of apparent intimal proliferation can, in extreme cases, be sufficient almost to occlude the vascular lumen. It may be noted that the term 'endarteritis' is a totally inapt one; however, it has attained some degree of respectability by becoming enshrined in the pathological literature, and to avoid confusion I will, with some reluctance, employ it in this account.

This vascular lesion was noted by many early students of placental pathology as occurring in the placentas of women with 'nephritis' (Wiedow, 1888; Fehling, 1891; Merttens, 1894; Eden, 1897; Williams, 1900), but thereafter was largely ignored and fell into neglect, its presence in the placenta of the woman with pre-eclampsia being only occasionally and sporadically noted (Riviere, 1930; Hunt et al, 1940; Sauramo, 1951). It was left to Paine (1957) and Isidor and Aubry (1957) to redescribe this lesion and to characterize it as a feature of the placenta in pre-eclampsia. It is perhaps typical of the history of placental studies that, in the same year as these papers appeared, Burstein et al (1957a) denied that any abnormality could be detected in the fetal vasculature of placentas from pre-eclamptic women.

Since then, a fetal obliterative endarteritis has also been described in placentas from cases of materno-fetal rhesus incompatibility (Repetti & Pescetto, 1951; Martius, 1956; de Cecco et al, 1962) and in those from diabetic women (Burstein et al, 1957b; Rolfini et al, 1963; Sani & Bottiglioni, 1964; Emmrich & Godel, 1972), whilst Robecchi and Aimone (1965), Holzl et al (1974) and Las Heras et al (1983) have confirmed that it is seen in many placentas from patients with pre-eclampsia. Thomsen and Schniewind (1961) and de Cecco et al (1963) have maintained that a fetal obliterative endarteritis occurs in placentas from prolonged, but otherwise normal, pregnancies, whilst Nezelof and Roussel (1954) have made a similar claim for placentas from patients with premature onset of labour. A fetal obliterative endarteritis has also been described in placentas from mothers smoking cigarettes during pregnancy (Lohr et al, 1972) and in placentas from low-birth-weight babies (Koenig, 1972; Koenig et al, 1973; Bender et al, 1976a).

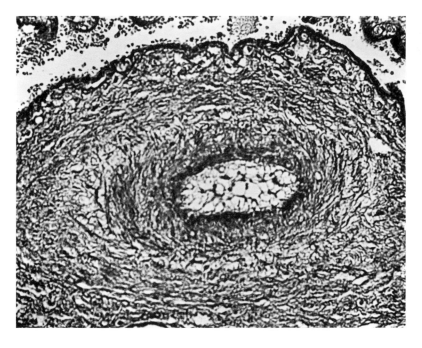

Figure 6.23. Obliterative endarteritis in a fetal stem artery. There is considerable swelling and proliferation of the endothelial cells (PAS ×150).

I have found (Fox, 1967c) that a very minor degree of fetal arterial obliterative endarteritis occurs in a small proportion of term placentas from uncomplicated pregnancies; the incidence or degree of this abnormality is not increased in placentas from prolonged pregnancies and it is absent from those from premature deliveries. There is a marked increase in the incidence of obliterative endarteritis in placentas from women with pre-eclampsia and in these circumstances the vascular lesion is always of greater severity than that found in placentas from uncomplicated pregnancies. In diabetic women it is largely, though admittedly not entirely, those with complicating pre-eclampsia or renal disease in whose placentas this vascular abnormality is seen. Overall the incidence of obliterative endarteritis is only slightly increased in placentas from cases of materno-fetal rhesus incompatibility though there is a definite excess of this abnormality in those from severely affected fetuses. A fetal stem vessel obliterative endarteritis is seen in some placentas from women who smoke and is a characteristic feature of many placentas from small-for-gestational-age infants.

The pathogenesis of fetal obliterative endarteritis is, after a long period of speculative discussion, now clear. Electron microscopy has shown that the apparent swelling of the endothelial cells is due to their partial displacement into the vascular lumen by herniations of medial smooth muscle cytoplasm into the intima (Fig. 6.24), a phenomenon indicating prolonged vasoconstriction of the fetal stem vessels (van der Veen et al, 1982). The probable stimulus for such vasoconstriction, certainly in cases of pre-eclampsia and idiopathic intrauterine fetal growth retardation, is uteroplacental ischaemia, whilst fetal hypoxia may be a stimulatory factor in cases of severe materno-fetal rhesus incompatibility. This belief is based on experimental studies which have shown that a reduction in maternal blood flow to the placenta and/or reduced oxygenation of placental tissue results in a marked decrease in fetal blood flow through the placenta and an increased fetal vascular resistance, almost certainly as a result of vasoconstriction (Dawes, 1969; Rudolph & Heymann, 1973; Stock et al, 1980; Howard et al, 1987; Kitagawa et al, 1987; Clapp, 1994; Read et al, 1995). The fetal stem vessels lack autonomic innervation and hence vasoconstriction must be achieved by humoral factors

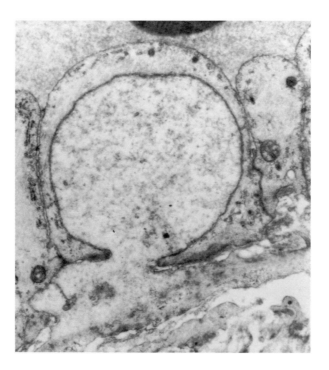

Figure 6.24. Electron micrograph of obliterative endarteritis in a fetal stem artery. What appeared to be a swollen endothelial cell on light microscopy is actually herniation of smooth muscle cytoplasm into the vascular lumen (EM ×11,050).

or autocrine/paracrine mechanisms, there being no shortage of possible candidates for playing such a role (Myatt, 1992; Howarth et al, 1995).

The significance of the obliterative changes in the fetal vessels is therefore that they are usually, though admittedly not invariably, an indication of uteroplacental ischaemia and/or fetal hypoxia. From a morphological viewpoint the arterial vasoconstriction leads to reduced fetal perfusion of the villi, which in turn results in stromal fibrosis and excessive formation of syncytial knots. In physiological terms the vasoconstriction is indicative of an attempt by the hypoxic fetus to divert blood to the cerebral and coronary circulations, the placental villous tissue being able to increase oxygen extraction when blood flow is decreased and being able to sustain a flow reduction of 50% without impairing fetal oxygenation (Istkovitz et al, 1983).

The above comments apply particularly to pregnancies complicated by pre-eclampsia or intrauterine growth retardation and it has to be admitted that the factor (or factors) responsible for the production of an endarteritis obliterans in some placentas from women with uncomplicated diabetes mellitus remains enigmatic. The vascular changes certainly cannot, however, be regarded as a manifestation of a diabetic vasculopathy.

Haemorrhagic Endovasculitis

This abnormality of the fetal placental vasculature was first described by Sander and her colleagues (Sander, 1980; Sander et al, 1986) as being characterized by obliteration of villous capillaries, thrombi in stem vessels, degeneration and fragmentation of capillary endothelial cells and extravasation of erythrocytes into the villous stroma. It was thought that this vascular lesion was commonly associated with a wide range of serious maternal and fetal complications of pregnancy and was frequently found in placentas from stillborn infants, a view with which Shen-Schwartz et al (1988) concurred. Silver et al (1988) showed, however, that this vascular lesion developed in cultured placental tissue when organ explants were allowed to degenerate and considered that haemorrhagic endovasculitis was commonly a post-mortem change. This view is now widely, though perhaps not universally, accepted and it is thought that when this lesion is found in a placenta from a live-born infant, it is usually in the vascular tree distal to an occluding thrombus.

HISTOPATHOLOGY OF THE MATERNAL UTEROPLACENTAL VESSELS

Two interrelated abnormalities of the maternal uteroplacental vasculature are of central importance in placental pathology, these being inadequate transformation of the spiral arteries of the placental bed into uteroplacental vessels and acute atherosis. For the sake of clarity these two abnormalities will, despite their close relationship, be considered separately.

Inadequate Transformation of Spiral Arteries

The physiological alterations occurring in the spiral arteries of the placental bed, which are a consequence of their invasion by extravillous cytotrophoblastic cells and which result in their transformation into uteroplacental vessels, have been described in Chapter 1. It will be recalled that this is a two-stage process, the first involving transformation of the intradecidual portions of the spiral arteries and the second leading to transformation of their intramyometrial segments. It has to be stressed that these changes are confined to the spiral arteries of the placental bed and are not seen in the spiral arteries of the decidua vera immediately adjacent to the placenta, in the spiral arteries of the decidua capsularis, or in the basal arteries.

It has been repeatedly shown, largely as a result of study of placental bed biopsies (Figs 6.25–6.27), that in women who are destined to develop pre-eclampsia, the second

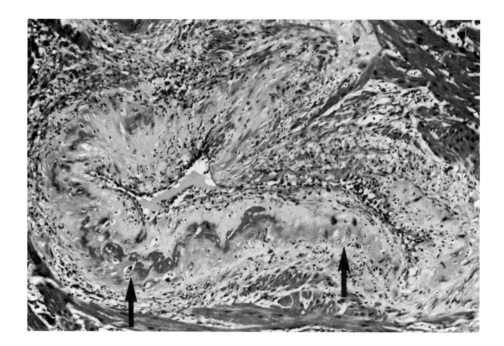

Figure 6.25. Placental bed biopsy showing the intramyometrial segment of a spiral artery from a normal pregnancy of 36 weeks' duration. The media has been largely replaced by fibrinoid, in which a few degenerate cytotrophoblastic cells (arrowed) can be seen, and the vessel has assumed a sac-like configuration (H & E ×125).

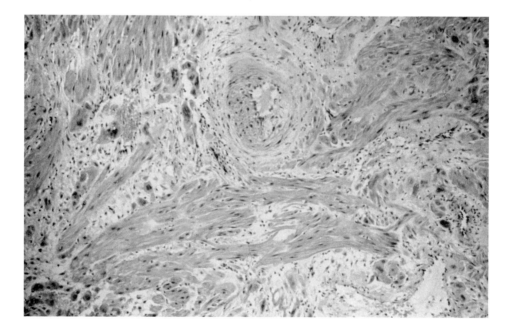

Figure 6.26. Placental bed biopsy showing the intramyometrial segment of a spiral artery from a patient with pre-eclampsia: there is no evidence of physiological change (H & E ×80).

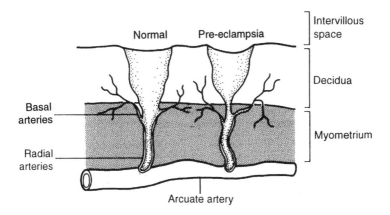

Figure 6.27. Diagrammatic representation of the spiral arteries in a normal pregnancy (left) and in a pregnancy complicated by pre-eclampsia (right). The spiral vessels are funnel-shaped, and in a normal pregnancy both the intradecidual and intramyometrial segments of the vessels are dilated: in pre-eclampsia the dilatation is confined to the decidual segment.

wave of intravascular cytotrophoblastic invasion does not occur and that the intramyometrial segments of the spiral arteries therefore retain their musculo-elastic media and do not dilate (Dixon & Robertson, 1958, 1961; Brosens, 1963, 1964; Renaer & Brosens, 1963; Robertson et al, 1967, 1975; Robertson & Dixon, 1969; Brosens et al, 1972; Robertson, 1976; Gerretsen et al, 1981; Hustin et al, 1983; Frusca et al, 1989; Wang, 1989; Olofsson et al, 1993). It subsequently became apparent that an identical abnormality is found, though less consistently, in cases of normotensive idiopathic fetal intrauterine growth retardation (Robertson et al, 1975, 1981, 1986; Sheppard & Bonnar, 1976, 1981; Brosens et al, 1977; De Wolf et al, 1980; Hustin et al, 1983; Althabe et al, 1985; Khong et al, 1986; McFadyen et al, 1986; Frusca et al, 1989; Khong & Robertson, 1992; Olofsson et al, 1993).

It was originally thought that this abnormality was uniform throughout the vessels of the placental bed and that the lack of trophoblastic invasion of the intramyometrial segments of the spiral arteries was an 'all or none' change but later studies have shown that these assumptions were incorrect. First, the extent to which failure of trophoblastic invasion occurs varies from vessel to vessel and in some of the spiral arteries there is a complete lack of trophoblastic invasion with absence of physiological changes throughout the entire length of both their intradecidual and intramyometrial segments (Khong et al, 1986). Secondly, the lack of physiological change within a segment of a vessel may be only partial and restricted to a portion of the circumference (Pijnenborg et al, 1991; Meekins et al, 1994).

The cause of the failure of trophoblast migration in patients who later develop pre-eclampsia or who, despite being normotensive, give birth to growth-retarded infants is unknown. It has been suggested that vascular invasion by trophoblast is regulated by the expression of cell adhesion molecules that permit interaction between endovascular trophoblast and decidual endothelial cells (Burrows et al, 1994), and Zhou et al (1993) considered that defective trophoblast migration is due to a failure of the extravillous cytotrophoblast to express cell adhesion molecules. By contrast, however, Labarrere and Faulk (1995) have found that whilst the endovascular cytotrophoblast in normal pregnancies reacts negatively for ICAM-1 antigens, those in pregnancies in which there is a failure of trophoblastic migration do express such antigens. Clearly, therefore, the role of cell adhesion molecules awaits clarification as does the role of cytokines, growth factors and immunological interactions between maternal and fetal tissues.

Despite our lack of knowledge of the pathogenesis of inadequate trophoblastic invasion of spiral arteries, this abnormality is the central factor in those pregnancies in which there is a reduced maternal blood flow to the placenta and it is therefore somewhat frustrating to the histopathologist that it is best identified and studied in placental bed biopsies. Such specimens are rarely available to the diagnostic pathologist who usually has to glean what information is available about the condition of these vessels from those contained within decidual fragments attached to the fetal surface of the placenta. Such fragments are, however, usually present and the fact that some vessels show no physiological change in their intradecidual segments can be recognized: the frequency with which such vessels are seen is increased if thin slices of the basal plate are taken perpendicular to the maternal surface (Khong & Chambers, 1992). Tissue distortion can, however, make these intradecidual vessels difficult to recognize and their identification can be facilitated by the use of immunocytochemical techniques, using antibodies to cytokeratins and smooth muscle actin, vessels showing physiological change being keratin positive and actin negative in contrast to uninvaded vessels which are keratin negative and actin positive (Labarrere & Faulk, 1994).

Acute Atherosis

This vascular abnormality was first described by Hertig (1945) and later elaborated on by Zeek and Assali (1950). It has since been the subject of many studies and reviews (Dixon & Robertson, 1958; Brosens, 1964; Maqueo et al, 1964; Robertson et al, 1967, 1975, 1976; De Wolf et al, 1975, 1981; Sheppard & Bonnar, 1976, 1980; Gerretsen et al, 1981; Althabe et al, 1985; Khong et al, 1987; Labarrere, 1988; Frusca et al, 1989; Khong, 1991). It was originally thought that this lesion was restricted to pregnancies complicated by pre-eclampsia but it is now known that it also occurs with considerable frequency in pregnancies complicated by fetal intrauterine growth retardation in normotensive pregnancies. There is, however, no convincing evidence that a true acute atherosis is ever seen in any other complication of pregnancy.

Acute atherosis is characterized by fibrinoid necrosis of the vessel wall, an accumulation of fat-containing macrophages, and a mononuclear perivascular infiltrate (Fig. 6.28): the appearance of lipophages marks a relatively late stage in the evolution of this lesion. This lesion is seen only in vessels that have not undergone physiological change as a result of trophoblastic invasion. Thus it is usually present in the intramyometrial

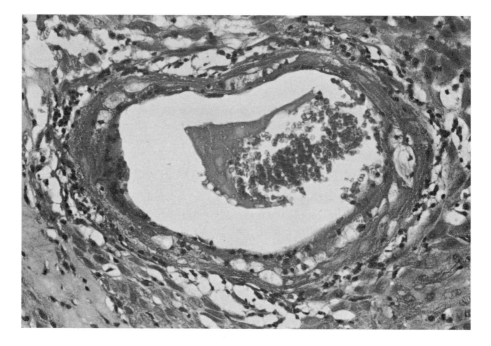

Figure 6.28. A placental bed biopsy from a patient with pre-eclampsia. There is an acute atherosis of a spiral artery. The necrotic vessel wall contains lipophages embedded in fibrinoid material, and there is a perivascular mononuclear cell infiltrate (H & E ×160).

segments of the spiral arteries of the placental bed, in the spiral arteries of the decidua parietalis and in the basal arteries; it is only apparent in the intradecidual portion of those spiral arteries of the placental bed in which there has been a complete lack of trophoblastic invasion. This apparently extraordinary finding is only explicable if the sequence of events that occurs in the evolution of acute atherosis is understood. Electron microscopic observations (de Wolf et al, 1975) have shown that the initial stage of this lesion is one of lipid accumulation in the muscle cells of the media and intima; these cells subsequently undergo necrosis, and the lipid thus released is then taken up by macrophages which accumulate in the wall of the damaged vessel. Arteries which have been invaded by cytotrophoblast have lost the muscular component of their wall and therefore cannot undergo this change. This is a satisfactory explanation for the restriction of atherosis to those vessels that have undergone physiological change.

The pathogenesis of acute atherosis is far from being fully understood. It has been commented on by Robertson and his colleagues that acute atherosis is remarkably similar to the vascular lesions seen in rejected renal allografts, and they have suggested that the atherosis may be the result, at least in part, of a delayed maternal hypersensitivity response to fetal antigens (Robertson et al, 1967). Others have also supported an immunological basis for this lesion (Kitzmiller & Benirschke, 1973; Labarrere et al, 1985; Laberrere, 1988) but proof of this view is still lacking.

REFERENCES

Aladjem, S. (1967) The syncytial knot: a sign of active syncytial proliferation. *American Journal of Obstetrics and Gynecology*, **99**, 350–358.

Althabe, O., Laberrere, C.A. and Telenta, M. (1985) Maternal vascular lesions in placentae of small for gestational age infants. *Placenta*, **6**, 265–276.

Altshuler, G. (1984) Chorangiosis: an important placental sign of neonatal morbidity and mortality. *Archives of Pathology and Laboratory Medicine*, **108**, 71–74.

Altshuler, G. (1991) The placenta. In *Surgical Pathology of the Female Reproductive System and Peritoneum*, Sternberg, S.S. and Mills, S.E. (Eds), pp. 17–36. New York: Raven Press.

Altshuler, G. (1993) A conceptual approach to placental pathology and pregnancy outcome. *Seminars in Diagnostic Pathology*, **10**, 204–221.

Alvarez, H. (1970) Prolifération du trophoblaste et sa relation avec l'hypertension artérielle de la toxémie gravidique. *Gynécologie et Obstétrique*, **69**, 581–588.

Alvarez, H., Sala, M.A. and Benedetti, W.L. (1972) Intervillous space reduction in the edematous placenta. *American Journal of Obstetrics and Gynecology*, **112**, 819–820.

Amalados, A.S. and Burton, G.J. (1985) Organ culture of human placental villi in hypoxic and hyperoxic conditions: a morphometric study. *Journal of Developmental Physiology*, **7**, 113–118.

Anderson, W.R. and McKay, D.G. (1966) Electron microscopic study of the trophoblast in normal and toxemic placentas. *American Journal of Obstetrics and Gynecology*, **95**, 1134–1148.

Arnholdt, H., Meisel, F., Fandrey, K. and Lohrs, U. (1991) Proliferation of villous trophoblast of the human placenta in normal and abnormal pregnancies. *Virchows Archives B Cellular Pathology*, **50**, 365–372.

Baker, B.L., Hook, S.J. and Severinghaus, A.E. (1944) The cytological structure of the human chorionic villus and decidua parietalis. *American Journal of Anatomy*, **74**, 291–325.

Bargmann, W. and Knoop, A. (1959) Elektronenmikroskopischen Untersuchungen an Placentarzotten des Menschen. Bemerkungen zum Synzytiumproblem. *Zeitschrift für Zellforschung und mikroskopische Anatomie*, **50**, 472–493.

Barker, G., Boyd, R.D.H., D'Souza, S.W. et al (1994) Placental water content and distribution. *Placenta*, **15**, 47–56.

Becker, V. (1963) Funktionelle Morphologie der Placenta. *Archiv für Gynäkologie*, **198**, 3–28.

Becker, V. (1971) Die Chronopathologie der Plazenta. Allgemeinpathologische Aspekte der Organreifung. *Deutsche medizinische Wochenschrift*, **96**, 1845–1849.

Becker, V. (1975) Abnormal maturation of villi. In *The Placenta and its Maternal Supply Line*, Gruenwald, P. (Ed.), pp. 232–243. Lancaster: Medical and Technical Publishing.

Becker, V. and Bleyl, U. (1961) Plazentarzotte bei Schwangerschaftstoxikose und fetaler Erythroblastose im fluoreszenzmikroskopischen Bilde. *Virchows Archiv für pathologische Anatomie und Physiologie und für klinische Medizin*, **334**, 516–527.

Becker, V. and Dolling, D. (1965) Gefässverschlüsse in der Plazenta bei Totgeborenen. *Virchows Archiv für pathologische Anatomie und Physiologie und für klinische Medizin*, **338**, 305–314.

Bender, H.G., Werner, C. and Horner, G. (1976a) Untersuchungen zum placentaren Reifenzustand bei Zwillingsschwangerschaften und seiner funktionellen Bedeutung. *Archiv für Gynäkologie*, **221**, 187–196.

Bender, H.G., Werner, C., Kortmann, H.R. and Becker, V. (1976b) Zur Endangitis obliterans der Plazentagefasse. *Archiv für Gynäkologie*, **221**, 145–159.

Benirschke, K. (1962) A review of the pathologic anatomy of the human placenta. *American Journal of Obstetrics and Gynecology*, **84**, 1595–1622.

Benirschke, K. (1994) Placenta pathology: questions to the perinatologist. *Journal of Perinatology*, **14**, 371–375.

Benirschke, K. and Kaufmann, P. (1995) *Pathology of the Human Placenta*, 3rd edn. New York: Springer-Verlag.

Bleyl, U. (1962) Histologische, histochemische und fluoreszenmikroskopische Untersuchungen an Hofbauer-Zellen. *Archiv für Gynäkologie*, **197**, 364–386.

Bleyl, U. and Stefek, E. (1965) Zur Morphologie und diagnostischen Bewertung der lockeren jungendlichen Zotten in reifen menschlichen Plazenten. *Beitrage zur pathologischen Anatomie und zur allgemeinen Pathologie*, **131**, 168–182.

Boyd, J.D. and Hamilton, W.J. (1970) *The Human Placenta*. Cambridge: W. Heffer and Sons.

Boyd, J.D. and Hughes, A.F.W. (1954) Observations on human chorionic villi using the electron microscope. *Journal of Anatomy*, **88**, 356–362.

Bremer, J.L. (1916) The interrelations of the mesonephros, kidney and placenta in different classes of mammals. *American Journal of Anatomy*, **19**, 179–209.

Brosens, I. (1963), Les artérioles spiralées de la cadaque basale dans les complications hypertensive de la grossesse: étude anatomo-clinique. *Bulletin de la Société Belge de Gynécologie et d'Obstétrique*, **33**, 61–70.

Brosens, I. (1964) A study of the spiral arteries of the decidua basalis in normotensive and hypertensive pregnancies. *Journal of Obstetrics and Gynaecology of the British Commonwealth*, **71**, 222–230.

Brosens, I., Robertson, W.B. and Dixon, H.G. (1972) The role of the spiral arteries in the pathogenesis of pre-eclampsia. *Obstetrics and Gynecology Annual*, **1**, 177–191.

Brosens, I., Dixon, H.G. and Robertson, W.B. (1977) Fetal growth retardation and the arteries of the placental bed. *British Journal of Obstetrics and Gynaecology*, **84**, 656–663.

Brzosko, W., Nowoslawski, A. and Pisarki, T. (1965) Analiza immunohistochemiczna mas wloknikowatych w lozysku ludzkim. (Immunohistochemical analysis of fibrinoid masses in human placenta.) *Ginekologica Polska*, **36**, 121–130.

Buckshee, K., Malkani, P.K. and Khatri, S. (1974) The villous cytotrophoblast as an index of placental dysfunction. In *Proceedings of the 6th Asian Congress of Obstetrics and Gynaecology, Kuala Lumpur, Malaysia*, pp. 223–235.

Burrows, T.D., King, A. and Loke, Y.W. (1994) Expression of adhesion molecules by endovascular trophoblast and decidual endothelial cells: implications for vascular invasion during implantation. *Placenta*, **15**, 21–33.

Burstein, R., Soule, S.D. and Blumenthal, H.T. (1957a) Histogenesis of pathological processes in placentas of metabolic disease in pregnancy. I. Toxemia and hypertension. *American Journal of Obstetrics and Gynecology*, **74**, 85–95.

Burstein, R., Soule, S.D. and Blumenthal, H.T. (1957b) Histogenesis of pathological processes in placentas of metabolic disease in pregnancy. II. The diabetic state. *American Journal of Obstetrics and Gynecology*, **74**, 96–104.

Burstein, R., Berns, A.W., Hirata, Y. and Blumenthal, H.T. (1963) A comparative histo- and immunopathological study of the placenta in diabetes mellitus and in erythroblastosis fetalis. *American Journal of Obstetrics and Gynecology*, **86**, 66–76.

Burton, G.J., Mayhew, T.M. and Robertson, L.A. (1989) Stereological re-examination of the effects of varying oxygen tensions on human placental villi maintained in organ culture for up to 12h. *Placenta*, **10**, 263–273.

Burton, G.J., Reshetnikova, O.S., Milaovanov, A.P. and Teleshova, O.V. (1996) Stereological evaluation of vascular adaptations in human placental villi to differing forms of hypoxic stress. *Placenta*, **17**, 49–55.

Busch, W. (1972) Die Placenta bei der fetalen Mangelentwicklung. Makroskopie und Mikroskopie von 150 Placenten fetaler Mangelentwicklungen. *Archiv für Gynäkologie*, **212**, 333–357.

Busch, W. (1974) Das fetale Risiko bei chronischer nutritiver Placentainsuffizienz unterschied-licher Pathogenese. *Archiv für Gynäkologie*, **216**, 167–174.

Castellucci, M., Celona, A., Bartels, H., et al (1987) Mitosis of the Hofbauer cell: possible implications for a fetal macrophage. *Placenta*, **8**, 65–76.

Cibils, L.A. (1974) The placenta and newborn infant in hypertensive conditions. *American Journal of Obstetrics and Gynecology*, **118**, 256–268.

Clapp, J.F. (1994) Physiological adaptation to intrauterine growth retardation. In *Early Fetal Growth and Development*, Ward, R.H.T., Smith, S.K. and Donnai, D. (Eds), pp. 371–383. London: RCOG Press.

Clavero-Nunez, J.A. (1962) Concepto actual de la anatomia placentaria. *Revista Espanola de Obstetricia y Ginecologia*, **20**, 80–99.

Clavero-Nunez, J.A. (1963) La placenta en la diabetes. *Revista Ibérica de Endocrinologia*, **10**, 73–80.

Dawes, G.S. (1969) Foetal blood gas homeostasis. In *Foetal Autonomy: CIBA Foundation Symposium*, Wolstenholme, G.E.N. and O'Connor, M. (Eds), pp. 162–172. London: J. & A. Churchill.

de Cecco, L., Ferrari, B., Niccolo, M. and Rolfini, G. (1962) Contributo allo studio della senescenza placentare. *Quaderni di Clinica Ostetrica e Ginecologica*, **17**, Supplement 12, 1055–1063.

de Cecco, L., Pavone, G. and Rolfini, G. (1963) La placenta umana nella isoimmunizzazione anti Rh. *Quaderni di Clinica Ostetrica e Ginecologica*, **18**, 675–682.

de Ikonicoff, L.K. (1970) Histologie et histochimie de la substance fibrinoide au niveau des villosités placentaires humaines. *Revue Francaise de Gynécologie et d'Obstétrique*, **66**, 139–146.

De Wolf, F., Robertson, W.B. and Brosens, I. (1975) The ultrastructure of acute atherosis in hypertensive pregnancy. *American Journal of Obstetrics and Gynecology*, **123**, 164–174.

De Wolf, F., Brosens, I. and Renaer, M. (1980) Fetal growth retardation and the maternal arterial supply of the human placenta in the absence of sustained hypertension. *British Journal of Obstetrics and Gynaecology*, **87**, 678–685.

Dixon, H.G. and Robertson, W.B. (1958) A study of the vessels of the placental bed in normotensive and hypertensive women. *Journal of Obstetrics and Gynaecology of the British Empire*, **65**, 803–810.

Dixon, H.G. and Robertson, W.B. (1961) Vascular changes in the placental bed. *Pathologia et Microbiologia*, **24**, 622–630.

Dring, W. and Kloos, K. (1964) Morphologische Routine-diagnostik der Placenta. *Munchener Medizinische Wochenschrift*, **106**, 1849–1855.

Eden, T.W. (1897) A study of the human placenta, physiological and pathological. *Journal of Pathology and Bacteriology*, **4**, 265–283.

Ehrhardt, G., Gerl, D. and Wasmund, B. (1972) Morphometrische Untersuchungen der Frühgeborenplazenta unter besonderer Berücksichtigung der Mikrofibrinoidablagerungen. *Zentralblatt für Gynäkologie*, **94**, 1110–1115.

Emmrich, P. (1966a) Zur Genese der fibrinoiden Zottenbuckel in der menschlichen Placenta. *Frankfurter Zeitschrift für Pathologie*, **75**, 66–73.

Emmrich, P. (1966b) Morphologie und Histochemie der Placenta bei intrauterinem Fruchttod mit Mazeration. *Gynaecologia*, **162**, 241–253.

Emmrich, P. and Godel, E. (1972) Morphologie der Plazenta bei mütterlichem Diabetes mellitus. *Zentralblatt für allgemeine Pathologie und pathologische Anatomie*, **116**, 56–63.

Emmrich, P. and Mülzer, G. (1968) Zur Morphologie der Plazenta bei Ubertragung. *Pathologia et Microbiologia*, **32**, 285–302.

Enders, A.C. and King, B.F. (1970) The cytology of Hofbauer cells. *Anatomical Record*, **167**, 231–252.

Faulk, W.P., Jeannet, M., Creighton, W.D. and Carbonara, A. (1974) Immunological studies of the human placenta: characterization of immunoglobulins on trophoblastic basement membranes. *Journal of Clinical Investigation*, **54**, 1011–1019.

Fehling, H. (1891) Weitere Beitrage zur klinischen Bedeutung der Nephritis in der Schwangerschaft. *Archiv für Gynäkologie*, **39**, 468–483.

Fox, H. (1964) The villous cytotrophoblast as an index of placental ischaemia. *Journal of Obstetrics and Gynaecology of the British Commonwealth*, **71**, 885–893.

Fox, H. (1965) The significance of villous syncytial knots in the human placenta. *Journal of Obstetrics and Gynaecology of the British Commonwealth*, **72**, 347–355.

Fox, H. (1967a) The incidence and significance of vasculo-syncytial membranes in the human placenta. *Journal of Obstetrics and Gynaecology of the British Commonwealth*, **74**, 28–33.

Fox, H. (1967b) The incidence and significance of Hofbauer cells in the mature human placenta. *Journal of Pathology and Bacteriology*, **93**, 710–717.

Fox, H. (1967c) Abnormalities of the foetal stem arteries in the human placenta. *Journal of Obstetrics and Gynaecology of the British Commonwealth*, **74**, 734–738.

Fox, H. (1968a) Fibrinoid necrosis of placental villi. *Journal of Obstetrics and Gynaecology of the British Commonwealth*, **75**, 448–452.

Fox, H. (1968b) Fibrosis of placental villi. *Journal of Pathology and Bacteriology*, **95**, 573–579.

Fox, H. (1968c) Basement membrane changes in the villi of the human placenta. *Journal of Obstetrics and Gynaecology of the British Commonwealth*, **75**, 302–306.

Fox, H. (1968d) Villous immaturity in the term placenta. *Obstetrics and Gynecology*, **31**, 9–12.

Fox, H. (1968e) Morphological changes in the human placenta following fetal death. *Journal of Obstetrics and Gynaecology of the British Commonwealth*, **75**, 839–843.

Fox, H. (1969) Histological features of placental senescence. In *The Foeto-Placental Unit*, Pecile, A. and Finzi, C. (Eds), pp. 3–7. Amsterdam: Excerpta Medica.

Fox, H. (1970) Effect of hypoxia on trophoblast in organ culture. *American Journal of Obstetrics and Gynecology*, **107**, 1058–1064.

Frusca, T., Morassi, L., Pecorelli, S., Grigolato, P. and Gastaldi, A. (1989) Histological features of uteroplacental vessels in normal and hypertensive patients in relation to birth weight. *British Journal of Obstetrics and Gynaecology*, **96**, 835–839.

Fujikura, T. and Benson, R.C. (1964) Placentitis and fibrous occlusion of fetal vessels in the placentas of still-born infants. *American Journal of Obstetrics and Gynecology*, **89**, 225–229.

Geier, G., Schuhmann, R. and Kraus, H. (1975) Regional unterschiedliche Zellproliferation innerhalb der Plazentone reifer menschlicher Plazenten: Autoradiographische Untersuchungen. *Archiv für Gynäkologie*, **218**, 31–37.

Geller, H.F. (1957) Über die sogennanten Hofbauerzellen in der reifen menschlichen Placenta. *Archiv für Gynäkologie*, **188**, 481–496.

Genest, D.R. (1992) Estimating the time of death in stillborn fetuses. II. Histologic evaluation of the placenta: a study of 71 stillborns. *Obstetrics and Gynecology*, **80**, 585–592.

Gerl, D., Eichhorn, H., Eichhorn, K.H. and Franke, H. (1973) Quantitative Messungen synzytialer Zellkernkonzentrationen der menschlichen Plazenta bei normalen und pathologischen Schwangerschaften. *Zentralblatt für Gynäkologie*, **95**, 263–266.

Gerretsen, G., Huisjes, H.J. and Elema, J.D. (1981) Morphological changes of the spiral arteries in the placental bed in relation to preeclampsia and fetal growth retardation. *British Journal of Obstetrics and Gynaecology*, **88**, 876–881.

Gershon, R. and Strauss, L. (1961) Structural changes in human placentas associated with fetal inanition or growth arrest (placental insufficiency syndrome) *American Journal of Diseases of Children*, **102**, 645–646.

Gille, J., Brner, P., Reinecke, J., Krause, P.-H. and Deicher, H. (1974a) Uber die Fibrinoidablagerungen in den Endzotten der menschlichen Placenta. *Archiv für Gynäkologie*, **217**, 263–271.

Gille, J., Brner, P., Reinecke, J., Krause, P.-H. and Deicher, H. (1974b) Light microscopical and immuno-histological studies of the placental barrier. In *Immunology in Obstetrics and Gynaecology*, Centaro, A. and Carretti, N. (Eds), pp. 275–278. Amsterdam: Excerpta Medica.

Gruenwald, P. (1961) Abnormalities of placental vascularity in relation to intrauterine deprivation and retardation of fetal growth: significance of avascular chorionic villi. *New York State Journal of Medicine*, **61**, 1508–1517.

Hall, W.E.B. (1949) The basement membrane of the fetal placental villus and its relation to toxic and pathological obstetrical states. *American Journal of Pathology*, **25**, 819.

Hertig, A.T. (1945) Vascular pathology in the hypertensive albuminuric toxemias of pregnancy. *Clinics*, **4**, 602–614.

Hofbauer, J. (1925) The function of the Hofbauer cells of the chorionic villus, particularly in relation to acute infection and syphilis. *American Journal of Obstetrics and Gynecology*, **10**, 1–14.

Holzl, M., Lüthje, D. and Seck-Ebersbach, K. (1974) Placentaveranderungen bei EPH-Gestose. Morphologischer Befund und Schweregrad der Erkrankung. *Archiv für Gynäkologie*, **217**, 315–334.

Horky, Z. (1964a) Die quantitativen Veranunderungen der Vaskularisation der Zotten in der diabetis-chen Plazenta. *Zentralblatt für Gynäkologie*, **86**, 8–15.

Horky, Z. (1964b) Beitrag zur Funktionsbedeutung der Hofbauer-Zellen (Beobachtungen in der Plazenta bei Diabetes mellitus). *Zentralblatt für Gynäkologie*, **86**, 1621–1626.

Horky, Z. (1965) Die Reifungsstörungen der Plazenta bei Diabetes mellitus. *Zentralblatt für Gynäkologie*, **87**, 1555–1564.

Hormann, G. (1947) Haben die sogenannten Horbauerzellen der Chorionzotten funktionelle Bedeutung? *Zentralblatt für Gynäkologie*, **69**, 1199–1205.

Hormann, G. (1948) Die Reifung der menschlichen Chorionzotte im Lichte konomischer Zweckmassigkeit. *Zentralblatt für Gynäkologie*, **70**, 625–631.

Hormann, G. (1953) Ein Beitrag zur funktionellen Morphologie der menschlichen Placenta. *Archiv für Gynäkologie*, **184**, 109–123.

Hormann, G. (1958a) Zur Systematik einer Pathologie der menschlichen Placenta. *Archiv für Gynäkologie*, **191**, 297–344.

Hormann, G. (1958b) Versuch einer Systematik plazenterer Entwicklungsstorungen. *Geburtshilfe und Frauenheilkunde*, **18**, 345–349.

Horn, V. and Horalek, F. (1961) Uber die sogenannte fibrinoide Substanz in der Placenta. *Zentralblatt für allgemeine Pathologie und pathologische Anatomie*, **102**, 514–521.

Howard, R.B., Hosokawa, T. and MacGuire, M.H. (1987) Hypoxia induced fetoplacental vasoconstriction in perfused human placental cotyledons. *American Journal of Obstetrics and Gynecology*, **157**, 1261–1266.

Howarth, S.R., Vallance, P. and Wilson, C.A. (1995) Role of thromboxane A$_2$ in the vasoconstrictor response to endothelin-1, angiotensin II and 5-hydroxytryptamine in human placental vessels. *Placenta*, **16**, 679–689.

Hunt, H.F., Patterson, W.B. and Nicodemus, R.E. (1940) Placental infarction and eclampsia. *American Journal of Clinical Pathology*, **10**, 319–331.

Hustin, J., Foidart, J.M. and Lambotte, R. (1983) Maternal vascular lesions in pre-eclampsia and intrauterine growth retardation: light microscopy and immunofluorescence. *Placenta*, **4**, 489–498.

Ikawa, A. (1959) Observations on the epithelium of human chorionic villi with the electron microscope. *Journal of the Japanese Obstetrical and Gynaecological Society*, **6**, 219–234.

Ilagan, N.B., Elias, E.G., Liang, K.C. et al (1990) Perinatal and neonatal significance of bacteria-related placental villous edema. *Acta Obstetricia et Gynecologica Scandinavica*, **69**, 287–290.

Isidor, P. and Aubry, B. (1957) A propos d'un type particulier d'artériopathie de la portion foetale du placenta. Essai d'explication pathogénique; ses rapports avec la toxemie gravidique et l'anoxie foetale. *Gynécologie et Obstétrique*, **56**, 152–166.

Istkovitz, J., LaGamma, E.F. and Rudolph, A.M. (1983) The effect of reducing umbilical blood flow on fetal oxygenation. *American Journal of Obstetrics and Gynecology*, **145**, 813–818.

Jakobovits, A. and Traub, A. (1972) Klinische Bedeutung der fibrinoiden Degeneration von Chorionzotten. *Zentralblatt für Gynäkologie*, **94**, 16–21.

Jones, C.P.J. (1976) *An ultrastructural and ultrahistochemical study of the human placenta in normal and abnormal pregnancy*. PhD Thesis, University of Manchester.

Jones, C.P.J. and Fox, H. (1976) An ultrastructural and ultrahistochemical study of the placenta of the diabetic woman. *Journal of Pathology*, **119**, 91–99.

Kaplan, C. (1993) Placental pathology for the nineties. *Pathology Annual*, **28(1)**, 15–95.

Kaufmann, P. (1972) Untersuchungen über die Langhans-Zellen in der menschlichen Placenta. *Zeitschrift für Zellforschung und mikroskopische Anatomie*, **128**, 283–302.

Kaufmann, P., Luckhardt, M., Schweikhart, G. and Cantle, S.J. (1987) Cross-sectional features and three-dimensional structure of human placental villi. *Placenta*, **8**, 235–247.

Khong, T.Y. (1991) Acute atherosis in pregnancies complicated by hypertension, small-for-gestational-stage infants, and diabetes mellitus. *Archives of Pathology and Laboratory Medicine*, **115**, 722–725.

Khong, T.Y. and Chambers, H.M. (1992) Alternative method of sampling placentas for the assessment of uteroplacental vasculature. *Journal of Clinical Pathology*, **45**, 925–927.

Khong, T.Y. and Robertson, W.B. (1992) Spiral artery disease. In *Immunological Obstetrics*, Coulam, C.B., Faulk, W.P. and McIntyre, J.A. (Eds), pp. 492–501. New York: Norton.

Khong, T.Y., de Wolf, F., Robertson, W.B. and Brosens, I. (1986) Inadequate maternal vascular response to placentation in pregnancies complicated by preeclampsia and by small for gestational age infants. *British Journal of Obstetrics and Gynaecology*, **93**, 1049–1059.

Khong, T.Y., Pearce, J.M. and Robertson, W.B. (1987) Acute atherosis in pre-eclampsia: maternal determinants and fetal outcome in the presence of the lesion. *American Journal of Obstetrics and Gynecology*, **157**, 360–363.

Khong, T.Y., Staples, A., Bendon, R.W. et al (1995) Observer reliability in assessing placental maturity by histology. *Journal of Clinical Pathology*, **48**, 420–423.

Kitigawa, H., Slegel, P.H. and MacGuire, M.H. (1987) Ischaemia induced vasoconstriction and adenosine release in perfused human placental cotyledons. *Pharmacologist*, **29**, 197.

Kitzmiller, J.L. and Benirschke, K. (1973) Immunofluorescent study of placental bed vessels in preeclampsia of pregnancy. *American Journal of Obstetrics and Gynecology*, **115**, 248–251.

Kliman, H.J., Perrotta, P.L. and Jones, D.C. (1995) The efficacy of placental biopsy. *American Journal of Obstetrics and Gynecology*, **173**, 1084–1088.

Kline, B.S. (1951) Microscopic observations of development of human placenta. *American Journal of Obstetrics and Gynecology*, **61**, 1065–1074.

Kloos, K. (1952) Zur Pathologie der Feten und Neugeborenen diabetischer Mütter. *Virchows Archiv für pathologische Anatomie und Physiologie und für klinische Medizin*, **321**, 177–227.

Kloos, K. and Vogel, M. (1968) Placentationsstörungen. Histologische Untersuchungen über Placentarreifungsstörungen am Routinematerial. *Virchows Archiv für pathologische Anatomie und physiologie und für klinische Medizin*, **343**, 245–257.

Koenig, U.D. (1972) Proliferative Gefassveränderungen der kindlichen Plazentargefasse und ihre Beziehung zur Plazentarinsuffizienz und Frühgeburt. *Zeitschrift für Geburtshilfe und Perinatologie*, **176**, 356–364.

Koenig, U.D., Mersmann, B. and Haupt, H. (1973) Proliferative plazentare Gefassveränderungen; Schwangerschaft und perinataler Verlauf beim Kind. *Zeitschrift für Geburtshilfe und Perinatologie*, **177**, 58–64.

Kovalovszki, L., Villanyi, E. and Banko, G. (1990) Placental villous edema: a possible cause of antenatal hypoxia. *Acta Paediatrica Hungarica*, **30**, 209–215.

Kubli, F. and Budliger, H. (1963) Beitrag zur Morphologie der insuffizienten Plazenta. *Geburtshilfe und Frauenheilkunde*, **23**, 37–43.

Labarrere, C.A. (1988) Acute atherosis: a histopathological hallmark of immune aggression? *Placenta*, **9**, 95–108.

Labarrere, C.A. and Faulk, W.P. (1992) Immunopathology of human extraembryonic tissues. In *Immunological Obstetrics*, Coulam, C.B., Faulk, W.P. and McIntyre, J.A. (Eds), pp. 439–463. New York: Norton.

Labarrere, C.A. and Faulk, W.F. (1994) Antigenic identification of cells in spiral artery trophoblastic invasion: validation of histologic studies by triple-antibody immunocytochemistry. *American Journal of Obstetrics and Gynecology*, **171**, 165–171.

Labarrere, C.A. and Faulk, W.P. (1995) Intercellular adhesion molecule-1 (ICAM-1) and HLA-DR antigens are expressed on endovascular cytotrophoblasts in abnormal pregnancies. *American Journal of Reproductive Immunology*, **33**, 47–53.

Labarrere, C.A., Alonso, J., Manni, J., Domenichini, E. and Althabe, O. (1985) Immunohistochemical findings in acute atherosis associated with intrauterine growth retardation. *American Journal of Reproductive Immunology and Microbiology*, **7**, 149–155.

Las Heras, J., Haust, M.D. and Harding, P.G. (1983) Morphology of fetal placental stem arteries in hypertensive disorders ('toxemia') of pregnancy. *Applied Pathology*, **1**, 301–309.

Lawrance, J.S. (1933) Concerning death of the fetus in pregnancy. *American Journal of Obstetrics and Gynecology*, **25**, 633–642.

Liebhart, M. (1968) Tkanka laczna lozysk pochodzacych z ciaz powiklanych przez cukrzyce matki. (The connective tissue in placenta samples collected from pregnancies complicated by diabetes mellitus.) *Ginekologica Polska*, **39**, 1353–1362.

Liebhart, M. (1969) Obrazy histopatologiczne lozysk w przpadkach niezgodnosci serologicznej i konfliktu serologicznego. (Microscopic patterns of placenta in cases of serological incompatibility and serological conflict.) *Ginekologica Polska*, **40**, 739–749.

Liebhart, M. (1970) Fibrinous necrosis of chorionic villi. *Acta Medica Polonica*, **11**, 121–125.

Liebhart, M. (1971) Some observations on so-called fibrinoid necrosis of placental villi: an electron-microscopic study. *Pathologia Europaea*, **6**, 217–220.

Liebhart, M. (1974) Ultrastructure of the stromal connective tissue of normal placenta and of placenta in diabetes mellitus of mother. *Pathologia Europaea*, **9**, 177–184.

Lohr, J., Ardelt, W. and Dehnhard, T. (1972) Nikotinarteriopathie der Plazenta? *Geburtshilfe und Frauenheilkunde*, **32**, 932–934.

McCormick, J.N., Faulk, W.P., Fox, H. and Fundenberg, H.H. (1971) Immunohistological and elution studies of the human placenta. *Journal of Experimental Medicine*, **91**, 1–13.

McFadyen, I.R., Price, A.B. and Geirsson, R.T. (1986) The relation to birthweight of histological appearances in vessels of the placental bed. *British Journal of Obstetrics and Gynaecology*, **93**, 476–481.

McKay, D.G., Hertig, A.T., Adams, E.C. and Richardson, M.V. (1958) Histochemical observations on the human placenta. *Obstetrics and Gynecology*, **12**, 1–36.

MacLennon, A.H., Sharp, F. and Shaw-Dunn, J. (1972) The ultrastructure of human trophoblast in spontaneous and induced hypoxia using a system of organ culture: a comparison with ultrastructural changes in pre-eclampsia and placental insufficiency. *Journal of Obstetrics and Gynaecology of the British Commonwealth*, **79**, 113–121.

Maqueo, M., Azuela, J.C. and de la Vega, M.D. (1964) Placental pathology in eclampsia and preeclampsia. *Obstetrics and Gynecology*, **24**, 350–356.

Martius, G. (1956) Histologische Untersuchungen der Plazenta zur Frage der Pathogenese des Morbus haemolyticus neonatorium. *Zentralblatt für Gynäkologie*, **78**, 2060–2065.

Mathews, R., Aikat, M. and Aikat, B.K. (1973) Morphological study of placenta in abnormal pregnancies. *Indian Journal of Pathology and Bacteriology*, **16**, 15–24.

Meekins, J.W., Pijnenborg, R., Hanssens, M, McFadyen, I.R. and van Assche, A. (1994) A study of placental bed spiral arteries and trophoblast invasion in normal and severe pre-eclamptic pregnancies. *British Journal of Obstetrics and Gynaecology*, **101**, 669–674.

Merrill, J.A. (1963) Common pathological changes of the placenta. *Clinical Obstetrics and Gynecology*, **6**, 96–109.

Merttens, I. (1894) Beitrage zur normalen und pathologischen Anatomie der menschlichen Placenta. *Zeitschrift für Geburtshilfe und Gynäkologie*, **30**, 1–22.

Moe, N. (1969) Deposits of fibrin and plasma proteins in the normal human placenta: an immunofluorescence study. *Acta Pathologica et Microbiologica Scandinavica*, **76**, 74–88.

Muller, G., Philippe, E., Lefakis, P. et al (1971) Les lesion placentaires de la gestose: étude anatomo-clinique. *Gynécologie et Obstétrique*, **70**, 309–316.

Mülzer, G., Emmrich, P., Birke, R. and Knaus, T. (1970) Diagnostik und Therapie der sogennanten Ubertragung im Vergleich zu typischen histologischen Placentabefunden. *Zeitschrift für Geburtschilfe und Gynäkologie*, **172**, 25–43.

Myatt, L. (1992) Current topic: control of vascular resistance in the human placenta. *Placenta*, **13**, 329–341.

Myers, R.A. and Fujikura, T. (1968) Placental changes after experimental abruptio placentae and fetal vessel ligation of rhesus monkey placenta. *American Journal of Obstetrics and Gynecology*, **100**, 846–851.

Naeye, R.L. (1989) Pregnancy hypertension, placental evidence of low uteroplacental blood flow and spontaneous term delivery. *Human Pathology*, **20**, 441–444.

Naeye, R.L. (1992) *Disorders of the Placenta, Fetus, and Neonate*. St Louis: Mosby Year Book.

Naeye, R.L., Maisels, J., Lorenz, R.P. and Botti, J.J. (1983) The clinical significance of placental villous edema. *Pediatrics*, **71**, 588–594.

Nagy, T., Boros, A. and Benko, K. (1965) Elektronmikropische Untersuchung junger und reifer menschlicher Placenten. *Archiv für Gynäkologie*, **200**, 428–440.

Nézelof, C. and Roussel, A. (1954) Le placenta des prématurés: étude de 75 cas. *Semaine des Hopitaux de Paris*, **30**, 3163–3167.

Olofsson, P., Laurini, R.N. and Marsal, K. (1993) A high uterine artery pulsatility index reflects a defective development of placental bed spiral arteries in pregnancies complicated by hypertension and fetal growth retardation. *European Journal of Obstetrics, Gynecology and Reproductive Biology*, **49**, 161–168.

Oswald, B. and Gerl, D. (1972) Die Mikrofibrinoidablagerungen in der menschlichen Placenta. *Acta Histochemica*, **42**, 356–359.

Paine, C.G. (1957) Observations on placental histology in normal and abnormal pregnancies. *Journal of Obstetrics and Gynaecology of the British Empire*, **64**, 668–672.

Panigel, M. and Anh, J.N.H. (1964a) Ultrastructure des villosités placentaires humaines. *Pathologie et Biologie*, **12**, 927–949.

Panigel, M. and Anh, J.N.H. (1964b) Ultrastructure des cellules de Hofbauer dans le placenta humain. *Compte Rendu des Séances de l'Académie des Sciences (Paris)*, **258**, 3556–3558.

Pijnenborg, R., Anthony, J., Davey, D.A. et al (1991) Placental bed spiral arteries in the hypertensive disorders of pregnancy. *British Journal of Obstetrics and Gynaecology*, **98**, 648–655.

Pisarki, T. (1967) Immunohistochemiczne badania nad rozmieszczeniem substancji bial-kowych w poplodzie i przechodzenia tych substancji od ciezarnej do plodu. (Immunohistochemical investigations upon the arrangement of proteinic substances in the afterbirth and the penetration of these substances from the pregnant to the foetus.) *Medycyna Doswiadczalna i Mikrobiologia*, **35**, 145–188.

Rayburn, W., Sander, C. and Compton, A. (1989) Histologic examination of the placenta in the growth-retarded fetus. *American Journal of Perinatology*, **6**, 58–61.

Read, M.A., Boura, A.L.A. and Walters, W.A.W. (1995) Effects of variation in oxygen tension on responses of the human fetoplacental vasculature to vasoactive agents *in vitro*. *Placenta*, **16**, 667–678.

Renaer, M. and Brosens, I. (1963) De spiraalvorige arteriolen van de decidua basalis bij de hypertensive verwikkelingen van de zwangerscuap. *Nederlands Tijdschrift voor Verloskunde en Gyneecologie*, **63**, 103–118.

Repetti, M. and Pescetto, G.C. (1951) Aspetti della placenta nella malattia emolitica. *Minerva Ginecologica*, **3**, 383–387.

Riviere, M. (1930) Contribution a l'étude microscopique comparée des placentas dits: albuminuriques et syphilitiques et des placentas normaux. *Gynécologie et Obstétrique*, **22**, 481–504.

Robecchi, E. and Aimone, V. (1965) Osservazioni istologiche sui vasi nella gestosi-albuimurica-ipertensiva-edemigena. *Minerva Ginecologica*, **17**, 994–1003.

Robertson, W.B. (1976) Uteroplacental vasculature. *Journal of Clinical Pathology*, **29**, Supplement (Royal College of Pathologists) 10, 9–17.

Robertson, W.B. and Dixon, H.G. (1969) Uteroplacental pathology. In *Foetus and Placenta*, Klopper, A. and Diczfalusy, E.(Eds), pp. 33–60. Oxford and Edinburgh: Blackwell Scientific.

Robertson, W.B., Brosens, I. and Dixon, H.G. (1967) The pathological response of the vessels of the placental bed to hypertensive pregnancy. *Journal of Pathology and Bacteriology*, **93**, 581–592.

Robertson, W.B., Brosens, I. and Dixon, H.G. (1975) Uteroplacental vascular pathology. *European Journal of Obstetrics, Gynecology and Reproductive Biology*, **5**, 47–65.

Robertson, W.B., Brosens, I. and Dixon, H.G. (1981) Maternal blood supply in fetal growth retardation. In *Fetal Growth Retardation*, Van Assche, A. and Robertson, W.B. (Eds), pp. 126–138. Edinburgh: Churchill Livingstone.

Robertson, W.B., Khong, T.Y., Brosens, I., De Wolf, F., Sheppard, B.L. and Bonnar, J. (1986) The placental bed biopsy: review from three European centers. *American Journal of Obstetrics and Gynecology*, **155**, 401–412.

Rodway, H.E. and Marsh, F. (1956) A study of Hofbauer's cells in human placenta. *Journal of Obstetrics and Gynaecology of the British Empire*, **63**, 111–115.

Rolfini, G., Pavone, G. and de Cecco, L. (1963) Studio comparativo pra gli aspetti microistofluoroscopiti della placenta nel diabete e della isoimmunizzazione anti Rh. *Recentia Medica*, **2**, 235–247.

Ruckhaberle, K.E. and Ruckhaberle, B. (1976) Der Zottentrophoblast in der Plazenten frühgeborener (eine enzym-histochemische Studie) *Zeitschrift für Geburtshilfe und Perinatologie*, **180**, 75–83.

Rudolph, A.M. and Heymann, M.A. (1973) Control of the foetal circulation. In *Foetal and Neonatal Physiology*, pp. 89–111. London: Cambridge University Press.

Salafia, C.M. (1992) Placental pathology in perinatal diagnosis. In *Gynecology and Obstetrics*, Sciarra, J.J. (Ed.), pp. 1–39. Philadelphia: Lippincott.

Salafia, C.M., Minior, V.K., Lopez-Zeno, J.A. et al (1995a) Relationship between placental histologic features and umbilical cord blood gases in preterm gestation. *American Journal of Obstetrics and Gynecology*, **173**, 1058–1064.

Salafia, C.M., Lopez-Zeno, J.A., Sherer, D.M. et al (1995b) Histologic evidence of old intrauterine bleeding is more frequent in prematurity. *American Journal of Obstetrics and Gynecology*, **173**, 1065–1070.

Salvatore, C.A. (1966) A placenta na toxemia de gravidez. *Maternidade e Infancia*, **25**, 87–116.

Salvatore, C.A. (1968) The placenta in toxemia: a comparative study. *American Journal of Obstetrics and Gynecology*, **102**, 347–353.

Sander, C.H. (1980) Hemorrhagic endovasculitis and hemorrhagic villitis of the placenta. *Archives of Pathology and Laboratory Medicine*, **104**, 371–373.

Sander, C.H., Kinnane, L., Stevens, N.G. and Echt, R. (1986) Haemorrhagic endovasculitis of the placenta: a review with clinical correlation. *Placenta*, **7**, 551–574.

Sani, G. and Bottiglioni, F. (1964) Studio istofunzionale della placenta nel diabete mellito. *Revista Italiana di Ginecologia*, **48**, 283–329.

Sauramo, H. (1951) Histology of the placenta in normal, premature and over-term cases, and in gestosis. *Annales Chirurgiae et Gynaecologiae Fenniae*, **40**, 164–188.

Sauramo, H. (1961) Histological and histochemical studies of the placenta and foetal membranes in pathological obstetrics. *Annales Chirurgiae et Gynaecologiae Fenniae*, **50**, 179–194.

Sawasaki, C., Nori, T., Inoue, T. and Shimni, K. (1957) Observations on the human placental membrane under the electron microscope. *Endocrinologia Japonica*, **4**, 1–11.

Sayeed, M., Chakrawarti, R.N. and Devi, P.K. (1976) A comparative study of placental villous changes in normal and abnormal pregnancy. *Journal of Obstetrics and Gynaecology of India*, **26**, 216–221.

Schroder, R. (1930) Die wieblichen Genitalorgane. In *Handbuch der Mikroskopische Anatomie des Menschen*, vol. 7/1, von Mollendorff, (Ed.), pp. 329–556. Berlin: Springer-Verlag.

Schuhmann, R. (1975) Reifungsstrungen der Plazenta. *Archiv für Gynäkologie*, **219**, 357–360.

Schuhmann, R. and Geier, G. (1972) Histomorphologische Placentabefunde bei EPH-Gestose. Ein Beitrag zur Morphologie der insuffizienten Placenta. *Archiv für Gynäkologie*, **213**, 31–47.

Schuhmann, R. and Wehler, V. (1971) Histologische Unterschiede an Placentazotten innerhalb der maternofetalen Stromungseinheit: Ein Beitrag zur funktionellen Morphologie der Placenta. *Archiv für Gynäkologie*, **240**, 425–439.

Schuhmann, R., Kraus, H., Borst, R. and Geier, G. (1976) Regional unterschiedliche Enzymaktivitt innerhalb der Placentone reifer menschlicher Placenten: Histochemische und biochemische Untersuchungen. *Archiv für Gynäkologie*, **220**, 209–226.

Schweikhart, G. Kaufmann, P. and Beck, T. (1986) Morphology of placental villi after premature delivery and its clinical relevance. *Archives of Gynecology and Obstetrics*, **239**, 101–114.

Sen, D.K. and Langley, F.A. (1974) Villous basement membrane thickening and fibrinoid necrosis in normal and abnormal placentas. *American Journal of Obstetrics and Gynecology*, **118**, 276–281.

Sermann, R. and Capria, V. (1965) Rillievi ultrastruttarali sul villi coriale umano nelle gestosi tardive. *Attualita di Ostetricia e Ginecologia*, **11**, 32–42.

Shanklin, D.R. (1958) The human placenta: a clinico-pathologic study. *Obstetrics and Gynecology*, **11**, 129–138.

Sheehan, M.M., Kealy, W.F. and Mundow, L.S. (1990) Placental chorangiosis associated with foetal death – a case report. *Irish Journal of Medical Sciences*, **159**, 249–250.

Shen-Schwartz, S., Macpherson, T.A. and Mueller-Heubach, E. (1988) The clinical significance of hemorrhagic endovasculitis of the placenta. *American Journal of Obstetrics and Gynecology*, **159**, 48–51.

Shen-Schwartz, S., Ruchelli, E. and Brown, D. (1989) Villous oedema of the placenta: a clinicopathological study. *Placenta*, **10**, 297–307.

Sheppard, B.L. and Bonnar, J. (1976) The ultrastructure of the arterial supply of the human placenta in pregnancy complicated by fetal growth retardation. *British Journal of Obstetrics and Gynaecology*, **83**, 948–959.

Sheppard, B.L. and Bonnar, J. (1980) Ultrastructural abnormalities of placental villi in placentae from pregnancies complicated by fetal growth retardation: their relationship to decidual spiral arterial lesions. *Placenta*, **1**, 145–156.

Sheppard, B.L. and Bonnar, J. (1981) An ultrastructural study of utero-placental arteries in hypertensive and normotensive pregnancy and fetal growth retardation. *British Journal of Obstetrics and Gynaecology*, **88**, 695–705.

Silver, M.M., Yeger, H. and Lines, L.D. (1988) Hemorrhagic endovasculitis-like lesion induced in placental organ culture. *Human Pathology*, **19**, 251–256.

Simpson, R.A., Mayhew, T.M. and Barnes, P.R. (1992) From 13 weeks to term, the trophoblast of human placenta grows by the continuous recruitment of new proliferative units: a study of nuclear number using the dissector. *Placenta*, **13**, 501–512.

Stieve, H. (1941) Die Entwicklung und der Bau der menschlichen Plazenta. 2. Zotten, Zottenraumgitter und Gefasse in der zweiten Hlfte der Schwangerschaft. *Zeitschrift für mikroskopich-anatomische Forschung*, **50**, 1–120.

Stock, M.K., Anderson, D.F., Phernetton, T.M., McLaughlin, M.K. and Rankin, J.H.G. (1980) Vascular response of the fetal placenta to local occlusion of the maternal placental vasculature. *Journal of Developmental Physiology*, **2**, 339–346.

Strachan, G.I. (1923) The development and structure of the human placenta. *Journal of Obstetrics and Gynaecology of the British Empire*, **30**, 611–642.

Tarjan, G. (1965) Placentördem in der Toxaemia. *Archiv für Gynäkologie*, **202**, 362–363.

Tenney, B. (1936) Syncytial degeneration in normal and pathologic placentas. *American Journal of Obstetrics and Gynecology*, **31**, 1024–1028.

Tenney, B. and Parker, F. (1940) The placenta in toxemia of pregnancy. *American Journal of Obstetrics and Gynecology*, **39**, 1000–1005.

Theuring, F. (1968) Fibröse Obliterationen an Deckplatten und Stammzottengefassen der Placenta nach Intrauterinem Fruchttod. *Archiv für Gynäkologie*, **206**, 237–251.

Thomsen, K. (1955) Placentarbefunde bei Spätgestosen und ihre ätiologische Zuordnung. *Archiv für Gynäkologie*, **185**, 476–503.

Thomsen, K. and Berle, P. (1960) Placentarbefunde bei Rh-Inkompatibilitat. *Archiv für Gynäkologie*, **192**, 628–643.

Thomsen, K. and Blankenburg, H. (1956) Über die Entwicklung und Rückbildung der Langhansschen Zellschicht in der menschlichen Placenta. *Archiv für Gynäkologie*, **187**, 638–649.

Thomsen, K. and Lieschke, G. (1958) Untersuchungen zur Placentarmorphologie bei Diabetes mellitus. *Acta Endocrinologica*, **29**, 602–614.

Thomsen, K. and Schniewind, H. (1961) Methodik und Ergebnisse der Perfusion normaler und übertragener menschlichen Placenten. *Archiv für Gynäkologie*, **195**, 463–467.

Tominaga, R. and Page, E.W. (1966) Accommodation of the human placenta to hypoxia. *American Journal of Obstetrics and Gynecology*, **94**, 679–685.

Traub, A., Jakobovits, A. and Szonagh, F.E. (1964) Ein Beitrag zur Nachweis der Langhanszellen in der Placenta ausgetragener unkomplizierter Schwangerschaften. *Zeitschrift für Geburtshilfe und Gynäkologie*, **162**, 314–320.

van der Veen, F., Walker, S. and Fox, H. (1982) Endarteritis obliterans of the fetal stem arteries of the human placenta: an electron microscopic study. *Placenta*, **3**, 181–190.

Vokaer, R. (1957) Critères histologiques et histochemiques de la senéscence placentaire. *Bulletin de la Fédération des Sociétés de Gynécologie et d'Obstétrique de Langue Francaise*, **9**, Supplement 1, 20–28.

Vracko, R. and Benditt, E. (1970) Capillary basal lamina thickening: its relationship to endothelial cell death and replacement. *Journal of Cell Biology*, **47**, 281–285.

Wang, T. (1989) Uterine Spiralarterien des Menschen bei Gestose, fetaler Wachstumsretardierung und Ubertragung. *Geburtshilfe und Frauenheilkunde*, **49**, 548–552.

Wentworth, P. (1967) The placenta in cases of hemolytic disease of the newborn. *American Journal of Obstetrics and Gynecology*, **98**, 283–289.

Wheeler, T., Elcock, C.L. and Anthony, F.W. (1995) Angiogenesis and the placental environment. *Placenta*, **16**, 289–296.

Wiedow, W. (1888) Uber den Zusammenhang zwischen Albuminurie and Placentarerkrankung. *Zeitschrift für Geburtshilfe und Gynäkologie*, **14**, 387–404.

Wigglesworth, J.S. (1962) The Langhans layer in late pregnancy: a histological study of normal and abnormal cases. *Journal of Obstetrics and Gynaecology of the British Commonwealth*, **69**, 355–365.

Wigglesworth, J.S. (1964) Morphological variations in the insufficient placenta. *Journal of Obstetrics and Gynaecology of the British Commonwealth*, **71**, 871–884.

Wilkin, P. (1965) *Pathologie du Placenta*. Paris: Masson et Cie.

Williams, J.W. (1990) The frequency and significance of infarcts of the placenta, based upon a microscopic examination of five hundred consecutive placentae. *American Journal of Obstetrics*, **41**, 775–801.

Wislocki, G.B. and Bennett, H.S. (1943) Histology and cytology of the human and monkey placenta with special reference to the trophoblast. *American Journal of Anatomy*, **73**, 335–449.

Wislocki, G.B. and Dempsey, E.W. (1955) Electron microscopy of the human placenta. *Anatomical Record*, **123**, 133–167.

Wynn, R.M. (1965) Electron microscopic contributions to placental physiology. *Journal of Obstetrics and Gynaecology of the British Commonwealth*, **72**, 955–963.

Wynn, R.M. (1967) Derivation and ultrastructure of the so-called Hofbauer cell. *American Journal of Obstetrics and Gynecology*, **97**, 235–248.

Zeek, P.M. and Assali, N.S. (1950) Vascular changes in the decidua associated with eclamptogenic toxemia of pregnancy. *American Journal of Clinical Pathology*, **20**, 1099–1109.

Zhou, Y., Damsky, C.H., Chiu, K., Roberts, J.M. and Fisher, S.J. (1993) Pre-eclampsia is associated with abnormal expression of adhesion molecules by invasive cytotrophoblasts. *Journal of Clinical Investigation*, **91**, 950–960.

7

THE PLACENTA IN PREGNANCIES OF ABNORMAL DURATION

The modal duration of pregnancy is approximately 40 weeks but there is, as with any biological parameter, a considerable scatter about this norm. For practical purposes, however, it would not be unreasonable for a pregnancy that extends to, or beyond, the 42nd week of gestation to be considered as prolonged, or for one in which delivery occurs before the 37th week to be regarded as having terminated prematurely.

THE PLACENTA IN PREMATURE ONSET OF LABOUR

Between 5 and 10% of babies are delivered prematurely; most of these are towards the mature end of the spectrum of preterm births, deliveries before the 32nd week of gestation accounting for about 1.5% of births and deliveries under 28 weeks accounting for only 0.2–0.6% of births. It is in this last group that prematurity poses its greatest threat because two-thirds of deaths in preterm infants occur in infants born at less than 28 weeks of gestation (Walkinshaw, 1995). In a considerable proportion of cases, early delivery is related to an obvious obstetrical complication such as twin pregnancy, abruptio placentae, cervical incompetence, placenta praevia or severe pre-eclampsia; obvious, that is, in the sense that they are easily diagnosed but in many cases far from obvious as to how and why these complications precipitate early labour. In a considerable proportion of the remainder, premature labour is a consequence of, and is secondary to, either chorioamnionitis or idiopathic premature rupture of the membranes. These conditions are discussed in Chapters 11 and 14 but it may be remarked here that the relationship between ascending infection and premature membrane rupture is a complex one because chorioamnionitis can cause premature membrane rupture whilst premature membrane rupture can be complicated by chorioamnionitis. Nevertheless it is now clear that chorioamnionitis, with or without membrane rupture, is the most important precipitating factor of very early preterm delivery, certainly before the 28th week of gestation and, though to a slightly lesser extent, before the 32nd week of gestation. True idiopathic primary premature onset of labour in women with intact, non-inflamed membranes is a relatively uncommon event, though not perhaps as uncommon as Lettieri et al (1993) have suggested, these workers being unable to find a potential aetiological factor in only 4% of preterm births.

Although observations on placentas from prematurely delivered babies have been few, several mutually contradictory findings have been reported. An important element in this disagreement has been the tendency, in some studies, to regard premature delivery as being the sole criterion for inclusion in the series. This has meant that placentas from uncomplicated pregnancies and those from pregnancies complicated by such conditions as pre-eclampsia or essential hypertension have been considered together as a single entity, a methodological and conceptual error that can only lead to contradictions and discrepancies. In this account I confine my comments to placentas from cases of premature delivery in otherwise fully normal pregnancies.

The prematurely delivered placenta is usually smaller and lighter than a term placenta but is otherwise generally unremarkable on naked-eye examination. There is not, in my experience, any excess of extrachorial placentation or of abnormal insertion of the cord and, despite claims to the contrary (Sauramo, 1951; Siegel & Rabanus, 1966), it has been the conclusion of most observers that infarcts, perivillous fibrin deposition and calcification are distinctly uncommon in these placentas, occurring with a much lower frequency than in the term placenta (Nézelof & Roussel, 1954; Wigglesworth, 1962; Wilkin, 1965; Fox, 1969a).

On histological examination the fetal stem arteries rarely show any abnormality and the villi are, in most instances, of apparently normal maturity for the length of the gestational period (Fig. 7.1). I use the word 'apparently' with some circumspection, because any comments as to the 'normal' maturity at this stage of gestation must be tempered by the fact that no normal control series is available for comparison, delivery during the early part of the third trimester being, by definition, invariably abnormal. It does not, however, seem unreasonable to adopt Wigglesworth's (1962) assumption that the structure of the placental villi at this time can be considered as lying somewhere between that of the second-trimester placenta and that of the normal placenta at term. It is almost invariably the case, however, that a proportion of prematurely delivered placentas depart from this pattern and have a villous morphology which is that of the fully mature term organ (Fig. 7.2). This proportion is about 10% in most series (Nézelof & Roussel, 1954; Becker, 1963, 1975; Fox, 1969a) but was significantly higher in the placentas examined by Aladjem (1968), Schweikhart et al (1986) and Suska et al (1990). The sceptic may argue that in such circumstances the estimate of the length of the

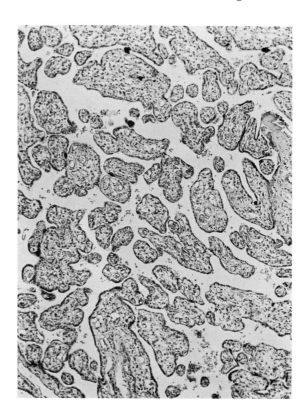

Figure 7.1. Histological appearances of the villi in a placenta from a pregnancy which terminated spontaneously at the 34th week of gestation. The villi have a uniform appearance and were considered to be of normal maturity for the length of the gestational period (H & E × 54).

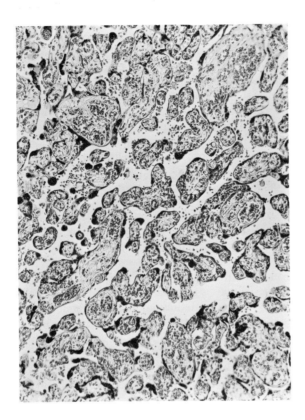

Figure 7.2. Histological appearances of the villi in a placenta from a pregnancy terminating spontaneously at the 35th week of gestation. The villi have a uniform appearance and are morphologically fully mature in all respects, this being an example of 'maturitas praecox placentae' (H & E × 90).

gestational period was faulty and that both the pregnancy and the placenta were at term; I have, however, encountered fully mature placentas from women who were undoubtedly only 30–32 weeks pregnant and who gave birth to babies whose weight and length were fully compatible with a pregnancy of this duration. These are then true examples of 'maturitas praecox placentae' and as such are a manifestation of an asynchrony between the rates of placental and fetal maturation, the cause of this being obscure. Naeye (1987, 1989, 1992) considers that premature placental maturation in such cases is evidence of chronic low uteroplacental blood flow and it is possible that this is at least partially true: nevertheless this remains as a speculative hypothesis which is unsupported by Doppler studies or placental bed biopsies. Rather less commonly the villi are unusually immature for the stage of pregnancy attained (Fig. 7.3).

Wigglesworth (1962) and Prata Martins (1964) have commented that in prematurely delivered placentas there is often a very marked variation in villous structure and maturity, but I would consider that in most instances this simply reflects the fact that fresh villous growth is more abundant in these placentas than in those delivered at term and that young, highly immature villi in the centre of the fetal lobules are unduly prominent. In my own series there was a rather high incidence of villous fibrinoid necrosis but no other lesion of the villi (Fig. 7.4). Syncytial knots and vasculo-syncytial membranes were infrequent, the cytotrophoblastic cells moderately prominent, the villous vessels often relatively small, the stroma quite abundant, and Hofbauer cells seen with some frequency, all these being normal characteristics of the immature villus. I have not encountered the villous atrophy and syncytial degeneration noted in placentas of prematurely delivered babies by Anghelescu et al (1962).

Salafia et al (1991) considered that three placental lesions were significantly related to preterm birth, these being umbilical–chorionic vasculitis, chronic villitis and decidual vascular abnormalities. In this study umbilical–chorionic vasculitis was used as a marker for ascending infection and the results were similar to those in other reports, evidence of infection being noted in 32–38% of cases delivered before the 33rd week of gestation and in 13% of cases delivered between the 33rd and 37th gestational weeks. Their claim

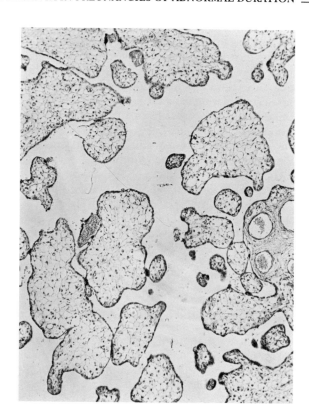

Figure 7.3. Villi in a placenta from a pregnancy terminating spontaneously at the 36th week of gestation. The villi are uniformly unduly immature for the length of the gestational period (H & E × 54).

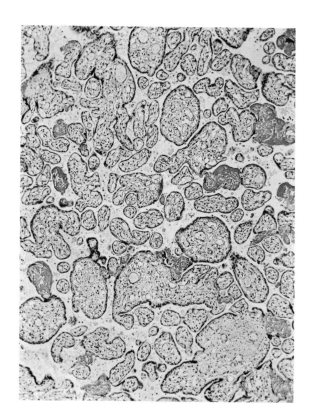

Figure 7.4. A placenta from a pregnancy terminating spontaneously at the 34th week of gestation. The villi are of normal maturity for the length of the gestational period, but an unduly high proportion show fibrinoid necrosis (H & E × 60).

that chronic villitis is significantly related to premature birth seems, however, more difficult to sustain because these workers noted a villitis in 4–9% of placentas from pregnancies terminating between the 22nd and 32nd weeks of gestation and in 16% of those from deliveries between the 33rd and 37th gestational weeks: These figures are, in general, either lower or not significantly higher than those usually noted in large series of unselected placentas (see Chapter 11) and were in fact below the incidence of villitis found in their placentas from term deliveries. The term 'decidual vascular abnormality' was used by Salafia and her co-workers to encompass absence of physiological change in the decidual vessels, chronic decidual vasculitis or thrombosis of decidual vessels, abnormalities of this type being found in a high percentage of cases of preterm birth, particularly those in which the fetus had a very low birth weight or was hypoxic (Salafia et al, 1995a,b). Salafia and Mill (1996) consider that the maternal vascular abnormalities seen in cases of non-pre-eclamptic preterm birth are qualitatively, though not quantitatively, identical to those found in pre-eclampsia and thus imply that defective placentation may be a factor in some cases of otherwise idiopathic premature onset of labour. This concept has won some support from Doppler studies (Strigini et al, 1995) and is certainly a feasible one because it is becoming increasingly clear that the spectrum of obstetrical disorders that may result from abnormal placentation is very wide.

Significance of Pathological Findings

What is the value of routine examination of placentas from prematurely delivered babies on a non-research basis? Clearly, the finding of a chorioamnionitis is important in terms of possible prophylaxis in succeeding pregnancies whilst, conversely and perhaps paradoxically, it is equally important to note the absence of a chorioamnionitis, thus guiding the obstetrician's attention to non-infective causes of preterm birth. Redline (1995), commenting on several studies that have appeared only in abstract form, has reviewed attempts to correlate placental lesions in preterm births with both short-term and long-term prognosis for the neonate. He noted that whilst some have found chorioamnionitis to be associated with an adverse fetal outcome, others have claimed that chorioamnionitis is usually associated with a good prognosis. He concurred with the latter view, which he considered to be explicable on the basis that chorioamnionitis causes preterm labour in otherwise normal pregnancies. It is my own view that the only real value of examining placentas from premature births in routine practice is to detect abnormalities that may recur in subsequent pregnancies. Attempts to correlate specific placental lesions with either neonatal death or long-term neurological damage are fraught with danger because they are, at best, only statistical associations. Further, in purely practical terms, the placental findings will not in any way influence the clinical management of the prematurely delivered neonate.

Does placental examination offer any pathogenetic clues to the cause of idiopathic premature onset of labour? If an excess of villous fibrinoid necrosis is found it is tempting to suggest that there has been an immune attack on the trophoblastic tissue and to regard the premature delivery as a form of graft rejection; unfortunately this temptation has to be resisted because there is, at the moment, no firm evidence to support this enticingly attractive hypothesis.

Those cases in which the placenta is, despite the short length of the gestational period, fully mature are of considerable interest and it is at least hypothetically possible that the accelerated maturation of the placenta may play some role in the initiation of premature labour. Currently, the placenta is not considered to be of great importance in the pathogenesis of preterm birth, much greater stress being placed on activation of decidual, cervical and fetal membrane factors (Lockwood, 1994). It is difficult to believe, however, that the placenta plays no role in the system of signalling that heralds the onset of labour and it is certainly possible that an unduly early attainment of placental maturity is of some importance in the pathogenesis of preterm birth.

Salafia et al (1995b) consider that the immature placenta is less capable of withstanding the stresses of labour than is the full-term placenta, largely because of the lack of functionally efficient terminal villi, and that fetal hypoxia is thus more likely to complicate preterm than term delivery. This is a plausible argument though this concept is not strictly relevant to the pathologist in most cases because this relative functional inefficiency is independent of any pathological lesions. They do, however, also suggest that placental lesions, such as perivillous fibrin deposition, syncytial knotting, cytotrophoblastic hyperplasia, villous fibrosis and decreased villous vascularity, may further decrease the functional capacity of the preterm placenta and thus adversely affect the fetus. For reasons elaborated upon in Chapters 5 and 6, this is a view with which I would disagree.

Finally, the intriguing possibility that at least some cases of premature onset of labour are a consequence of inadequate placentation is one that requires further exploration by placental bed biopsies and Doppler studies.

THE PLACENTA IN PROLONGED PREGNANCY

In the past it was thought that between 10 and 12% of pregnancies extended to, or beyond, the 42nd week of gestation, whilst 5% persisted for 43 weeks or more (Bolte et al, 1972; Perkins, 1974). It hardly needs stating, of course, that many of these were actually miscalculated term pregnancies and the introduction of a routine ultrasound examination in early pregnancy reduced the incidence of prolonged pregnancies to about 6% (Eik-Nes et al, 1984; Cardozo et al, 1986). Indeed, it is claimed that with very accurate dating studies the incidence of prolonged gestations does not exceed 1% (Boyd et al, 1988). Some cases of prolongation of pregnancy must represent the expected normal scatter around the modal time of delivery of 40 weeks; probably only a proportion of prolonged pregnancies are therefore truly pathological and any explanation for the failure to go into labour in such patients awaits clarification of the still poorly understood, but undoubtedly complex, factors controlling the onset of labour (Johnson et al, 1995; Turnbull, 1995).

It is not my intention to discuss in any detail the clinical aspects of prolonged pregnancy, as these have been considered at length by Vorherr (1975a,b) and it will suffice here to outline and summarize his review which, despite the passage of time and despite his insistence on the role played by 'placental insufficiency', remains authoritative. In most, but not all, studies of prolonged pregnancy there has been a considerably elevated perinatal mortality which rises almost geometrically as the gestational period extends to the 43rd or 44th week. There is an increased incidence of clinically detectable intrauterine hypoxia in cases of prolonged pregnancy, whilst there is a tendency for mean birth weight to level off at 42 weeks and then decline slightly, though in this latter respect it should be noted that the proportion of unduly heavy (macrosomic) infants is significantly higher in prolonged than in term pregnancies. A proportion of infants from prolonged pregnancies, probably between 20 and 40%, appear to suffer from intrauterine malnutrition and develop various degrees of the 'postmaturity' syndrome; this, in its full-blown state, is characterized by dehydration and loss of subcutaneous fat, with the development of dry, wrinkled, parchment-like skin, loss of vernix caseosa and languo hair, maceration of skin creases, increased hardness of the skull bones, long, thin limbs and, perhaps not surprisingly, an 'apprehensive' look. This syndrome is commonly associated with oligohydramnios and, with increased fetal surveillance, is much less commonly encountered today than during the period reviewed by Vorherr.

Placental Ageing

It is considered by many that the ill-effects of prolonged pregnancy are due largely to 'placental insufficiency', it being supposed that during the course of a normal pregnancy the placenta progressively ages and that the term organ is in, or on the verge of, a decline into morphological and functional senescence, a state that is fully attained in prolonged pregnancies. The villi of the term placenta are often described as showing all the morphological hallmarks of senescence but this view is based almost entirely on a misunderstanding and misinterpretation of the histological manifestations of the normal processes of maturation of the villous tree and of functional trophoblastic differentiation and there are no light or electron microscopic features in the placenta that can be considered as indicative of an ageing process (Fox, 1979; Haigh et al, 1989). A claim (Parmley et al, 1981) that lipofuscin pigment progressively accumulates in the villous syncytiotrophoblast (a change generally accepted to be a feature of ageing cells) has been fully refuted (Haigh et al, 1984).

It is often suggested that a feature of placental ageing is the cessation of DNA synthesis and of organ growth that has been claimed to occur during the later weeks of gestation (Winick et al, 1967). More recent studies, however, have shown that total placental DNA content continues to rise in a linear fashion until, and beyond, the 40th week of pregnancy (Sands & Dobbing, 1985). This finding is in accord with histological evidence of fresh villous growth in the term placenta, with autoradiographic and cytometric studies that have demonstrated continuing DNA synthesis in the term organ (Geier et al, 1975; Hustin et al, 1984; Iversen & Farsund, 1985) and with morphometric studies that have shown persistent villous growth, continuing expansion of the villous surface area and progressive branching of the villous tree up to, and beyond, term (Boyd, 1984; Jackson et al, 1992). Placental growth certainly slows during the last few weeks of gestation though this decline is neither invariable nor irreversible. Those arguing that a decreased placental growth rate during late pregnancy is evidence of senescence often appear to be comparing the placenta to an organ such as the gut in which continuing viability is dependent on a constantly replicating stem cell population producing short-lived post-mitotic cells. A more apt comparison would be with an organ such as the liver, which is formed principally of long-lived post-mitotic cells and which, once an optimal size has been attained to meet the metabolic demands placed on it, shows little evidence of cell proliferation whilst retaining a latent capacity for growth activity. Certainly there seems no good reason why the placenta, once it has reached a size sufficient to meet adequately its transfer function, should continue to grow and the term placenta, with its considerable functional reserve capacity, has more than met this aim.

The view that the functional capacity of the placenta declines towards term is based on evidence that is, at best, equivocal and there are in fact no changes indicative of any decline in intrinsic placental functions such as replicative ability and microsomal protein synthetic capacity (Fox, 1979). There is undoubtedly a decrease in placental oxygen consumption during the later months of pregnancy but this is not necessarily evidence of ageing because the metabolic demands of the term placenta are considerably lower than are those of the first-trimester organ, largely because of completion of architectural remodelling and a reduced growth activity.

Morphological Changes in the Placenta

No uniformity of opinion exists as to whether there are specific morphological changes in placentas from prolonged pregnancies. Some have denied that any structural abnormality can be detected in such placentas (McKiddie, 1949; Merrill, 1963; Wigglesworth, 1964) but this has not been the general experience and most workers have found histological abnormalities in a proportion of placentas from prolonged pregnancies, though amongst these there has been no agreement on the nature of the abnormal findings.

The naked-eye appearances of placentas from prolonged pregnancies are in no way characteristic, though several (those associated with fetal macrosomia) are unusually heavy. There is a widespread impression that these placentas are often extensively infarcted and heavily calcified (Buscemi, 1957; Clavero-Nunez, 1962; Kubli & Budliger, 1963; Siegel, 1963; Siegel & Rabanus, 1966), but it has been my experience that this is not the case, placentas from prolonged pregnancies being no more frequently calcified and containing no greater numbers of infarcts than term placentas (Fox, 1969b).

Furthermore, there is no excess of perivillous fibrin deposition, fetal artery thrombosis or retroplacental haematoma formation.

On histological examination of placentas from prolonged but otherwise uncomplicated pregnancies, the stem arteries are usually normal and do not show an excess, or any increased degree, of 'obliterative endarteritis'. It is true that there have been reports of an increased incidence of this arterial lesion in placentas from prolonged pregnancies (Thomsen & Schniewind, 1961; de Cecco et al, 1962; Salvatore, 1971) but this was certainly not the case in my own series (Fox, 1969b), and I believe these claims to be based on faulty selection of material or misinterpretation of data (the latter is certainly the case in Salvatore's series, because his results, as detailed, offer no support for his conclusion). This is an important point, as it is my opinion that the most characteristic feature of placentas from prolonged pregnancies is reduced villous perfusion (Fig. 7.5) which is not secondary to a lesion of the fetal stem arteries. There appears to be a primary collapse of the villous fetal vessels, which, instead of being sinusoidally dilated, are small and inconspicuous (Fox, 1967); these poorly perfused villi are richly endowed with syncytial knots and have an increased amount of stromal fibrosis (Fig. 7.6), such changes being, as discussed in Chapter 6, an invariable consequence of a reduced fetal blood flow through the villi. These changes have, of course, been noted by many others (Arienzo, 1955; Buscemi, 1957; Carenza & Coppola, 1957; Durst, 1963; Clavero et al, 1964; Vanrell-Cruells & Comas-Funallet, 1965; Alvarez et al, 1966; Emmrich & Malzer, 1968; Malzer et al, 1970; Justus et al, 1971; Liebhart & Kuczynska-Sicinska, 1971; Novitsky et al, 1976), though there has often been a tendency to overemphasize the significance of the profusion of syncytial knots and the villous fibrosis at the expense of the more important primary change of decreased villous perfusion. Occasional villi that are poorly perfused are seen in placentas from uncomplicated term pregnancies, but they are rarely, if ever, present in the abundance with which they occur in those from protracted gestations, and I would regard the particular combination of normal fetal stem arteries and inadequately perfused fibrotic villi bearing numerous syncytial knots as being highly characteristic of, indeed almost specific for, prolonged pregnancy.

I have never seen any evidence of either the compensatory regenerative growth of villi or the delayed villous maturation that have been described in placentas from prolonged pregnancies (Zhemkova & Topchieva, 1964; Zaliznyak, 1967; Hitschold et al, 1989), but the villi of some such placentas do show a mild or moderate cytotrophoblastic proliferation (Fig. 7.7) and some degree of thickening of the trophoblastic basement membrane, changes indicative of a minor degree of placental ischaemia. Not

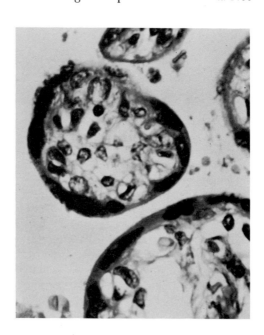

Figure 7.5. A villus in a placenta from a pregnancy that was terminated at the 43rd week of gestation. The villous vessels are small and inconspicuous (H & E × 800).

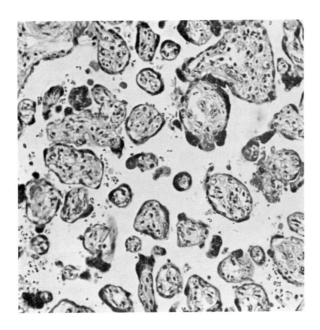

Figure 7.6. Villi in a placenta from a woman delivered at the 42nd week of gestation. The villi are poorly perfused, fibrotic and show excessive syncytial knot formation (H & E × 110).

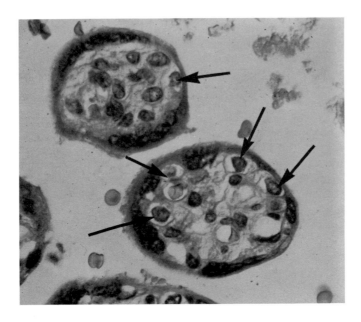

Figure 7.7. Villi in a placenta from a woman delivered at the 43rd week of gestation. The villi are poorly perfused and also contain an excessive number of cytotrophoblastic cells (arrowed) (H & E × 800).

all placentas from prolonged pregnancies show these histological changes and in a considerable proportion the villous morphology is normal and indistinguishable from that seen in normal term placentas.

Ultrastructural studies of placentas from prolonged pregnancies have been few (de Palo, 1967; Devizorova & Shvirst, 1970; Kemnitz & Theuring, 1974; Jones & Fox, 1978; Ito et al, 1984) and have tended to show a decrease in the number of syncytial microvilli on the outer surface of the syncytium, a decline in the number of pinocytotic vesicles in the syncytium, vacuolation of the endoplasmic reticulum, and a decrease in the number of mitochondria, Golgi bodies and secretory droplets in the trophoblast. Thickening of the trophoblastic basement membrane has also been confirmed (Fig. 7.8). Jones and Fox (1978) further noted small foci of syncytial necrosis, which were presumed to be due to ischaemia (Fig. 7.9).

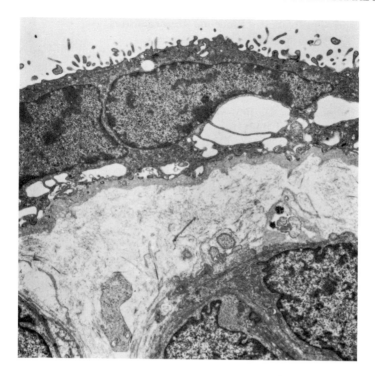

Figure 7.8. Ultrastructure of villous syncytiotrophoblast in a placenta from a prolonged pregnancy. The syncytiotrophoblast shows very little pinocytotic activity, is depleted of microvilli and shows dilatation of the rough endoplasmic reticulum. The trophoblastic basement membrane is slightly thickened (×12,500).

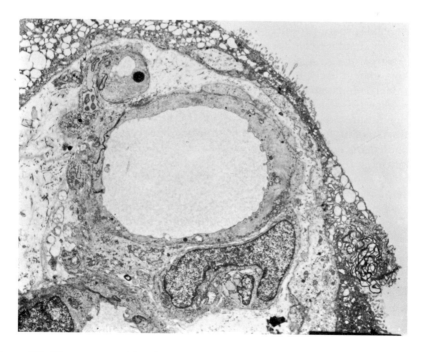

Figure 7.9. Ultrastructure of the placenta from a prolonged pregnancy. There is a loss of syncytial microvilli and a focal area of syncytial necrosis (×5000).

Pathogenesis and Significance of Placental Abnormalities

Many placentas from prolonged pregnancies are normal in all respects, but in the remainder the principal abnormality is diminished fetal perfusion of the placental villi. This occurs in the presence of normal stem arteries and is, in my view, a consequence of the oligohydramnios and fetal dehydration that is seen in a significant proportion of prolonged gestations. Doppler flow velocimetry studies have, in general though not unanimously, indicated that there is no increased fetal vascular resistance in the placenta in prolonged pregnancies (Guidetti et al, 1987; Stokes et al, 1991; Zimmermann et al, 1995) and the lack of any structural abnormality in the villous vessels has been confirmed by their normal histological appearance after perfusion fixation (Larsen et al, 1995). Further, umbilical vein flow studies have shown that fetal blood flow through the placenta is often reduced in cases of oligohydramnios (Gill et al, 1993). Diminished placental villous perfusion is therefore a consequence of the ill-effects of prolonged pregnancy and is unlikely, in itself, to be responsible for the fetal complications encountered in prolonged gestations, because the ability of the placental tissue to increase oxygen extraction when blood flow is decreased allows it to sustain a fetal flow reduction of 50% without impairing fetal oxygenation (Itskovitz et al, 1983).

Evidence of mild to moderate uteroplacental ischaemia is also found in a proportion of placentas from prolonged pregnancies, occasionally in isolation but often in association with diminished villous perfusion. This is in accord with the long-standing observation that the uteroplacental blood flow tends to diminish after the 40th week of gestation is passed (Browne, 1963; Dixon et al, 1963; Robertson & Dixon, 1969), a finding that has received experimental support from studies of artificially prolonged pregnancies in rats (Yamagushi et al, 1975). The cause of this is, however, thoroughly obscure: Magnin and Gabriel (1966) could find no histological abnormality in the maternal decidual vessels in prolonged pregnancies though Wang (1989) has, rather unconvincingly, described intimal swelling in the spiral vessels in such cases. One speculative possibility is that the reduced flow is a consequence of the diminished villous vascularity, because ten Berge (1955, 1956) has suggested that there is, in the normal placenta, a villous 'pulse' that plays a role in the circulation of the maternal blood through the intervillous space. Reduced villous vascularity may therefore lead to a loss of this pulse, with subsequent stagnation of maternal blood in the intervillous space, a rise in intervillous space pressure, and a consequent reduction in maternal blood flow. This is a rather simplistic concept but one that is not therefore necessarily incorrect.

The degree of uteroplacental ischaemia suffered in prolonged pregnancy is not very striking and unlikely, by itself, to cause fetal embarrassment. It is possible, however, that the combination of diminished fetal villous perfusion and mild uteroplacental ischaemia allows two individually unimportant abnormalities to summate and thus attain a significant status. It has been suggested that the ill-effects on the fetus of prolonged pregnancy, at least in terms of fetal distress, are due to cord compression, this being a consequence of oligohydramnios (Leveno et al, 1984) but Silver et al (1988), whilst confirming that cord compression was indeed common in prolonged gestations, were unable to correlate such compression with fetal distress. It should be noted that these claims and counter-claims were based on fetal heart rate tracings and cord blood analyses and not on pathological studies: possibly greater attention should be paid by pathologists to the cord in prolonged gestations and less attention devoted to the fruitless task of defining placental senescence.

REFERENCES

Aladjem, S. (1968) Placenta of the premature infant. *American Journal of Obstetrics and Gynecology*, **102,** 311–312.

Alvarez, H., Benedetti, W.L. and de Leonis, V.K. (1966) La placenta del embarazo prolongado. *V Congreso Latinoamericano de Obstetricia y Ginecologia*, **2,** 636–640.

Anghelescu, V., Gheorghiu, C., Tirnoveanu, G., Chiva, P. and Cohn, D. (1962) Aspesti morfopatologie ale placentei si prematuritatia. *Morfologia Normala si Patologica*, **7,** 137–142.

Arienzo, F. (1955) Studio anatomo-patologo delle placente nella gravidanza protratta. *Quaderni di Anatomia Pratica*, **10**, 418–431.

Becker, V. (1963) Funktionelle Morphologie der Placenta. *Archiv für Gynäkologie*, **198**, 3–28.

Becker, V. (1975) Abnormal maturation of the villi. In *The Placenta and its Maternal Supply Line*, Gruenwald, P. (Ed.), pp. 232–243. Lancaster: Medical and Technical Publishing.

Bolte, A., Bachmann, K.D., Hofmann, E., Röhricht, J. and Strothmann, G. (1972) Verlängerte Schwangerschaftsdauer und Placentadysfunktion. I. Häufigkeit und Diagnostik bei den Geburtsjahrgängen 1955–1966. *Deutsche Medizinische Wochenschrift*, **97**, 671–675.

Boyd, M.E., Usher, R.H., McLean, F.H. and Kramer, M.S. (1988) Obstetric consequences of post maturity. *American Journal of Obstetrics and Gynecology*, **157**, 334–338.

Boyd, P.A. (1984) Quantitative studies of the normal human placenta from 10 weeks of gestation to term. *Early Human Development*, **9**, 297–307.

Browne, J.C.McC. (1963) Placental insufficiency. *Scottish Medical Journal*, **8**, 459–465.

Buscemi, C. (1957) Ricerche istologiche ed istochemiche sulla placenta di gravidanze sesotine. *Rivista di Ostetricia e Ginecologia*, **12**, 281–230.

Cardozo, L., Fysh, J. and Pearce, J.M. (1986) Prolonged pregnancy: the management debate. *British Medical Journal*, **293**, 1059–1063.

Carenza, L. and Coppola, G. (1957) Studio istologico della placenta nelle gravidanza il termine. *Clinica Ostetrica e Ginecologica*, **59**, 241–252.

Clavero, J.A., Montalvo, L., Ayala, M.J. and Corredera y Velasco, J. (1964) Estudio placentario y citologia vaginal en los embarazos prolongados. *Acta Ginecologica*, **15**, 635–646.

Clavero-Nunez, J.A. (1962) Patologia placentaria. *Revista Española de Obstetricia y Ginecologia*, **20**, 208–215.

de Cecco, L., Ferrari, B., Niccolo, M. and Rolfini, G. (1962) Contributo allo studio della senescenza placentare. *Quaderni di Clinica Ostetrica e Ginecologica*, **17**, Supplement 12, 1055–1063.

de Palo, G.M. (1967) L'ipersenescenza placentare nella gravidanza oltre il termine con feto ipodistrofico: studio al microscopio elettronico. *Rivista di Ostetricia e Ginecologia*, **22**, 829–836.

Devizorova, A.S. and Schvirst, E.M. (1970) Ultrastructural characteristics of placental villi in prolonged pregnancy. *Akusherstvo i Ginekologiya* (Moscow), **46**, 49–55.

Dixon, H.G., Browne, J.C.McC. and Davey, D.A. (1963) Choriodecidual and myometrial blood-flow. *Lancet*, **ii**, 369–373.

Durst, B. (1963) Histoloske promjene u placent kod produljene trubnoce. (Histological findings in placenta of protracted pregnancy.) *Radovi Medicinskog Fakulteta u Zacrebu*, **11**, 119–129.

Eik-Nes, S.H., Oakland, O., Aure, J.C. and Ulstein, M. (1984) Ultrasound screening in pregnancy: a randomised controlled trial. *Lancet*, **i**, 1347–1349.

Emmrich, P. and Malzer, G. (1968) Zur Morphologie der Plazenta bei Übertragung. *Pathologia et Microbiologia*, **32**, 285–302.

Fox, H. (1967) Senescence of placental villi. *Journal of Obstetrics and Gynaecology of the British Commonwealth*, **74**, 881–885.

Fox, H. (1969a) The placenta in premature onset of labour. *Journal of Obstetrics and Gynaecology of the British Commonwealth*, **76**, 240–244.

Fox, H. (1969b) Histological features of placental senescence. In *The Foeto-Placental Unit*, Pecile, A. and Finzi, C. (Eds), pp. 3–7. Amsterdam: Excerpta Medica.

Fox, H. (1979) The placenta as a model for organ aging. In *Placenta – A Neglected Experimental Animal*, Beaconsfield, P. and Villee, C. (Eds), pp. 351–378. Oxford: Pergamon.

Geier, G., Schuhmann, R. and Kraus, H. (1975) Regionale unterschliedliche Zellproliferation innerhalb der Plazentome reifer menschlicher Plazenten: autoradiographische Untersuchungen. *Archiv für Gynäkologie*, **218**, 31–37.

Gill, R.W., Warren, P.S., Garrett, W.J., Kossoff, G. and Stewart, A. (1993) Umbilical vein blood flow. In *Ultrasound in Obstetrics and Gynecology*, Chervenak, F.A., Isaacson, G.C. and Campbell, S. (Eds), pp. 587–595. Boston: Little, Brown.

Guidetti, D.A., Divon, M.Y., Cavalieri, R.L., Langer, O. and Merkatz, I.R. (1987) Fetal umbilical artery flow velocimetry in postdate pregnancies. *American Journal of Obstetrics and Gynecology*, **157**, 1521–1523.

Haigh, M., Chawner, L.E. and Fox, H. (1984) The human placenta does not contain lipofuscin pigment. *Placenta*, **5**, 459–464.

Haigh, M., Fox, H. and Taylor, C.J. (1989) A morphometric analysis of age-related changes in villous syncytiotrophoblastic subcellular organelles in the human placenta using a computerised image analysis system. *Fetus*, **1**, 27–34.

Hitschold, T., Weiss, E., Berle, P. and Muntefering, H. (1989) Histologische Placentabefunde bei Terminüberschreitung: Korrelation zwischen placentarer Reifungsretardierung, Fetaloutcome und dopplersonographischen Befunden der Nabelarterie. *Zeitschrift für Geburtshilfe und Perinatologie*, **193**, 42–46.

Hustin, J., Foedart, J.M. and Lambotte, R. (1984) Cellular proliferation in villi of normal and pathological pregnancies. *Gynecologic and Obstetric Investigation*, **17**, 1–9.

Ito, H., Tanaka, T., Watanabe, H. and Ito, K. (1984) Ultrastructural observation of the placenta in prolonged pregnancy. *Asia and Oceania Journal of Obstetrics and Gynaecology*, **10**, 211–216.

Itskovitz, J., LaGamma, E.F. and Rudolph, A.M. (1983) The effect of reducing umbilical blood flow on fetal oxygenation. *American Journal of Obstetrics and Gynecology*, **145**, 813–818.

Iversen, O.E. and Farsund, T. (1985) Flow cytometry in the assessment of human placental growth. *Acta Obstetricia et Gynecologica Scandinavica*, **64**, 605–607.Jackson, M.R., Mayhew, T.M. and Boyd, P.A. (1992) A quantitative description of the elaboration and maturation of villi from 10 weeks of gestation to term. *Placenta*, **13**, 357–370.

Johnson, M.R., Bennett, P.R. and Steer, P.J. (1995) An update on the endocrine control of labour. In *Turnbull's Obstetrics*, 2nd edn, Chamberlain, G. (Ed.), pp. 545–550. Edinburgh: Churchill Livingstone.

Jones, C.J.P. and Fox, H. (1978) Ultrastructure of the placenta in prolonged pregnancy. *Journal of Pathology*, **126**, 173–179.

Justus, B., Justus, J. and Holtoroff, J. (1971) Übertragene dystrophische Neugeborene und dazugahörige morphologische Plazentabefunde. *Zeitschrift für Geburtshilfe und Gynäkologie*, **175**, 44–54.

Kemnitz, P. and Theuring, F. (1974) Makroskopische, licht- und elektronmikroskopische Plazentabefunde bei Übertragung. *Zentralblatt für allgemeine Pathologie und pathologische Anatomie*, **118**, 82–89.

Kubli, F. and Budliger, H. (1963) Beitrag zur Morphologie der insuffizienten Placenta. *Geburtshilfe und Frauenheilkunde*, **23**, 37–43.

Larsen, L.G., Clausen, H.V., Andersen, B. and Graem, N. (1995) A stereologic study of postmature placentas fixed by dual perfusion. *American Journal of Obstetrics and Gynecology*, **175**, 500–507.

Lettieri, L., Vintzileos, A.M., Rodis, J.F., Albini, S.M. and Salafia, C.M. (1993) Does 'idiopathic' preterm labor resulting in preterm birth exist? *American Journal of Obstetrics and Gynecology*, **160**, 1480–1485.

Leveno, K.J., Quirk, J.G. Jr, Cunningham, F.G. et al (1984) Prolonged pregnancy. I. Observations concerning the causes of fetal distress. *American Journal of Obstetrics and Gynecology*, **150**, 465–473.

Liebhart, M. and Kuczynska-Sicinska, J. (1971) Ocena histopatologiczna lozyska w ciazy przetermi-nowanej. (Microscopic evaluation of the placenta in protracted pregnancy.) *Ginekologia Polska*, **42**, 883–890.

Lockwood, C.J. (1994) Recent advances in elucidating the pathogenesis of preterm delivery, the detection of patients at risk, and preventative therapies. *Current Opinion in Obstetrics and Gynecology*, **6**, 7–18.

McKiddie, J.M. (1949) Foetal mortality in postmaturity. *Journal of Obstetrics and Gynaecology of the British Empire*, **56**, 386–392.

Magnin, P. and Gabriel, H. (1966) Les scléroses vasculaires de la cadaque profonde. *Gynécologie et Obstétrique*, **65**, 37–56.

Mälzer, M., Emmrich, P., Birke, R. and Knaus, T. (1970) Diagnostik und Therapie der soggenanten Ubertragung im Vergleich zu typisch histologischen Placentabefunden. *Zeitschrift für Geburtshilfe und Gynäkologie*, **172**, 25–43.

Merrill, J.A. (1963) Common pathological changes of the placenta. *Clinical Obstetrics and Gynecology*, **6**, 96–109.

Naeye, R.L. (1987) Functionally important disorders of the placenta, umbilical cord and fetal membranes. *Human Pathology*, **17**, 680–691.

Naeye, R.L. (1989) Pregnancy hypertension, placental evidences of low uteroplacental blood flow and spontaneous preterm delivery. *Human Pathology*, **20**, 441–444.

Naeye, R.L. (1992) *Disorders of the Placenta, Fetus, and Neonate: Diagnosis and Clinical Significance*. St Louis: Mosby Year Book.

Nézelof, C. and Roussel, A. (1954) Le placenta des prématurés: étude de 75 cas. *Semaine des Hopitaux de Paris*, **30**, 3163–3167.

Novitsky, I.S., Belomestnova, L.N. and Chernykh, A.P. (1976) The influence of over-term pregnancy on the state of the placenta and the fetus. *Akusherstvo i Ginekologiya* (Moscow), **1**, 29–32.

Parmley, T.H., Gupta, P.K. and Walker, M.A. (1981) 'Aging' pigments in term human placenta. *American Journal of Obstetrics and Gynecology*, **139**, 760–763.

Perkins, R.P. (1974) Antenatal assessment of fetal maturity: a review. *Obstetrical and Gynecological Survey*, **29**, 369–384.

Prata Martins, J.A. (1964) Patologia placentaria en les partus prematuros. *Acta Ginecologica*, **15**, 83–88.

Redline, R.W. (1995) Placental pathology: a neglected link between basic disease mechanisms and untoward pregnancy outcome. *Current Opinion in Obstetrics and Gynecology*, **7**, 10–15.

Robertson, W.B. and Dixon, H.G. (1969) Utero-placental pathology. In *Foetus and Placenta*, Klopper, A. and Diczfalusy, E. (Eds), pp. 33–60. Oxford and Edinburgh: Blackwell Scientific.

Salafia, C.M., Vogel, C.A., Vintzileos, A.M. et al (1991) Placental pathologic findings in preterm birth. *American Journal of Obstetrics and Gynecology*, **165**, 934–938.

Salafia, C.M., Ernst, L., Pezzullo, J.C. et al (1995a) The very low birth weight infant: maternal complications leading to preterm birth, placental lesions, and intrauterine growth. *American Journal of Perinatology*, **12**, 106–110.

Salafia, C.M., Minior, V.K., Lopez-Zeno, J.A. et al (1995b) Relationship between placental histologic features and umbilical cord blood gases in preterm gestations. *American Journal of Obstetrics and Gynecology*, **173**, 1058–1064.

Salafia, C.M. and Mill, J.F. (1996) The value of placental pathology in studies of spontaneous prematurity. *Current Opinion in Obstetrics and Gynecology*, **8**, 89–95.

Salvatore, C.A. (1971) The placenta in prolonged gestation. *Maternidade e Infancia*, **30**, 71–77.

Sands, J. and Dobbing, J. (1985) Continuing growth and development of third-trimester human placenta. *Placenta*, **6**, 13–22.

Sauramo, H. (1951) Histology of the placenta in normal, premature and overterm cases, and in gestosis. *Annales Chirurgiae et Gynaecologia Fenniae*, **40**, 164–188.

Schweikhart, G., Kaufmann, P. and Beck, T. (1986) Morphology of placental villi after premature delivery and its clinical relevance. *Archives of Gynecology*, **239**, 101–114.

Siegel, P. (1963) Die Placenta beim übertragenen dystropischen Neugeborenen. *Archiv für Gynäkologie*, **198**, 67–71.

Siegel, P. and Rabanus, W. (1966) Die Häufigkeit der sogenannten Plazentarinfarkte bei Übertragungen, Frühgeburten und Schwangerschaftsspezifischen Erkrankungen. *Zentralblatt für Gynäkologie*, **88**, 345–350.

Silver, R.K., Dooley, S.L., MacGregor, S.N. and Depp, R. (1988) Fetal acidosis in prolonged pregnancy cannot be attributed to cord compression alone. *American Journal of Obstetrics and Gynecology*, **159**, 666–669.

Stokes, H.J., Roberts, R.V. and Newnham, J.P. (1991) Doppler flow velocity waveform analysis in post-date pregnancies. *Australian and New Zealand Journal of Obstetrics and Gynaecology*, **31**, 27–30.

Strigini, F.A.L., Lancioni, G., de Luca, G. et al (1995) Uterine artery velocimetry and spontaneous preterm delivery. *Obstetrics and Gynecology*, **85**, 374–377.

Suska, P., Jakubovsky, J. and Polak, S. (1990) Premature delivery and placenta: a morphological study. *Czechoslovak Medicine*, **13**, 193–212.

ten Berge, B.S. (1955) Capillaraktion in der Placenta. *Archiv für Gynäkologie*, **186**, 253–256.

ten Berge, B.S. (1956) L'activité capillaire dans les villosités placentaires. *Bulletin de la Société Belge de Gynécologie et d'Obstétrique*, **26**, 210–216.

Thomsen, K. and Schniewind, H. (1961) Methodik und Ergebnisse der Perfusion normaler und übertragener Placenten. *Archiv für Gynäkologie*, **195**, 463–467.

Turnbull, A. (1995) The endocrine control of labour. In *Turnbull's Obstetrics*, 2nd edn, Chamberlain, G. (Ed.), pp. 529–545. Edinburgh: Churchill Livingstone.

Vanrell-Cruells, J. (1963) Pathologische Vernderungen bei der übertragenen Placenta. *Archiv für Gynäkologie*, **198**, 71–72.

Vanrell-Cruells, J. and Comas-Funallet, J. (1965) La placenta de los fetos hipermaduros. *Revista de Genetica y Sexologica*, **1**, 3–9.

Vorherr, H. (1975a) Placental insufficiency and postmaturity. *European Journal of Obstetrics, Gynecology and Reproductive Biology*, **5**, 109–122.

Vorherr, H. (1975b) Placental insufficiency in relation to postterm pregnancy and fetal postmaturity: evaluation of fetoplacental function; management of the postterm gravida. *American Journal of Obstetrics and Gynecology*, **123**, 67–103.

Walkinshaw, S.A. (1995) Preterm labour and delivery of the preterm infant. In *Turnbull's Obstetrics*, 2nd edn, Chamberlain, G. (Ed.), pp. 609–632. Edinburgh: Churchill Livingstone

Wang, T. (1989) Uterine Spiralarterien des Menschen bei Gestose, fëtaler Wachstumretardierung und Übertragung. *Geburtshilfe und Frauenheilkunde*, **49**, 548–552.

Wigglesworth, J.S. (1962) The gross and microscopic pathology of the prematurely delivered placenta. *Journal of Obstetrics and Gynaecology of the British Commonwealth*, **69**, 934–943.

Wigglesworth, J.S. (1964) Morphological variations in the insufficient placenta. *Journal of Obstetrics and Gynaecology of the British Commonwealth*, **71**, 871–884.

Wilkin, P. (1965) *Pathologie du Placenta*. Paris: Masson.

Winick, M., Coscia, A. and Noble, A. (1967) Cellular growth in human placenta. I. Normal cellular growth. *Pediatrics*, **39**, 248–251.

Yamagushi, R., Ushioda, E., Nishakawa, Y. and Shintani, M. (1975) Uteroplacental blood flow in normal and prolonged pregnancies pursued with tracer microspheres. *Acta Obstetrica Gynaecologica Japonica*, **22**, 175–181.

Zaliznyak, V.A. (1967) Regenerative processes in the placenta in overdue pregnancy. *Arkhiv Patologii*, **29**, 51–56.

Zhemkova, Z.P. and Topchieva, O.I. (1964) Compensatory growth of villi in post-mature human placenta. *Nature*, **204**, 703–704.

Zimmermann, P., Alback, T., Koskinen, J. et al (1995) Doppler flow velocimetry of the umbilical artery, uteroplacental arteries and fetal middle cerebral artery in prolonged pregnancy. *Ultrasound in Obstetrics and Gynecology*, **5**, 189–197.

8

THE PLACENTA IN MATERNAL DISORDERS

There is a voluminous literature that concerns itself with the effects on the placenta of maternal disease, e.g. pre-eclampsia, essential hypertension, diabetes mellitus, etc., but those with the tenacity to read through this will be left with a well-founded impression of confusion and chaos, the various reports being awash with contradictions, rebuttals and incompatible findings. The reasons for this are worth examining because they highlight some of the problems that are encountered in attempting to establish a systematic pathology of the placenta.

Many of the studies of the effects of maternal disease on the placenta have suffered from serious methodological defects and these may be summarized thus:

1. Too few placentas were examined. The placental changes may be very variable and a cohesive picture may emerge only after a large series of placentas has been examined.
2. The lack of a control group. As most placental pathology is quantitative rather than qualitative it is clear that the incidence of any lesion in placentas from abnormal pregnancies must be contrasted with that found in placentas from women whose pregnancies were uncomplicated. The omission of this precaution from many studies has often led to unwarranted conclusions being drawn.
3. The consideration of placentas from pregnancies of varying duration as a homogeneous group. Thus, for example, many pregnancies from women with pre-eclampsia terminate, or are terminated, prematurely; the placentas from such cases should be, but rarely are, compared with placentas from uncomplicated pregnancies of the same gestational length.
4. The failure to examine a maternal complication in isolation. Thus, for instance, studies of placentas from diabetic women have often considered as a single entity those from women whose pregnancies were otherwise uncomplicated and those from patients suffering from both diabetes mellitus and superimposed pre-eclampsia.
5. A failure to take into account the changes that occur in the placenta after fetal death; these are considerable and have often either been disregarded or misinterpreted.

The comments in the following sections of this chapter are based on studies in which these various pitfalls have, as far as is possible, been avoided.

PRE-ECLAMPSIA

Pre-eclampsia is a pregnancy-specific syndrome that may terminate in eclampsia and is characterized by a group of signs of which hypertension is one (Redman, 1995). Regrettably, the terms 'pregnancy-induced hypertension' and 'pre-eclampsia' are often used as interchangeable synonyms, a laxity not only of terminology but also of thought which, as Redman (1995) has remarked, further muddles an already muddled subject. Pregnancy-induced hypertension describes hypertension that appears for the first time after the 20th week of gestation and which resolves after the pregnancy has terminated: pregnancy-induced hypertension by itself does not indicate that the patient has pre-eclampsia, a syndrome that can only be diagnosed if at least one more sign is present, the second sign being, by convention, proteinuria (Davey & MacGillivray, 1988). Oedema is not a defining feature of pre-eclampsia because whilst women with eclampsia do have oedema (particularly facial oedema) the vast majority of pregnant women with oedema (usually peripheral in distribution) do not have pre-eclampsia (Rubin, 1988).

The definitions of 'mild', 'moderate' and 'severe' pre-eclampsia are, at best, arbitrary but it is useful to define mild pre-eclampsia as being characterized by a diastolic blood pressure of less than 100 mmHg in association with slight (trace or 1+) proteinuria and to regard patients with a diastolic blood pressure of 110 mmHg or higher who also have well-marked (2+ or more) proteinuria as having severe pre-eclampsia (Cunningham & Leveno, 1988). These definitions clearly leave room for an intermediate group of patients with moderate pre-eclampsia.

Pre-eclampsia is a syndrome characterized by a variable cluster of signs and symptoms and there is increasingly strong evidence that diffuse endothelial damage is a fundamental factor in the pathogenesis of the maternal syndrome (Roberts et al, 1989). Equally, however, there is strong evidence that the endothelial damage is a secondary phenomenon and that the primary pathology of pre-eclampsia is to be found in the placenta (Redman, 1991, 1995; Roberts & Redman, 1993).

Morphological Changes in the Placenta in Pre-eclampsia

Macroscopic Findings

Placentas from women with pre-eclampsia tend, on average, to be smaller than those from uncomplicated pregnancies; the decrease is, however, only slight. A proportion of placentas from pre-eclamptic women are unduly large, and the placental/fetal weight ratio is often increased (Thomson et al, 1969; Nummi, 1972; Holzl et al, 1974; Soma et al, 1982). Very occasionally a hydropic placenta may be encountered.

There is, in my experience, no excess of extrachorial placentation or of abnormal insertion of the cord in placentas from pre-eclamptic patients; the only gross lesions that occur more commonly than in placentas from uncomplicated pregnancies are infarction and retroplacental haematomas. The relationship between placental infarction and pre-eclampsia is a straightforward one which has been made unnecessarily complicated and confused. It has at various times been claimed that placental infarcts are pathognomonic of pre-eclampsia and are, furthermore, the cause of the disease (Bartholomew & Kracke, 1932; Hunt et al, 1940; Bartholomew et al, 1961), that placental infarction occurs no more commonly in pre-eclampsia than in uncomplicated pregnancies (Haffner, 1921; Clements, 1934; Shanklin, 1958, 1959; Werner et al, 1974), and that, although the incidence of placental infarction is increased in pre-eclampsia, this lesion is neither a specific nor an invariable feature of the disease (Traut & Kuder, 1934; Hill & Trimble 1944; Falkiner & Apthorp, 1944; Thomsen, 1955; Nesbitt, 1958; Little, 1960, 1961; Gregor, 1961; Maqueo et al, 1964; Torpin & Swain, 1966; Wentworth, 1967; Wallenburg, 1969). There is no doubt that the claims of the third group are correct; the overall incidence of placental infarction is much higher than in uncomplicated pregnancies (Fig. 8.1), rising from about 33% in women with mild pre-eclampsia to 60% in patients with the severe form of the disease (Fox, 1967). Furthermore, the extent of the infarcted area is often greater than that ever found in uncomplicated

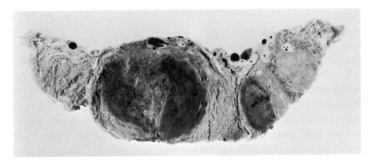

Figure 8.1. Multiple fresh infarcts in a placenta from a patient with severe pre-eclampsia. This is a characteristic but by no means universal finding.

pregnancies; extensive infarction (i.e. involving 5–10% of the placental parenchyma) is rarely found in placentas from uncomplicated pregnancies, is noted only exceptionally in those from women with mild pre-eclampsia, and is present in 30% of placentas from cases of severe pre-eclampsia. It will be appreciated, however, that 40% of placentas from women with the severe form of the disease are not infarcted at all and that a further 30% of such placentas are not infarcted to any significant or important extent. It will also be apparent that placentas from patients with mild pre-eclampsia have only a slightly increased incidence of infarction and are very rarely extensively infarcted.

Retroplacental haematomas are found unduly frequently in placentas from pre-eclamptic women, being present in between 12 and 15%. The relationship between this lesion and the maternal disease is far from being fully clarified because, as discussed in Chapter 5, whilst there are many who would maintain that the retroplacental bleeding occurs as a complication of pre-eclampsia, there are others who argue equally adamantly that the haematoma causes the pre-eclampsia.

Otherwise these placentas show no excess of gross lesions; fetal artery thrombosis and perivillous fibrin deposition do not occur with any undue frequency whilst calcification is distinctly uncommon.

Histological Findings

I have usually found the villi in most placentas from pre-eclamptic women to be of normal maturity for the length of the gestational period. In a small proportion there is some delay in villous maturation and morphometric studies have indicated that this delay in, or failure of, formation of terminal villi is largely restricted to women with severe pre-eclampsia who have given birth to markedly growth-retarded infants (Teasdale, 1985a, 1987). On the other hand, a proportion of placentas from patients suffering from this disease show premature formation of terminal villi and thus appear unduly mature for the period of gestation. Villous oedema is sometimes seen and may occasionally be sufficiently marked for the villi to be considered as hydropic.

The most striking and characteristic features of the villi in pre-eclampsia are an undue number and prominence of the villous cytotrophoblastic cells (Fig. 8.2) and irregular thickening of the trophoblastic basement membrane (Fig. 8.3), the intensity of these changes being related to the severity and duration of the maternal pre-eclampsia.

The villi are often normally vascularized, but in a significant proportion of placentas they are hypovascular, with small, non-dilated and relatively inconspicuous vessels (Fig. 8.4). This change is associated with, and parallels in severity the degree of, an 'obliterative endarteritis' of the fetal stem arteries (Las Heras et al, 1983, 1985), a lesion that is found, to a greater or lesser extent, in about a third of placentas from pre-eclamptic patients (Fig. 8.5). The hypovascular villi, but not those that are adequately perfused from the fetal side, have an abundance of syncytial knots, usually lack vasculo-syncytial membranes, and have an increased content of stromal collagen. I have never, with the light microscope, been able to observe any degenerative changes in the villous

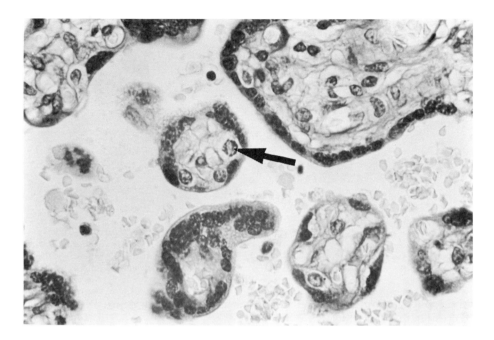

Figure 8.2. Villi in a placenta from a woman with pre-eclampsia. The syncytiotrophoblast shows no obvious degenerative changes, but the cytotrophoblastic cells (one of which is arrowed) are unduly numerous and prominent (PAS ×500).

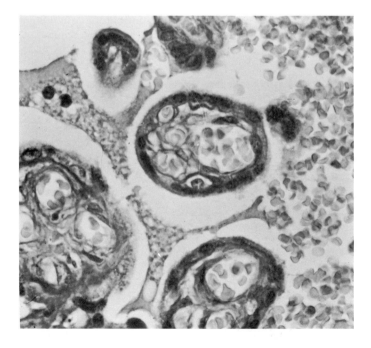

Figure 8.3. Villi in a placenta from a patient with pre-eclampsia. There is marked focal thickening of the villous trophoblastic basement membrane (PAS ×670).

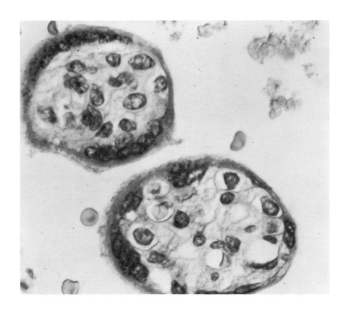

Figure 8.4. Poorly vascularized villi in a placenta from a woman with pre-eclampsia (H & E ×840).

syncytiotrophoblast, but there is a tendency for an excessive incidence of villous fibrinoid necrosis in these placentas.

If decidua is found attached to the basal plate of the placenta it may be possible to observe the characteristic changes that occur in the maternal decidual arteries. These are, as discussed in Chapter 5, a failure of some of the spiral arteries of the placental bed to undergo physiological change, even in their intradecidual segments (Khong et al, 1986), and an atherosis characterized by a fibrinoid necrosis of the arterial wall together with an intramural accumulation of lipid-laden macrophages and a perivascular lymphocytic cuffing. It has to be emphasized that atherosis only occurs in the minority of spiral arteries which have not undergone physiological change in their intradecidual segments and in basal arteries (Khong & Robertson, 1992). If the

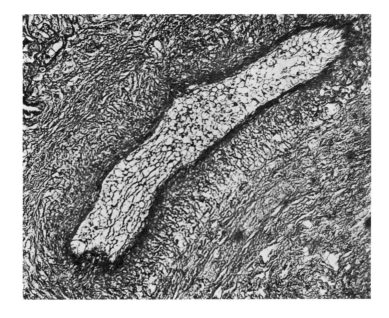

Figure 8.5. A well-marked 'obliterative endarteritis' in a fetal stem artery in a placenta from a woman with pre-eclampsia (H & E ×70).

vessels directly underlying an area of infarction are seen, it is often possible to detect occluding thrombi.

Redline and Patterson (1995) have recently described an excess of hyperproliferative extravillous cytotrophoblastic cells in the implantation site in cases of preeclampsia, a finding that requires both confirmation and assessment of its significance.

Ultrastructural Findings

There have been relatively few studies of the fine structure of the placenta in maternal pre-eclampsia (Sermann & Capria, 1965; Anderson & McKay, 1966; Pudda & Lecca, 1969; Salvatore, 1970; Franke et al, 1971; Jones & Fox, 1980; Soma et al, 1982; Hirano, 1989; Sankawa, 1990) but these, whilst disagreeing on minor points of detail, have yielded a more clear-cut picture than that obtained by light microscopists. Ultrastructural studies have, in general, confirmed the presence of villous cytotrophoblastic hyperplasia and trophoblastic basement membrane thickening and have further demonstrated dilatation of the syncytial rough endoplasmic reticulum (Fig. 8.6) and a decrease in the pinocytotic and secretory activity of the trophoblast. Damage to, and localized loss of, syncytial microvilli are also apparent, whilst small, scattered, focal areas of syncytial necrosis are sometimes seen (Fig. 8.7); these latter have also been noted on scanning electron microscopy (Fig. 8.8) as circumscribed foci of syncytial ulceration (Fox & Agrofojo-Blanco, 1974).

General Comment on Morphological Changes

Although there is a combination of gross and histological changes that is characteristic of placentas from pre-eclamptic women, it will be apparent that there is no single lesion which is invariably found in such placentas and that there are no placental abnormalities which are specific to this complication of pregnancy. It is by no means unusual to encounter a placenta from a pre-eclamptic woman that is virtually normal, particularly if the disease has been of a mild nature and of short duration. Placental

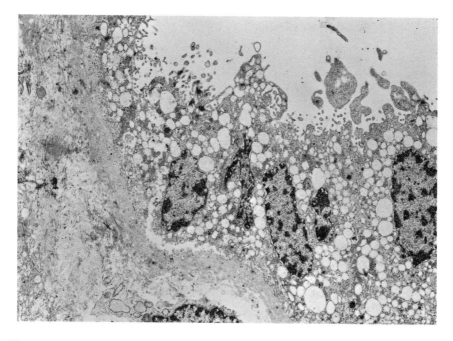

Figure 8.6. Electron micrograph of villous syncytiotrophoblast in a placenta from a woman with pre-eclampsia. There is dilatation of the rough endoplasmic reticulum, distortion of the surface and loss of microvilli. The trophoblastic basement membrane is thickened (EM ×6250).

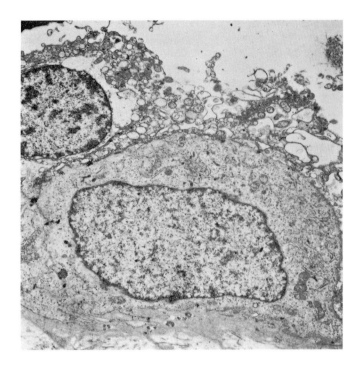

Figure 8.7. Electron micrograph of villous trophoblast in a placenta from a woman with pre-eclampsia. The syncytiotrophoblast is necrotic but the underlying cytotrophoblast is normal (EM ×10,000).

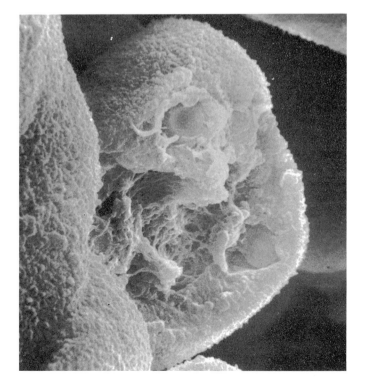

Figure 8.8. Scanning electron micrograph of villi in a placenta from a woman with pre-eclampsia. Two areas of focal syncytial ulceration are evident (×1050).

lesions are usually accentuated and more conspicuous in cases of severe pre-eclampsia, but the duration of the disease process is probably equally important in this respect. This indicates, of course, that changes in the placenta are a response to, rather than a cause of, the pre-eclamptic process, but before discussing the nature of this response it is necessary to question some of the concepts of placental pathology in pre-eclampsia that are entrenched in the minds of many pathologists and obstetricians.

It is often stated that in this disease the placenta characteristically shows syncytial degeneration and evidence of premature ageing (Tenney, 1936; Tenney & Parker, 1940; Wislocki & Dempsey, 1946; Page, 1948; Paine, 1957; Shanklin, 1958, 1959; Sauramo, 1961; Maqueo et al, 1964, 1965; Salvatore, 1966, 1968; Cibils, 1974), but I have never been persuaded that either of these two phenomena is a feature of the placenta in pre-eclampsia. The term 'syncytial degeneration' is a somewhat nebulous one and those who claim to have detected this abnormality have rarely specified their precise findings. It is true that small foci of syncytial necrosis are seen on electron microscopic examination of these placentas, but such lesions are far too small to be visible on light microscopy and I remain unconvinced that any widespread syncytial degeneration occurs in pre-eclampsia. I am equally unconvinced that morphological evidence of premature senescence is seen in these placentas. As discussed in Chapter 7, it is impossible to define structural changes in the placenta that are indicative of ageing and it is therefore equally impossible to delineate premature or accelerated ageing in morphological terms, it being probable that the excess of syncytial knots and stromal collagen that is often present has been wrongly interpreted as evidence of senescence rather than as a consequence of inadequate fetal perfusion. It is not simply a verbal nuance to distinguish between premature ageing and accelerated villous maturation and there is no doubt that a proportion of placentas from pre-eclamptic patients show this latter feature. As the fully mature placental tree, with its rich perfusion of terminal villi, is optimally adapted for materno-fetal transfer mechanisms it can be seen that accelerated maturation is, in teleological terms, a compensatory mechanism to increase the transfer capacity of the placenta in the face of an adverse maternal environment. Accelerated villous maturation is certainly a feature of some placentas from pre-eclamptic women but I would not agree with those who maintain that premature maturation is an extremely common and virtually specific feature of the placenta in maternal pre-eclampsia (Schuhmann & Geier, 1972; Holzl et al, 1974).

It has been suggested that the undue prominence of the cytotrophoblastic cells in placentas from pre-eclamptic women is due to a maturational arrest (Ruckhaberle & Ruckhaberle, 1976) but the presence of mitotic figures in this cellular population, the autoradiographic evidence of DNA synthesis and the high proliferation index as determined by immunocytochemical staining for Ki67 (Kaltenbach et al, 1974; Hustin et al, 1984; Arnholdt et al, 1991) clearly indicate that their increased number is due to a true proliferation. Whilst cytotrophoblastic hyperplasia is certainly a feature of these placentas I have never seen any convincing evidence of the syncytial hyperplasia that has also been noted (Riviere, 1930; Rindi, 1950; Alvarez et al, 1967, 1969; Slomko & Pisarki, 1967; Alvarez, 1970).

Pathogenesis of Morphological Changes

It is my view, indeed most people's view, that all the changes seen in the placenta in maternal pre-eclampsia are, with the sole exception of the increased incidence of villous fibrinoid necrosis, secondary to, and are caused by, an abnormal maternal uteroplacental vasculature. It has, of course, been well established for many years that the maternal blood flow to the placenta is reduced in pre-eclampsia (Browne & Veall, 1953; Morris et al, 1956; Browne, 1958; Dixon et al, 1963; Lippert et al, 1980; Lunell et al, 1982) and more recently this has been confirmed by Doppler studies (Campbell et al, 1983; Cohen-Overbeek et al, 1985; Trudinger et al, 1985b; Arduini et al, 1987; Leiberman et al, 1989; Trudinger & Cook, 1990). Over the past 20 years it has been clearly shown that this limitation of the maternal blood supply to the placenta is due to restricted trophoblastic invasion of the spiral arteries of the placental bed with sub-sequent inadequate conversion of the spiral arteries into uteroplacental vessels. This topic is discussed fully in Chapter 6 but it is worth noting that there is, in pre-eclampsia, a clear correlation between inadequate development of the uteroplacental arteries, as noted in placental bed biopsies, and an abnormal uterine flow velocity waveform in Doppler studies (Voigt & Becker, 1992; Olofsson et al, 1993; Lin et al, 1995).

The increased incidence of infarction in placentas from patients with pre-eclampsia is almost certainly a consequence of the atherosis that is seen in spiral arteries in which there is either no physiological change or only partial physiological change (Brosens & Renaer, 1972) whilst virtually all the villous abnormalities represent a response, either directly or indirectly, to the ischaemia which is a consequence of the arterial abnorm-alities. Cytotrophoblastic hyperplasia is a specific response, and trophoblastic basement membrane thickening a non-specific response, to placental ischaemia (see Chapter 6) and they are therefore a direct consequence of the reduced maternal blood flow. The excess of syncytial knots and of villous stromal fibrosis are not due to uteroplacental ischaemia but are a consequence of the reduced villous perfusion that is caused by the stem vessel lesion often referred to as 'obliterative endarteritis' but which is in fact the morphological hallmark of prolonged vasoconstriction of these vessels (see Chapter 6). This vasoconstriction leads to a significant increase in placental vascular resistance (Trudinger et al, 1985a) and almost certainly represents a fetal haemodynamic response to the uteroplacental ischaemia, as it has been clearly shown in experimental studies that restriction of maternal uteroplacental blood flow and/or reduced oxygenation of pla-cental tissue results in a marked decrease in fetal blood flow through the placenta, presumably as a result of vasoconstriction (Barcroft, 1947; Born et al, 1956; Reynolds & Paul, 1958; Dawes, 1969; Rudolph & Heymann, 1973; Stock et al, 1980; Howard et al, 1987; Clapp, 1994). This diminished placental perfusion is part of a fetal haemodynamic response to diminished oxygen supply and which results in a preferential diversion of blood to the vitally important cerebral and cardiac circulations. As is discussed in Chapter 9, although it may seem paradoxical to reduce placental blood flow under these circumstances, the villous tissue can increase oxygen extraction when blood flow is decreased and can sustain a flow reduction of 50% without impairing fetal oxygenation (Itskovitz et al, 1983).

The view that all, or virtually all, the villous abnormalities seen in pre-eclampsia are due solely to uteroplacental ischaemia is strengthened by the fact that very similar changes may be reproduced *in vitro* by culturing villi under conditions of low oxygen tension (Fox, 1970; MacLennan et al, 1972) and by the demonstration that the lesions induced in the rabbit placenta by constriction of the terminal aorta mimic those seen in the human placenta in pre-eclampsia (Abitbol et al, 1976). The only villous lesion that cannot be attributed to ischaemia is fibrinoid necrosis, which is certainly seen in excess in many placentas from pre-eclamptic women; however, the significance of this finding remains enigmatic.

It has to be said that not everyone agrees that inadequate conversion of spiral arter-ies to uteroplacental vessels is invariably a feature of pre-eclampsia. Salafia et al (1995) consider that in cases in which pre-eclampsia occurs before the 33rd week of gestation, maternal vascular abnormalities are present in only a proportion of cases, the remainder being associated with inflammatory or coagulative lesions of the placenta. This belief, however, is based on a study of the basal plate vessels in delivered placentas and not on placental bed biopsies: it is only the latter that reveal the true and full picture of the adequacy or otherwise of maternal vascular adaptation to the gravid state.

Functional Significance of Placental Changes

The functional significance of the placental changes in pre-eclampsia is open to debate. It is often assumed that uteroplacental ischaemia damages the placenta and impairs its function to a degree that it is no longer able adequately to transfer oxygen and nutrients to the fetus, but my view would be that under conditions of ischaemia the placenta, far from failing in its allotted function, is in fact performing its task as effectively as the unfavourable maternal milieu will allow and, indeed, attempts to compensate for the restriction of maternal blood supply. Thus, there seems little doubt that the syncytiotrophoblast suffers ischaemic damage in pre-eclampsia, but the response to this insult is a hyperplasia of the cytotrophoblastic cells, which undergo this change in an attempt to repair and replace the injured syncytial tissue. In this respect the attempt at syncytial repair appears eminently successful, because it requires prolonged searching on both transmission and scanning electron microscopy to find small foci of syncytial necrosis, and it therefore seems that the reparative ability of the placenta functions with great efficiency in pre-eclampsia. Hence there is no reason to believe that, except under extreme circumstances, the placenta is irretrievably damaged in pre-eclampsia. Indeed, the fact that the placental/fetal weight ratio is often increased in this condition suggests that there is compensatory growth of placental villi in an attempt to overcome the unfavourable maternal environment, although admittedly, this suggestion has not been confirmed in morphometric studies (Boyd & Scott, 1985).

Some placental products or activities, such as placental activation and inhibition of plasminogen, are reduced in pre-eclampsia but others, such as release into the maternal circulation of hCG and placental corticotrophin – releasing hormone, are increased (Redman, 1993). There does not appear to be any reduction in placental energy supply in pre-eclampsia (Bloxham et al, 1987) whilst the ability of the placenta to transfer free fatty acids to the fetus is probably increased in placentas from pre-eclamptic women (Biale, 1985).

It seems unreasonable to postulate, therefore, that the apparent ill-effects of pre-eclampsia on the fetus, e.g., low birth weight, intrauterine hypoxia or intrauterine death, are due to placental insufficiency rather than being a direct result of the inability of the mother to supply her fetus with an adequate amount of oxygen and nutrients.

The Placenta and the Maternal Syndrome of Pre-eclampsia

As previously mentioned there is strong evidence that the maternal features of pre-eclampsia are due to widespread endothelial damage and it is currently thought that this is due to the release from the ischaemic placenta of a factor, or of factors, which directly damage endothelial cells. In pre-eclamptic women there are circulating factors that inflict injury on endothelium (Rodgers et al, 1988; Tsukimori et al, 1992) and it has been shown that there is a protein in the syncytiotrophoblastic microvillous plasma membrane which, in culture, specifically inhibits endothelial cell proliferation and disrupts endothelial cell monolayers (Smarason et al, 1993). It has been known for some time that in pregnancies complicated by pre-eclampsia there is, as compared with uncomplicated gestations, an increased content of trophoblastic tissue in uterine venous blood (Jaameri et al, 1965) and this increased trophoblastic entry has recently been confirmed in a study using modern cell labelling techniques (Chua et al, 1991). It seems reasonable to suggest therefore that in pre-eclampsia the ischaemic placenta sheds excessive trophoblastic tissue into the maternal circulation and that this results in widespread endothelial cell dysfunction and the development of the maternal signs and symptoms of pre-eclampsia. Why there should be excessive loss of trophoblastic tissue into the maternal circulation from the ischaemic placenta is unclear. Certainly, the view that this could be a result of a deficiency of cell adhesion molecules cannot be sustained because such molecules appear to be normally expressed in placentas from pregnancies complicated by pre-eclampsia (Divers et al, 1995; Lyall et al, 1995).

Whatever the pathogenesis of the maternal syndrome of pre-eclampsia may be, it is not an inevitable result of a diminished maternal uteroplacental blood flow because such a reduction occurs in most cases of idiopathic intrauterine fetal growth retardation without the development of a pre-eclamptic syndrome.

ESSENTIAL HYPERTENSION

Very few specific studies have been made of placentas from women with essential hypertension without superimposed pre-eclampsia, although Paine (1957) described such placentas as showing premature senescence, whilst Wilkin (1965) noted an excess of villous syncytial knots and cytotrophoblastic cells. Salafia et al (1990) noted a high incidence of infarction in placentas from patients with chronic hypertension though this occurred less frequently than in placentas from pre-eclamptic patients. In my own experience the changes seen in the hypertensive woman's placenta are qualitatively, but not quantitatively, similar to those seen in placentas from pre-eclamptic patients. Thus the incidence and extent of infarction is closely similar to that found in placentas from pre-eclamptic women, and the villi also show the same characteristic combination of histological changes, i.e. cytotrophoblastic hyperplasia and basement membrane thickening. An obliterative endarteritis of the fetal stem arteries is, however, encountered much less frequently in the placenta of hypertensive patients and is rarely of as marked a degree as in placentas from pregnancies complicated by pre-eclampsia; hence there is a considerably lesser tendency for there to be an excess of villous syncytial knots or stromal collagen. The only qualitative difference between the hypertensive and the pre-eclamptic woman's placenta is the absence of any excess of villous fibrinoid necrosis in the former.

The similarity between the hypertensive and the pre-eclamptic woman's placenta is not confined to their light microscopic appearances but is equally apparent at the electron microscopic level. Fox and Jones (1982) made a study of the fine structure of the placenta in maternal essential hypertension, and confirmed the hyperplasia of the cytotrophoblastic cells and the thickening of the trophoblastic basement membrane. They also noted a reduction in syncytial secretory and pinocytotic activity, a diminution in the number of syncytial microvilli, dilatation of the syncytial rough endoplasmic reticulum, and focal syncytial necrosis. The ultrastructural changes are thus very similar to those noted in pre-eclampsia but are less marked and less extensive.

As in pre-eclampsia, it would appear that all the changes seen in the placenta in pregnancies complicated by essential hypertension are due, either directly or indirectly, to uteroplacental ischaemia and that there are no lesions which are specific to this disease. The uteroplacental ischaemia is a direct consequence of the hypertensive changes in the maternal vasculature and there seems no reason for postulating that any other factor plays a role in the production of the placental lesions.

The general comments made earlier in this chapter on the placenta in pre-eclampsia apply with equal force to the placenta in essential hypertension. There are no grounds for believing that the placenta is irretrievably damaged or functionally inefficient in essential hypertension and, indeed, though some have found an increased incidence of intrauterine fetal growth retardation in pregnancies complicated by essential hypertension (Wildschut et al, 1983), in most studies the neonate has usually been either of normal weight (Chamberlain et al, 1978; MacGillivray & Campbell, 1980) or somewhat larger than neonates from normotensive women (Salafia et al, 1990). This favourable fetal outcome, together with the histological findings, indicates that the degree of uteroplacental ischaemia in essential hypertension is considerably less than that experienced in pre-eclampsia and it is also possible that the elevated blood pressure may help to compensate for the increased vascular resistance: certainly, antihypertensive therapy has no effect on fetal growth or welfare (Meekins et al, 1995).

DIABETES MELLITUS

Diabetes mellitus is an important and complex complication of pregnancy. This topic has been the subject of several excellent recent reviews (Hagay & Reece, 1992; de Swiet, 1995; Garner, 1995) and it is noteworthy that despite improvements in diabetic control there is still a high incidence of congenital malformations in the infants of diabetic mothers, and that macrosomia and late intrauterine death, though drastically reduced in incidence during recent years, still persist; there is also an increased risk of developing pre-eclampsia.

In this section I use the term 'diabetes mellitus complicating pregnancy' to refer to pregnancies occurring in women who were known to be diabetic before the pregnancy began, the subject of gestational diabetes being considered in a later section. About 50% of diabetics who become pregnant will be suffering from the insulin-dependent form of the disease. I exclude from discussion those diabetic pregnancies that are complicated by pre-eclampsia.

Macroscopic Appearances

The traditional belief that the placenta of the diabetic woman is unusually bulky and oedematous is correct in only a very small minority of cases. The mean weight of the diabetic woman's placenta is only slightly (and certainly not significantly) higher than the mean weight of placentas from uncomplicated pregnancies (Thomson et al, 1969; Nummi, 1972; Clarson et al, 1989). The range of weights encountered, however, is wide and most placentas from diabetic women fall well within the normal placental weight range found in non-diabetic pregnancies. Placentas from diabetic women are usually unremarkable on macroscopic examination. Fetal artery thrombosis occurs with undue frequency in these placentas but there is otherwise no excess of gross lesions: in particular, neither infarction nor calcification is seen with any greater frequency than in placentas from uncomplicated pregnancies.

Histological Findings

The placenta of the diabetic woman has, during the last 45 years, served as the subject of an impressively large number of histopathological studies and reports (Kloos, 1952; Knopp, 1955; Burstein et al, 1957; Thomsen & Lieschke, 1958; Clavero-Nunez, 1963a; Rolfini et al, 1963; Dashkevich & Sechonov, 1964; Horky, 1964, 1965; Sani & Bottiglioni, 1964; Driscoll, 1965, 1975; Holzner & Thalhammer, 1965; Maqueo et al, 1965; Vogel, 1967; Liebhart, 1968a,b, 1973; Emmrich & Godel, 1972a,b,c; Werner & Schneiderhan, 1972; Emmrich et al, 1974a,b, 1975a,b; Holzl et al, 1975; Salzberger & Liban, 1975; Haust, 1981; Bjork & Persson, 1982; Laurini et al, 1987; Semmler & Emmrich, 1989). It would be agreeable to be able to record that this plethora of investigations has yielded a clear and coherent picture of the pathological changes that occur in the diabetic's placenta, but the truth is that they have succeeded only in painting a blurred and confused canvas. Little point would be served in attempting to review or collate this mass of contradictory data and I shall simply present my own findings (Fox, 1969), not because I have been vouchsafed with any greater insight into the effects of the diabetic state on the human placenta than has any other observer, but because my findings are based on a study which was, as far as is possible, free of the methodological defects that have been at the root of most of the disagreement which has characterized this facet of placental pathology.

About 40% of placentas from diabetic patients have villi that show a normal degree of morphological maturity for the length of the gestational period. In the remaining 60% the villous maturity is at odds with the length of the pregnancy, although, unfortunately, there is no stereotyped pattern of abnormality: about half of these placentas have villi that are unduly immature (Fig. 8.9) and about half show an accelerated villous maturation. Villous oedema is common (Fig. 8.10), albeit usually of slight degree, and hence stromal Hofbauer cells are seen frequently and with some ease. There is a tendency, by no means manifest in all these placentas, for the villous stroma to be unusually fibrotic and for there to be an excessive number of syncytial knots; villous cytotrophoblastic cells are often numerous and prominent, whilst the trophoblastic basement membrane not uncommonly shows a moderate degree of focal or diffuse

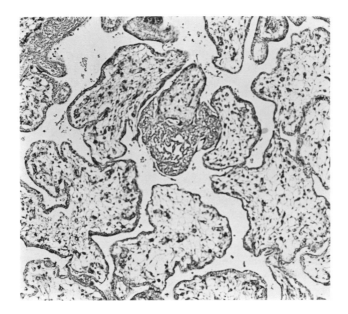

Figure 8.9. Villi in a placenta from a diabetic woman: the pregnancy was terminated at the 36th week of gestation and the villi are considered to be unduly immature for the length of gestational period (H & E ×90).

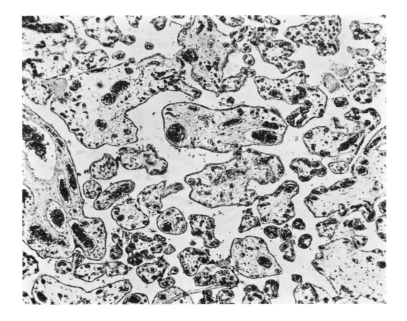

Figure 8.10. Villous oedema in a placenta from a diabetic woman (H & E ×70).

thickening. Villous vascularity is very variable: in many placentas the villi are normally vascularized, in some they are hypovascular and poorly perfused, whilst in others the villous vessels are prominent and strikingly congested (Fig. 8.11). A notable feature of the placenta of diabetic patients is the frequent presence of an excessive number of villi that have undergone fibrinoid necrosis (Fig. 8.12).

A 'proliferative endarteritis' of the fetal stem arteries is found in about a quarter of placentas from diabetic women and this is often of a quite marked degree. I have never seen any change in these vessels that could be considered as a manifestation of diabetic angiopathy.

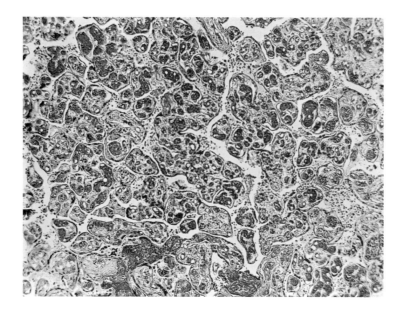

Figure 8.11. Villous congestion in a placenta from a diabetic woman (H & E ×90).

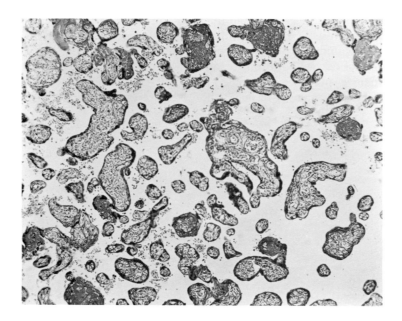

Figure 8.12. Villi in a placenta from a diabetic woman. A high proportion show fibrinoid necrosis (H & E ×90).

Morphometric Findings

The placenta of the diabetic woman has been the focus of several morphometric studies. Singer et al (1981) were unable to detect any quantitative difference between such placentas and those from uncomplicated pregnancies but Teasdale (1983, 1985b) showed that placentas from women with White's classes B and C diabetes had an increased amount of both parenchymal and non-parenchymal tissue and an increased materno-fetal exchange area. Boyd et al (1986) also noted an increased villous surface area in placentas from diabetic women whilst Stoz et al (1987, 1988b) considered that the morphometric changes observed by them were indicative of retarded placental development, though this change was least apparent in those from women with White's class D diabetes. Mayhew et al (1993) found a higher diffusive conductance in diabetic placentas than in those from uncomplicated pregnancies, i.e. morphometric changes which they considered facilitated oxygen transfer across the placenta. This finding is in accord with the observation, based on a morphometric study, that the basement membrane of the villous fetal capillaries is significantly thinner in the diabetic woman's placenta than in the placenta of healthy women (Jirkovska, 1991).

Ultrastructural Findings

The relatively few studies of the fine structure of the placenta in pregnancies complicated by diabetes mellitus have yielded results almost as disconcertingly contradictory as have been the reports of light microscopists (Zacks & Blazar, 1963; Hirota & Strauss, 1964; Lister, 1965; Okudaira et al, 1966; Widmaier, 1970; Liebhart, 1971; Asmussen, 1982a; Bobkov & Bobkova, 1984). In an electron-optical study of our own material (Jones and Fox, 1976a) the main findings were an increased number of villous cytotrophoblastic cells (which were often of the 'intermediate' type and in which mitotic figures were not uncommon), small scattered foci of syncytial necrosis (Fig. 8.13), an increased number of secretory droplets, mitochondria and Golgi bodies in the syncytiotrophoblast (Fig. 8.14) and thickening of the trophoblastic basement membrane. Pinocytotic vesicles were seen with increased frequency and the syncytial rough endoplasmic reticulum was dilated and contained flocculent material. Syncytial surface microvilli were of normal appearance and appeared to be present in normal density. In a quantitative ultrastructural study, Teasdale and Jean-Jaques (1986) noted, however, an increased density of microvilli on the free surface of the villous syncytiotrophoblast.

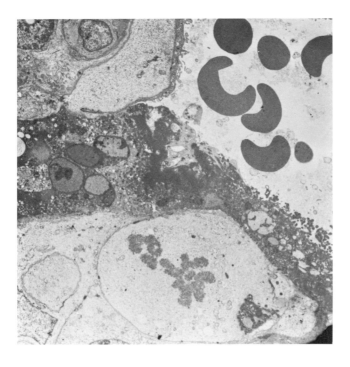

Figure 8.13. Electron micrograph of villous trophoblast in a placenta from a diabetic woman. A focal area of syncytial necrosis is seen and below this a cytotrophoblastic cell is undergoing mitotic division (EM ×5000).

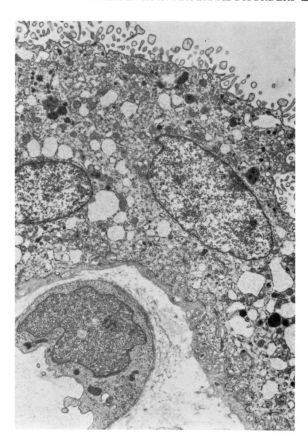

Figure 8.14. Electron micrograph of villous trophoblast in a placenta from a diabetic woman. There is abundant secretory and absorptive activity (EM ×10,000).

Relationship Between Placental Abnormalities, Severity of Diabetic State and Degree of Diabetic Control

I have been unable to detect any obvious or consistent correlation between the degree and extent of the abnormalities noted in the placenta of the diabetic woman and either the severity of the diabetic state or the degree of metabolic control. Semmler and Emmrich (1989) also thought that the placental abnormalities were unrelated to the severity of the maternal diabetes but did consider them to be related to the degree of control of the hyperglycaemic state. Bjork and Persson (1982) could not, however, find any relationship between the placental abnormalities noted in their study and the level of blood glucose control attained in late gestation, but thought that there was a significant correlation between the placental abnormalities and the degree of metabolic control achieved in early pregnancy.

The definitive demonstration that the degree of metabolic control, at any stage of pregnancy, does not influence in any way the development of placental abnormalities in maternal diabetes mellitus has, however, come from a study by Laurini et al (1987). These workers studied a group of insulin-dependent diabetic women (White classes B–D) who were treated by continuous subcutaneous insulin infusion. This form of control was instituted before conception in some of the patients, before the 16th week of gestation in others and, in one patient, at the 23rd gestational week. Very tight metabolic control was achieved in all patients but placental abnormalities, at both light and electron microscopic level, were totally unrelated to either the degree of control of blood sugar levels or the stage of pregnancy at which rigid control was achieved. Thus quite marked abnormalities were found in the placentas of some women who were normoglycaemic in the periconceptual period and throughout pregnancy whilst there were no significant differences noted between placentas from patients in whom periconceptual control was attained and those in whom control was achieved post-conceptually. Even more strikingly, placentas from some women whose blood glucose levels were rigidly controlled throughout pregnancy by insulin infusion showed the same abnormalities as were found in placentas from the same women during previous pregnancies in which metabolic control was poor.

Pathogenesis of Placental Abnormalities

None of the abnormalities found in the placenta of the diabetic woman is in any way specific to the diabetic state though when taken together the spectrum of abnormalities forms a very characteristic pattern. There is, however, no single all-embracing patho-genetic hypothesis that can be evoked to explain this particular combination of findings.

It is not known if the abnormalities of villous maturation are due to abnormal fetal 'messages' or to an intrinsic placental growth disturbance. Similarly the factors control-ling villous vascularization are unknown but it is highly unlikely that the excess villous vascularization noted in a proportion of cases is, as maintained by Asmussen (1982a,b), a manifestation of diabetic microangiopathy: the fetus is not diabetic and the vascular appearances do not remotely resemble those of a diabetic microangiopathy.

It seems clear that the syncytiotrophoblast of these placentas suffers some degree of damage and shows focal necrosis: it is also clear that this damage is efficiently repaired and that residual lesions within the syncytiotrophoblast are focal, few and detectable only on electron microscopy. It has often been suggested, either directly or by implication, that the placenta suffers hypoxic damage in maternal diabetes either because of reduced uteroplacental blood flow (Driscoll, 1965; Emmrich et al, 1975a,b) or because large immature villi encroach upon and narrow the intervillous space (Aladjem, 1967; Jacomo et al, 1976). The syncytial necrosis is unlikely to be due to uteroplacental ischaemia, because the maternal decidual arteries in diabetic women are, if there is no complicating hypertensive disorder, morphologically normal (Pinkerton, 1963; Magnin & Gabriel, 1966; Khong, 1991) and there is fully normal physiological conversion of the spiral arteries of the placental bed into uteroplacental vessels (Robertson, 1979; Bjork et al, 1984; Wilkinson et al, 1997). This observation is in accord with Doppler studies which have shown that uterine and arcuate arterial flow velocity waveforms are normal in otherwise uncomplicated diabetic pregnancies (Hutter et al, 1993a,b; Salveson et al, 1993) though there may be a slightly increased vascular resistance in patients with a known vasculopathy (Zimmermann et al, 1994). It is therefore unlikely that uteroplacental ischaemia plays any significant role in the pathogenesis of the syncytial damage in the diabetic's placenta whilst the concept of intervillous space reduction has been disposed of by Teasdale (1983, 1985b) who showed that the volume of this space is either normal or increased in these placentas. Some other explanation for the syncytial necrosis must therefore be sought, and it seems at least possible that the tissue damage is a consequence of the abnormal metabolic milieu to which the syncytiotrophoblast is exposed, as this could cause an alteration in intracellular pH with subsequent activation of lysosomes.

The undue prominence of villous cytotrophoblastic cells in the placenta of diabetic women has been thought to be due largely to a failure of cytotrophoblastic regression, this being considered to be one facet of the tendency for the villi to be unduly imma-ture. It is certainly the case that in some of these placentas failure of regression is the principal reason for the excessive number of cytotrophoblastic cells. It is now clear, however, that there is also a hyperplasia of the cytotrophoblastic cells in most placentas from diabetic women, because electron microscopy shows that many of these cells are of the 'intermediate' type and that mitotic activity occurs with some frequency. This prolif-eration is a response to the syncytial necrosis and is a repair-hyperplasia phenomenon in which the cytotrophoblastic cells, being the stem cells of the syncytiotrophoblast, pro-liferate in an attempt to repair and replace the damaged syncytiotrophoblast, an attempt that appears to be largely successful insofar as residual evidence of syncytial damage is slight indeed and is only detected after prolonged searching.

Most of the other pathological features of these placentas are less open to rational discussion, and no obvious explanation is available for the abnormalities of villous maturation or for the 'obliterative endarteritis' of the fetal stem arteries. It has been suggested that this arterial abnormality, the fibrinoid necrosis of villi, and the thickening of the trophoblastic basement membrane are all due to an immunological reaction in which immune complexes of insulin and anti-insulin antibodies are deposited or formed at these sites (Burstein et al, 1963), but a prolonged electron microscopic search for evidence of such complexes in the thickened trophoblastic basement membrane has proved fruitless (Jones and Fox, 1976a). (The immunopathological findings in the placentas of diabetic women are discussed in Chapter 12.)

Functional Significance of Placental Changes

Despite the mystery in which many features of the diabetic patient's placenta are shrouded, there seems no reason for believing that placental function is impaired; indeed, the converse appears more likely, as there is much to suggest that the placenta of diabetic patients is functioning with above-average efficiency. The mere fact that the diabetic's child is often unusually heavy, as a result of the growth stimulating effect of fetal hyperinsulinaemia, is an indication in itself that there is no serious impairment of placental transfer function whilst morphological indicators of trophoblastic functional activity indicate that the trophoblast is functioning at a normal, or enhanced, level. The dilatation of the syncytial rough endoplasmic reticulum and the increased number of secretory droplets indicate increased secretory and synthetic activity whilst the normal appearance of the synctial microvilli, their increased density, the increased number of sycytial pinocytotic vesicles, the increased diffusive conductance and the greater area available for materno-fetal transfer all indicate that placental transfer function is at least maintained and, indeed, almost certainly augumented. It is therefore very unlikely that any ill-effects suffered by the fetus of a diabetic patient are due to placental dysfunction.

GESTATIONAL DIABETES

There is some confusion as to the definition of gestational diabetes. The term was originally applied to a condition in which glycosuria and hyperglycaemia develop during pregnancy with a reversion to normal glucose tolerance after delivery. Currently, however, the term is used to describe all patients who are shown to be diabetic for the first time in pregnancy without any reference being made to persistence or otherwise of the diabetic state after the pregnancy. In this section the term 'gestational diabetes' is used in its original sense.

Little attention has been paid to the placental changes that may be encountered in women with gestational diabetes, although Aladjem (1967) did examine a group of such placentas by phase-contrast microscopy and described focal syncytial detachment or rupture. We have examined a small sample of placentas from women with excellently controlled transitory gestational diabetes by both light and electron microscopy and have found that, whilst occasionally such placentas are virtually normal, the majority show changes identical in character to those found in placentas from women with well-established overt diabetes mellitus (Jones & Fox, 1976b). Although the pathological changes tend to be less marked and to occur with decreased frequency than in placentas from frankly diabetic women patients, there is, nevertheless, a not inconsiderable degree of overlap, and it is not possible to tell by examining a placenta histologically whether it is from a woman with excellently controlled mild, transitory gestational diabetes or from one with moderately controlled overt diabetes of long standing. Teasdale (1981) found that on morphometric examination, placentas from women with White's class A diabetes (gestational diabetes) showed changes very similar to those with Class B diabetes. Stoz et al (1988a) considered, however, that the changes detectable on morphometric study of placentas from women with gestational diabetes lay somewhere between those found in placentas from non-diabetic patients and those noted in placentas from women with overt insulin-dependent diabetes.

Salafia and Silberman (1989) have specifically commented on the presence of an umbilical vasculitis in a proportion of placentas from women with gestational diabetes. They correlate this lesion with abnormal fetal heart rate patterns and consider that the vasculitis affects umbilical haemodynamics and causes fetal hypoxia. However, there is no convincing evidence that fetal hypoxia occurs with undue frequency in pregnancies complicated by gestational diabetes.

HAEMATOLOGICAL DISORDERS

Anaemia

Several observers, working in tropical countries, have noted that the placenta tends to be unduly heavy in pregnancies complicated by severe maternal anaemia (Beischer et al, 1970; Mathews et al, 1973; Parikh & Parikh, 1974; Agboola, 1975), the fetus often being small and the placental/fetal weight ratio increased: the only histological abnormality seen in these placentas, and that inconsistently, was a minor degree of villous oedema. The increased size of the placenta in these cases has been interpreted as a compensatory mechanism to overcome the diminished content of oxygen in the maternal blood, a concept supported in the very large studies of Wingerd et al (1976) and Godfrey et al (1991) in which the weight of the placenta was found to vary inversely with the maternal haemoglobin concentration.

Recently, however, Reshetnikova et al (1995) found that the placentas of women suffering from iron deficiency anaemia were, if anything, slightly smaller than those from normal women and, using a stereological technique, demonstrated diminished growth of the placental villous tree in the placentas of anaemic women.

It is, rather obviously, difficult to reconcile these conflicting results but Reshetnikova and her co-workers, working in the Ukraine, studied only 10 placentas and the degree of anaemia in their maternal population was much less profound than that encountered in patients in tropical areas such as India, West Africa and Papua New Guinea. On the other hand there are, in these latter patients, many confounding factors such as malnutrition and infection.

Folic acid deficiency

The placenta shows no specific abnormalities in megaloblastic anaemia resulting from folic acid deficiency during pregnancy, though this statement is based on experience in the UK, in which a severe anaemia of this type is rarely seen. I have not noted any abnormality in the very few placentas I have seen from patients with pernicious anaemia, though, again, this is rarely, if ever, encountered in a severe form during gestation.

Sickle cell disease

Placentas from women with sickle cell disease have been reported as showing an excess of infarction and perivillous fibrin deposition (Anderson et al, 1960; Anyaegbunam et al, 1994) but in the few examples that I have seen, the only feature of note has been that the maternal erythrocytes in the intervillous space showed well-marked sickling (Fig. 8.15).

CARDIAC DISEASE

In women with a well-compensated heart disorder during pregnancy the placenta is usually normal in all respects, but in those with decompensated cardiac disease the placenta tends to be larger than usual (Clavero and Botella Llusia, 1963). This can

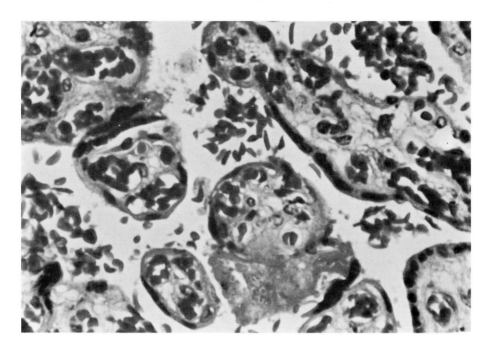

Figure 8.15. A placenta from a woman with sickle cell disease. The maternal red cells in the intervillous space show well-marked sickling (H & E ×350).

again be considered as a compensatory mechanism, as there is a true increase in placental size. Clavero-Nunez (1963b) has noted that the only histological abnormalities seen in these placentas are slight villous oedema and marked congestion of the villous vessels.

HEPATIC DISEASE

Liebhart and Wojcicka (1970) have commented that in any patient with jaundice during pregnancy there is an accumulation of haemosiderin-laden macrophages in the membranes, chorionic plate and, occasionally, the villi. Khudr and Benirschke (1972) also noted pigment-laden macrophages in placentas from women with infective hepatitis during pregnancy but thought that the pigment was bilirubin. Women with severe liver disease rarely become pregnant and hence little is known about the possible effects of hepatic dysfunction on the placenta.

Liebhart and Wojcicka (1970) studied placentas from women with intrahepatic cholestasis of pregnancy and maintained that there is a tendency towards poor villous vascularization, stromal fibrosis and an excessive formation of syncytial knots. By contrast, the only histological abnormality in the placentas of such cases reviewed by Fisk and Storey (1988) was relatively frequent meconium staining. Costoya et al (1980) undertook an electron-optical examination of placentas from patients with gestational intrahepatic cholestasis and noted an apparent maturational arrest of the villous cytotrophoblastic cells, dilatation of the rough endoplasmic reticulum of the villous syncytiotrophoblast and a marked increase in the number of syncytial osmiophilic bodies. The cause of these trophoblastic abnormalities in a condition now considered to represent an exaggerated response to oestrogens (MacSween, 1995) is, to say the least, uncertain.

MATERNAL EXPOSURE TO TOXIC SUBSTANCES

Very little is known about the effects on the placenta of maternal exposure to drugs, toxic chemicals, environmental pollutants or food additives. The only example of possible toxic damage which has so far received anything more than the most scanty attention has been cigarette smoking but in all accounts of the effects of cigarette smoking, alcohol ingestion and drug usage on the placenta, it has to be borne in mind that the use of these substances is often interrelated and it is almost impossible, for instance, to study the placentas of heroin users who do not also indulge in tobacco and alcohol.

Cigarette smoking

Cigarette smoking is associated with a decrease in fetal weight but has no significant effect on placental weight, this resulting in a decreased feto-placental weight ratio (Wingerd et al, 1976; Christianson, 1979; Salafia et al, 1992). Placentas from smoking mothers do not, in my experience, show any excess of gross lesions though, as discussed in Chapter 5, an association has been found between smoking and an increased incidence of abruptio placentae in many, though not all, studies. The only reasonably consistent findings on light microscopy are an excess of villous cytotrophoblastic cells and irregular thickening of the trophoblastic basement membrane (Naeye, 1978, 1979; van der Veen & Fox, 1982; van der Welde et al, 1983). Morphometric analysis of the placentas of smokers has either shown few changes of note (Teasdale & Ghislaine, 1989) or an increased thickness of the villous membrane (Burton et al, 1989) but electron microscopy confirms the presence of a villous cytotrophoblastic hyperplasia, most of these cells being of the intermediate type and some showing mitotic activity, and of trophoblastic basement membrane thickening (Asmussen, 1978, 1980; van der Veen & Fox, 1982; Demir et al, 1994): however, occasional cytotrophoblastic cells show marked degenerative changes. Much of the villous syncytiotrophoblast has a normal fine structure but small areas of syncytial necrosis are often present while focal areas are seen in which there is a markedly complicated infolding of the surface plasma membrane with local loss and malformation of the microvilli (Fig. 8.16). Syncytial pinocytic activity tends to be reduced and the number of syncytial secretory droplets is decreased.

Many of the abnormalities seen in the placentas of cigarette smokers suggest ischaemic damage and it does appear highly probable that uteroplacental blood flow is reduced in these women. It has been shown experimentally that infusion of nicotine into pregnant animals results in a sharp decrease in uterine blood flow (Resnik et al, 1979; Suzuki et al, 1980) whilst in the pregnant human the smoking of a single cigarette causes an acute reduction in intervillous blood flow (Lehtorvirta & Forss, 1978). These effects of nicotine are presumably mediated by its ability to induce vasoconstriction of the uterine vasculature but not all the placental abnormalities are explicable solely on the basis of ischaemia, this applying particularly to the degenerative changes seen in the villous cytotrophoblastic cells and to the curious focal infoldings of the syncytial plasma membrane. Damage of this latter type could be due to any of the multitude of chemical substances found in tobacco smoke but a good case can be made for the toxic role of cadmium. Cadmium is a known constituent of tobacco smoke, has been shown experimentally to have a particular propensity for causing placental necrosis in pregnant animals (Levin et al, 1981; Di Sant' Agnese et al, 1983) and is present in much higher concentration in placentas from smokers than in those from non-smokers (Peereboom et al, 1979). It is also possible, however, that exposure of the placenta to the polycyclic hydrocarbons present in tobacco smoke may lead to inhibition of trophoblastic oxidative enzyme systems (Longo, 1980).

Irrespective of the exact manner by which the placenta suffers injury in smokers, it seems highly unlikely that the damage inflicted could be held responsible for the increased incidence of low-birth-weight babies amongst the infants of smoking mothers. Any ischaemic damage suffered by the villous trophoblast appears to be readily and efficiently repaired, most of the trophoblast appearing fully normal. Any presumed loss of placental function would be of a degree unlikely to dissipate the functional reserve capacity of the organ and reduced fetal growth is probably partly due to an inadequate

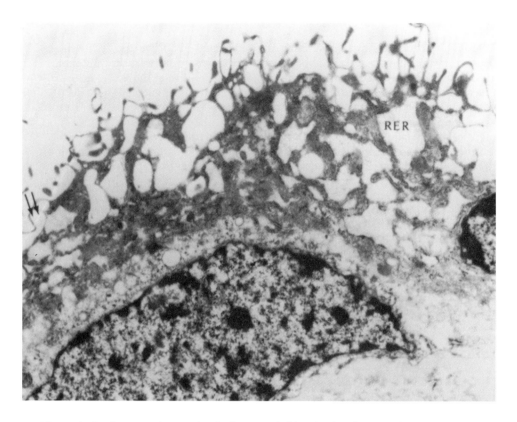

Figure 8.16. Electron micrograph of villous trophoblast in the placenta of a cigarette-smoking woman. This shows a focal area of infolding of the free plasma membrane. The underlying cytotrophoblastic cell is of the intermediate type. RER, rough endoplasmic reticulum (EM ×12,850).

maternal supply of oxygen and nutrients and partly due to the effects of transmitted carbon monoxide.

Alcohol

Rather surprisingly, in view of the well-known fetal alcohol syndrome, there appears to have been only one detailed study of placental morphology in cases of maternal alcohol abuse (Baldwin et al, 1982). The only findings that were clearly independent of low socioeconomic status were an excess of placental infarcts and of plaques of perivillous fibrin (neither of extensive degree) and features, such as villous stromal fibrosis and excesss syncytial knot formation, suggestive of reduced fetal perfusion of the villi. This study was not adequately controlled for smoking or drug usage but the findings were possibly a reflection of the ill-effects of alcohol, which readily traverses the placenta, on the fetus.

Cocaine

The quite extensive litany of the possible complications of pregnancy caused by, and the ill-effects on the fetus of, maternal cocaine usage has been extensively discussed by Slutsker (1992). As discussed in Chapter 5 the relationship between cocaine intake during pregnancy and an increased incidence of abruptio placentae remains controversial whilst a detailed study of 13 placentas from maternal cocaine users failed to reveal any characteristic morphological changes (Gilbert et al, 1990).

Dioxin

The placental changes occurring after maternal exposure to dioxin have been studied in cases therapeutically aborted after the Seveso disaster in Italy (Remotti et al, 1981). At the light-microscopic level no abnormality was seen but electron microscopy revealed the presence of numerous osmiophilic microprecipitates in, and deep to, the villous trophoblastic basement membrane. These bodies contained calcium, iron, sulphur and potassium and it has been suggested that they are evidence of a toxic impairment of the metabolic systems for transtrophoblastic transfer of mineral elements. The truth or otherwise of this contention and the possible functional significance, if any, of this morphological finding are currently unknown.

MISCELLANEOUS MATERNAL DISORDERS

Scleroderma

Benirschke and Kaufmann (1995) described two placentas from women with scleroderma and noted extensive fibrin deposition giving the appearance of maternal floor infarction; in one there was also extensive infarction. I have seen only one placenta from a patient with scleroderma and this was normal in all respects.

SYSTEMIC LUPUS ERYTHEMATOSUS

There have been several studies of the placenta in pregnancies complicated by maternal lupus erythematosus, these being prompted by the high incidence of abortion and preterm fetal death associated with this disease (Benirschke & Driscoll, 1967; Haustein, 1973; Abramowsky et al, 1980; Hanley et al, 1988; Erlendsson et al, 1993; Di et al, 1994), and from these has emerged a mixed picture, some placentas being virtually normal and others showing a necrotizing arteritis of the vessels of the placental bed and extensive infarction of the placental parenchyma. This problem reflects the difficulty in disentangling the effects on the placenta of systemic lupus erythematosus *per se* and the effects of anti-phospholipid antibodies which are, of course, often present in patients with this disease. There is a widespread view that the vascular lesions, and the associated placental infarction, are specifically associated with the presence of anti-phospholipid antibodies (De Wolf et al, 1982; Hanley et al, 1988; Out et al, 1991; Silver et al, 1992; Erlendsson et al, 1993; Branch, 1994) though, as is briefly discussed in Chapter 10, this is not a universally held concept. Whether or not systemic lupus erythematosus uncomplicated by the presence of anti-phospholipid antibodies is associated with placental lesions is a moot point, especially as many cases are complicated by pre-eclampsia. Immunopathological abnormalities of the placenta have, however, been described in this condition and these are discussed in Chapter 12.

Sarcoidosis

Non-caseating epithelioid granulomas of sarcoid type have been noted in placentas from women suffering from sarcoidosis (Kelerman & Mandi, 1969).

REFERENCES

Abitbol, M., Driscoll, S.G. and Ober, W.M. (1976) Placental lesions in experimental toxemia in the rabbit. *American Journal of Obstetrics and Gynecology*, **125**, 942–948.
Abramowsky, C.R., Vegas, M.E., Swinehart, G. and Gyves, M.T. (1980) Decidual vasculopathy of the placenta in lupus erythematosus. *New England Journal of Medicine*, **303**, 668–672.
Agboola, A. (1975) Placental changes in patients with a low haematocrit. *British Journal of Obstetrics and Gynaecology*, **82**, 225–227.

Aladjem, S. (1967) Morphologic aspects of the placenta in gestational diabetes seen by phase-contrast microscopy: an anatomicoclinical correlation. *American Journal of Obstetrics and Gynecology*, **99**, 341–349.

Alvarez, H. (1970) Prolifération du trophoblaste et sa relation avec l'hypertension artérielle de la toxémie gravidique. *Gynécologie et Obstétrique*, **69**, 581–588.

Alvarez, H., Benedetti, W.L. and de Leonis, V.K. (1967) Syncytial proliferation in normal and toxemic pregnancies. *Obstetrics and Gynecology*, **29**, 637–643.

Anderson, M., Went, L.N., MacIver, J.E. and Dixon, H.G. (1960) Sickle cell disease in pregnancy. *Lancet*, **ii**, 516–521.

Anderson, W.R. and McKay, D.G. (1966) Electron microscopic study of the trophoblast in normal and toxemic placentas. *American Journal of Obstetrics and Gynecology*, **95**, 1134–1148.

Anyaegbunam, A., Mikhail, M., Axioitis, C., Morel, M.I. and Merkatz, I.R. (1994) Placental histology and placental/fetal weight ratios in pregnant women with sickle cell disease: relationship to pregnancy outcome. *Journal of the Association of Academic Minority Physicians*, **5**, 123–125.

Arduini, D., Rizzo, G., Romanini, C. and Mancuso, S. (1987) Utero-placental blood flow velocity waveforms as predictors of pregnancy-induced hypertension. *European Journal of Obstetrics, Gynecology and Reproductive Biology*, **26**, 335–341.

Arnholdt, H., Meisel, F., Fandrey, K. and Lohrs, U. (1991) Proliferation of villous trophoblast of the human placenta in normal and abnormal pregnancies. *Virchows Archives B Cell Pathology*, **60**, 365–372.

Asmussen, I. (1978) Ultrastructure of the human placenta at term: observations on placentas from newborn children of smoking and non-smoking mothers. *Acta Obstetricia et Gynecologica Scandinavica*, **56**, 119–126.

Asmussen, I. (1980) Ultrastructure of the villi and fetal capillaries in placentas delivered by smoking and non-smoking mothers. *British Journal of Obstetrics and Gynaecology*, **87**, 239–245.

Asmussen, I. (1982a) Ultrastructure of the villi and fetal capillaries of the placentas delivered by non-smoking diabetic women (White group D) *Acta Pathologica, Microbiologica et Immunologica Scandinavica Section A*, **90**, 95–101.

Asmussen, I. (1982b) Vascular morphology in diabetic placentas. *Contributions to Gynecology and Obstetrics*, **9**, 76–85.

Baldwin, V.J., MacLeod, P.M. and Benirschke, K. (1982) Placental findings in alcohol abuse in pregnancy. *Birth Defects Original Article Series*, **18**, 89–94.

Barcroft, T. (1947) *Researches in Pre-Natal Life*. Springfield, Illinois: Charles C. Thomas.

Bartholomew, R.A., Colvin, E.D., Grimes, W.H., Fish, J.S., Lester, W.M. and Galloway, W.H. (1961) Criteria by which toxemia of pregnancy may be diagnosed from unlabelled formalin-fixed placentas. *American Journal of Obstetrics and Gynecology*, **82**, 277–290.

Bartholomew, R.A. and Kracke, R.R. (1932) The relation of placental infarcts to eclamptic toxemia: a clinical, pathologic and experimental study. *American Journal of Obstetrics and Gynecology*, **24**, 797–819.

Beischer, N.A., Sivasamboo, R., Vohra, S., Silpisornkosal, S. and Reid, S. (1970) Placental hypertrophy in severe pregnancy anaemia. *Journal of Obstetrics and Gynaecology of the British Commonwealth*, **77**, 398–409.

Benirschke, K. and Driscoll, S.G. (1967) *The Pathology of the Human Placenta*. Berlin: Springer-Verlag.

Benirschke, K. and Kaufmann, P. (1995) *Pathology of the Human Placenta*, 3rd edn. New York: Springer-Verlag.

Biale, Y. (1985) Lipolytic activity in the placentas of chronically deprived fetuses. *Acta Obstetricia et Gynecologica Scandinavica*, **64**, 111–114.

Bjork, O. and Persson, B. (1982) Placental changes in relation to the degree of metabolic control in diabetes mellitus. *Placenta*, **3**, 367–378.

Bjork, O., Persson, B., Stranenborg, M. and Baclavinkova, V. (1984) Spiral artery lesions in relation to metabolic control in diabetes mellitus. *Acta Obstetricia et Gynecologica Scandinavica*, **63**, 123–127.

Bloxham, D.L., Bullen, B.E., Walters, B.N.J. and Lao, T.T. (1987) Placental glycolysis and energy metabolism in preeclampsia. *American Journal of Obstetrics and Gynecology*, **157**, 97–101.

Bobkov, V.M. and Bobkova, S.A. (1984) Placental ultrastructure in women with impaired glucose tolerance during pregnancy. *Problem Endokrinol Moscau*, **30**, 22–25.

Born, G.V.R., Dawes, G.S. and Mott, J.C. (1956) Oxygen lack and autonomic nervous control of the foetal circulation in the lamb. *Journal of Physiology*, **134**, 149–166.

Boyd, P.A. and Scott, A. (1985) Quantitative structural studies on human placentas associated with preeclampsia, essential hypertension and intrauterine growth retardation. *British Journal of Obstetrics and Gynaecology*, **92**, 714–721.

Boyd, P.A., Scott, A. and Keeling, J.W. (1986) Quantitative structural studies on placentas from pregnancies complicated by diabetes mellitus. *British Journal of Obstetrics and Gynaecology*, **93**, 31–35.

Branch, D.W. (1994) Thoughts on the mechanism of pregnancy loss associated with the antiphospholipid syndrome. *Lupus*, **3**, 275–280.

Brosens, I. and Renaer, M. (1972) On the pathogenesis of placental infarcts in pre-eclampsia. *Journal of Obstetrics and Gynaecology of the British Commonwealth*, **79**, 794–799.

Browne, J.C.M. (1958) The uterine circulation in toxemia. *Clinical Obstetrics and Gynecology*, **1**, 341–348.

Browne, J.C.M. and Veall, N. (1953) The maternal placental blood flow in normotensive and hypertensive women. *Journal of Obstetrics and Gynaecology of the British Empire*, **60**, 141–147.

Burstein, R., Soule, S.D. and Blumenthal, H.T. (1957) Histogenesis of pathological processes in placentas of metabolic disease in pregnancy. II. The diabetic state. *American Journal of Obstetrics and Gynecology*, **74**, 96–104.

Burstein, R., Berns, A.W., Hirata, Y. and Blumenthal, H.T. (1963) A comparative histo- and immunopathological study of the placenta in diabetes mellitus and in erythroblastosis fetalis. *American Journal of Obstetrics and Gynecology*, **86**, 66–76.

Burton, G.J., Palmer, M.E. and Dalton, K.J. (1989) Morphometric differences between the placental vasculature of non-smokers, smokers and ex-smokers. *British Journal of Obstetrics and Gynaecology*, **96**, 907–915.

Campbell, S., Griffin, D.R., Pearce, J.M. et al. (1983) New Doppler technique for assessing uteroplacental blood flow. *Lancet*, **1**, 675–677.

Chamberlain, G., Phillip, E., Howlett, B. and Masters, K. (1978) *British Births 1970 Volume 2 Obstetric Care*. London: Heinemann.

Christianson, R.E. (1979) Gross differences observed in the placentas of smokers and non-smokers. *American Journal of Epidemiology*, **110**, 178–187.

Chua, S., Wilkins, T., Sargent, I.L. and Redman, C.W.G. (1991) Trophoblast deportation in pre-eclamptic pregnancy. *British Journal of Obstetrics and Gynaecology*, **98**, 973–979.

Cibils, L.A. (1974) The placenta and newborn infant in hypertensive conditions. *American Journal of Obstetrics and Gynecology*, **118**, 256–268.

Clapp, J.F. (1994) Physiological adaptation to intrauterine growth retardation. In *Early Fetal Growth and Development*, Ward, R.H.T., Smith, S.K. and Donnai, D. (Eds), pp. 371–383. London: RCOG Press.

Clarson, C., Tevaarwerk, G.J., Harding, P.G., Chance, G.W. and Haust, M.D. (1989) Placental weight in diabetic pregnancies. *Placenta*, **10**, 275–281.

Clavero, J.A. and Botella Llusia, J. (1963) Measurements of the villus surface in normal and pathologic pregnancies. *American Journal of Obstetrics and Gynecology*, **86**, 234–240.

Clavero-Nunez, J.A. (1963a) La placenta en la diabetes. *Revista Iberica de Endocrinologia*, **10**, 73–80.

Clavero-Nunez, J.A. (1963b) La placenta de las cardiacas. *Revista Espanola de Obstetricia y Ginecologia*, **22**, 129–134.

Clements, A.B. (1934) Placental necrosis. *American Journal of Obstetrics and Gynecology*, **27**, 84–89.

Cohen-Overbeek, T., Pearce, J.M. and Campbell, S. (1985) The antenatal assessment of utero-placental and feto-placental blood flow using Doppler ultrasound. *Ultrasound in Medicine and Biology*, **11**, 329–339.

Costoya, A.L., Leontic, E.A., Rosenberg, H.G. and Delgada, M.A. (1980) Morphological study of placental terminal villi in intrahepatic cholestasis. *Placenta*, **1**, 361–368.

Cunningham, F.G. and Leveno, K.J. (1988) Management of pregnancy-induced hypertension. In *Handbook of Hypertension. Volume 10. Hypertension in Pregnancy*, Rubin, P.C. (Ed.), pp. 290–319. Amsterdam: Elsevier.

Dashkevich, O.V. and Sechonov, I.M. (1964) The morphology of the placenta in diabetes mellitus. *Arkhiv Patologii*, **26**, 71–74.

Davey, D.A. and MacGillivray, I. (1988) The classification and definition of the hypertensive disorders of pregnancy. *American Journal of Obstetrics and Gynecology*, **158**, 892–898.

Dawes, G.S. (1969) Foetal blood gas homeostasis. In *Foetal Autonomy: CIBA Foundation Symposium*, Wolstenholme, G.E.N. and O'Connor, M. (Eds), pp. 162–172. London: J. & A. Churchill.

Demir, R., Demir, A.Y. and Yinanc, M. (1994) Structural changes in the placental barrier of the smoking mother: a quantitative and ultrastructural study. *Pathology Research and Practice*, **190**, 656–667.

de Swiet, M. (1995) Medical disorders in pregnancy: diabetes, thyroid disease, epilepsy. In *Turnbull's Obstetrics*, 2nd edn, Chamberlain, G. (Ed.), pp. 383–405. Edinburgh: Churchill Livingstone.

De Wolf, F., Carreras, L.O., Moerman, P., Vermylen, J., van Assche, A. and Renaer, M. (1982) Decidual vasculopathy and extensive placental infarction in a patient with repeated thromboembolic accidents, recurrent fetal loss and a lupus anticoagulant. *American Journal of Obstetrics and Gynecology*, **142**, 829–834.

Di, W., Hong, S.Y. and Yan, J.H. (1994) Pathological study on placenta from pregnancies with systemic lupus erythematosus. *Chinese Journal of Obstetrics and Gynecology*, **29**, 708–710.

Di Sant' Agnese, P.A., Jenson, K.D., Levin, A. and Miller, R.K. (1983) Placental toxicity of cadmium in the rat: an ultrastructural study. *Placenta*, **4**, 149–164.

Divers, M.J., Bulmer, J.N., Miller, D. and Lilford, R.J. (1995) Beta 1 integrins in third trimester human placentae: no differential expression in pathological pregnancy. *Placenta*, **16**, 245–260.

Dixon, H.G., Browne, J.C.M. and Davey, D.A. (1963) Choriodecidual and myometrial blood flow. *Lancet*, **ii**, 369–373.

Driscoll, S.G. (1965) The pathology of pregnancy complicated by diabetes mellitus. *Medical Clinics of North America*, **49**, 1053–1067.

Driscoll, S.G. (1975) Placental structure and maternal diabetes mellitus. In *Early Diabetes in Early Life*, Camerini-Davalos, R.A. and Cole, H.S. (Eds), pp. 227–230. New York, San Francisco, London: Academic Press.

Emmrich, P. and Gödel, E. (1972a) Morphologie der Placenta bei mütterlichem Diabetes mellitus. *Zentralblatt für allgemeine Pathologie und pathologische Anatomie*, **116**, 56–63.

Emmrich, P. and Godel, E. (1972b) Morphologie der Plazenta bei mütterlichem Diabetes mellitus: Vorschlag einer einheitlichen morphologischen Plazentadiagnostik unter Berücksichtigung internistischer geburtshilflicher und pädiatrischer Gesichtspunkte sowie Literaturubersicht. *Zentralblatt für Gynäkologie*, **94**, 881–887.

Emmrich, P. and Godel, E. (1972c) Plazentabefunde bei Neugeborenen diabetischer Mütter mit einem Geburtsgewicht unter 3000g. *Pathologia et Microbiologia*, **38**, 107–117.

Emmrich, P., Amendt, P. and Gödel, E. (1974a) Morphologie der Plazenta und neonatale Azidose bei mütterlichem Diabetes mellitus. *Pathologia et Microbiologica*, **49**, 100–114.

Emmrich, P., Amendt, P. and Gödel, E. (1974b) Klinische Parameter zum Plazentaboden bei mütterlichem Diabetes mellitus. *Zentralblatt für Gynäkologie*, **96**, 1493–1498.

Emmrich, P., Birke, R. and Gödel, E. (1975a) Beitrag zur Morphologie der myometrialen und dezidualen Arterien bei normalen Schwangerschaften, EPH-Gestosen und mütterlichem Diabetes mellitus. *Pathologia et Microbiologia*, **43**, 38–61.

Emmrich, P., Godel, E., Amendt, P. and Müller, G. (1975b) Schwangerschaft bei Diabetikerinnen mit diabetischer Angiolopathie. Klinische Ergebnisse in Korrelation zu morphologischen Befunden an der Plazenta. *Zentralblatt für Gynäkologie*, **97**, 875–883.

Erlendsson, K., Steinsson, K., Johansson, J.H. and Geirssson, R.T. (1993) Relation of antiphospholipid antibody and placental bed inflammatory vascular changes to the outcome of pregnancy in successive pregnancies of two women with systemic lupus erythematosus. *Journal of Rheumatism*, **20**, 1779–1785.

Falkiner, N.M. and Apthorp, J.O.E. (1944) The placenta in eclampsia and nephritic toxaemia. *Journal of Obstetrics and Gynaecology of the British Empire*, **51**, 30–37.

Fisk, N.M. and Storey, G.N.B. (1988) Fetal outcome in obstetric cholestasis. *British Journal of Obstetrics and Gynaecology*, **95**, 1137–1143.

Fox, H. (1967) The significance of placental infarction in perinatal morbidity and mortality. *Biologia Neonatorum*, **11**, 87–105.

Fox, H. (1969) Pathology of the placenta in maternal diabetes mellitus. *Obstetrics and Gynecology*, **34**, 792–798.

Fox, H. (1970) Effect of hypoxia on trophoblast in organ culture: a morphologic and autoradiographic study. *American Journal of Obstetrics and Gynecology*, **107**, 1058–1064.

Fox, H. and Agrofojo-Blanco, A. (1974) Scanning electron microscopy of the human placenta in normal and abnormal pregnancies. *European Journal of Obstetrics, Gynecology and Reproductive Biology*, **4**, 45–50.

Fox, H. and Jones, C.J.P. (1982) Ultrastructure of the human placenta in maternal essential hypertension. In *Pregnancy Hypertension*, Sammour, M., Symonds, M., Zuspan, F. and El-Tomi, N. (Eds), pp. 323–331. Cairo: Ain Shams University Press.

Franke, H., Gerl, D. and Stoessner, I. (1971) Die Feinstruktur der Chorionzotten bei Spätgestose unterschiedlicher Schweregrade. *Zeitschrift für Geburtshilfe und Gynäkologie*, **175**, 226–244.

Garner, P. (1995) Type 1 diabetes mellitus and pregnancy. *Lancet*, **345**, 157–161.

Gilbert, W.M., Lafferty, C.M., Benirscke, K. and Resnik, R. (1990) Lack of specific placental abnormality associated with cocaine use. *American Journal of Obstetrics and Gynecology*, **163**, 998–999.

Godfrey, K.M., Redman, C.W.G., Barker, D.J.P. and Osmond, C. (1991) The effect of maternal anaemia and iron deficiency on the ratio of fetal weight to placental weight. *British Journal of Obstetrics and Gynaecology*, **98**, 886–891.

Gregor, F. (1961) Histologische Veränderungen der Plazenta bei Spättoxikosen. *Zeitschrift für Geburtshilfe und Gynäkologie*, **157**, 325–340.

Haffner, R. (1921) Les soi-disant infarctus placentaires et leur relation avec l'albuminurie de grossesse. *Gynécologie et Obstétrique*, **3**, 81–89.

Hagay, Z.J. and Reece, E.A. (1992) Diabetes mellitus in pregnancy. In *Medicine of the Fetus and Mother*, Reece, E.A., Hobbins, J.C., Mahoney, M.J. and Petrie, R.H. (Eds), pp. 982–1020. Philadelphia: Lippincott.

Hanley, J.G., Gladman, D.D., Rose, T.H., Laskin, C.A. and Urowitz, M.B. (1988) Lupus pregnancy: a prospective study of placental changes. *Arthritis and Rheumatism*, **31**, 358–366.

Haust, M.D. (1981) Maternal diabetes mellitus: effects on the fetus and newborn. In *Perinatal Diseases*, Naeye, R.L., Kissane, J.M. and Kaufman, N. (Eds), pp. 201–285. Baltimore: Williams & Wilkins.

Haustein, U.F. (1973) Elektronmikroscopische Untersuchungen der Plazenta bei Lupus erythematodes visceralis. *Zentralblatt für Gynäkologie*, **95**, 1818–1823.

Hill, J.H. and Trimble, W.K. (1944) Placental infarction as a diagnostic criterion of maternal toxemia. *American Journal of Obstetrics and Gynecology*, **48**, 622–629.

Hirano, M. (1989) Ultrastructural study on human placental villi in toxemia of pregnancy – characteristic features obtained by a quick quenching and freezing. *Acta Obstetricia et Gynecologica Japonica*, **41**, 550–556.

Hirota, K. and Strauss, L. (1964) Electron microscopic observations on the human placenta in maternal diabetes. *Federation Proceedings*, **23**, 575.

Hölzl, M., Lüthje, D. and Dietrich, H. (1975) Placentaveränderungen bei Diabetes mellitus unter besonderer Beruchsichtigung von Zottenreifungsstorungen. *Zentralblatt für Gynäkologie*, **97**, 846–858.

Hölzl, M., Lüthje, D. and Seck-Ebersbach, K. (1974) Placentaveränderungen bei EPH-Gestose: morphologischer Befund und Schweregrad der Erkrankung. *Archiv für Gynäkologie*, **217**, 315–334.

Holzner, J. and Thalhammer, O. (1965) Zur Histologie und Histochemie des Plazenta bei Diabetes mellitus und Schwangerschaft Glykosurie. *Wiener klinische Wochenschrift*, **77**, 1024–1025.

Horky, Z. (1964) Die quantitativen Veränderungen der Vaskularisation der Zotten in der diabetischen Plazenta. *Zentralblatt für Gynäkologie*, **86**, 8–15.

Horky, Z. (1965) Die Reifungsstrungen der Plazenta bei Diabetes mellitus. *Zentralblatt für Gynäkologie*, **87**, 1555–1564.

Howard, R.B., Hosokawa, T. and Maguire, M.H. (1987) Hypoxia-induced fetoplacental vasoconstriction in perfused human placental cotyledons. *American Journal of Obstetrics and Gynecology*, **157**, 1261–1266.

Hunt, H.F., Patterson, W.B. and Nicodemus, R.E. (1940) Placental infarction and eclampsia. *American Journal of Clinical Pathology*, **10**, 319–331.

Hustin, J., Foedart, J.M. and Lambotte, R. (1984) Cellular proliferation in villi of normal and pathological pregnancies. *Gynecological and Obstetrical Investigation*, **17**, 1–9.

Hutter, W., Grab, D., Ehmann, J., Stoz, F. and Wolf A. (1993a) Der diagnostische Stellenwert der Continuous-wave (cw) Dopplersonographie bei mütterlichem Diabetes mellitus. *Ultrschall Medizin*, **14**, 169–174.

Hutter, W., Grab, D., Ehmann, J., Stoz, F. and Wolf, A. (1993b) Die Wertigkeit doppelsonographischer Untersuchungen bei insulinplichtige Diabetikerinnen. *Zeitschrift fur Geburtshilfe und Gynäkologie*, **197**, 38–42.

Istkovitz, J., LaGamma, E.F. and Rudolph, A.M. (1983) The effect of reducing umbilical blood flow on fetal oxygenation. *American Journal of Obstetrics and Gynecology*, **145**, 813–818.

Jaameri, K.E.U., Koivuniemi, A.P. and Carpen, E.O. (1965) Occurrence of trophoblasts in the blood of toxaemic patients. *Gynaecologia*, **160**, 315–320.

Jacomo, K.H., Benedetti, W.L., Sala, M.A. and Alvarez, H. (1976) Pathology of the trophoblast and fetal vessels of the placenta in maternal diabetes mellitus. *Acta Diabetolica Latinica*, **13**, 216–235.

Jiang, L., Luo, Y., Xia, Y. and Yan, Y. (1984) Ultrastructure findings in pre-eclamptic placentas. *Chinese Medical Journal*, **97**, 825–830.

Jirkovska, M. (1991) Comparison of the thickness of the capillary basement membrane of the human placenta under normal conditions and in type 1 diabetes. *Functional and Developmental Morphology*, **1**, 9–16.

Jones, C.J.P. and Fox, H. (1976a) An ultrastructural and ultrahistochemical study of the placenta of the diabetic woman. *Journal of Pathology*, **119**, 91–99.

Jones, C.J.P. and Fox, H. (1976b) Placental changes in gestational diabetes: an ultrastructural study. *Obstetrics and Gynaecology*, **48**, 274–280.

Jones, C.J.P. and Fox, H. (1980) An ultrastructural and ultrahistochemical study of the human placenta in maternal pre-eclampsia. *Placenta*, **1**, 61–76.

Kaltenbach, F.J., Fettig, O. and Krieger, M.L. (1974) Autoradiographische Untersuchungen über das Proliferationsverhalten der menschlichen Placenta unter normalen und pathologischen Bedingungen. *Archiv für Gynäkologie*, **216**, 369–386.

Kelerman, J.T. and Mandi, L. (1969) Sarcoidose in der Placenta. *Zentralblatt für allgemeine Pathologie und pathologische Anatomie*, **112**, 18–21.

Khong, T.Y. (1991) Acute atherosis in pregnancies complicated by hypertension, small-for-gestational-age infants, and diabetes mellitus. *Archives of Pathology and Laboratory Medicine*, **115**, 722–725

Khong, T.Y. and Robertson, W.B. (1992) Spiral artery disease. In *Immunological Obstetrics*, Coulam, C.B., Faulk, W.P. and McIntyre, J. (Eds), pp. 492–501. New York: Norton.

Khong, T.Y., De Wolf, F., Robertson, W.B. and Brosens, I. (1986) Inadequate maternal response to placentation in pregnancies complicated by pre-eclampsia and by small-for-gestational-age infants. *British Journal of Obstetrics and Gynaecology*, **93**, 1049–1059.

Khudr, G. and Benirschke, K. (1972) Placental lesions in viral hepatitis. *Obstetrics and Gynecology*, **40**, 381–384.

Kloos, K. (1952) Zur Pathologie der Feten und Neugeborenen diabetischer Mütter. *Virchows Archiv für pathologische Anatomie und Physiologie und für klinische Medizin*, **321**, 177–227.

Knopp, J. (1955) Morphologie reifer Chorionzotten bei behandleter Lues und bei Diabetes mellitus. *Verhandlungen der Deutschen Gesellschaft für Pathologie*, **39**, 158–162.

Las Heras, J., Haust, M.D. and Harding, P.G. (1983) Morphology of fetal placental stem arteries in hypertensive disorders ('toxemia') of pregnancy. *Applied Pathology*, **1**, 301–309.

Las Heras, J., Baskerville, J.C., Harding, P.G. and Haust, M.D. (1985) Morphometric studies of fetal placental stem arteries in hypertensive disorders ('toxaemia') of pregnancy. *Placenta*, **6**, 217–227.

Laurini, R.N., Visser, G.H.A., van Ballegooie, E. and Schoots, C.J.F. (1987) Morphological findings in placentae of insulin-dependent diabetic patients treated with continuous subcutaneous insulin infusion (CSII) *Placenta*, **8**, 153–165.

Lehtorvirta, P. and Forss, M. (1978) The acute effect of smoking on intervillous blood flow of the placenta. *British Journal of Obstetrics and Gynaecology*, **85**, 720–731.

Leiberman, J.R., Meizner, I., Maimon, E. and Hagay, Z.J. (1989) Unilateral and bilateral increase in resistance to blood flow in arcuate arteries during hypertensive disorders of pregnancy. *Clinical and Experimental Hypertension*, **B8**, 603–611.

Levin, A.A., Plautz, J.R., di Sant' Agnese, P.A. and Miller, R.K. (1981) Cadmium: placental mechanisms of fetal toxicity. *Placenta*, Supplement **3**, 303–318.

Liebhart, M. (1968a) Zmiany histopatologiczne w lozyskach matck chorych na cukrzyce jawna. (Microscopic changes in the placenta specimens from women with manifest diabetes mellitus.) *Ginekologia Polska*, **39**, 977–981.

Liebhart, M. (1968b) Thanka laczna lozysk pochodzacych z ciaz powiklanych przez cukrzyce matki. (The connective tissue in placenta samples collected from pregnancies complicated by diabetes mellitus.) *Ginekologia Polska*, **39**, 1353–1362.

Liebhart, M. (1971) The electron-microscopic pattern of placental villi in diabetes of the mother. *Acta Medica Polonica*, **12**, 133–137.

Liebhart, M. (1973) Badania porownawcze lozysk z ciaz powiklanych cukrzyca matki i konfliktem serologicznym. (A comparative study of the placental villi in pregnancy complicated by diabetes in the mother and serologic conflict.) *Patologia Polska*, **24**, 127–138.

Liebhart, M. and Wojcicka, J. (1970) Microscopic patterns of placenta in cases of pregnancy complicated by intrahepatic cholestasis (idiopathic jaundice) *Polish Medical Journal*, **9**, 1589–1600.

Lin, S., Shimizu, I., Suehara, N., Nakayama, M. and Aono, T. (1995) Uterine artery Doppler velocimetry in relation to trophoblast migration into the myometrium of the placental bed. *Obstetrics and Gynecology*, **85**, 760–765.

Lippert, T.H., Cloeren, S.F., Kidess, E. and Fridrich, R. (1980) Assessment of uteroplacental haemodynamics in pre-eclampsia. In *Pregnancy Hypertension*, Bonnar, J., MacGillivray, I. and Symonds E.M. (Eds), pp. 267–270. Lancaster: MTP Press.

Lister, U.M. (1965) The ultrastructure of the placenta in abnormal pregnancy. I. Preliminary observations on the fine structure of the human placenta in cases of maternal diabetes. *Journal of Obstetrics and Gynaecology of the British Commonwealth*, **72**, 203–214.

Little, W.A. (1960) Placental infarction. *Obstetrics and Gynecology*, **15**, 109–129.

Little, W.A. (1961) Clinical aspects of placental infarction and fibrin deposition. *New York State Journal of Medicine*, **61**, 1496–1499.

Longo, L.D. (1980) Environmental pollution and pregnancy: risks and uncertainties for the fetus and infant. *American Journal of Obstetrics and Gynecology*, **137**, 162–175.

Lunell, N.O., Nylund, L., Lewander, R. and Sarby, B. (1982) Uteroplacental blood flow in pre-eclampsia: measurement with indium-113m and a computer linked gamma camera. *Clinical and Experimental Hypertension*, **B1**, 105–117.

Lyall, F., Greer, I.A., Boswell, F. et al (1995) Expression of cell adhesion molecules in placentae from pregnancies complicated by pre-eclampsia and intrauterine growth retardation. *Placenta*, **16**, 579–587.

MacGillivray, I. and Campbell, D.M. (1980) The effect of hypertension and oedema on birth weight. In *Pregnancy Hypertension*, Bonnar, J., MacGillivray, I. and Symonds, E.M. (Eds), pp. 307–311. Lancaster: MTP Press.

MacLennan, A.H., Sharp, F. and Shaw-Dunn, J. (1972) The ultrastructure of human trophoblast in spontaneous and induced hypoxia using a system of organ culture: a comparison with ultrastructural changes in pre-eclampsia and placental insufficiency. *Journal of Obstetrics and Gynaecology of the British Commonwealth*, **79**, 113–121.

MacSween, R.N.M. (1995) Pathology of the liver and gall bladder in pregnancy. In *Haines and Taylor: Obstetrical and Gynaecological Pathology*, 4th edn, Fox, H. (Ed.), pp 1735–1758. New York: Churchill Livingstone.

Magnin, P. and Gabriel, H. (1966) Les scléroses vasculaires de la cadaque profonde. *Gynécologie et Obstétrique*, **65**, 37–56.

Maqueo, M., Azuela, J.C. and Vega, M.D. de la (1964) Placental pathology in eclampsia and pre-eclampsia. *Obstetrics and Gynecology*, **24**, 350–356.

Maqueo, M., Azuela, J.C., Karchmer, S. and Arenas, J.C. (1965) Placental morphology in pathologic gestations with or without toxemia: observations in cases of diabetes mellitus, hydrops fetalis, twin pregnancy, placenta previa, and hydatidiform mole. *Obstetrics and Gynecology*, **26**, 184–191.

Mathews, R., Aikat, M. and Aikat, B.K. (1973) Morphological study of placenta in abnormal pregnancies. *Indian Journal of Pathology and Bacteriology*, **16**, 15–24.

Mayhew, T.M., Sorensen, F.B., Klebe, J.G. and Jackson, M.R. (1993) Oxygen diffusive conductance in placentae from control and diabetic women. *Diabetologia*, **36**, 955–960.

Meekins, W., Pijnenborg, R., Hanssens, M., McFadyen, I.R. and Van Assche, F.A. (1995) Spiral artery morphology in pregnancies complicated by chronic hypertension: the relation to antihypertensive therapy and to superimposed preeclampsia. *Hypertension in Pregnancy*, **14**, 67–80.

Morris, N., Osborn, S.B., Wright, H.P. and Hart, A. (1956) Effective uterine blood flow during exercise in normal and pre-eclamptic pregnancies. *Lancet*, **ii**, 481–484.

Naeye, R.L. (1978) Effects of maternal cigarette smoking on the fetus and placenta. *British Journal of Obstetrics and Gynaecology*, **85**, 732–737.

Naeye, R.L. (1979) The duration of maternal cigarette smoking, fetal and placental disorders. *Early Human Development*, **3**, 229–237.

Nesbitt, R. (1958) Pathology of placenta in toxemia. *Clinical Obstetrics and Gynecology*, **I**, 349–357.

Nummi, S. (1972) Relative weight of the placenta and perinatal mortality: a retrospective clinical and statistical analysis. *Acta Obstetrica et Gynecologica Scandinavica*, Supplement **17**.

Okudaira, Y., Hirota, K., Cohen, S. and Strauss, L. (1966) Ultrastructure of the human placenta in maternal diabetes mellitus. *Laboratory Investigation*, **15**, 910–926.

Olofsson, P., Laurini, R.N. and Marsal, K. (1993) A high uterine pulsatility index reflects a defective development of placental bed spiral arteries in pregnancies complicated by hypertension and fetal growth retardation. *European Journal of Obstetrics, Gynecology and Reproductive Biology*, **49**, 161–168.

Out, H.J., Kooijman, C.D., Bruinse, H.W. and Derksen, R.H. (1991) Histopathological findings in placentas from patients with intra-uterine death and anti-phospholipid antibodies. *European Journal of Obstetrics, Gynecology and Reproductive Biology*, **41**, 179–186.

Page, E.W. (1948) Placental dysfunction in eclamptogenic toxemias. *Obstetrical and Gynecological Survey*, **3**, 615–628.

Paine, G.C. (1957) Observations on placental histology in normal and abnormal pregnancy. *Journal of Obstetrics and Gynaecology of the British Empire*, **64**, 668–672.

Parikh, K. and Parikh, S.R. (1974) Placental hypertrophy in pregnancy anaemia. *In Proceedings of the 6th Asian Congress of Obstetrics and Gynaecology, Kuala Lumpur, Malaysia*, pp. 244–250.

Peereboom, J.W.C., de Voogt, P., de Hatten, B., van der Welde, W. and Peereboom-Stegenan, J.H.J.C. (1979) The use of the human placenta as a biological indicator for cadmium exposure. In *Proceedings of the Second Conference on the Management of Control of Heavy Metals in the Environment*, pp. 7–9. Edinburgh: CPC Consultants.

Pinkerton, J.H.M. (1963) The placental bed arterioles in diabetes. *Proceedings of the Royal Society of Medicine*, **56**, 1021–1022.

Pudda, E. and Lecca, U. (1969) Rilievi ultrastrutturali su placente gestosiche. *Rivista Italiana di Ginecologia*, **53**, 152–161.

Redline, R.W. and Patterson, P. (1995) Pre-eclampsia is associated with an excess of proliferative immature intermediate trophoblast. *Human Pathology*, **26**, 594–600.

Redman, C.W.G. (1991) Current topic: pre-eclampsia and the placenta. *Placenta*, **12**, 301–308.

Redman, C.W.G. (1993) The placenta, pre-eclampsia and chronic villitis. In *The Human Placenta*, Redman, C.W.G., Sargent, I.L. and Starkey, P.M. (Eds), pp. 433–467. Oxford: Blackwell.

Redman, C.W.G. (1995) Hypertension in pregnancy. In *Turnbull's Obstetrics*, 2nd edn, Chamberlain, G. (Ed.), pp. 441–470. Edinburgh: Churchill Livingstone.

Remotti, G., de Virgilis, G., Bioanco, V. and Candiani, R. (1981) The morphology of early trophoblast after dioxin poisoning in the Seveso area. *Placenta*, **2**, 55–62.

Reshetnikova, O.S., Burton, G.J. and Teleshova, O.V. (1995) Placental histomorphometry and morphologic diffusing capacity of the villous membrane in pregnancies complicated by iron-deficiency anemia. *American Journal of Obstetrics and Gynecology*, **173**, 724–727.

Resnik, R., Brisk, G.W. and Wilkes, M. (1979) Catecholamine-mediated reduction in uterine blood flow after nicotine infusion in the pregnant ewe. *Journal of Clinical Investigation*, **63**, 1133–1136.

Reynolds, S.R.M. and Paul, W.M. (1958) Relation of bradycardia and blood pressure of the fetal lamb in utero to mild and severe hypoxia. *American Journal of Physiology*, **193**, 249–259.

Rindi, V. (1950) Ulteriores contributo alla definizione morfologica della barriera placentare nella gravidanza normale e patologica. *Rivista Italiana di Ginecologia*, **33**, 488–503.

Riviere, M. (1930) Contribution a l'étude microscopique comparée des placentas dits: albuminuriques et syphilitiques et des placentas normaux. *Gynécologie et Obstétrique*, **22**, 481–504.

Roberts, J.M. and Redman, C.W.G. (1993) Pre-eclampsia: more than pregnancy-induced hypertension. *Lancet*, **341**, 1447–1451.

Roberts, J.M., Taylor, R.N., Musci, T. et al (1989) Preeclampsia: an endothelial cell disorder. *American Journal of Obstetrics and Gynecology*, **161**, 1200–1204.

Robertson, W.B. (1979) Utero-placental blood supply in maternal diabetes. In *Carbohydrare Metabolism in Pregnancy and the Newborn, 1978*, Sutherland, H.W. and Stowers, J.M. (Eds), pp. 63–75. Berlin: Springer-Verlag.

Rolfini, G., Pavone, G. and de Cecco, L. (1963) Studio fragli aspetti microistofluoroscopici della placenta nel diabete e nella isoimmunizzazione anti Rh. *Recentia Medica*, **11**, 235–242.

Rubin, P.C. (1988) Hypertension in pregnancy: clinical features. In *Handbook of Hypertension. Volume 10. Hypertension in Pregnancy*, Rubin, P.C. (Ed.), pp. 10–15. Amsterdam: Elsevier.

Ruckhaberle, K.E. and Ruckhaberle, B. (1976) Der Zottentrophoblast in der Plazenten frühgeborener (einer enzymhistochemische Studie) *Zeitschrift für Geburtshilfe und Perinatologie*, **180**, 75–83.

Rudolph, A.M. and Heymann, M.A. (1973) Control of the foetal circulation. In *Foetal and Neonatal Physiology*, pp. 89–111. London: Cambridge University Press.

Salafia, C.M. and Silberman, L (1989) Placental pathology and abnormal fetal heart rate patterns in gestational diabetes. *Pediatric Pathology*, **9**, 513–520.

Salafia, C.M., Xenophon, J., Vintzileos, A.M., Lerer, T. and Silberman, L. (1990) Fetal growth and placental pathology in maternal hypertensive diseases. *Clinical and Experimental Hypertension*, **B9**, 27–41.

Salafia, C.M., Vintzileos, A.M., Lerer, T. and Silberman, L. (1992) Relationships between maternal smoking, placental pathology, and fetal growth. *Journal of Maternal-Fetal Medicine*, **1**, 90–95.

Salafia, C.M., Pezzullo, J.C., Lopez-Zeno, J.A. et al (1995) Placental pathologic features of preterm eclampsia. *American Journal of Obstetrics and Gynecology*, **173**, 1097–1105.

Salvatore, C.A. (1966) A placenta na toxemia de gravidez. *Maternidade e Infancia*, **25**, 87–116.

Salvatore, C.A. (1968) The placenta in toxemia: a comparative study. *American Journal of Obstetrics and Gynecology*, **102**, 347–353.

Salvatore, C.A. (1970) Ultrastructure of chorionic villi of the toxemic placenta. *Anais Brasileiros de Ginecologia*, **67**, 207–220.

Salveson, D.R., Higueras, M.T., Mansur, C.A. et al (1993) Placental and fetal Doppler velocimetry in pregnancies complicated by maternal diabetes mellitus. *American Journal of Obstetrics and Gynecology*, **168**, 645–652.

Salzberger, M. and Liban, E. (1975) Diabetes and ante-natal fetal death. *Israel Journal of Medical Sciences*, **11**, 623–628.

Sani, G. and Bottiglioni, F. (1964) Studio istofunzionale della placenta nel diabete mellito. *Rivista Italiana di Ginecologia*, **48**, 283–329.

Sankawa, T. (1990) Studies of structural changes in toxemic placentas. *Acta Obstetricia et Gynecologica Japonica*, **42**, 1291–1297.

Sauramo, H. (1961) Histological and histochemical studies of the placenta and foetal membranes in pathological obstetrics. *Annales Chirurgiae et Gynaecologiae Fenniae*, **50**, 179–194.

Schuhmann, R. and Geier, G. (1972) Histomorphologische Placentabefunde bei EPH-Gestose: ein Beitrag zur Morphologie dur insuffizienten Placenta. *Archiv für Gynäkologie*, **213**, 31–47.

Semmler, K. and Emmrich, P. (1989) Morphologie der Plazenta in Relation zur Glykamielage in der Schwangerschaft beim Diabetes mellitus. *Zeitschrift für Geburtshilfe und Gynäkologie*, **193**, 124–128.

Sermann, R. and Capria, V. (1965) Rillievi ultrastrutturali sul villo coriale umano nelle gestosi tardive. *Attualita di Ostetricia e Ginecologia*, **11**, 32–42.

Shanklin, D.R. (1958) The human placenta: a clinico-pathologic study. *Obstetrics and Gynecology*, **11**, 129–138.

Shanklin, D.R. (1959) The human placenta with especial reference to infarction and toxemia. *Obstetrics and Gynecology*, **13**, 325–336.

Silver, M.M., Laxer, R.M., Laskin, C.A., Smallhorn, J.F. and Gare, D.J. (1992) Association of fetal heart block and massive placental infarction due to maternal autoantibodies. *Pediatric Pathology*, **12**, 131–139.

Singer, D.B. (1984) The placenta in pregnancies complicated by diabetes mellitus. *Perspectives in Pediatric Pathology*, **8**, 199–212.

Slomko, A. and Pisarki, T. (1967) The placenta in toxaemia of pregnancy. *Bulletin Société des Amis des Sciences et des Lettres de Poznan*, **16**, 159–165.

Slutsker, L. (1992) Risks associated with cocaine use during pregnancy. *Obstetrics and Gynecology*, **79**, 778–789.

Smarason, A.K., Sergent, I.L., Starkey, P.M. and Redman, C.W.G. (1993) The effect of placental syncytiotrophoblast microvillous membranes from normal and pre-eclamptic women on the growth of endothelial cells in vitro. *British Journal of Obstetrics and Gynaecology*, **100**, 943–949.

Soma, H., Yoshida, K., Mulkaida, T. and Tabuchi, Y. (1982) Morphologic changes in the hypertensive placenta. *Contributions to Gynecology and Obstetrics*, **9**, 58–75.

Stock, M.K., Anderson, D.F., Phernetton, T.M., McLaughlin, M.K. and Rankin, J.H.G. (1980) Vascular response of the fetal placenta to local occlusion of the maternal placental vasculature. *Journal of Developmental Physiology*, **2**, 339–346.

Stoz, F., Schuhmann, R.A. and Schmid, A. (1987) Morphometric investigations of terminal villi of diabetic placentas in relation to the White classification of diabetes mellitus. *Journal of Perinatal Medicine*, **15**, 193–198.

Stoz, F., Schuhmann, R.A. and Haas, B. (1988a) Morphohistometric investigations in placentas of gestational diabetes. *Journal of Perinatal Medicine*, **16**, 205–209.

Stoz, F., Schuhmann, R.A. and Schultz, R. (1988b) Morphohistometric investigations of placentas of diabetic patients in correlation to the metabolic adjustment of the disease. *Journal of Perinatal Medicine*, **16**, 211–216.

Suzuki, K., Minei, I.J. and Johnson, E.E. (1980) Effect of nicotine on uterine blood flow in the pregnant rhesus monkey. *American Journal of Obstetrics and Gynecology*, **136**, 1009–1013.

Teasdale, F. (1981) Histomorphometry of the placenta of the diabetic woman: class A diabetes mellitus. *Placenta*, **2**, 242–252.

Teasdale, F. (1983) Histomorphometry of the human placenta in class B diabetes mellitus. *Placenta*, **4**, 1–12.

Teasdale, F. (1985a) Histomorphometry of the human placenta in maternal preeclampsia. *American Journal of Obstetrics and Gynecology*, **152**, 25–31.

Teasdale F. (1985b) Histomorphometry of the human placenta in class C diabetes mellitus. *Placenta*, **6**, 69–82.

Teasdale, F. (1987) Histomorphometry of the human placenta in pre-eclampsia associated with severe intrauterine growth retardation. *Placenta*, **8**, 119–128.

Teasdale, F. and Ghislaine, J.J. (1989) Morphological changes in the placentas of smoking mothers: a histomorphometric study. *Biology of the Neonate*, **55**, 251–259.

Teasdale, F. and Jean-Jacques, G. (1986) Morphometry of the microvillous membrane of the human placenta in maternal diabetes mellitus. *Placenta*, **7**, 81–88.

Tenney, B. (1936) Syncytial degeneration in normal and pathologic placentas. *American Journal of Obstetrics and Gynecology*, **31**, 1024–1028.

Tenney, B. and Parker, F. (1940) The placenta in toxemia of pregnancy. *American Journal of Obstetrics and Gynecology*, **39**, 1000–1005.

Thomsen, K. (1955) Placentarbefunde bei Spätgestosen und ihre ätiologische Zuordnung. *Archiv für Gynäkologie*, **185**, 476–503.

Thomsen, K. and Lieschke, G. (1958) Untersuchungen zur Placentarmorphologie bei Diabetes mellitus. *Acta Endocrinologica*, **29**, 602–614.

Thomson, A.M., Billewicz, W.Z. and Hytten, F.E. (1969) The weight of the placenta in relation to birthweight. *Journal of Obstetrics and Gynaecology of the British Commonwealth*, **76**, 865–872.

Torpin, R. and Swain, B. (1966) Placental infarction in 1000 cases; correlated with clinical findings. *American Journal of Obstetrics and Gynecology*, **94**, 284–285.

Traut, H.E. and Kuder, A. (1934) The lesions of fifteen hundred placentas considered from a clinical point of view. *American Journal of Obstetrics and Gynecology*, **27**, 552–558.

Trudinger, B.J. and Cook, C.M. (1990) Doppler umbilical and uterine flow waveforms in severe pregnancy hypertension. *British Journal of Obstetrics and Gynaecology*, **97**, 142–148.

Trudinger, B.J., Giles, W.B., Cook, C.M., Bombardieri, J. and Collins, L. (1985a) Fetal umbilical artery flow velocity waveforms and placental resistance: clinical significance. *British Journal of Obstetrics and Gynaecology*, **92**, 23–30.

Trudinger, B.J., Giles, W.B. and Cook, C.M. (1985b) Uteroplacental blood flow velocity waveforms in normal and complicated pregnancy. *British Journal of Obstetrics and Gynaecology*, **92**, 39–45.

Tsukimori, K., Maeda, H., Shingu, M. et al (1992) The possible role of endothelial cells in hypertensive disorders during pregnancy. *Obstetrics and Gynecology*, **80**, 229–233.

van der Veen, F. and Fox, H. (1982) The effects of cigarette smoking on the human placenta: a light and electron microsopic study. *Placenta*, **3**, 243–256.

van der Welde, W.J., Copius-Peereboom-Stegeman, J.H.J., Trefffers, P.E. and James, J. (1983) Structural changes in the placenta of smoking mothers: a quantitative study. *Placenta*, **4**, 181–190.

Vogel, M. (1967) Plakopathia diabetica: Entwicklungsstörungen der Placenta bei Diabetes mellitus der Mutter. *Virchows Archiv für pathologische Anatomie und Physiologie und für klinische Medizin*, **343**, 51–63.

Voigt, H.J. and Becker, V. (1992) Doppler flow measurements and histomorphology of the placental bed in uteroplacental insufficiency. *Journal of Perinatal Medicine*, **20**, 139–147.

Wallenburg, H.C.S. (1969) Uber den Zusammenhang zwischen Spatgestose und Placentar-infarkt. *Archiv für Gynäkologie*, **208**, 80–90.

Wentworth, P. (1967) Placental infarction and toxemia of pregnancy. *American Journal of Obstetrics and Gynecology*, **99**, 318–326.

Werner, C. and Schneiderhan, W. (1972) Plazentamorphologie und Plazentafunktion in Abhängigkeit von der diabetischen Stoffwechselführung. *Geburtshilfe und Frauenheilkunde*, **32**, 959–966.

Werner, C., Bender, H.C. and Klunsch, H. (1974) Morphologische Placentabefunde in Abhängigkeit von Schweregradder EPH-Gestose. *Geburtshilfe und Frauenheilkunde*, **34**, 168–174.

Widmaier, G. (1970) Zur Ultrastruktur menschlicher Placentazotten beim Diabetes mellitus. *Archiv für Gynäkologie*, **208**, 396–409.

Wilkin, P. (1965) *Pathologie du Placenta*. Paris: Masson.

Wilkinson, J., Fox, H. and Jauniaux, E. (1997) A study of placental bed biopsies in pregnancies complicated by maternal diabetes mellitus (in preparation).

Wingerd, J., Christianson, R.A., Lovitt, W.V. and Schoen, E.J. (1976) Placental ratio in white and black women: relation to smoking and anemia. *American Journal of Obstetrics and Gynecology*, **124**, 671–675.

Wislocki, G.B. and Dempsey, E.W. (1946) Histochemical age-changes in normal and pathological placental villi (hydatidiform mole, eclampsia) *Endocrinology*, **38**, 90–109.

Zacks, S.I. and Blazar, A.S. (1963) Chorionic villi in normal pregnancy, pre-eclamptic toxemia, erythroblastosis and diabetes mellitus. *Obstetrics and Gynecology*, **22**, 149–167.

Zimmermann, P., Kujansuu, E. and Tuimala, R. (1994) Doppler flow velocimetry of the uterine and uteroplacental circulation in pregnancies complicated by insulin-dependent diabetes mellitus. *Journal of Perinatal Medicine*, **22**, 137–147.

9

THE PLACENTA IN ABNORMALITIES AND DISORDERS OF THE FETUS

INTRAUTERINE FETAL DEATH

There is some debate as to where the line should be drawn between an abortion and a stillbirth but for the purposes of this discussion it will be assumed that an intrauterine fetal death after the 22nd week of gestation is a stillbirth.

It is a time-honoured cliché that examination of the placenta is an integral component of an autopsy on a stillborn infant. It is surprising, however, how little hard, factual, critically evaluated information was available, until very recently, about the diagnostic value of autopsies on stillbirths, whilst the extent to which placental examination helps in elucidating the cause of intrauterine demise is still a matter of dispute.

This is not the place to discuss at length the value of autopsies on stillbirths but estimates as to the percentage of such deaths for which a cause can be identified have ranged from 20% to over 90% (Hovatta et al, 1983; Rayburn et al, 1985; Kalousek & Barrett, 1994; Pauli et al, 1994; Stanley, 1995). To a very considerable extent these differing figures reflect the fact that there are two distinct populations of stillbirths, one at a peak gestational age of 24 weeks and the other with a peak at, or near, term (Pauli et al, 1994). Stillbirths at 24 weeks are, in reality, late abortions and in this group chromosomal abnormalities, malformations and infections are the most common causes of death (Pauli & Reiser, 1994). Those series in which it is claimed that a cause for intrauterine death can be identified in a high proportion of stillbirths tend to be heavily skewed towards this late abortion group (Redline, 1995). By contrast, intrauterine deaths at term are commonly of obscure aetiology though fetal hydrops, feto-maternal haemorrhage and umbilical cord accidents account for a proportion of cases (Redline, 1995).

Opinions vary as to the value of placental examination in establishing the cause of intrauterine fetal death and this reflects disparate views as to the importance of placental lesions or abnormalities as a cause, either direct or contributory, of fetal demise. Hovatta et al (1983) studied 243 stillbirths and considered that just over 50% of these were due to placental factors and that nearly 12% resulted from cord complications. Included, however, as instances of 'placental failure' were, *inter alia*, pre-eclampsia, twin births, preterm labour and uterine anomalies, conditions for which terminology indicating a functional failure of the placenta seems quite inappropriate. Further, death was attributed in just over 25% of cases to abruptio placentae or large placental infarcts without adequate consideration of the many live infants whose placentas show such lesions. Rayburn et al (1985) claimed that they were able to establish the cause of fetal death in 88 of 89 stillbirths examined. Placental histological abnormalities were the sole abnormal findings in 11% of these cases and these consisted of vascular insufficiency and haemorrhagic endovasculitis, either alone or in combination. The importance of haemorrhagic endovasculitis is a matter of dispute (see Chapter 6) but I would certainly not consider it to be a causal factor in fetal death. The definition of vascular insuff- iciency used by these authors is one with which I would not agree, including as it does an increase in the number of syncytial knots, and whilst these authors conclude that routine histological examination of the placenta after fetal death is of diagnostic value in pinpointing the cause of fetal death, I would not think that they have proved their claim. Volker (1992) considers that 50% of stillbirths are directly due to placental causes and lists delayed villous maturation, 'endarteritis obliterans' of the placental stem ves- sels and placental infarction as causes of a 'chronic placental insufficiency' which leads to fetal demise, a viewpoint that ignores the fact that such abnormalities can be found in many placentas from live births. It seems often to be the case that pathologists sieze on any abnormality, no matter how functionally unimportant, that is present in the placenta and attribute fetal death to this, thus effectively disguising the true cause of death or, perhaps even more importantly, concealing our ignorance, in many cases, of the factors that have led to the adverse pregnancy outcome. Any claim that a particular placental lesion has been the direct cause of fetal demise must be stringently evaluated, a procedure that tends to reduce dramatically the proportion of such deaths due to placental causes.

Macroscopic Features

Macroscopic examination of the placenta is of clear value in considering the par- ticular problem of a stillbirth in a multiple gestation (see Chapter 4), examination of the umbilical cord may also yield important, sometimes critical, clues as to the cause of death (see Chapter 15) whilst study of the membranes may help to identify such lesions as a severe chorioamnionitis or a ruptured vasa praevia (see Chapter 16).

Macroscopic examination of the placenta of a non-hydropic singleton stillbirth is clearly of some value though it would be over-optimistic to expect such an examination to yield a causal factor for fetal death in anything more than a small minority of cases. It is true that, on occasion, inspection of the placenta may reveal an obvious presump- tive cause for fetal demise, e.g., massive infarction, a very large retroplacental haematoma, a huge haemangioma, very extensive fetal artery thrombosis or well- marked placental floor infarction, but such a finding is very much the exception rather than the rule. It is of particular importance not to overstress the significance of gross lesions and to bear in mind that even quite extensive infarction or perivillous fibrin deposition is compatible with continuing fetal viability (see Chapter 5).

Histological Examination

Those undertaking histological examination of the placenta from a stillborn fetus must take into account the time interval that has elapsed between fetal demise and delivery. After fetal death in utero the placenta remains fully viable, is still a living, func- tioning organ, and can, indeed invariably does, undergo a series of morphological changes. These changes, which are now well documented, show a consistent pattern and are progressive (Wilkin, 1965; Emmrich, 1966a,b, 1992; Davies & Glasser, 1967; Fox, 1968; Theuring, 1968; Holzl & Luthje, 1974; Hustin & Gaspard, 1977).

There is a considerable increase in the number of villous syncytial knots (Fig. 9.1), though the syncytiotrophoblast of the villi usually appears otherwise normal; the villous cytotrophoblastic cells become more numerous and prominent, whilst the trophoblastic basement membrane undergoes a gradual thickening. The villous stroma becomes

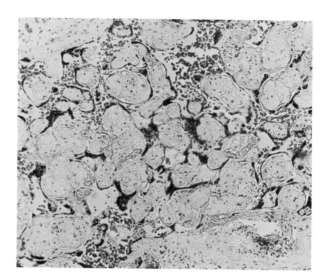

Figure 9.1. Villi in a placenta from a macerated stillbirth. The villi show many syncytial knots and are avascular and fibrotic (H & E ×90).

increasingly dense and fibrotic, and the villous fetal vessels undergo a progressive sclerosis (Fig. 9.2), which leads eventually to their obliteration. A degree of villous oedema is not uncommon (Fig. 9.3) and hence Hofbauer cells may often be seen. There is nothing to suggest that gross calcification occurs as a post-mortem change in the placenta, indeed the reverse is the case and calcium is lost from the placenta, but nevertheless calcification of scattered terminal villi is encountered quite commonly (Fig. 9.4). The fetal stem vessels show striking changes, with their lumina becoming greatly narrowed, and eventually obliterated, by a process of fibromuscular sclerosis.

Genest (1992) has recently re-examined the placental changes that occur after fetal death in an attempt to relate them with a greater degree of precision to the duration of intrauterine retention of the dead fetus. His findings were very similar to those described above but, in addition, he noted villous intravascular karyorrhexis, probably of leucocytic nuclei, as the earliest post-mortem change, a feature that I admittedly did not look for in my earlier study. He also failed to detect an increase in syncytial knots or

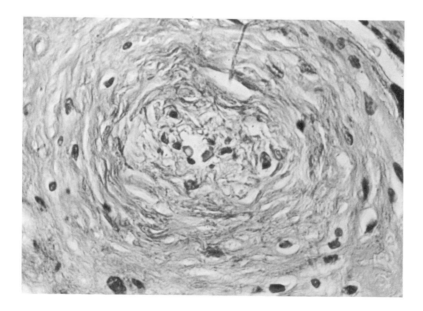

Figure 9.2. Fibromuscular sclerosis of a fetal stem artery in a placenta from a baby who had been dead *in utero* for 8 days before delivery (H & E ×220).

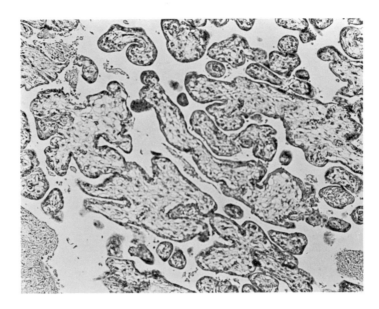

Figure 9.3. A moderate degree of villous oedema in a placenta from a stillborn infant who had been dead *in utero* for 1 week before delivery (H & E ×90).

in villous cytotrophoblastic cells. It should be noted, however, that the placentas I studied were largely from near-term stillbirths whilst those he examined had a mean gestational age of 26.7 weeks, a stage in gestation when cytotrophoblastic proliferation is less easy to determine, particularly as he did not use a PAS stain. Possibly the earlier age of the placentas in his study was also a factor in his inability to find an increasing number of syncytial knots, a change that in my experience is one of the most obvious and striking features of post-mortem changes in the term placenta. Genest showed that three histological features can be used to determine the approximate time interval between death and delivery, these being villous intravascular karyorrhexis, changes in the villous stem arteries and villous fibrosis. Thus if none of these changes is present the fetus has been dead for less than 6 hours whilst if karyorrhexis is the only change noted, the time interval is between 6 and 48 hours. The presence of this change together with stem vessel abnormalities and fibrosis of 50% or less, of the villi indicates that fetal demise had occurred between 2 and 14 days before delivery whilst changes more marked than these indicate a retention period of over 14 days.

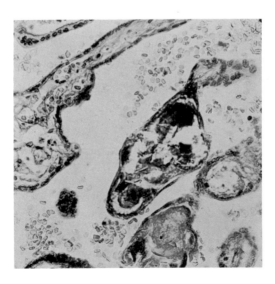

Figure 9.4. Calcification of a villus in a placenta from a macerated stillbirth (PAS ×300).

The pathogenesis of these post-mortem changes in villous morphology is reasonably clear. The death of the fetus is, of course, followed by a complete cessation of the fetal circulation through the placenta, and this will lead to fibromuscular sclerosis of the fetal stem arteries, obliteration of the villous capillaries, villous stromal fibrosis, and a proliferation of villous syncytial knots. The trophoblastic basement membrane thickening and the cytotrophoblastic hyperplasia are, on the other hand, a response to a reduced maternal blood flow to the placenta. It is known that maternal uteroplacental blood flow decreases notably after fetal death (Browne & Veall, 1953), though the decrease is not of a degree such as to impair the continuing viability of the trophoblast. The teleological advantages of this reduction in uteroplacental blood flow are obvious, but the mechanism by which it is produced is obscure. One possibility is that it is a consequence of the loss of the fetal circulation through the villi, because ten Berge (1955) has described a villous 'pulse' which may help the circulation of maternal blood through the intervillous space, and a loss of this could lead to the stagnation of blood in the intervillous space, a rise in intervillous space pressure and a consequent decrease in uteroplacental blood flow. This is, of course, a somewhat simplistic (though not necessarily incorrect) view as there must be many feto-maternal 'messages' which are interrupted by fetal death. The villous oedema is possibly due to the accumulation of fluid transferred across the trophoblast, and the villous calcification may also reflect an accumulation of transferred calcium.

These post-mortem alterations in the placenta of the dead fetus are of no importance in themselves but do have two unfortunate consequences. The first is that they may be wrongly considered to have been present at the time of, and to have contributed to, fetal demise; this is particularly the case with the changes in the fetal stem arteries, which have not infrequently been invoked as an aetiological factor in fetal death (Fujikura & Benson, 1964; Becker & Dolling, 1965). The second is that histological examination of these placentas is of limited value; examination of a placenta from a stillbirth dead *in utero* for less than 48 hours is just as valid and worthwhile as is examination of a placenta from a live-born infant. If the retention period is longer than this, however, the ability to detect villous changes resulting from alterations in either uteroplacental or fetoplacental blood flow progressively diminishes whilst histological examination of the placental tissue from a fetus dead *in utero* for more than 14 days is largely a worthless procedure in this respect. Histological study of the villous tissue of a macerated fetus may yield limited information, such as confirming the presence of a maternal floor infarction or similar gross lesion or detecting the presence of a severe or widespread villitis, but is very often unrewarding.

THE SMALL-FOR-GESTATIONAL-AGE INFANT

Until comparatively recently, all babies weighing less that 2500 g at birth were regarded as a single group – 'the low-birth-weight baby'. It has gradually become clear, however, that these infants do not form a homogeneous entity and that they can be divided into two quite separate categories: the first comprises babies who have been delivered prematurely but who are of a normal weight for the length of the period of gestation, whilst the second is formed of babies who are unduly small for the stage of pregnancy attained, irrespective of its duration. In this chapter, consideration is afforded only to the second group, entry into which is decided, not by the yardstick of an arbitrary and absolute weight level, but by the neonate's failure to achieve the tenth percentile of the weight normally expected for its gestational age. These babies have been variously categorized as 'small for dates', 'small for gestational age', 'pseudopremature' or 'dysmature', and the syndrome of low birth weight for gestational age has been called 'chronic fetal distress', 'intrauterine growth retardation', 'intrauterine malnutrition' and 'placental insufficiency'. I prefer the terms 'intrauterine growth retardation' to describe the process and 'small for gestational age' to describe the fetus or neonate, as these are factually accurate and free of aetiological connotations.

A baby may be small for a variety of reasons, but there are certain overt maternal and fetal factors that may lead to, or are associated with, a poor fetal growth rate. Pre-eminent amongst the maternal factors is severe pre-eclampsia, and in women with this disease the smallness of the baby is almost certainly due to the inadequacy of the utero-placental circulation; the pathological basis for this is discussed in Chapters 6 and 8. Other maternal factors of importance are cigarette smoking, drug abuse and certain infections, such as malaria. The most obvious fetal factors associated with a low birth weight are congenital malformations and chromosomal abnormalities, and here the failure of the fetus to achieve a normal weight is clearly an expression of a generalized disorder of growth and is unrelated to the adequacy or otherwise of the placenta. If cases such as these are removed from consideration there remains an important residue of unduly small infants who are delivered after an apparently uncomplicated pregnancy, are free from congenital malformations and have a normal karotype; it is this group which is considered here.

The placenta of the idiopathically small-for-gestational-age infant has been the subject of many pathological studies which have used light microscopy (Botella-Llusia, 1961; Gershon & Strauss, 1961; Gruenwald, 1961, 1963; Rumbolz et al, 1961; Kubli & Budliger, 1963; Wigglesworth, 1964; Bazso & Gaal, 1965; Tremblay et al, 1965; Wilkin, 1965; Wong & Latour, 1966; Schuhmann, 1969; Younoszai & Haworth, 1969; Emmrich & Lassker, 1970, 1971; Schrodt, 1970; Busch, 1972, 1974; Schuhmann et al, 1972; Scott & Jordan, 1972; Bender, 1974; Altshuler et al, 1975; Koenig et al, 1975; Spaczynski et al, 1976; Driscoll, 1979; Garcia, 1982; Rayburn et al, 1989; Liu, 1990; Salafia et al, 1992), electron microscopy (Lister, 1969; Theuring & Kemnitz, 1974; Sandstedt, 1979; Sheppard & Bonnar, 1980; Van der Veen & Fox, 1983) and stereology (Aherne & Dunnill, 1966; Clavero-Nunez et al, 1971; Teasdale, 1984; Boyd & Scott, 1985; Li, 1992; Shen, 1992).

It cannot be said that the efforts of these many workers have been crowned with success in terms of any characteristic or consistent pathological picture having emerged. This lack of agreement has been due to many factors amongst which can be included differing definitions of fetal growth retardation, the inclusion of cases caused by pre-eclampsia, a common disregard of maternal smoking habits, a failure to exclude cases in which the neonate has a low birth weight but is not small for gestational age, a neglect of possible maternal drug abuse and a failure to distinguish between those cases of growth retardation in which the neonate has a normal ponderal index and those in which the ponderal index is abnormal. Quite apart from these methodological defects there have been two conceptual deficiencies. The first of these is the partially recognized but commonly ignored fact that idiopathic fetal growth retardation is almost certainly, even after exclusion of all known predisposing fetal and maternal factors, a heterogeneous condition which is unlikely to yield a stereotyped pattern of placental findings. Second, in many of these studies there has been a background assumption, either stated or implied, that placental abnormalities, lesions or damage result in a state of 'placental insufficiency' which is responsible for the defective fetal growth. As pointed out in Chapter 5, the placenta has a very considerable physiological reserve capacity and in only very rare cases does it suffer damage of such an extent that it becomes functionally inadequate.

Placental Size

Most, though not all, small babies have small placentas and this commonplace observation has been quantified by morphometric studies (Teasdale, 1984; Boyd & Scott, 1985; Shen, 1992). It is therefore often assumed that the baby is small *because* the placenta is small, a point of view which implies that fetal size is rigidly limited by placental mass. If, however, fetal growth was narrowly limited by placental mass this would, of necessity, imply that the placenta has little or no functional reserve capacity. As pointed out in Chapter 5, simple pathological studies indicate that the placenta can withstand functional inactivation of 30–40% of its villous population without any discernible effect on fetal growth or development; thus the placenta does have a considerable functional reserve capacity, a finding confirmed by experiments involving surgical reduction of placental mass (Robinson et al, 1979), artificially increased fetal oxygen consumption (Lorijn & Longo, 1980) or microsphere embolization of maternal uteroplacental vessels (Charlton & Johengen, 1988). Furthermore, the placenta has a normally unrealized potential for increased compensatory growth when in an unfavourable maternal milieu from the start of pregnancy as is shown by the unduly large placentas seen in pregnancy at high altitude (Kruger & Arias Stella, 1970), in cases of severe maternal anaemia (Beischer et al, 1970; Agboola, 1975; Godfrey et al, 1991), in pregnancies in women with congestive cardiac failure (Clavero-Nunez, 1963) and in many experimental studies which have subjected the placenta to chronic hypoxia (Robinson & Owens, 1993).

The fact that the placenta does have a very considerable reserve capacity together with a potential for compensatory growth makes it unlikely that placental mass restricts fetal growth and I agree fully with Gruenwald (1975) when he makes the point that the placenta is a fetal organ and therefore shares in any depression of fetal growth, the small fetus not only having a small liver and a small heart but also a small placenta. Thus, the placenta is small because the fetus is small, rather than the reverse.

Gross Abnormalities

Circumvallate placentation is associated with an increased incidence of low birth weight but, as discussed in Chapter 3, most of the neonates so classified only just fall within the defined category of small for gestational age.

The overall incidence of infarction tends to be increased in placentas from growth-retarded infants (Bjoro, 1981; Suska et al, 1989; Salafia et al, 1992) and Laurini et al (1994) have claimed that infarction is the only placental lesion which correlates with growth retardation. In my experience the infarcts in placentas from growth-retarded infants are usually small and most placentas from these infants show no infarction at all. Maternal floor infarction, very extensive perivillous fibrin deposition, widespread thrombosis of fetal arteries and unusually large, or multiple, placental haemangiomas may all be associated with diminished fetal growth (see Chapters 5 and 13) but such lesions are found in only a small minority of placentas from small-for-gestational-age infants, the vast majority of such placentas showing no significant gross lesions.

Histological Abnormalities

Histological examination of placentas from small-for-gestational-age infants reveals no constant or diagnostic pathological picture. Many, probably about 25%, are histologically normal in all respects for the length of the gestational period. The remainder either show the features of poor fetal perfusion, with villous hypovascularity, villous stromal fibrosis and an excessive formation of syncytial knots, evidence of having been subjected to ischaemia with hyperplasia of the villous cytotrophoblastic cells and a variable degree of thickening of the trophoblastic basement membrane or, most commonly, an admixture of both ischaemic and diminished perfusion patterns. A few placentas show a delay in villous maturation, though this latter feature is not common, the villi in most cases appearing fully mature for the length of the gestational period.

Villitis of unknown aetiology is seen with undue frequency in placentas from small-for-gestational-age infants, though the reported proportion of such placentas in which this lesion has been found has been very variable, ranging from 7.5% to 86% (Altshuler et al, 1975; Labarrere et al, 1982, 1986; Bjoro & Myhre, 1984; Mortimer et al, 1985; Nordenvall & Sandstedt, 1990; Salafia et al, 1992). Most authors, however, have found an incidence in the region of 30%.

Maternal Vasculature

The finding of ischaemic changes in many placentas of idiopathic intrauterine growth-retarded fetuses suggests that there may be diminished maternal blood flow in such cases and this suggestion has been confirmed by Doppler studies of the utero-placental circulation (Trudinger et al, 1985a,b; McCowan et al, 1988; Jacobson et al, 1990; Bewley et al, 1991; Iwata et al, 1993; Schulman, 1993). Ferrazzi et al (1994) further showed that there was a clear correlation between an abnormal uteroplacental waveform and the presence of ischaemic changes in the placenta. The basis for this diminished blood flow is inadequate conversion of the spiral arteries of the placental bed into uteroplacental vessels because of failure of the extravillous trophoblast to extend into their intramyometrial segments (Sheppard & Bonnar, 1976, 1981; Brosens et al, 1977; Robertson et al, 1981, 1986; Hustin et al, 1983; Khong et al, 1986; Khong & Robertson, 1992), the defect in placentation being identical to that found in patients with pre-eclampsia (see Chapters 6 and 8) and being specifically associated with abnormal uterine flow velocity waveforms (Lin et al, 1995). There must be strong grounds for presuming that this ischaemia is an important factor in the failure of fetal growth because in animal studies experimentally induced limitation of placental blood flow will result in an unduly small fetus (Robinson & Owens, 1993; Clapp, 1994). A further vascular lesion, acute atherosis (see Chapter 6), may also be present in the maternal vessels in cases of idiopathic intrauterine growth retardation (Sheppard & Bonnar, 1976, 1981; De Wolf et al, 1980; Hustin et al, 1983; Althabe et al, 1985; Khong, 1991; Khong & Robertson, 1992) and in two studies birth weight was most markedly reduced in those cases in which acute atherosis complicated inadequate physiological change in the placental bed vasculature (McFadyen et al, 1986; Frusca et al, 1989).

Abnormal Fetal Perfusion

Histological examination of placentas from small-for-gestational-age infants often shows evidence of diminished fetal perfusion of the villous vessels but it was only with the introduction of Doppler studies of umbilical artery blood flow velocity waveforms and umbilical vein blood flow that serious attention was paid to the possible role played by abnormalities of the placental fetal vasculature in idiopathic intrauterine growth retardation. Trudinger et al (1985b,c) showed that in many pregnancies complicated by idiopathic fetal growth retardation there were abnormal waveforms in the fetal umbilical arteries which were indicative of an increased resistance in the placental vascular bed, the inference being that fetal perfusion of the placenta was decreased in such cases. This finding was subsequently confirmed in other studies (McCowan et al, 1987; Gudmundsson & Marsal, 1988; Bracero et al, 1989; Ritchie, 1991; Zacutti et al, 1992; Hitschold et al, 1993) and Doppler studies of umbilical vein blood flow have confirmed the diminished fetal perfusion of the placenta of many growth-retarded fetuses (Gill et al, 1993).

The morphological basis for the increased resistance in the fetal vasculature of growth-retarded fetuses is a matter for dispute. Giles et al (1985) found widespread obliteration of small muscular arteries in the tertiary stem villi in such cases and others have reported similar findings (McCowan et al, 1987; Bracero et al, 1989; Fok et al, 1990). Hitschold et al (1993) thought, however, that the basic abnormality was a reduction in the vascularity of the terminal villi whilst Macara et al (1995) did not think that there was any selective loss of small stem villous vessels and also suggested that the increased vascular impedance was at the level of the capillaries in the terminal villi. Because placental vascular resistance increased progressively in serial studies of growth-retarded fetuses in the cases studied by Giles et al (1985), it was thought that the vascular lesion was a progressive one and probably secondary to uteroplacental ischaemia. Bracero et al (1989) noted, however, that in some cases placental vascular resistance, although still remaining abnormal, decreased as pregnancy progressed and thought that in such cases there may have been a primary defect, or arrested development, of placental angiogenesis. Jackson et al (1995) agreed, on the basis of a morphometric study, with this view and suggested that the increased vascular resistance was due to reduced villous tree elaboration with a global reduction in placental vascularity. In a not dissimilar study, Kreczy et al (1995) concluded that the high resistance in the fetal vasculature was due to a decreased number of arteries in the tertiary stem villi, a deficiency they also attributed to an early developmental arrest of placental angiogenesis.

It has been my experience that a characteristic feature of many placentas from small-for-gestational-age fetuses is an 'endarteritis obliterans' in the large stem arteries (Van der Veen & Fox, 1983), a finding also noted by others (Koenig, 1972; Koenig et al, 1973; Bender et al, 1976) and now known to be the hallmark of a prolonged vasoconstriction (see Chapter 6). This will, if sustained, lead to a progressive sclerosis and eventual obliteration of the more distal vasculature with diminished vascularization of the terminal villi. This dynamic vascular change is probably a response to uteroplacental ischaemia because experimental studies have clearly shown that a reduction in maternal blood flow to the placenta is followed by an increased vascular resistance within the fetal placental vasculature and decreased fetal perfusion of the villi (Stock et al, 1980; Clapp, 1994). In teleological terms this response to placental ischaemia is part of an attempt by the deprived fetus to divert blood to the cerebral and coronary circulations. Though it may seem paradoxical to reduce placental blood flow, the placental tissue can increase oxygen extraction from the maternal blood when the fetal blood flow is decreased and can sustain a flow reduction of 50% without impairing fetal oxygenation (Itskovitz et al, 1983). This haemodynamic view of the basis for an increased fetal vascular resistance in the placenta of low-birth-weight infants is conceptually more appealing than the alternative concept of arrested angiogenesis because it is difficult both to reconcile this latter view with the proven inadequate placentation in many such cases and to suggest an aetiological factor for arrested vascular development. Furthermore, the concept of a fixed vascular deficiency accords ill with the observation that in many, though not all, cases of fetal growth retardation maternal hyperoxygenation decreases fetal intraplacental vascular resistance (Bilardo et al, 1991; de Rochembeau et al, 1992).

Cytogenetic Abnormalities

Fetal cytogenetic abnormalities are, of course, well known to be associated with diminished fetal growth but only within recent years has it been recognized that the chromosomal constitution of the placenta is not necessarily the same as that of the fetus, discrepancies between fetus and placenta being usually due to a mosaicism which is not present in the fetus. The abnormal cell line in the placenta is usually a trisomy of chromosomes 7, 16 or 18 and in such cases the zygote is often trisomic with postzygotic loss of the extra chromosomal material in the embryonic, but not the trophoblastic, precursor cells. It is a majority view that this condition of confined placental mosaicism is associated with a high incidence of intrauterine fetal growth retardation (Kalousek et al, 1987; Kalousek, 1990, 1994; Post & Nijhuis, 1992; Kalousek & Langlois, 1994; Wolstenholme et al, 1994) though this has admittedly not been everyone's experience (Schwinger et al, 1989; Kennerknecht et al, 1993; Roland et al, 1994); paradoxically, confined placental mosaicism also appears to be associated with an increased incidence of unusually high birth weight (Wolstenholme et al, 1994). The quantitative contribution of confined placental mosaicism to the overall incidence of intrauterine fetal growth retardation remains to be established, though it is unlikely to be high, and it has not yet been shown that this chromosomal abnormality is associated with any histological changes in the placenta (Kalousek, personal communication).

General Comments

There must be a strong suspicion that the most important factor in many cases of intrauterine fetal growth retardation is faulty placentation with inadequate conversion of spiral ateries into uteroplacental blood vessels and a consequent restraint upon the ability of the mother to supply the fetus with nutrients and oxygen, this eventually resulting in a secondary reduction in fetal villous perfusion. Histological evidence of ischaemia is frequently encountered in placentas from growth-retarded infants whilst attempts to induce experimental fetal growth retardation rely heavily on techniques that reduce maternal placental blood flow (Carter, 1993; Robinson & Owens, 1993; Clapp, 1994).

The cause of the inadequate placentation is just as obscure in cases of idiopathic fetal growth retardation as it is in pre-eclampsia (see Chapter 8) but during placentation there be some immunological interaction between trophoblastic and maternal tissues that probably limits the migratory capacity of the trophoblast. It could therefore be postulated that inadequate placentation is often due to an abnormal maternal–trophoblastic immune reaction (King & Loke, 1994) and that the frequently seen villitis of unknown aetiology in placentas from growth-retarded fetuses is a further hallmark of this abnormal immunological interaction. Further, as discussed in Chapter 10, there is evidence that in many cases of first-trimester abortion there is inadequate placentation and it has been suggested that defective trophoblastic migration and invasion may be secondary to a fetal chromosomal abnormality. It is therefore possible that there is a similar defect in cases of restricted placental mosaicism though the inadequacy of placentation may be less marked than that due to a non-mosaic chromosomally abnormal trophoblast and result in fetal growth retardation rather than first-trimester loss.

Inadequate placentation, restricted placental mosaicism and villitis of unknown aetiology can therefore be linked into a unitary hypothesis, one which is admittedly speculative but which nevertheless serves to emphasize the dominant role played by a reduced maternal uteroplacental blood flow in many, but certainly not all, pregnancies which result in a child that is not only small for its gestational age but which is at increased risk of coronary artery disease, hypertension and diabetes when it attains middle age (Barker, 1994).

It has, in all fairness, to be mentioned that this view of the major importance of a restricted maternal uteroplacental flow in intrauterine fetal growth retardation has recently been challenged, especially for those cases in which Doppler studies show absent end-diastolic flow velocity. It has been suggested that under such circumstances there may be a primary defect in placental nutrient and gas transfer, this view being based upon an ultrastructural study (Macara et al, 1996). However, it is difficult to envisage any metabolic abnormality that could cause a global reduction in placental transfer mechanisms and the suggestion that the thickening of the trophoblastic basement membrane, noted in this study, plays a significant role in reducing villous transfer efficiency lacks conviction. Nevertheless this concept merits further study, which no doubt it will receive.

PRENATAL BRAIN DAMAGE

The particular problem of antenatal brain damage in monochorionic twins is discussed in Chapter 4 and the comments in this section apply only to singleton gestations.

If one excludes cerebral damage caused by maldevelopment or infection, a residue of cases remains which is thought to be due to ischaemic or hypoxic damage to the developing brain. Infants with brain damage of this type are often referred to as suffering from 'cerebral palsy' but 'hypoxic-ischaemic encephalopathy' is a preferable, and less emotionally laden, term. Ischaemia is, however, certainly not the only factor involved in the production of these brain lesions because carbon dioxide retention, acidosis, hypotension and hypoglycaemia may also be of importance (Squier, 1993) but, nevertheless, the term ischaemic damage is usually used as a convenient and brief portmanteau description. The number of such cases caused by intrapartum hypoxia is disputed but it is currently widely felt that these represent only a small minority (10–15%) and that the brain damage usually occurs before the onset of labour, though at what stage of gestation is unknown (Freeman & Nelson, 1988; Adamson et al, 1995; Palmer et al, 1995). It is also not known whether the insult to the cerebral tissues is usually an acute or a chronic one.

Altshuler (1993a) has commented that placental pathology frequently reveals the pathogenesis of cerebral palsy, mental retardation and other neurodevelopmental disorders, but despite this confident assertion, for which adequate documentation is lacking, the value of placental examination in cases of prenatal brain damage is a contentious subject. To some extent, attempts to correlate brain damage with placental abnormalities represent attempts at correlating lesions of unknown aetiology with abnormalities of unproven or uncertain significance. Naeye (1988, 1991, 1992) has studied extensively the relationship between placental and umbilical cord lesions and neurological abnormalities in living children and, whilst demonstrating associations between many placental lesions, particularly villous oedema, and subsequent evidence of neurological damage, has placed considerable emphasis upon the role played by meconium, citing the experimental study of Altshuler and Hyde (1989) which showed that meconium is capable of causing vasoconstriction in umbilical vessels. It has to be stressed, however, that the demonstration of an *in vitro* capacity to cause umbilical vasoconstriction does not prove that this actually occurs *in vivo* and that the vast majority of infants with meconium staining of their placentas show no evidence of neurological damage. Bejar et al (1988) found that the only variable associated with antenatal white matter necrosis in singleton pregnancies was chorioamnionitis and funisitis and Cooke (1990) also found chorioamnionitis to be related to this form of cerebral damage.

In a recent study, Grafe (1994) attempted to correlate prenatal brain damage with placental pathology in infants who were either stillborn or died within 1 hour of birth, dividing the cerebral lesions into the three groups of germinal matrix/intraventricular haemorrhage, white matter gliosis/necrosis and neuronal necrosis. The only placental correlate of germinal matrix/intraventricular haemorrhage was a funisitis but both white matter necrosis and neuronal necrosis were found to be significantly associated with placental chronic vascular problems, cord complications and old placental infarcts; white matter necrosis, but not neuronal necrosis, was also associated with meconium staining whilst surface vessel thrombosis in the placenta was associated only with neuronal necrosis. It was noteworthy that there was no association between chorioamnionitis and any form of prenatal cerebral damage in this series and that there was a similar lack of any association with villous oedema. This study suffered from a lack of precise definition of the placental lesions, a deficiency freely admitted by the author. Thus, the extent of the placental infarction was not quantitated and whilst velamentous insertion of the cord features as an associated factor it is not indicated whether there had been any tearing of these vessels. It is therefore difficult to know what to make of these findings: their implication is that antenatal cerebral damage tends to be associated with cord abnormalities and with evidence of ischaemic or thrombotic lesions in the placenta but as the author states 'these placental findings could either produce or reflect chronic hypoxia or ischaemia in the fetus' and there is no doubt that most instances of placental infarcts or thrombi are not associated with fetal brain damage.

Burke and Tannenberg (1995) studied ischaemic cerebral injuries in stillborn infants, mainly damage to the periventricular white matter, and found these to be significantly related to placental infarction, a lesion that they equate with reduced maternal uteroplacental blood flow.

It is my view that whilst it is undoubtedly of interest and importance to study placentas from brain-damaged infants, we currently know too little about the true nature of antenatal cerebral injury to be able to draw any conclusions from these studies. It is fully acceptable to place emphasis on cord lesions as possible aetiological factors in antenatal brain damage. I would not, however, regard it as a scientifically tenable hypothesis to suggest that the placental lesions noted in these studies caused the brain damage whilst if it is implied that the placental lesions are, in many cases, simply the visible hallmark of an inadequate or compromised maternal uteroplacental circulation, it is surprising that none of the women in Grafe's study suffered from pre-eclampsia. Indeed, there is no clear relationship between cerebral damage and pre-eclampsia.

FETAL HYPOXIA

Obstetricians (and unfortunately sometimes lawyers) not uncommonly pose three questions to pathologists who undertake examination of a placenta from cases in which there has been definite or suspected fetal hypoxia. These are:

1. Does placental examination reveal evidence of fetal hypoxia?
2. If there is evidence of fetal hypoxia does placental examination indicate whether this is acute or chronic?
3. Is there a placental lesion present which could be considered as a causal factor in the development of fetal hypoxia?

In the past it was thought that meconium staining of the placenta and extra-placental membranes was indicative of intrauterine fetal hypoxia but, as discussed in Chapter 16, this view is no longer tenable, there being no clear correlation between the passage of meconium and fetal blood gas levels. A more realistic indicator of fetal hypoxia is the presence of a significant number of nucleated red blood cells in the fetal blood in the villous vessels. It is, of course, the case that nucleated erythrocytes are often present in the fetal blood in pregnancies complicated by fetal hydrops, in cases of feto-maternal haemorrhage and in some infections but in the absence of such complications any obvious excess of nucleated fetal red blood cells in a term placenta is usually, probably invariably, an indication of fetal hypoxia. Anderson (1941) counted 1000 fetal red cells in each of 260 placentas from uncomplicated pregnancies and found nucleated erythrocytes in 16.5% of term placentas, the number of such cells being one, or at most two, per 1000 red blood cells. He noted an increased number of nucleated red cells in the placentas of fresh stillbirths and commented that a 'decided increase points to pathologic states'. In my own study I found that nucleated erythrocytes were present in a quite high proportion of placentas from term infants but that in the absence of clinically detectable fetal hypoxia there was rarely more than one such cell per 1000 erythrocytes, a high nucleated red blood cell count being clearly associated with fetal hypoxia (Fox, 1967a).

Since then it has been widely accepted that an excess of nucleated fetal erythrocytes in the fetal vessels of the placenta is, in the absence of other factors that might cause increased haematopoietic activity, an indication of fetal hypoxia (Altshuler & Herman, 1989; Green & Mimouni, 1990; Salafia, 1992; Altshuler, 1993b; Benirschke, 1994; Benirschke & Kaufmann, 1995). The question then arises as to the duration of the time interval between an episode of fetal hypoxia and the appearance of nucleated red cells in the fetal blood. It is usually assumed that the release of nucleated erythrocytes into the fetal circulation is mediated by a rise in fetal serum erythropoietin levels (Maier et al, 1993) and in experimental studies fetal serum erythropoietin levels begin to rise at about 3 hours after an episode of induced fetal hypoxia (Widness et al, 1993). Salafia (1992) claims that the fetal bone marrow is relatively sluggish in its response to stress and that it takes at least 24 hours for nucleated erythrocytes to appear in the circulation, their presence therefore being indicative of chronic rather than acute hypoxia. It is, however, by no means certain that the appearance of nucleated erythrocytes in the fetal circulation is mediated entirely by increased erythropoietin levels. Benirschke (1994) has recorded a case in which nucleated red cells appeared within the fetal circulation within 1 hour of an episode of fetal bleeding. It is extremely unlikely that the appearance of these cells within such a short period could be mediated by erythropoietin and it is likely that there had been a sudden hypoxia-induced release of nucleated red cells sequestrated within the spleen and liver, this being perhaps not an unexpected process. Hence although the presence of nucleated red cells in fetal blood is a good indicator of fetal hypoxia it does not, in my view, provide any reliable information about the timing, or the duration, of such hypoxia.

Placental lesions can be held responsible for fetal hypoxia under some circumstances, all in my opinion rare. Thus maternal floor infarction, very extensive fetal artery thrombosis, large chorangiomas and large retroplacental haematomas can all, on occasion, be regarded as causal factors in the production of fetal hypoxia as can, probably much more importantly, umbilical cord lesions. It is, however, doubtful if any other intrinsic placental abnormalities can be held responsible for inadequate fetal oxygenation. Fetal hypoxia occurs most commonly in association with uteroplacental ischaemia due to inadequate conversion of placental bed spiral arteries to uteroplacental vessels and under these circumstances the decreased ability of the mother to supply an adequate supply of oxygen to the fetus is almost certainly the major factor in the production of fetal hypoxia. It is true that not everyone shares this opinion because Salafia et al (1995) found no correlation between a decidual vasculopathy and fetal hypoxia, considering that it is the placental damage caused by the uteroplacental ischaemia, and not the vascular abnormality itself, which is responsible for the fetal hypoxia. This view tends to ignore the massive functional reserve capacity of the placenta, the ability of the placenta to mount compensatory mechanisms to an unfavourable maternal milieu and the fact that relying on the examination of basal plate vessels, rather than placental bed biopsies, is a suboptimal method of assessing the adequacy of the maternal uteroplacental circulation.

IMMUNE HYDROPS: HAEMOLYTIC DISEASE OF THE NEONATE AS A RESULT OF MATERNO-FETAL RHESUS INCOMPATIBILITY

The first detailed and accurate description of placental morphology in materno-fetal rhesus incompatibility was written by Hellman and Hertig nearly 60 years ago (Hellman & Hertig, 1938). Subsequent reports of the placental changes in this condition included those of Henderson (1942), Javert (1942), Schmidt (1949), Bichenbach and Kivel (1950), King (1951), Respetti and Pescetto (1951), Martius (1956), Chernyak and Rabtsevich (1959), Thomsen and Berle (1960), Becker and Bleyl (1961), Marziale (1961), Calderon et al (1963), de Cecco et al (1963), Zacks and Blazar (1963), Wentworth (1967), Liebhart (1969, 1973), Busch and Vogel (1972), and Holzl et al (1975) and these succeeded in achieving a considerable, though not absolutely complete, measure of agreement about the outstanding characteristics of the placenta (this being by no means a common occurrence in studies of placental pathology). In recent years the successful prophylaxis of this disease, allied to the effective intrauterine treatment of those cases that escape immunoprophylaxis, has resulted in a marked decrease in interest in the placenta in materno-fetal rhesus isoimmunization with a corresponding decline in the number of studies devoted to this topic.

The description given here is of the placental changes in materno-fetal rhesus isoimmunization but identical changes are seen in placentas from cases of other types of immune hydrops such as those due to ABO isoimmunization or anti-Kell antibodies.

Macroscopic Features

Many placentas from cases of materno-fetal rhesus incompatibility appear normal to the naked eye, whilst others, though of normal size and weight, show a varying degree of pallor which may occasionally be of an extreme degree (Fig. 9.5). A proportion are unduly heavy and bulky, and although these are usually strikingly pale and often overtly oedematous, they may be of virtually normal colour and texture. Those placentas that are unduly pallid may present a homogeneous appearance, but they more commonly have a rather variegated pattern in which there is a patchwork of alternating dark and pale areas. It is usual to class the very bulky, oedematous placentas as 'hydropic', and there is no doubt that placentas meriting this description are encountered. However, it has been my experience that there is an uninterrupted spectrum of placental appearances in this disease and that it is exceedingly difficult to separate a discrete group of hydropic placentas by the drawing of any sharp dividing line.

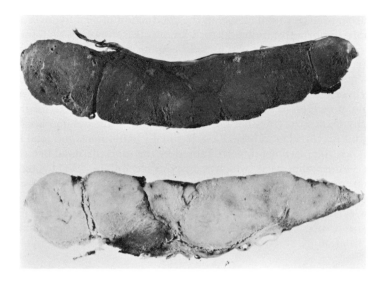

Figure 9.5. Above is a slice of placenta from an uncomplicated pregnancy, whilst below is a similar slice from a case of severe materno-fetal rhesus incompatibility; the latter shows the characteristic appearance of marked pallor.

The only gross lesion that occurs with undue frequency in these placentas is intervillous thrombosis; thrombi of this type are present in almost 50% of cases and are frequently multiple. Septal cysts are often encountered, particularly in the large oedematous placentas.

Histological Abnormalities

In a proportion of placentas from cases of materno-fetal rhesus incompatibility the villi are histologically normal in all respects, but in the majority the villi show, to a variable degree, a combination of abnormalities which, whilst being in no way specific for this disease, are nevertheless characteristic of it.

A generalized delay in villous maturation is common but is rarely of an extreme degree (Fig. 9.6); however, this is compounded by the frequent presence of groups of extremely immature villi scattered throughout the placental substance in excessive numbers. The villous syncytiotrophoblast usually appears normal on light microscopy but the cytotrophoblastic cells tend to be numerous and conspicuous; some degree of thickening of the trophoblastic basement membrane is not uncommonly seen. The villi are usually normally vascularized for their degree of maturity and I have never seen any evidence of the villous 'haemangiomatosis' which figures prominently in some descriptions of these placentas. The villous stroma is frequently oedematous (Fig. 9.7) but this change is very variable in degree, not only from placenta to placenta but from one area to another in any given placenta (Fig. 9.8); because of the oedema the stromal Hofbauer cells are easily apparent but I would not, unlike others (Pilz et al, 1980), consider that their number is increased. Stromal oedema is by no means, however, an invariable finding in these placentas (Fig. 9.9), and quite often the stroma has a curiously glazed or 'glassy' appearance or is unusually cellular (though not fibrotic). Indeed, one of the most striking features of the placenta in rhesus incompatibility is how much the villi can vary in a single placenta, it being by no means unusual to find an intermingling of oedematous villi, villi with a glazed appearance and villi with a hypercellular stromal core. One other feature of note is the relatively frequent occurrence of villous fibrinoid necrosis, this lesion being present in excess in about a quarter of these placentas.

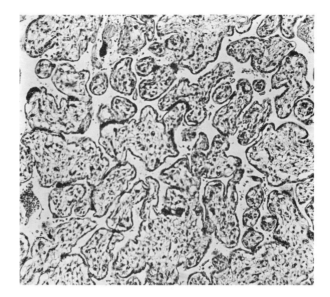

Figure 9.6. Villi in a placenta from a case of materno-fetal rhesus incompatibility. The pregnancy was terminated at the 38th week of gestation but the villi show a markedly immature appearance. There is only a minor degree of villous oedema but the villous stroma is rather cellular (H & E ×90).

Nucleated erythrocytes are commonly seen in the fetal vessels, whilst what at first sight appear to be foci of erythropoiesis may occasionally be noted. These foci are within the fetal capillaries rather than in the villous stroma (Fig. 9.10) and it is probable that they are just aggregates of highly immature fetal red cells rather than true areas of erythropoiesis.

It has often been claimed that the fetal stem arteries show an 'obliterative endarteritis' in rhesus incompatibility (Sansone & Pescetto, 1953; Martius, 1956; Burstein & Blumenthal, 1962; de Cecco et al, 1963), but in my own material the incidence of this vascular abnormality was not significantly higher than in placentas from uncomplicated pregnancies (Fox, 1967b).

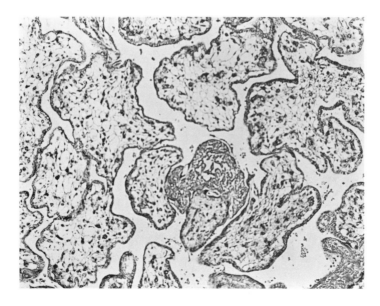

Figure 9.7. Villous oedema in a placenta from a case of materno-fetal rhesus incompatability (H & E ×90).

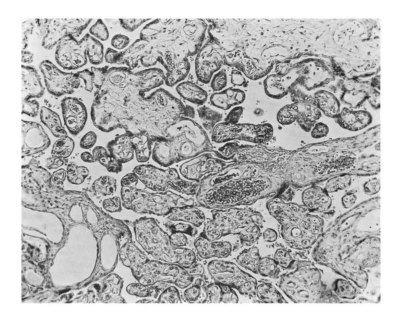

Figure 9.8. Villi in a placenta from a case of materno-fetal rhesus incompatability. In this placenta there was marked regional variation in the degree of villous oedema; thus the villi in the lower part of the field are virtually oedema-free, whilst those in the upper part of the field are markedly oedematous (H & E ×90).

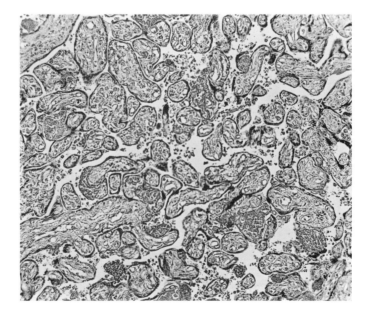

Figure 9.9. Villi in a placenta from a case of severe haemolytic disease of the neonate resulting from materno-fetal rhesus incompatibility. The pregnancy was terminated at the 37th week of gestation but, despite the severity of the haemolytic disease, the villi are not oedematous (H & E ×90).

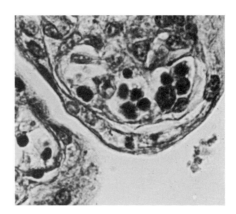

Figure 9.10. A focus of 'erythropoiesis' in a fetal villous vessel in a placenta from a case of materno-fetal rhesus incompatibility (H & E ×700).

Ultrastructural Changes

Placentas from cases of materno-fetal rhesus incompatibility have been infrequently submitted to electron-optical examination (Arnold et al, 1961; Zacks & Blazar, 1963; Widmaier, 1969; Liebhart, 1971). Jones and Fox (1978), in an electron microscopic study, noted occasional small foci of syncytial necrosis, local loss or distortion of the syncytial microvilli, focal dilatation of syncytiotrophoblastic endoplasmic reticulum, an abundance of villous cytotrophoblastic cells (some showing mitotic activity) and irregular thickening of the trophoblastic basement membrane: no evidence was seen of immune complex deposition.

General Comments

The pathogenesis of the placental changes in materno-fetal rhesus incompatibility is, for the most part, wreathed in obscurity. In cases in which the fetus is hydropic it seems reasonable to assume that the placental oedema is simply a manifestation of the generalized accumulation of fluid in the fetal tissues, presumably as a result of heart failure. Having said that, the nature of the other changes must be largely a matter for speculation. In many cases, much of the increased bulk of the placenta is independent of oedema and appears to be due to a true hyperplasia of the villous tree. Thus, histological examination shows an abundance of very young, freshly formed villi, and this impression of burgeoning growth has been confirmed by microdissection studies (Crawford, 1959) and by autoradiographic analysis of trophoblastic DNA synthesis (Kaltenbach et al, 1974). It is clearly tempting to regard this increased growth activity as a mechanism to compensate for the fetal anaemia, especially as the placental findings in rhesus incompatibility may be closely mimicked in cases of fetal anaemia due to other causes, e.g., chronic feto-maternal haemorrhage or alpha-thalassaemia. Similar placental changes can, however, be encountered in other circumstances in which the fetus is not necessarily anaemic, e.g., syphilis, toxoplasmosis and metastasizing neuroblastoma, and it is difficult to understand how many of the other features of the placenta in rhesus incompatibility, such as syncytial necrosis or trophoblastic basement thickening, could be attributed to fetal anaemia. There are no grounds for believing that the maternal uteroplacental vasculature is in any way abnormal in rhesus incompatibility but the possibility that the increase in villous size (resulting from immaturity and oedema) decreases the capacity of the intervillous space and thus limits the maternal blood flow through the placenta has been canvassed (Alvarez et al, 1972): this is, I suppose, possible but unlikely.

Haemolytic disease of the neonate due to rhesus incompatibility is, of course, an immunological disease, and the question therefore arises as to whether some, or even all, of the placental changes in this condition are immunologically mediated. It is possible to envisage the placenta as containing D-antigen and thus serving as a site for antibody attack, and over the years there have been several claims to have detected D-antigen in placental tissue (Boorman & Dodd, 1943; Kaser, 1947; Preisler, 1958; Bazso & Gyongyossy, 1959; Pozzi & Marzetti, 1962). Burstein et al (1963) have maintained that fluorescein-labelled anti-D localizes on villous basement membranes and the walls of the fetal stem arteries of placentas from rhesus-positive infants of rhesus-negative mothers. Martius (1956) and Dordelmann (1963), however, were unable to detect D-antigen in placental tissue. Most of the studies claiming positive results used techniques that would not nowadays be classed as technically immaculate, and today it is widely accepted that rhesus antigens are found only on erythrocytes and are thus tissue-specific alloantigens (Bagshawe & Lawler, 1975). A possible alternative could be that immune complexes are deposited in the placenta from the fetal circulation, but Jones and Fox (1978) made a specific ultrastructural search for such complexes, which proved fruitless.

Irrespective of how the placental abnormalities are produced, there must be an assumption that the placenta is probably not functioning at an optimal capacity in materno-fetal rhesus incompatibility, if only because the villi so often show a delay in maturation. I doubt, however, if I would go as far as Bender (1974), who considers that the placenta in this condition can be taken as a model for 'placental insufficiency', and I would be surprised if any inadequacy of placental function contributed to the relatively high fetal death rate which used to be the rule in materno-fetal rhesus incompatibility. This statement is based largely on the fact that any defects in trophoblastic capacity resulting from an arrest of villous maturation are probably sufficiently compensated for by the increased growth of the placenta.

NON-IMMUNE HYDROPS

There are numerous causes of non-immune fetal hydrops, these including cardiac lesions, chromosomal abnormalities, infections, fetal neoplasms, metabolic disorders and haemoglobinopathies (Mostoufi-Zadeh et al, 1985; Machin, 1989; Harahan et al, 1991; Boyd & Keeling, 1992; Keeling, 1993; McCoy et al, 1995): in a significant proportion of cases, however, no cause for the hydrops can be identified. In such cases the placenta is usually, though not invariably, also hydropic and, irrespective of aetiology, the placental appearances resemble closely those seen in severe materno-fetal rhesus isoimmunization, apart from the absence in some cases of nucleated red blood cells. In some instances specific features, such as neuroblastomatous cells in fetal villous vessels or the intranuclear inclusions of parvovirus in fetal red cells, may serve as aetiological clues but in most cases the pathologist will not be able either to achieve a specific diagnosis or make a distinction, on purely morphological grounds, from an immune hydrops.

Alpha-thalassaemia

The placenta of a child afflicted with this condition can show a variety of appearances, ranging from near normality to a very close mimicry of the appearances seen in severe erythroblastosis fetalis. Sometimes the degree of hydropic change in the placenta is extreme.

Congenital Nephrosis

Placentas from infants with this form of renal disease are usually, but far from invariably, bulky, pale and oedematous. Histological examination (Fig. 9.11) confirms the well-marked villous oedema and shows that the villi are usually unduly immature for the length of the gestational period (Kouvalainen et al, 1962; Faulk et al, 1974; Hung et al, 1977). Inferrera et al (1980) studied a placenta from an infant with this

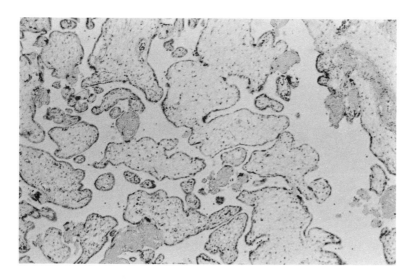

Figure 9.11. Villi in a placenta from a child with congenital nephrotic syndrome. The villi are immature and oedematous (H & E ×60).

form of renal disease in which the villi appeared immature but otherwise normal on light microscopy. At the ultrastructural level the only abnormality was an irregular nodular thickening of the trophoblastic basement membrane. This prompted their suggestion that in this condition there is production of abnormal basement membranes both in the placenta and in the renal glomeruli. Kaplan et al (1985), however, found no abnormality, apart from mild villous oedema, on light and electron microscopy of several placentas from congenitally nephrotic infants.

METABOLIC STORAGE DISEASES

Several fetal metabolic storage diseases can be detected on placental examination. At the light microscopic level these usually present a non-specific appearance (or, at least, a non-diagnostic appearance) with foamy vacuolation of the villous trophoblast, stromal cells and Hofbauer cells. Cozzutto (1983) has suggested that care must be taken to distinguish this change from non-specific pseudo-vacuolation caused by placental oedema but Benirschke and Kaufmann (1995) have maintained, correctly in my view, that this type of fine vacuolation is never seen in oedematous placentas from infants without a storage disorder. A specific diagnosis of the particular type of fetal metabolic storage disease rests, however, upon electron microsopy, biochemical analysis and the use of molecular probes directed specifically against the storage material.

Sphingomyelin Lipidosis

Niemann–Pick Disease

Sarrut and Belamich (1983) reported syncytial vacuolation in placentas from infants with Niemann–Pick disease and Jones et al (1990), in their electron microscopic study, described gross accumulations of material in the form of laminated inclusions or myelin bodies in all components of the placental villi, including cytotrophoblast, syncytiotrophoblast, stromal cells and Hofbauer cells (Fig. 9.12). The number of these accumulations was such as to cause marked cellular swelling and distortion. These myelin bodies stain positively for unesterified cholesterol with filipin (Vanier et al, 1989).

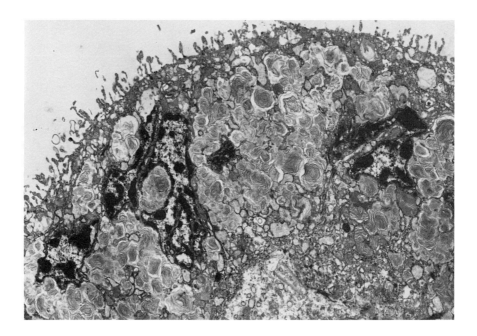

Figure 9.12. Electronmicrograph of villous syncytiotrophoblast in a placenta from a fetus with Niemann–Pick disease. Numerous laminated inclusions are present in the syncytial cytoplasm (×3610).

GM₁ Gangliosidosis

Lowden et al (1973) described vacuolation of the villous syncytiotrophoblast in the placenta of a fetus with GM$_1$-gangliosidosis, and thought that this was indicative of storage of ganglioside within the villous syncytiotrophoblast. They identified the absence of beta-galactosidase within the villous tissue. Roberts et al (1991) noted vacuolation of the syncytiotrophoblast, cytotrophoblast and Hofbauer cells in a similar case but Benirschke and Kaufmann (1995) consider that the characteristic feature of this disease is amniotic, rather than syncytial, vacuolation.

GM₂ Gangliosidoses

Tay–Sachs' Disease (Type I)

Electron microscopy of the placenta in cases of Tay–Sachs' disease shows marked syncytial vacuolation (Fig. 9.13) with the apical vacuoles containing membranous inclusions (Jones et al, 1990).

Sandhoff's Disease (Type II)

The most striking feature on electron-optical examination of a placenta from a fetus with this disease was the occurrence of multiple parallel arrays in occasional lysosomes within stromal cells. The villous syncytiotrophoblast was vacuolated and contained occasional myelin bodies (Fig. 9.14).

Glycogenosis

Glycogen Storage Disease Type II (Pompe's)

Bendon and Hug (1985) described vacuolated glycogen-containing amniotic stromal cells on light microscopy of a placenta from a child with type II glycogen storage

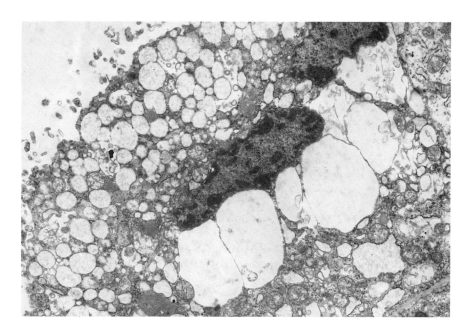

Figure 9.13. Electronmicrograph of villous trophoblast in a placenta from a fetus with Tay–Sachs' disease: the syncytium is highly vacuolated (×5740).

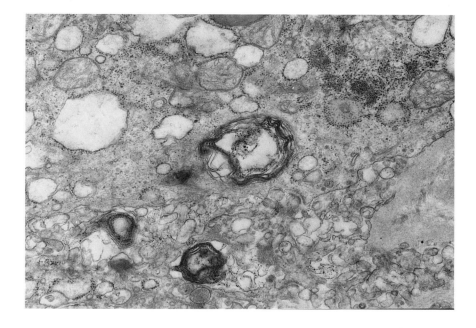

Figure 9.14. Electronmicrograph of villous syncytial cytoplasm in a placenta from a fetus with Sandhoff's disease. The cytoplasm is vacuolated and occasional myelin bodies are present (×25,500).

disease. Electron microsopy of this placenta, and of material from other cases, showed membrane-bound vacuoles full of glycogen in villous stromal, cytotrophoblastic and endothelial cells whilst unbound cytoplasmic rosettes were also seen. Jones et al (1990) confirmed the accumulation of glycogen within lysosomes in these sites (Fig. 9.15).

Mucopolysaccharidoses

Hurler's Disease (Type I)

On electron-optical examination the principal feature of placentas from fetuses with this disease is vacuolation of stromal fibroblasts (Fig. 9.16) and pericytes (Jones et al, 1990): syncytial vacuolation is also seen.

Sanfilippo Disease (Type IIIA)

Jones et al (1990) studied a placenta from a term infant with this disorder and noted vacuolated syncytial cytoplasm and membranous whorls on the basal surface of the syncytiotrophoblast. This was a poorly fixed placenta, however, and this changes may have been degenerative in nature.

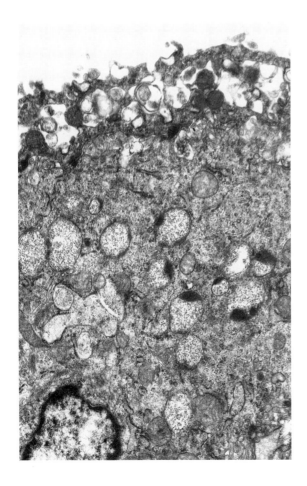

Figure 9.15. Electronmicrograph of villous trophoblast in a placenta from a fetus with Pompe's disease. Intralysosomal accumulations of glycogen are present in a cytotrophoblastic cell (×14,450).

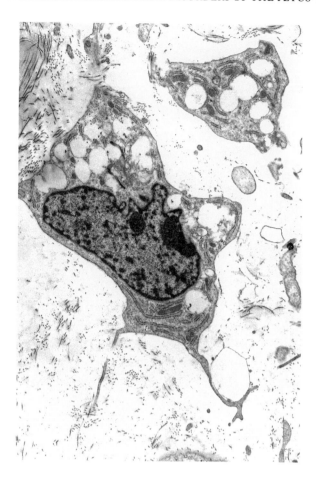

Figure 9.16. Electron-micrograph of a vacuolated villous stromal cell in a placenta from a fetus with Hurler's disease (×5780).

Morquio's Disease (Type IVA)

Marked villous oedema has been noted in the placenta of a child with this disease but there were no features suggestive of storage products in the trophoblast (Applegarth et al, 1987).

Beta-Glucuronidase Deficiency (Type VII)

Nelson et al (1993) described cytoplasmic vacuolation of the villous Hofbauer cells in a hydropic placenta from a stillborn fetus thought to have beta-glucuronidase deficiency.

Sialic Acid Storage Disease

In this fetal disorder the syncytiotrophoblast is packed with membrane-bound vacuoles which contain amorphous or fibrillary material (Fig. 9.17). Similar inclusions are also present in the Hofbauer and endothelial cells (Jauniaux et al, 1987; Jones et al, 1990).

Mucolipidoses

Mucolipidosis Type I (Sialidosis)

Foamy changes in the syncytiotrophoblast and stromal cells in a term placenta from an infant suffering from sialidosis were noted by Riches and Smuckler (1983)

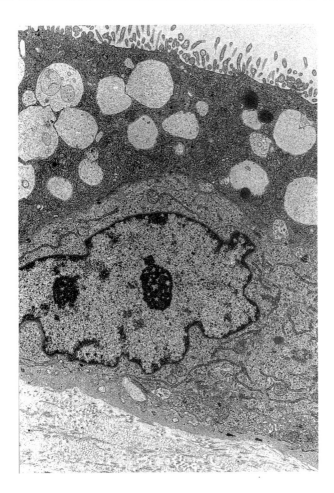

Figure 9.17. Electron-micrograph of villous trophoblast in a placenta from a fetus with sialic acid storage disease. The syncytium is packed with vacuoles whilst the cytotrophoblastic cell is not affected (×6170).

whilst Laver et al (1983) and Mahmood and Haleem (1989) described vacuolation of the syncytiotrophoblast and Hofbauer cells in similar cases.

Mucolipidosis Type II (I Cell Disease)

Powell et al (1976) noted foamy changes in the cytoplasm of the syncytiotrophoblast, extravillous cytotrophoblast and villous Hofbauer cells in the large, pale placenta of a fetus with mucolipidosis type II: no vacuolation was seen in decidual cells. Similar findings were noted by Sarrut and Belamich (1983) whilst Rapola and Aula (1977) demonstrated extensive fine vacuolation of the villous syncytiotrophoblast on electron microscopy of a placenta from a 19-week gestation.

Mucolipidosis Type IV

Sekeles et al (1978) described foamy villous stromal cells in a placenta from a fetus with this condition and also noted the presence of lamellar inclusions within villous endothelial cells.

Neuronal Ceroid Lipofuscinosis

Ultrastructural studies of placentas from cases of infantile and juvenile neuronal ceroid lipofuscinosis have demonstrated typical fingerprint inclusions in membrane-bound vacuoles in amniotic cells, endothelial cells of the villous capillaries and syncytiotrophoblast (Rapola et al, 1988; Conradi et al, 1989).

Fabry's Disease

Popli et al (1990) studied a placenta from a woman considered to be a hetero-zygous carrier of Fabry's disease. On light microscopy the only abnormality was the presence of argyrophilic granules in decidual cells. Electrom microscopy showed these to be lysosomes containing densely packed concentric lamellar inclusions.

MISCELLANEOUS DISORDERS OF THE FETUS

Anencephaly

Ten Berge (1965) has described syncytial degeneration, oedema and cavitation of the stroma in the placentas of anencephalic babies. In my own experience of such placentas, many have been fully normal, a few have been oedematous, and a small proportion have shown some degree of failure of villous maturation.

Feto-maternal Haemorrhage

Minor degrees of non-traumatic fetal bleeding into the maternal circulation occur with considerable frequency during the last trimester (Renaer et al, 1976), but there may occasionally be a spontaneous massive transfusion of fetal blood into the maternal circulation and this can lead to intrauterine death, intrauterine hypoxia, abnormal fetal heart rhythyms, fetal hydrops or neonatal anaemia (Renaer et al, 1976; Laube & Schauberger, 1982; Fay, 1983; Clark & Miller, 1984; Bacevice et al, 1985; Fliegner et al, 1987; Willis & Foreman, 1988; Catalano & Capeless, 1990; Fischer et al, 1990; Rouse & Weiner, 1990; Kosasa et al, 1993; Almeida & Bowman, 1994). The placenta is of normal size and appearance in many such cases, but in a small proportion it is hydropic and may resemble that of the infant with erythroblastosis fetalis. There is a statistical rela-tionship between feto-maternal bleeding and the presence of intervillous thrombi, pla-cental infarcts and retroplacental haematomas (Wentworth, 1964; Banti Devi et al, 1968) whilst feto-maternal bleeding can complicate a large chorangioma. It is very unusual, however, to be able to detect any obvious direct source for a massive feto-maternal haemorrhage.

Beckwith–Wiedemann Syndrome

Lage (1991) described four placentas with massive hydrops of the stem villi: one placenta was from an infant with Beckwith–Wiedemann syndrome whilst two were from infants with features suggestive of this syndrome, the fourth fetus being frag-mented. Subsequently McCowen and Becroft (1994) described placentomegaly in three cases of Beckwith–Wiedemann syndrome. Histologically there was stromal expansion of the villous tree and in one placenta there was cystic change in many of the stem villi. These changes appear to be characteristic of, possibly specific for, Beckwith–Wiedemann syndrome, to the extent that they allow for ultrasound diagnosis of this condition (Hillstrom et al, 1995).

REFERENCES

Adamson, S.J., Alessandri, L.M., Badawi, P.R. et al (1995) Predictors of neonatal encephalopathy in full term infants. *British Medical Journal*, **311**, 598–602.
Agboola, A. (1975) Placental changes in patients with a low haematocrit. *British Journal of Obstetrics and Gynaecology*, **82**, 225–227.
Aherne, W. and Dunnill, M.S. (1966) Quantitative aspects of placental structure. *Journal of Pathology and Bacteriology*, **91**, 123–139.
Almeida, V. de and Bowman, J.M. (1994) Massive fetomaternal hemorrhage: Manitoba experience. *Obstetrics and Gynecology*, **83**, 323–328.

Althabe, D., Laberrere, C. and Telenta, M. (1985) Maternal vascular lesions in placentae of small-for-gestational-age infants. *Placenta*, **6**, 369–373.

Altshuler, G. (1993a) Some placental considerations related to neurodevelopmental and other disorders. *Journal of Child Neurology*, **8**, 78–94.

Altshuler, G. (1993b) A conceptual approach to placental pathology and pregnancy outcome. *Seminars in Diagnostic Pathology*, **10**, 204–221.

Altshuler, G. and Herman, A.A. (1989) The medicolegal imperative: placental pathology and epidemiology. In *Fetal and Neonatal Brain Injury: Mechanisms, Management and the Risks of Practice*, Stevenson, D.K. and Sunshine, P. (Eds), pp. 250–263. Philadelphia: Decker.

Altshuler G. and Hyde, S. (1989) Meconium induced vasoconstriction: a potential cause of cerebral and other fetal hypo-perfusion and of poor pregnancy outcome. *Child Neurology*, **4**, 137–142.

Altshuler, G., Russell, P. and Ermocilla, R. (1975) The placental pathology of small-for-gestational age infants. *American Journal of Obstetrics and Gynecology*, **121**, 351–359.

Alvarez, H., Sala, M.A. and Benedetti, W.L. (1972) Intervillous space reduction in the edematous placenta. *American Journal of Obstetrics and Gynecology*, **112**, 819–820.

Anderson, G.W. (1941) Studies on the nucleated red cell count in the chorionic capillaries and the cord blood of various ages of pregnancy. *American Journal of Obstetrics and Gynecology*, **42**, 1–14.

Applegarth, D.A., Toone, J.R., Wilson, R.D., Long, S.L. and Baldwin, V.J. (1987) Morquio disease presenting as hydrops fetalis and enzyme analysis of chorionic villus tissue in a subsequent pregnancy. *Pediatric Pathology*, **7**, 593–599.

Arnold, M., Geller, H.F. and Sasse, D. (1961) Beitrag zur elektronenmikroskopischen Morphologie der menschlichen Placenta. *Archiv für Gynäkologie*, **196**, 238–253.

Bacevice, A.E., Dierker, L.J. and Wolfson, R.N. (1985) Intrauterine atrial fibrillation associated with feto-maternal hemorrhage. *American Journal of Obstetrics and Gynecology*, **153**, 81–82.

Bagshawe, K. and Lawler, S. (1975) The immunogenicity of the placenta and trophoblast. In *Immunobiology of Trophoblast*, Edwards, R.G., Howe, C.W.S. and Johnson, M.H. (Eds), pp. 171–182. London: Cambridge University Press.

Banti Devi, Jennison, R.F. and Langley, F.A. (1968) Significance of placental pathology in transplacental haemorrhage. *Journal of Clinical Pathology*, **21**, 322–331.

Barker, J.D.P. (1994) Fetal growth and adult disease. In *Early Fetal Growth and Development*, Ward, R.H.T., Smith, S.K. and Donnai, D. (Eds), pp. 197–209. London: RCOG Press.

Bazso, J. and Gaal, J. (1965) Histologische Untersuchungen der Plazenta bei im intrauterinen Wachstum zuruckgebliebenen Neugeborenen. *Zentralblatt für Gynäkologie*, **87**, 1356–1366.

Bazso, J. and Gyongyossy, A. (1959) Experimentelle Untersuchungen über den Rh-antigen-Gehalt der Plazenta. *Zentralblatt für Gynäkologie*, **81**, 1507–1513.

Becker, V. and Bleyl, U. (1961) Placentarzotte bei Schwangerschaftstoxikose und fetaler Erythroblastose im fluorescenzmikroskopischen Bilde. *Virchows Archiv für pathologischen Anatomie und Physiologie und für klinische Medizin*, **334**, 516–527.

Becker, V. and Dolling, D. (1965) Gefässverschlüsse in der Placenta von Totgeborenen. *Virchows Archiv für pathologischen Anatomie und Physiologie und für klinische Medizin*, **338**, 305–314.

Beischer, N.A., Sivasamboo, R., Vohra, S., Silpisornkosal, S. and Reid, S. (1970) Placental hypertrophy in severe pregnancy anaemia. *Journal of Obstetrics and Gynaecology of the British Commonwealth*, **77**, 398–409.

Bejar, R., Wozniak, P., Alard, M. et al (1988) Antenatal origin of neurologic damage in newborn infants. *American Journal of Obstetrics and Gynecology*, **159**, 357–363.

Bender, H.G. (1974) Placenta-Insuffizienz: morphometrische Untersuchungen am Modell der Rhesus-Placenta. *Archiv für Gynäkologie*, **216**, 289–300.

Bender, H.G., Werner, C., Kortmann, H.R. and Becker, V. (1976) Zue Endangitisobliterans der Plazentagefässe. *Archiv für Gynäkologie*, **221**, 145–159.

Bendon, R.W. and Hug, G. (1985) Morphologic characteristics of the placenta in glycogen storage disease type II (alpha-1,4-glucosidase deficiency) *American Journal of Obstetrics and Gynecology*, **152**, 1021–1026.

Benirschke, K. (1994) Placenta pathology: questions to the perinatologist. *Journal of Perinatology*, **14**, 371–375.

Benirschke, K. and Kaufmann, P. (1995) *Pathology of the Human Placenta*, 3rd edn. New York: Springer-Verlag.

Bewley, S.M., Cooper, D. and Campbell, S. (1991) Doppler investigation of uteroplacental blood flow resistance in the second trimester: a screening study for pre-eclampsia and intrauterine growth retardation. *British Journal of Obstetrics and Gynaecology*, **98**, 871–879.

Bichenbach, W. and Kivel, F. (1950) Mikroskopische Untersuchungen an Erythroblastose-Placenten. *Archiv für Gynäkologie*, **177**, 559–566.

Bilardo, C.M., Snijders, R.M., Campbell, S. and Nicolaides, K. (1991) Doppler study of the fetal circulation during long-term maternal hyperoxygenation for severe early onset intrauterine growth retardation. *Ultrasound in Obstetrics and Gynecology*, **1**, 250–257.

Bjoro, K.J. (1981) Gross pathology of the placenta in intrauterine growth retardation. *Annales Chirurgiae et Gynecologiae Fennae*, **70**, 316–322.

Bjoro, K.J. and Myhre, E. (1984) The role of chronic non-specific inflammatory lesions of the placenta in intrauterine growth retardation. *Acta Pathologica Microbiologica et Immunologica Scandinavica*, **92**, 133–137.

Boorman, K.E. and Dodd, B.E. (1943) The group specific substances A, B, M, N, and Rh: their occurrence in tissues and body fluids. *Journal of Pathology and Bacteriology*, **55**, 329–339.

Botella-Llusia, J. (1961) Über das Syndrom der Plazentarinsuffizienz und seine Bedeutung für die praktische Geburtshilfe. *Deutsches Medizinisches Journal*, **12**, 543–546.

Boyd, P.A. and Keeling, J.W. (1992) Fetal hydrops. *Journal of Medical Genetics*, **29**, 91–97.

Boyd, P.A. and Scott, A. (1985) Quantitative structural studies on human placentae associated with preeclampsia, essential hypertension and intrauterine growth retardation. *British Journal of Obstetrics and Gynaecology*, **92**, 714–721.

Bracero, L.A., Beneck, D., Kirshenbaum, N. et al (1989) Doppler velocimetry and placental disease. *American Journal of Obstetrics and Gynecology*, **161**, 388–393.

Brosens, I., Dixon, H.G. and Robertson, W.B. (1977) Fetal growth retardation and the vasculature of the placental bed. *British Journal of Obstetrics and Gynaecology*, **84**, 656–664.

Browne, J.C.M. and Veall, N. (1953) The maternal-placental blood flow in normotensive and hypertensive women. *Journal of Obstetrics and Gynaecology of the British Empire*, **60**, 141–147.

Burke, C.J. and Tannenberg, A.E. (1995) Prenatal brain damage and placental infarction – an autopsy study. *Developmental Medicine and Childhood Neurology*, **37**, 555–562.

Burstein, R.H. and Blumenthal, H.T. (1962) Vascular lesions of the placenta of possible immunogenic origin in erythroblastosis fetalis. *American Journal of Obstetrics and Gynecology*, **83**, 1062–1068.

Burstein, R., Berns, A.W., Hirata, Y. and Blumenthal, H.T. (1963) A comparative histo- and immunopathological study of the placenta in diabetes mellitus and in erythroblastosis fetalis. *American Journal of Obstetrics and Gynecology*, **86**, 66–76.

Busch, W. (1972) Die Placenta bei der fetalen Mangelentwicklung. Makroskopie und Mikroskopie von 150 Placenten fetaler Mangelentwicklungen. *Archiv für Gynäkologie*, **212**, 333–357.

Busch, W. (1974) Das fetale Risiko bei chronischer nutritiver Placentainsuffizienz unterschiedlicher Pathogenese. *Archiv für Gynäkologie*, **216**, 167–174.

Busch, W. and Vogel, M. (1972) Die Plazenta beim 'Morbus haemolyticus neonatorum'. *Zeitschrift für Geburtshilfe und Perinatologie*, **176**, 17–28.

Calderon, M.J.J., Maqueo, T.M. and Torres, T. (1963) Correlacion entre alteraciones placentarias y del producto en eritroblastosis fetal. *Ginecologia y Obstetricia de México*, **18**, 373–382.

Carter, A.M. (1983) Current topic: restriction of placental and fetal growth in the guinea-pig. *Placenta*, **14**, 125–135.

Catalano, P.M. and Capeless, E.L. (1990) Fetomaternal bleeding as a cause of recurrent fetal morbidity and mortality. *Obstetrics and Gynecology*, **76**, 972–973.

Charlton, V. and Johenge, M. (1988) Fetal intravenous nutritional supplements ameliorates the development of embolized induced growth retardation in sheep. *Pediatric Research*, **22**, 55–61.

Chernyak, A.A. and Rabtsevich, T.S. (1959) Pathomorphological changes in the placenta in Rhesus incompatibility of maternal and fetal blood. *Akusherstvo i Ginekologiya* (Moscow), **1**, 30–34.

Claap, J.F. (1994) Physiological adaptation to intrauterine growth retardation. In *Early Fetal Growth and Development*, Ward, R.H.T., Smith, S.K. and Donnai, D. (Eds), pp. 371–383. London: RCOG Press.

Clark, S.L. and Miller, F.C. (1984) Sinusoidal fetal heart rate pattern associated with massive fetomaternal transfusion. *American Journal of Obstetrics and Gynecology*, **149**, 97–99.

Clavero-Nunez, J.A. (1963) La placenta de las cardiacas. *Revista Espanola de Obstetricia y Ginecologia*, **22**, 129–134.

Clavero-Nunez, J.A., Negueruela, J. and Botella-Llusia, J. (1971) Placental morphometry and placental circulometry. *Journal of Reproductive Medicine*, **6**, 23–31.

Conradi, N.G., Uvebrant, P., Hokegard, K.-H., Wahlstrom, J. and Mellqvist, L (1989) First trimester diagnosis of juvenile neuronal ceroid lipofuscinosis by demonstration of fingerprint inclusions in chorionic villi. *Prenatal Diagnosis*, **9**, 283–287.

Cooke, R.W.I. (1990) Cerebral palsy in very low birth weight infants. *Archives of Disease in Childhood*, **65**, 201–206.

Cozzutto, C. (1983) Foamy degeneration of placenta. *Virchows Archiv A Pathological Anatomy and Histopathology*, **401**, 363–368.

Crawford, J.M. (1959) A study of human placental growth with observations on the placenta in erythroblastosis foetalis. *Journal of Obstetrics and Gynaecology of the British Empire*, **66**, 885–896.

Davies, J. and Glasser, S.R. (1967) Light and electron microscopic observations on a human placenta 2 weeks after fetal death. *American Journal of Obstetrics and Gynecology*, **98**, 1111–1124.

de Cecco, L., Pavone, G. and Rolfini, G. (1963) La placenta umana nella isoimmunizzazione anti Rh. (Studio comparative fra gli aspetti istologici comuni e quelli microfluoroscopici.) *Quaderni di Clinica Ostetrica e Ginecologica*, **18**, 675–682.

de Rochembeau, B., Poix, D. and Mellier, G. (1992) Maternal hyperoxygenation: a fetal blood flow velocity prognosis test in small-for-gestational-age fetuses. *Ultrasound in Obstetrics and Gynecology*, **2**, 279–282.

De Wolf, F., Brosens, I. and Renaer, M. (1980) Fetal growth retardation and the maternal arterial supply of the human placenta in the absence of sustained hypertension. *British Journal of Obstetrics and Gynaecology*, **87**, 678–685.

Dordelmann, P. (1963) Zur Pathogenese des Morbus haemolyticus neonatorium. *Zeitschrift für Geburtshilfe und Gynäkologie*, **160**, 19–49.

Driscoll, S.G. (1979) Placental lesions. *Clinical Perinatology*, **6**, 397–402.

Emmrich, P. (1966a) Untersuchungen an Placenten mazerierter Totgeburten im Hinblick auf die mogliche Ursache des intrauterinen Fruchttodes. *Zeitschrift für Geburtshilfe und Gynäkologie*, **165**, 185–194.

Emmrich, P. (1966b) Morphologie und Histochemie der Placenta bei intrauterinem Fruchttod mit Mazeration. *Gynaecologia*, **162**, 241–253.

Emmrich, P. (1992) Pathologie der Plazenta. IX. Intrauteriner Fruchttod. Regression, Odem und Fibrosierung des Zotten- stromas. *Zentralblat für Pathologie*, **138**, 1–8.

Emmrich, P. and Lassker, G. (1970) Morphologische Plazentabefunde in Abhangigkeit vom Grad der intrauterinen Wachstumsretardierung bei Mangelgeburten. *Kinderärztliche Praxis*, **38**, 537–539.

Emmrich, P. and Lassker, G. (1971) Morphologische Plazentabefunde bei Neugeborenen mit intrauteriner Mangelentwicklung. *Pathologia et Microbiologia*, **37**, 57–72.

Faulk, W.P., van Loghem, E. and Stickler, G.B. (1974) Maternal antibody to fetal light chain (Inv) antigens. *American Journal of Medicine*, **56**, 393–397.

Fay, R.A. (1983) Feto-maternal haemorrhage as a cause of fetal morbidity and mortality. *British Journal of Obstetrics and Gynaecology*, **90**, 443–446.

Ferrazzi, E., Antonio, B., Gaetano, B., Laura, M. and Alessandra, P. (1994) Ischemic haemorrhagic placental damage and vascular lesions are associated with abnormal uteroplacental Doppler waveform in growth retarded fetuses. *Journal of Perinatal Medicine*, **22** (supplement 1), 73–78.

Fischer, R.L., Kuhlman, K., Grover, J., Montgomery, O. and Wapner, R.J. (1990) Chronic massive fetomaternal hemorrhage treated with repeated fetal intravascular transfusions. *American Journal of Obstetrics and Gynecology*, **162**, 203–204.

Fliegner, J.R.H., Fortune, D.W. and Barrie, J.U. (1987) Occult fetomaternal haemorrhage as a cause of fetal mortality and morbidity. *Australian and New Zealand Journal of Obstetrics and Gynaecology*, **27**, 158–161.

Fok, R.Y., Pavlova, Z., Benirschke, K., Paul, R.H. and Platt, T.D. (1990) The correlation of arterial lesions with umbilical artery Doppler velocimetry in the placentas of small-for-dates pregnancies. *Obstetrics and Gynecology*, **75**, 578–583.

Fox, H. (1967a) The incidence and significance of nucleated erythrocytes in the foetal vessels of the mature human placenta. *Journal of Obstetrics and Gynaecology of the British Commonwealth*, **74**, 40–43.

Fox, H. (1967b) Abnormalities of the fetal stem arteries in the human placenta. *Journal of Obstetrics and Gynaecology of the British Commonwealth*, **74**, 734–738.

Fox, H. (1968) Morphological changes in the human placenta following fetal death. *Journal of Obstetrics and Gynaecology of the British Commonwealth*, **75**, 839–843.

Freeman, J.M. and Nelson, K.B. (1988) Intrapartum asphyxia and cerebral palsy. *Paediatrics*, **82**, 240–249.

Frusca, T., Morassi, L., Pecorelli, S., Grigolata, P. and Gastaldi, A. (1989) Histological features of uteroplacental vessels in normal and hypertensive patients in relation to birthweight. *British Journal of Obstetrics and Gynaecology*, **96**, 835–839.

Fujikura, T. and Benson, R.C. (1964) Placentitis and fibrous occlusion of fetal vessels in the placentas of stillborn infants. *American Journal of Obstetrics and Gynecology*, **89**, 225–229.

Garcia, A.G.P. (1982) Placental morphology of low-birth-weight infants born at term: gross and microscopic study of 50 cases. *Contributions to Gynecology and Obstetrics*, **9**, 100–112.

Genest, D.R. (1992) Estimating the time of death in stillborn fetuses. II. Histologic evaluation of the placenta; a study of 71 stillborns. *Obstetrics and Gynecology*, **80**, 585–592.

Gershon, R. and Strauss, L. (1961) Structural changes in human placentas associated with fetal inanition or growth arrest ('placental insufficiency syndrome') *American Journal of Diseases of Children*, **102**, 645–646.

Giles, W.B., Trudinger, B.J. and Baird, P.J. (1985) Fetal umbilical artery flow velocity wavelengths and placental resistance: pathologic correlation. *British Journal of Obstetrics and Gynaecology*, **92**, 31–38.

Gill, R.W., Warren, P.S., Garrett, W.J., Kossoff, G. and Stewart, A. (1993) Umbilical vein blood flow. In *Ultrasound in Obstetrics and Gynecology*, Chervenak, F.A., Isaacson, G.C. and Campbell, S. (Eds), pp. 587–595. Boston: Little, Brown.

Godfrey, K.M., Redman, C.W.G., Barker, D.J.P. and Osmond C. (1991) The effect of maternal anaemia and iron deficiency on the ratio of fetal weight to placental weight. *British Journal of Obstetrics and Gynaecology*, **98**, 886–891.

Green, D.W. and Mimouni, F. (1990) Nucleated eryhthrocytes in healthy infants and in infants of diabetic mothers. *Journal of Pediatrics*, **116**, 129–131.

Gruenwald, P. (1961) Abnormalities of placental vascularity in relation to intrauterine deprivation and retardation of fetal growth: significance of avascular chorionic villi. *New York State Journal of Medicine*, **61**, 1508–1513.

Gruenwald, P. (1963) Chronic fetal distress and placental insufficiency. *Biologia Neonatorum*, **5**, 215–265.

Gruenwald, P. (1975) The supply line of the fetus: definitions relating to fetal growth. In *The Placenta and its Maternal Supply Line*, Gruenwald, P. (Ed.), pp. 1–17. Lancaster: Medical and Technical Publishing.

Gudmundsson, S. and Marsal, K. (1988) Umbilical and uteroplacental blood flow velocity waveforms in pregnancies with fetal growth retardation. *European Journal of Obstetrics, Gynecology and Reproductive Biology*, **27**, 187–196.

Harahan, D., Murphy, J.F., O'Brien, N. et al (1991) Clinico-pathological findings in non-immune hydrops fetalis. *Irish Medical Journal*, **84**, 62–63.

Hellman, L.M. and Hertig, A.T. (1938) Pathological changes in the placenta associated with erythro-blastosis of the fetus. *American Journal of Pathology*, **14**, 111–120.

Henderson, J.L. (1942) Erythroblastosis or syphilis: observations on erythroblastosis and its differential diagnosis from congenital syphilis. *Journal of Obstetrics and Gynaecology of the British Empire*, **49**, 499–511.

Hillstrom, M.M., Brown, D.L., Wilkins-Haug, L. and Genest, D.L. (1995) Sonographic appearance of placental villous hydrops associated with Beckwith–Wiedemann syndrome. *Journal of Ultrasound Medicine*, **14**, 61–64.

Hitschold, T., Weiss, E., Beck, T., Hunterfering, H. and Berle, P. (1993) Low target birthweight or growth retardation? Umbilical Doppler flow velocity waveforms and histometric analysis of the feto-placental vascular tree. *American Journal of Obstetrics and Gynecology*, **168**, 1260–1264.

Holzl, M. and Lüthje, D. (1974) Die Bedeutung pathologischer Plazentabefunde bei intrauterinem Fruchttod. *Zentralblatt für Gynäkologie*, **95**, 1481–1491.

Holzl, M., Lüthje, D. and Dietrich, H. (1975) Placentaveranderungen bei Rh Inkompatibilitat unter besonderer Berucksichtigung von Zottenreifungsstorungen. *Zentralblatt für Gynäkologie*, **97**, 859–870.

Hovatta, O., Lipasti, A., Rapola, J. and Karjalainen, O. (1983) Causes of stillbirth: a clinicopathological study of 243 patients. *British Journal of Obstetrics and Gynaecology*, **90**, 691–696.

Hung, P.L., Huang, C.C. and Huang, T.S. (1977) Nephrotic syndrome in a Chinese infant. *American Journal of Diseases of Children*, **131**, 557–559.

Hustin, J. and Gaspard, U. (1977) Comparison of histological changes seen in placental tissue cultures and in placentae obtained after fetal death. *British Journal of Obstetrics and Gynaecology*, **84**, 210–215.

Hustin, J., Foidart, J.M. and Lambotte, R. (1983) Maternal vascular lesions in pre-eclampsia and intrauterine growth retardation: light microscopy and immunofluorescence. *Placenta*, **4**, 489–498.

Inferrara, C., Barresi, G., Chimicata, S. et al. (1980) Morphologic considerations on the placenta in congenital nephrotic syndrome of Finnish type. *Virschows Archiv A Pathological Anatomy and Histology*, **389**, 13–26.

Itskovitz, J., LaGamma, E.F. and Rudolph, A.M. (1983) The effect of reducing umbilical blood flow on fetal oxygenation. *American Journal of Obstetrics and Gynecology*, **145**, 813–818.

Iwata, M., Matsuzaki, N., Shimizu, I. et al (1993) Prenatal detection of ischemic changes in the placenta of the growth-retarded fetus by Doppler flow velocimetry of the maternal uterine artery. *Obstetrics and Gynecology*, **82**, 494–499.

Jackson, M.R., Walsh, A.J., Morrow, R.J. et al (1995) Reduced placental villous tree elaboration in small-for-gestational-age newborn pregnancies: relationship with umbilical artery Doppler waveforms. *American Journal of Obstetrics and Gynecology*, **172**, 518–525.

Jacobson, S.-L., Imhof, R., Manning, M. et al (1990) The value of Doppler assessment of the uteroplacental circulation in predicting preeclampsia or intrauterine growth retardation. *American Journal of Obstetrics and Gynecology*, **162**, 110–114.

Jauniaux, E., Vamos, E., Libert, J. et al (1987) Placental electron microscopy and histochemistry in a case of sialic acid storage disease. *Placenta*, **8**, 433–442.

Javert, C.T. (1942) Erythroblastosis neonatorium: an obstetrical–pathological study of 47 cases. *Surgery, Gynecology and Obstetrics*, **74**, 1–19.

Jones, C.J.P. and Fox, H. (1978) An ultrastructural study of the placenta in materno-fetal rhesus incompatibility. *Virchows Archiv A Pathological Anatomy and Histology*, **379**, 229–241.

Jones, C.J.P., Lendon, M., Chawner, L.E. and Jauniaux, E. (1990) Ultrastructure of the human placenta in metabolic storage disease. *Placenta*, **11**, 395–411.

Kalousek, D.K. (1990) Confined placental mosaicism and intrauterine development. *Pediatric Pathology*, **10**, 69–77.

Kalousek, D.K. (1994) Current topic: confined placental mosaicism and intrauterine fetal development. *Placenta*, **15**, 219–230.

Kalousek, D.K. and Barrett, I. (1994) Confined placental mosaicism and stillbirth. *Pediatric Pathology*, **14**, 151–159.

Kalousek, D.K. and Langlois, S. (1994) The effects of placental and somatic chromosomal mosaicism on fetal growth. In *Early Fetal Growth and Development*, Ward, R.H.T., Smith, S.K. and Donnai, D. (Eds), pp. 245–256. London: RCOG Press.

Kalousek, D.K., Dill, F.J., Pantzar, D. et al (1987) Confined chorionic mosaicism in prenatal diagnosis. *Human Genetics*, **77**, 163–167.

Kaltenbach, F.J., Fettig, O. and Krieger, M.L. (1974) Autoradiographische Untersuchungen über das Proliferationsverhalten der menschlichen Placenta unter normalen und pathologischen Bedingungen. *Archiv für Gynäkologie*, **216**, 369–386.

Käser, O. (1947) Neuere Erkentnisse aus dem Gebiet der Blutgruppen und Blutfaktoren. *Gynaecologia*, **123**, 345–379.

Keeling, J.W. (1993) Fetal hydrops. In *Fetal and Neonatal Pathology*, 2nd edn, Keeling J.W. (Ed.), pp. 253–270. London: Springer-Verlag.

Kennerknecht, I., Kramer, S., Grab, D., Terinde, R. and Vogel, W. (1993) A prospective cytogenetic study of third-trimester placentae in small-for-date but otherwise normal newborns. *Prenatal Diagnosis*, **13**, 257–269.

Khong, T.Y. (1991) Acute atherosis in pregnancies complicated by hypertension, small-for-gestational-age infants and diabetes mellitus. *Archives of Pathology and Laboratory Medicine*, **115**, 722–725.

Khong, T.Y. and Robertson, W.B. (1992) Spiral artery disease. In *Immunological Obstetrics*, Coulam, C.B., Faulk, W.P. and McIntyre J.A. (Eds), pp. 492–501. New York: Norton.

Khong, T.Y., De Wolf, F., Robertson, W.B. and Brosens, I. (1986) Inadequate maternal vascular response to placentation in pregnancies complicated by pre-eclampsia and by small-for-gestational-age infants. *British Journal of Obstetrics and Gynaecology*, **93,** 1049–1059.

King, A. and Loke, Y.W. (1994) Unexplained fetal growth retardation: what is the cause? *Archives of Disease in Childhood*, **70,** F225–F227.

King, E.B. (1951) The placental findings associated with erythroblastosis fetalis. *Western Journal of Surgery, Obstetrics and Gynecology*, **59,** 192–198.

Koenig, U.D. (1972) Proliferative Gefässveranderüngen der kindlichen Plazentargefässe und ihre Beziehung zur Plazentarinsuffizienz und Frühgeburt. *Zeitschrift für Geburtshilfe und Perinatologie*, **176,** 356–364.

Koenig, U.D., Mersmann, B. and Haupt, H. (1973) Proliferative plazentare Gefässveranderüngen: Schwangerschaft und perinateler Verlauf bein Kind. *Zeitschrift für Geburtshilfe und Perinatologie*, **177,** 58–64.

Koenig, U.D., Paulussen, F. and Hansmann, M. (1975) Placentamorphologie und intrauterine Wachstummretardierung. *Archiv für Gynäkologie*, **219,** 377–378.

Kosasa, T.S., Ebesugawa, I., Nakayama, R.T. and Hale, R.W. (1993) Massive fetomaternal hemorrhage preceded by decreased fetal movement and a nonreactive fetal heart rate pattern. *Obstetrics and Gynecology*, **82,** 711–714.

Kouvalainen, K., Hjett, L. and Hallman, N. (1962) Placenta in the congenital nephrotic syndrome. *Annales Paediatrici Fenniae*, **8,** 181–188.

Kreczy, A., Fusi, L. and Wigglesworth, J.S. (1995) Correlation between umbilical arterial flow and placental morphology. *International Journal of Gynecological Pathology*, **14,** 306–309.

Kruger, H. and Arias-Stella, J. (1970) The placenta and the newborn infant at high altitudes. *American Journal of Obstetrics and Gynecology*, **106,** 586–591.

Kubli, F. and Budliger. H. (1963) Beitrag zur Morphologie der insuffizienten Placenta. *Geburtshilfe und Frauenheilkunde*, **23,** 37–43.

Labarrere, C., Althabe, O. and Telenta, M. (1982) Chronic villitis of unknown aetiology in placentae of idiopathic small for gestational age infants. *Placenta*, **3,** 309–318.

Labarrere, C., Althabe, O., Calenti, E. and Musculo, D. (1986) Deficiency of blocking factors in intrauterine growth retardation and its relationship with chronic villitis. *American Journal of Reproductive Immunology and Microbiology*, **10,** 14–19.

Lage, J.M. (1991) Placentomegaly with massive hydrops of placental stem villi, diploid DNA content, and fetal omphaloceles: possible association with Beckwith–Wiedemann syndrome. *Human Pathology*, **22,** 591–597.

Laube, D.W. and Schauberger, C.W. (1982) Fetomaternal bleeding as a cause for 'unexplained' fetal death. *Obstetrics and Gynecology*, **60,** 649–651.

Laurini, R., Laurin, J. and Marsal, K. (1994) Placental histology and fetal blood flow in intrauterine growth retardation. *Acta Obstetricia et Gynecologica Scandinavica*, **73,** 529–534.

Laver, J., Fried, K., Beer, S.I. et al (1983) Infantile lethal neuraminidase deficiency (sialidosis) *Clinical Genetics*, **23,** 97–101.

Li, B.Z. (1992) The stereological study on normal and intrauterine growth retardation (IUGR) placentae. *Chinese Journal of Pathology*, **21,** 227–228.

Liebhart, M. (1969) Obrazy histopatologiczne lozysk w przpadkach niezgodnosci serologicznej i konfliktu serologicznego. (Microscopic patterns of placenta in cases of serological incompatibility and serological conflict.) *Ginekologia Polska*, **40,** 739–749.

Liebhart, M. (1971) The ultrastructure of placental villi in cases of serological conflict in Rh-incompatibility. *Pathologia Europaea*, **6,** 415–421.

Liebhart, M. (1973) Badania porownawcze lozysk z ciaz powiklanych cukrzyca matki i konfliktem serologicznym. (A comparative study of the placental villi in pregnancy complicated by diabetes in the mother and serologic conflict.) *Patologia Polska*, **24,** 127–138.

Lin, S., Shimizu, I., Suehara, N., Nakayama, M. and Aono, T. (1995) Uterine artery Doppler velocimetry in relation to trophoblast migration into the myometrium of the placental bed. *Obstetrics and Gynecology*, **85,** 760–765.

Lister, U.M. (1969) Placental ultrastructure in dysmaturity. In *The Foeto-Placental Unit*, Pecile, A. and Finzi, C. (Eds), pp. 8–17. Amsterdam: Excerpta Medica.

Liu, Q.X. (1990) Pathology of the placenta from small for gestational age infants. *Chinese Journal of Obstetrics and Gynecology*, **25,** 331–334.

Lorijn, R.H.W. and Longo, L.D. (1980) Clinical and physiologic implications of increased fetal oxygen consumption. *American Journal of Obstetrics and Gynecology*, **136,** 451–457.

Lowden, J.A., Cutz, E., Conen, P.E., Rudd, N. and Doran, T.A. (1973) Prenatal diagnosis of Gm_1 gangliosidosis. *New England Journal of Medicine*, **288,** 225–228.

Macara, L., Kingdom, J.C.P., Kohnen, G. et al (1995) Elaboration of stem villous vessels in growth restricted pregnancies with abnormal umbilical artery Doppler waveforms. *British Journal of Obstetrics and Gynaecology*, **102,** 807–812.

Macara, L., Kingdom, J.C.P., Kaufmann, P. et al (1996) Structural analysis of placental terminal villi from growth-restricted pregnancies with abnormal umbilical artery Doppler waveforms. *Placenta*, **17,** 37–48.

McCowan, L.M., Mullen, B.M. and Ritchie, K. (1987) Umbilical artery flow velocity waveforms and the placental vascular bed. *American Journal of Obstetrics and Gynecology*, **157**, 900–902.

McCowan, L.M., Ritchie, K., Mo, L.Y. et al (1988) Uterine artery flow velocity waveforms in normal and growth retarded pregnancies. *American Journal of Obstetrics and Gynecology*, **158**, 499–504.

McCoy, M.C., Katz, V.L., Gould, N. and Kuller, J.A. (1995) Non-immune hydrops after 20 weeks' gestation: review of 10 years' experience with suggestions for management. *Obstetrics and Gynecology*, **85**, 578–582.

McFadyen, I.R., Price, A.B. and Geirsson, R.T. (1986) The relation of birth weight to histological appearances in vessels of the placental bed. *British Journal of Obstetrics and Gynaecology*, **93**, 47–51.

Machin, G.A. (1989) Hydrops revisited: literature review of 1414 cases published in the 1980s. *American Journal of Medical Genetics*, **34**, 366–390.

Mahmood, K. and Haleem, A. (1989) Placental morphology in sialidosis: report of a case. *Annals of Saudi Medicine*, **9**, 302–304.

Maier, R.F., Bohme, K., Dudenhausen, J.W. et al (1993) Cord blood erythropoietin in relation to different markers of fetal hypoxia. *Obstetrics and Gynecology*, **81**, 575–580.

Martius, G. (1956) Histologische Untersuchungen der Plazenta zur Frage der Pathogeneses des Morbus haemolyticus neonatorium. *Zentralblatt für Gynäkologie*, **78**, 2060–2065.

Marziale, P. (1961) La placenta sulla mallatia emolitica del neonato. *Clinica Ostetrice e Ginecologica*, **63**, 155–168.

Mortimer, G., MacDonald, D.J. and Smeeth, A. (1985) A pilot study of the incidence and significance of placental villitis. *British Journal of Obstetrics and Gynaecology*, **92**, 629–633.

Mostoufi-Zadeh, M., Weiss, L.M. and Driscoll, S.G. (1985) Nonimmune hydrops fetalis: a challenge in perinatal pathology. *Human Pathology*, **16**, 785–789.

Naeye, R.L. (1988) How and when does antenatal hypoxia damage fetal brains? In *Perinatal Events and Brain Damage in Surviving Children*, Kubli, F., Paten, N., Schmidt, W. and Linderkamp, O. (Eds), pp. 70–80. New York: Springer-Verlag.

Naeye, R.L. (1991) Acute chorioamnionitis and the disorders that produce placental insufficiency. In *Pathology of Reproductive Failure*, Kraus, F.T., Damjanov, I. and Kaufman, N. (Eds), pp. 286–307. Baltimore: Williams & Wilkins.

Naeye, R.L. (1992) *Disorders of the Placenta, Fetus, and Neonate: Diagnosis and Clinical Significance.* St Louis: Mosby.

Nelson, J., Kenny, B., O'Hara, D., Harper, A. and Broadhead, D. (1993) Foamy changes of placental cells in probable beta glucuronidase deficiency associated with hydrops fetalis. *Journal of Clinical Pathology*, **46**, 370–371.

Nordenvall, M. and Sandstedt, B. (1990) Placental villitis and intrauterine growth retardation in a Swedish population. *Acta Pathologica Microbiologica et Immunologica*, **98**, 19–24.

Palmer, L., Blair, E., Petterson, B. and Burton, P. (1995) Antenatal antecedents of moderate and severe cerebral palsy. *Paediatric and Perinatal Epidemiology*, **9**, 171–184.

Pauli, R.M., Reiser, C.A., Lebovitz, R.M. and Kirkpatrick, S.J. (1994) Wisconsin stillbirth service program. I. Establishment and assessment of a community-based program for etiologic investigation of intrauterine deaths. *American Journal of Medical Genetics*, **50**, 116–134.

Pauli, R.M. and Reiser, C.A. (1994) Wisconsin stillbirth service program. II. Analysis of diagnoses and diagnostic categories in the first 1000 referrals. *American Journal of Medical Genetics*, **50**, 135–153.

Pilz, I., Schweikhart, G. and Kaufmann, P. (1980) Zur Abgrenzung normaler, artefizieller und pathologischer Strukturen in reifen Plazentarzotten. III. Morphometrische Untersuchungen bei Rhesus-Inkompabilitat. *Archives of Gynecology*, **229**, 137–154.

Popli, S., Leehey, D.J., Molnar, Z.V., Nawab, Z.M. and Ing, T.S. (1990) Demonstration of Fabry's disease deposits in placenta. *American Journal of Obstetrics and Gynecology*, **162**, 464–465.

Post, J.G. and Nijhuis, J.G. (1992) Trisomy 16 confined to the placenta. *Prenatal Diagnosis*, **12**, 1001–1007.

Powell, H.C., Benirschke, K., Favara, B.E. and Pfluoger, O.H. Jr (1976) Foamy changes of placental cells in fetal storage disorders. *Virchows Archiv A Pathological Anatomy and Histology*, **369**, 191–196.

Pozzi, V. and Marzetti, L. (1962) Fattore Rh e placenta: nota preliminare. *Minerva Ginecologica*, **14**, 1007–1008.

Preisler, O. (1958) Zum Nachweis des Antigen Rh im Gewebe. *Zentralblatt für Gynäkologie*, **80**, 238–242.

Rapola, J. and Aula, P. (1977) Morphology of the placenta in fetal I-cell disease. *Clinical Genetics*, **11**, 107–113.

Rapola, P., Santavuori, P. and Heiskala, H. (1988) Placental pathology and pre-natal diagnosis of infantile type of neuronal ceroid-lipofuscinosis. *American Journal of Medical Genetics*, **5** (Suppl.), 99–103.

Rayburn, W., Sander, C., Barr, M. Jr and Rygiel, R. (1985) The stillborn fetus: placental histologic examination in determining a cause. *Obstetrics and Gynecology*, **65**, 637–641.

Rayburn, W., Sander, C. and Compton, A. (1989) Histologic examination of the placenta in the growth-retarded fetus. *American Journal of Perinatology*, **6**, 58–61.

Redline, R.W. (1995) Placental pathology: a neglected link between basic disease mechanisms and untoward pregnancy outcome. *Current Opinion in Obstetrics and Gynecology*, **7**, 10–15.

Renaer, M., van de Putte, I. and Vermylen, C. (1976) Massive feto-maternal hemorrhage as a cause of perinatal mortality and morbidity. *European Journal of Obstetrics, Gynecology and Reproductive Biology*, **6**, 125–140.

Respetti, M. and Pescetto, G. (1951) Aspetti della placenta nella malattia emolitica del neonate. *Minerva Ginecologica*, **5**, 389–393.

Riches, W.G. and Smuckler, E.A. (1983) A severe infantile mucolipidosis: clinical, biochemical and pathological features. *Archives of Pathology and Laboratory Medicine*, **107**, 147–152.

Ritchie, J.W. (1991) Use of Doppler technology in assessing fetal health. *Journal of Developmental Physiology*, **15**, 121–123.

Roberts, D.J., Ampola, M.G. and Lage, J.M. (1991) Diagnosis of unsuspected fetal metabolic storage disease by routine placental examination. *Human Pathology*, **11**, 647–656.

Robertson, W.B., Brosens, I. and Dixon, H.G. (1981) Maternal blood supply in fetal growth retardation. In *Fetal Growth Retardation*, Van Assche, A. and Robertson, W.B. (Eds), pp. 126–138. Edinburgh: Churchill Livingstone.

Robertson, W.B., Khong, T.Y., Brosens, I. et al (1986) The placental bed biopsy: review from three European centers. *American Journal of Obstetrics and Gynecology*, **155**, 401–412.

Robinson, J.S. and Owens, J. (1993) The placenta and intrauterine growth retardation. In *The Human Placenta*, Redman, C.W.G., Sargent, I.L. and Starkey, P.M. (Eds), pp. 558–578. Oxford: Blackwell Scientific.

Robinson, J.S., Kingston, E.J., Jones, C.T. and Thornburn, G.D. (1979) Studies on experimental growth retardation in sheep: the effect of removal of endometrial caruncles on fetal size and metabolism. *Journal of Developmental Physiology*, **1**, 379–398.

Roland, B., Lynch, L., Berkowitz, G. and Zinberg, R. (1994) Confined placental mosaicism in CVS and pregnancy outcome. *Prenatal Diagnosis*, **14**, 589–593.

Rouse, D. and Weiner, C. (1990) Ongoing fetomaternal hemorrhage treated by serial fetal intravascular transfusions. *Obstetrics and Gynecology*, **76**, 974–975.

Rumbolz, W.L., Edwards, M.C. and McGoogan, L.S. (1961) The small full term infant and placental insufficiency. *Western Journal of Surgery*, **69**, 53–61.

Salafia, C.M. (1992) Placental pathology in perinatal diagnosis. In *Gynecology and Obstetrics (Revised)*, Sciarra, J. (Ed.), pp. 1–39. Philadelphia: Lippincott.

Salafia, C.M., Vintzileos, A.M., Silberman, L., Bantham, K.F. and Vogel, C.A. (1992) Placental pathology of idiopathic intrauterine growth retardation at term. *American Journal of Perinatology*, **9**, 179–184.

Salafia, C.M., Minior, V.K. and Lopez-Zeno, J.A. (1995) Relationship between placental histologic features and umbilical cord blood gases in preterm gestations. *American Journal of Obstetrics and Gynecology*, **173**, 1058–1064.

Sandstedt, B. (1979) The placenta and low birthweight. *Current Topics in Pathology*, **66**, 1–55.

Sansone, G. and Pescetto, G. (1953) Considerazione su di un caso di malattia emolitica del neonata con particolare riguardo allo studio della placenta. *Minerva Ginecologica*, **5**, 389–393.

Sarrut, S. and Belamich, P. (1983) Etude du placenta dans trois observations de dyslipide a revelation neonatale. *Archives d'Anatomie et de Cytologie Pathologiques*, **31**, 187–189.

Schmidt, A.L.C. (1949) De placenta bij erythroblastosis. *Nederlands Tijdschrift voor Geneeskunde*, **93**, 3732–3747.

Schrodt, U. (1970) Morphometrische Untersuchungen der Placenta bei dystrophen Neuegeborenen. *Zentralblatt für Gynäkologie*, **92**, 671–673.

Schuhmann, R. (1969) Hypotrophes reifes Kind am Termin aus placentarer Ursache (sogenannter placentarer Zwerg) *Beitrage zur pathologischen Anatomie und zur allgemeinen Pathologie*, **138**, 426–435.

Schuhmann, R., Lehmann, W.D. and Geier, G. (1972) Beziehungen zwischen Plazentamorphologie und Ostrogenwerten im letzten Schwangerschaftstrimonen. Ein Beitrag zur Morphologie der insuffizienten Plazenta. *Zeitschrift für Geburtshilfe und Perinatologie*, **176**, 379–390.

Schulman, H. (1993) Uteroplacental flow velocity. In *Ultrasound in Obstetrics and Gynecology*, Chervenak, F.A., Isaacson, G.C. and Campbell, S. (Eds), pp. 569–577. Boston: Little, Brown.

Schwinger, E., Seidl, E., Klink, F. et al (1989) Chromosome mosaicism of the placenta – a cause of developmental failure of the fetus? *Prenatal Diagnosis*, **9**, 639–647.

Scott, J.M. and Jordan, J.M. (1972) Placental insufficiency and the small-for-dates baby. *American Journal of Obstetrics and Gynecology*, **113**, 823–832.

Sekeles, E., Ornoy, A., Cohen, R. and Kohn, G. (1978) Mucolipidosis IV: fetal and placental pathology: a report on two subsequent interruptions of pregnancy. *Monographs in Human Genetics*, **10**, 47–50.

Shen, Y. (1992) Stereological study of the placentae in intrauterine growth retardation with different ponderal index. *Chinese Journal of Obstetrics and Gynecology*, **27**, 351–354.

Sheppard, B.L. and Bonnar, J. (1976) The ultrastructure of the arterial supply of the human placenta in pregnancy complicated by fetal growth retardation. *British Journal of Obstetrics and Gynaecology*, **83**, 948–959.

Sheppard, B. and Bonnar, J. (1980) Ultrastructural abnormalities of placental villi in placentae from pregnancies complicated by intrauterine fetal growth retardation: their relationship to decidual spiral arterial lesions. *Placenta*, **1**, 145–156.

Sheppard, B. and Bonnar, J. (1981) An ultrastructural study of uteroplacental spiral arteries in hypertensive and normotensive pregnancy and fetal growth retardation. *British Journal of Obstetrics and Gynaecology*, **88**, 695–705.

Spaczynski, M., Pisarki, T. and Glyda, A. (1976) Zmiany morfologiczne w plytach podstawowych lozysk od plodow z niska waga urodzeniowa. (Morphological changes in the basal plates of placenta in deliveries of low weight fetuses.) *Ginekologia Polska*, **41**, 721–726.

Squier, M.V. (1993) Acquired diseases of the nervous system. In *Fetal and Neonatal Pathology*, 2nd edn, Keeling, J.W. (Ed.), pp. 571–593. London: Springer-Verlag.

Stanley, F.J. (1995) Obstetrical responsibility for abnormal fetal outcome. In *Turnbull's Obstetrics*, 2nd edn,. Chamberlain, G. (Ed.), pp. 833–846. Edinburgh: Churchill Livingstone.

Stock, M.K., Anderson, D.F., Phernetton, T.M., McLaughlin, M.K. and Rankin, J.H.G. (1980) Vascular response of the fetal placenta to local occlusion of the maternal placental vasculature. *Journal of Developmental Physiology*, **2**, 339–346.

Suska, P., Vierik, J., Handzo, I. and Krizko, M. (1989) Vyskyt makroskopickych zmien placent u intrauterinne rastovo retardovanych novorodencov. (Incidence of macroscopic changes in the placenta in intrauterine growth retardation in neonates.) *Bratislaske Lekarske Listy*, **90**, 604–607.

Teasdale, F. (1984) Idiopathic intrauterine growth retardation: histomorphometry of the human placenta. *Placenta*, **5**, 83–92.

ten Berge, B.S. (1955) Capillaraktion in der Placenta. *Archiv für Gynäkologie*, **186**, 253–256.

ten Berge, B.S. (1965) The placenta in anencephaly. *Gynaecologia*, **159**, 359–364.

Theuring, F. (1968) Fibröse Obliterationen an Deckplatten und Stammzottengefassen der Placenta nach intrauterinem Fruchttod. *Archiv für Gynäkologie*, **206**, 237–251.

Theuring, F. and Kemnitz, P. (1974) Elektronenmikroskopische Plazentabefunde bei fetaler intrauteriner Wachstumretardierung (sog. small for dates babies) *Zentralblatt für allgemeine Pathologie und pathologische Anatomie*, **118**, 82–89.

Thomsen, K. and Berle, P. (1960) Placentarbefunde bei Rh-Inkompatibilitat. *Archiv für Gynäkologie*, **192**, 628–643.

Tremblay, P.C., Sybulski, S. and Maughan, G.B. (1965) Role of the placenta in fetal malnutrition. *American Journal of Obstetrics and Gynecology*, **91**, 597–605.

Trudinger, B.J., Giles, W.B. and Cook, C.M. (1985a) Uteroplacental blood flow velocity–time waveforms in normal and complicated pregnancy. *British Journal of Obstetrics and Gynaecology*, **92**, 39–45.

Trudinger, B.J., Giles, W.B. and Cook, C.M. (1985b) Flow velocity waveforms in the maternal uteroplacental and fetal umbilical placental circulations. *American Journal of Obstetrics and Gynecology*, **152**, 155–163.

Trudinger, B.J., Giles, W.B., Cook, C.M., Bombardieri, J. and Collins, L. (1985c) Fetal umbilical artery flow velocity waveforms and placental resistance: clinical significance. *British Journal of Obstetrics and Gynaecology*, **92**, 23–30.

Van der Veen, F. and Fox, H. (1983) The human placenta in idiopathic intrauterine growth retardation: a light and electron microscopic study. *Placenta*, **4**, 65–78.

Vanier, M.T., Rousson, R.M., Mandon, G. et al (1989) Diagnosis of Niemann–Pick disease type C on chorionic villus biopsy. *Lancet*, **i**, 1014–1015.

Volker, U. (1992) Gewichts- und Grossenvergleich von Plazenten und Feten bei intrauterinem Fruchttod. *Perinatal Medizin*, **4**, 8–16.

Wentworth, P. (1964) A placental lesion to account for foetal haemorrhage into the maternal circulation. *Journal of Obstetrics and Gynaecology of the British Commonwealth*, **71**, 379–387.

Wentworth, P. (1967) The placenta in cases of hemolytic disease of the newborn. *American Journal of Obstetrics and Gynecology*, **98**, 283–289.

Widmaier, G. (1969) Beitrag zur Ultrastruktur der menschlichen Placentazotten beim Morbus haemolyticus neonatorum. *Archiv für Gynäkologie*, **207**, 528–538.

Widness, J.A., Teramo, K.A., Clemons G.K. et al (1993) Temporal response of immunoreactive erythropoietin to acute hypoxemia in fetal sheep. *Pediatric Research*, **20**, 15–19.

Wigglesworth, J.S. (1964) Morphological variations in the insufficient placenta. *Journal of Obstetrics and Gynaecology of the British Commonwealth*, **71**, 871–884.

Wilkin, P. (1965) *Pathologie du Placenta*. Paris: Masson.

Willis, C. and Foreman, C.S. (1988) Chronic massive fetomaternal hemorrhage: a case report. *Obstetrics and Gynecology*, **71**, 459–461.

Wolstenholme, J., Rooney, D.E. and Davison, E.V. (1994) Confined placental mosaicism, IUGR, and adverse pregnancy outcome: a controlled retrospective UK collaborative study. *Prenatal Diagnosis*, **14**, 345–361.

Wong, T.C. and Latour, J.P.A. (1966) Microscopic measurement of the placental components in an attempt to assess malnourished newborn infants. *American Journal of Obstetrics and Gynecology*, **94**, 942–950.

Younoszai, M.K. and Haworth, J.C. (1969) Placental dimensions and relations in preterm, term and growth retarded infants. *American Journal of Obstetrics and Gynecology*, **103**, 265–271.

Zacutti, A., Borruto, F., Bottacci, G. et al (1992) Umbilical blood flow and placental pathology. *Clinical and Experimental Obstetrics and Gynecology*, **19**, 63–69.

Zacks, S.I. and Blazar, A.S. (1963) Chorionic villi in normal pregnancy, pre-eclamptic toxemia, erythroblastosis and diabetes mellitus. *Obstetrics and Gynecology*, **22**, 149–167.

10

THE PLACENTA IN ABORTION

SPONTANEOUS ABORTION

There has in the past been much pedantic quibbling as to the definition of a spontaneous abortion, but for practical purposes any pregnancy that terminates before the fetus is viable is an abortion. The most widely used definition is that employed by the World Health Organization (1977) which defines an abortion as 'expulsion of an embryo or fetus weighing 500 grams or less'; using this definition, pregnancies that terminate in a spontaneous abortion will always do so before the 22nd week of gestation. It will be noted that this definition evades the issue as to whether a live-born infant weighing less than 500 g should be considered as an abortion and whilst including some cases of partial hydatidiform mole, excludes complete moles. In reality, of course, most abortions occur during the first trimester or in the early second trimester and thus pose no difficulties of recognition or definition.

Because spontaneous abortion is so common, and because most abortions are followed by a perfectly normal subsequent pregnancy, early pregnancy loss only becomes a real clinical problem in women who recurrently, or 'habitually', abort. There are, however, differing views as to what exactly constitutes 'recurrent' abortion because it is certainly possible for a woman to have two consecutive abortions simply by pure chance. The odds against abortion occurring in three successive pregnancies simply by chance are, however, very high and therefore a woman who aborts in three successive pregnancies can be regarded as suffering recurrent pregnancy loss (Berry et al, 1995), although in fact this will occur in 0.3% of women as a result of bad luck alone (Hatasaka, 1994).

Incidence

It is widely agreed that about 15% of recognized pregnancies spontaneously abort (Alberman, 1988; Daya, 1994; Hatasaka, 1994; Berry et al, 1995); there is no doubt, however, that a significant proportion of conceptuses are lost without the woman being aware that she is, or has been, pregnant. Roberts and Lowe (1975), with the aid of an ingenious mathematical formula, calculated that 78% of conceptuses in women aged 20–29 years in England and Wales abort whilst Edmonds et al (1982), using highly sensitive beta-hCG assays, found that the rate of clinically undetectable early pregnancy loss was as high as two-thirds of all conceptions. Later studies have yielded more conservative estimates, suggesting that 18–22% of conceptions fail to survive as a clinically recognizable pregnancy (Sweeney et al, 1988; Wilcox et al, 1988). Most of these early pregnancy failures occur prior to, or very soon after, implantation and possible causes of pregnancy loss at this stage include a failure of gene activation, a chromosomal abnormality or errors of cytokinesis and karyokinesis (Chard, 1991).

Aetiological Factors

Any attempt to categorize the factors responsible for spontaneous abortion must, in our present state of knowledge, be both riddled with lacunae of ignorance and, at least partially, based on hypotheses or unproven assumptions. Amongst the suggested aetiological factors are the following.

Infections

Any infection in early pregnancy that is accompanied by a severe maternal systemic disturbance, e.g., lobar pneumonia, can cause abortion without there being any direct involvement of the placenta or fetus (Kline et al, 1985). Several organisms appear, however, to have a specifically abortifacient effect although producing few or no systemic symptoms in the mother. The organisms that have been particularly stigmatized in this respect include rubella virus, *Listeria monocytogenes*, cytomegalovirus, *Toxoplasma gondii*, *Campylobacter* sp. and, possibly, herpes simplex virus and coxsackie virus (Charles & Larsen, 1990). These infections are discussed more fully in Chapter 11, where it is pointed out that fetal death in such circumstances is probably a direct consequence of fetal infection and not a reflection of placental dysfunction caused by inflammatory damage. *Chlamydia trachomatis* and *Mycoplasma hominis* have not, despite some claims to the contrary (Stray-Peterson et al, 1978; Quinn et al, 1987; Witkin & Ledger, 1992), been clearly linked to abortion (Charles & Larsen, 1990; Rae et al, 1994; Summers, 1994) but a high incidence of positive cultures for *Ureaplasma urealyticum* has been obtained from spontaneously aborted placental tissue (Joste et al, 1994).

The actual quantitative contribution of infections to sporadic human abortion is unknown but is probably low (Summers, 1994) whilst infection appears to play little role in recurrent abortion (Plouffe et al, 1992).

Physical Factors

Claims that uterine leiomyomas, especially those in a submucous site, are associated with a high incidence of early pregnancy loss and that myomectomy results in a much improved reproductive performance (Buttram & Reiter, 1981; Garcia & Tureck, 1984) are difficult to evaluate as they are based on uncontrolled studies: the most that can be said is that leiomyomas *may* be a very infrequent cause of abortion (Treffers, 1990).

It has been widely conceded that uterine malformations are a cause of early pregnancy loss and that they may be an important factor in cases of recurrent abortion (Bennett, 1987). The foundations for this belief, however, are not as firm as is generally thought to be the case. Treffers (1990) reviewed critically the then available evidence for a causal relationship between uterine malformations and abortion and came to the iconoclastic but scientifically impeccable conclusion that the statistical basis for such a belief was weak and largely explicable in terms of selective reporting. Nevertheless, reports continue to appear claiming a very high incidence of abortion, often recurrent, both generally for women with uterine anomalies (Ludmir and March, 1990; Stein and March, 1990; Golan et al, 1992; Makino et al, 1992) and specifically in unicornuate uteri (Donderwinkel et al, 1992; Moutos et al, 1992) and septate uteri (Kovacevic et al, 1990; Manchesi et al, 1991; Michalas, 1991). It is difficult to draw any firm conclusions from these conflicting views but, on balance, it does appear that the incidence of abortion is increased in women with uterine malformations, though probably not dramatically. The association with early pregnancy loss appears to be strongest for septate uteri (Patton, 1994) and it is of interest that this is only true if the placenta is actually implanted on the septum (Fedele et al, 1989).

Cervical incompetence is widely believed to be a well-documented cause of second-trimester abortion but in fact there is no agreement about the criteria for the diagnosis of this abnormality, no agreement about its incidence and no agreement about the value of cervical cerclage (Treffers, 1990; Quinn, 1993).

External trauma to the uterus occupies a much lower place in the aetiological hierarchy of abortion than that which would be afforded to it by the general public (Baker, 1982; Sorensen et al, 1986)

Endocrinological Abnormalities

Luteal phase deficiency has been thought to be an important factor in the pathogenesis of early pregnancy loss and this concept served as the basis for the administration of progesterone to prevent spontaneous abortion. There is now considerable scepticism about the validity of this diagnosis, however, and even greater doubt about the value, in terms of management of recurrent abortion, of treating it (Stirrat, 1990; Simpson, 1992; Coulam & Stern, 1994; Dawood, 1994).

An increased incidence of spontaneous abortion has been noted in pregnancies following conception during a cycle in which the levels of luteinizing hormone (LH) were elevated during the follicular phase (Regan et al, 1990; Balen et al, 1993a). Because tonic elevation of LH occurs in women with the polycystic ovary syndrome it was postulated that the raised hormone levels were simply acting as a surrogate for clinically covert ovarian disease. It is, indeed, the case that women with the polycystic ovary syndrome have a high incidence of spontaneous, commonly recurrent, abortion (Sagle et al, 1988; Balen et al, 1993b) but it is the high levels of LH that determine the risk of pregnancy loss, not the polycystic ovary syndrome *per se*. The high abortion rate is also found in women with normal ovaries and raised LH levels and the polycystic ovary syndrome is a risk factor for abortion simply because there is a high incidence of elevated LH levels in this condition (Watson et al, 1993). The mechanism of LH hypersecretion in women with normal ovaries is unknown but it has been suggested that the adverse effect of LH is mediated by its effect on theca cells, the resulting high androgen levels affecting oocyte quality. The adverse effect of androgens also appears to apply to women with the polycystic ovary syndrome because it is only those patients with high androgen levels that suffer early pregnancy loss (Tulppala et al, 1993).

There is no increased risk of spontaneous abortion in women with well-controlled diabetes mellitus but there is an excess incidence of early pregnancy loss in diabetic women with inadequate glucose control (Simpson, 1992; Clifford & Regan, 1994). Neither hypo- nor hyperthyroidism is currently considered a risk factor for spontaneous abortion (Huisjes, 1990; Coulam & Stern, 1994).

Psychological Factors

There is evidence, convincing to psychiatrists, that psychogenic factors may be of aetiological importance in a small proportion of first-trimester abortions (Michel-Wolfromm, 1967; Silverman, 1970; Hertz, 1973); but this evidence is anecdotal, uncontrolled and based on the study of women who had already suffered repeated pregnancy failures, no information being available about the prior personality or psychological status of women who subsequently suffer recurrent abortion (Huisjes, 1990; Keye, 1994).

Immunological Factors

This subject is considered in greater detail in Chapter 12 and only a broad summary of immunological factors in early pregnancy loss will be outlined here. The concept of abortion being due, in some instances, to an immune-mediated graft rejection process is seductively attractive; indeed, many have succumbed to the temptation and have supported this view on purely conjectural grounds. There is, in fact, no convincing evidence that cytotoxic antibodies, serum blocking factors or HLA-sharing influence pregnancy outcome and no direct scientific evidence that alloimmune factors play any role in early pregnancy loss (Stirrat, 1990, 1992; Silver & Branch, 1994; Berry et al, 1995).

The role played by autoimmune mechanisms has been explored at length and has centred, in recent years, on antiphospholipid antibodies. It has long been recognized that women suffering from systemic lupus erythematosus have a high incidence of spontaneous abortion and it later became apparent that pregnancy loss in this disease is related to the presence of antiphospholipid antibodies (lupus anticoagulant and anti-cardiolipin antibody) which, it is now recognized, are not confined to patients with lupus but can also occur in women who are otherwise apparently well. There is no relationship between sporadic abortion and the presence of antiphospholipid antibodies (Infante-Rivard et al, 1991), which contrasts with the apparently clear-cut association of these antibodies with recurrent early pregnancy loss (Triplett, 1992; Silver & Branch, 1994). There have been wide differences, however, in the reported incidence of these antibodies in both women with uncomplicated pregnancies and in patients suffering repeated abortions. This probably reflects both patient selection bias and variations in laboratory testing but not everybody has been convinced that there is a real correlation between antiphospholipid antibodies and early, as opposed to late, fetal loss (Petri et al, 1987; Simpson, 1992; Melk et al, 1995). Even allowing for a causal role of antiphospholipid antibodies in recurrent abortion, the mechanism by which they cause fetal loss is disputed because the finding of a decidual vasculopathy and extensive placental infarction in some studies has not been confirmed in others (Branch, 1994; Silver & Branch, 1994). Experimental studies have suggested that antiphospholipid antibodies may, in fact, have a direct embryotoxic effect (Sthoeger et al, 1993).

Evidence that antinuclear antibodies are associated with recurrent pregnancy loss is, at best, flimsy but there does seem to be an increased risk of early fetal loss in women who, though euthyroid, have thyroid autoantibodies (Stagnaro-Green et al, 1990). There is, however, no convincing evidence that such antibodies play a role in the aetiology of recurrent abortion (Gleicher et al, 1993; Pratt et al, 1993; Silver & Branch, 1994).

Congenital Abnormalities

This term is used here to denote anatomical abnormalities in karotypically normal embryos. It is difficult, however, to disentangle these two variables because whilst, for instance, cleft lip and palate is found three times as commonly in aborted embryos than in live-born infants, these abnormalities are not uncommon in chromosomal abnormalities. Despite this codicil it is clear that the incidence of anatomical malformations in spontaneous abortions is unduly high; thus, for example, the incidence of isolated neural tube defects, which are not usually associated with an abnormal karotype, is very much higher in spontaneously aborted fetuses than in either live newborns or in therapeutically aborted fetuses (Fantel et al, 1980; Byrne & Warburton, 1986; McFadden & Kalousek, 1989).

Genetic Abnormalities

There is little doubt that chromosomal abnormalities are the single most important factor in spontaneous abortion, because at least 50% of early spontaneous abortions are cytogenetically abnormal (Boué et al, 1975; Lauritsen, 1976; Hassold et al, 1980; Warburton et al, 1980; Simpson & Bombard, 1987; Creasy, 1988; Davison & Burn, 1990; Eiben et al, 1990; Ohno et al, 1991; Cowchock et al, 1993; Kalousek et al, 1993). There has been fairly general agreement that autosomal trisomy, 45XO monosomy, triploidy and tetraploidy account, respectively, for about 45–55%, 20–30%, 15–20% and 5% of abnormal karyotypes in spontaneous abortions (Creasy, 1988; Davison & Burn, 1990; Simpson, 1992; Byrne & Ward, 1994). Trisomies involving every chromosome have been described in spontaneous abortions with the exceptions of number 1 and the Y chromosome: between a third and a half of such trisomies involve chromosome 16 whilst chromosomes 2, 7, 13, 14, 15, 21 and 22 each account for between 5 and 10% of trisomic pregnancy losses. It is of interest that the incidence of abortion varies considerably amongst the various types of chromosomal abnormality but that each particular karotypic abnormality is associated with a specific and consistent incidence of pregnancy loss. Thus, for instance, 98% of monosomy OX embryos are aborted and whilst virtually all cases of trisomy 16 abort this is only true for 70% of those with trisomies 17–18 or 21–22 (Rushton, 1995).

Most cytogenetic abnormalities associated with abortion arise *de novo* but a small number of abnormal karotypes result from parental abnormalities, most commonly balanced translocations, and these may be associated with recurrent pregnancy loss (Simpson et al, 1981; de Braekeleer & Dao, 1990).

A particular form of chromosomal abnormality, confined placental mosaicism, appears to be associated with an increased risk of spontaneous abortion (Kalousek et al, 1992; Wang et al, 1993) but this is a double-edged weapon because, as discussed below, confined placental mosaicism may also actually prevent abortion.

It is probable that consideration only of cytogenetic abnormalities underestimates the genetic contribution to spontaneous abortion. The application of DNA technology will almost certainly reveal a range of genetic deletions and rearrangements that are not detectable by standard cytogenetic techniques. It has, indeed, been suggested that molecular research will reveal that early pregnancy loss is, with few exceptions, related entirely to genetic causes (Byrne & Ward, 1994) though this is, perhaps, the view of enthusiasts for a particular approach.

Pathogenesis

A mere listing of possible aetiological factors in abortion gives no indication as to why and how early pregnancy loss actually occurs. To say that a conceptus has aborted *because of* a neural tube defect or a 45 XO monosomy is an easy but overfacile explanation, because, quite obviously, many fetuses with similar abnormalities do not abort but attain viability. Furthermore we have very little knowledge as to how a chromosomal abnormality is recognized and of the mechanisms by which such an abnormality results in abortion.

Some light has, however, been shed on the pathogenesis of spontaneous abortion in recent years. Khong et al (1987) and Michel et al (1990) suggested that there is, in many cases of early pregnancy loss, inadequate placentation with a failure of extravillous trophoblast to invade adequately the spiral arteries of the placental bed. This was confirmed by Hustin et al (1990) who found absent or reduced physiological change in the placental bed spiral arteries in over 60% of early spontaneous abortions and Hustin and Jauniaux (1992) have suggested that inadequate trophoblastic migration and invasion may be secondary to a fetal chromosomal abnormality or a severe fetal abnormality. This view is consistent with the finding that a confined placental mosaicism may prevent abortion of an aneuploid fetus. Thus, whilst the vast majority of cases of fetal trisomy 13 or 18 abort, those with an associated confined placental mosaicism, in which a proportion of the cytotrophoblastic cells have a normal diploid chromosomal complement, survive (Kalousek et al, 1989; Kalousek, 1993, 1994). This suggests that placental function, rather than maternal recognition of a trisomic fetus, determines survival in trisomic conceptuses and is entirely compatible with the concept that the presence of a diploid cytotrophoblastic cell line allows for adequate trophoblastic invasion and migration.

If inadequate placentation is a common feature in many spontaneous abortions, why should it result in pregnancy failure at this early stage? One view has been that the abortion is due to uteroplacental ischaemia as a result of inadequate conversion of spiral arteries into uteroplacental vessels (Rushton, 1988). It is extremely unlikely, however, that ischaemia could be held responsible for fetal demise at a stage of pregnancy when there is little or no true perfusion of the intervillous space by maternal blood (Hustin & Schaaps, 1987; Exalto, 1995). The alternative view, championed by Hustin and his colleagues (Hustin et al, 1990; Hustin & Jauniaux, 1992; Jauniaux et al, 1994), and one that has much to recommend it, is that abortion is due to premature entry of maternal blood into the intervillous space. They argue that the migrating extravillous trophoblast normally forms intravascular cellular plugs in the placental bed vessels which restrict free passage of maternal blood into the intervillous space. If these plugs are not adequately formed, maternal blood will enter the intervillous space prematurely and disrupt the trophoblastic shell with resultant abortion.

Pathology

General Anatomico-Pathological Classification of Material from Abortions

The pathologist will find that the tissue presented for the study of an abortus ranges from a complete placenta and fetus to a few scanty curettings. It is therefore necessary to adopt an overall anatomical classification of abortion material; several such classifications have been suggested (Mall & Meyer, 1921; Geneva Conference, 1966; Hertig, 1968, Laurini, 1990) but the one suggested by Fujikura et al (1966) is, with slight modifications, probably the most useful in practice. Abortion material is grouped as follows:

1. Incomplete specimen
   (a) Villi only
   (b) Villi and decidua
   (c) Decidua and trophoblastic cells
2. Ruptured empty sac
   (a) With cord stump
   (b) Without cord stump
3. Intact empty sac
4. Fetus present
   (a) With chorionic sac
       i. Normal non-macerated fetus
       ii. Normal macerated fetus
       iii. Grossly disorganized fetus
       iv. Focal abnormality of fetus
   (b) Without chorionic sac
       i. Normal non-macerated fetus
       ii. Normal macerated fetus
       iii. Grossly disorganized fetus
       iv. Focal abnormality of fetus

In this classification the term 'focal abnormality' refers to a defect such as spina bifida, whilst the expression 'grossly disorganized' is applied to those fetuses which are so ill-formed that they can only be classed as 'nodular' or 'cylindrical'. Most of the other terms used in this classification are self-explanatory, though it should be noted that 'intact empty sac' is used instead of 'blighted ovum', this latter expression being open to widely differing interpretations and being, in itself, meaningless. The term 'anembryonic pregnancy' is also synonymous with 'intact empty sac' and is, when applied to conventional abortions, quite a useful terminology: unfortunately this description has also been applied, misleadingly, to complete hydatidiform moles. These latter are not included in this classification though they are simply an unusual form of abortion. This omission is deliberate, because a mole is a distinctive entity which falls outside the general group of run-of-the-mill abortions and merits the separate attention that it is afforded in Chapter 14.

Although the above classification has many merits, the reality of the situation is that most abortion material reaching the pathologist either consists only of decidua and placental tissue or is decidual tissue which contains a placental site reaction; fetal tissues may or may not be present but it is uncommon to receive an intact fetus or a complete sac. The embryo is, therefore, not considered further in this account and those requiring information on this aspect of the pathology of early pregnancy failure are referred to specialist texts on embryonic and fetal pathology (Kalousek et al, 1990).

Macroscopic Abnormalities of the Cord and Placenta

Abnormalities of the cord

Javert and Barton (1952) and Javert (1957) have, with considerable justification, maintained that abnormalities of the umbilical cord have been largely ignored in studies of spontaneous abortion. However, they have trod the path of many enthusiasts by espousing their cause beyond the limits of credibility, claiming that lesions or abnormalities of the cord are a (or even the) major aetiological factor in spontaneous abortion. They have, in this respect, laid particular stress on the importance of achordia, whilst also emphasizing that excessive length, undue shortness, stricture, knots or torsion of the cord all play significant roles in the causation of early pregnancy failure.

A critical analysis of their results suggests, however, that they have overplayed their hand, because in their series of 1000 abortions any real knowledge of the state of the cord was available in only 297 cases; in 104 of these a cord lesion was present. The most common single abnormality of the cord was 'achordia without fetus', a term that is synonymous with an intact empty sac. Few would agree that under such circumstances it is justifiable to regard the absence of the cord as *the* primary abnormality, most preferring to regard these cases as being examples of extreme embryonic abnormality with defective development of the embryonic cell mass. A further nine instances of 'achordia with fetus' were noted, the fetus being invariably grossly disorganized; again it would be more logical to regard these as examples of a gross defect in embryonic differentiation rather than as primary cord abnormalities. Unduly short or excessively long cords are, in themselves, not fully acceptable as a cause of abortion, but torsion, stricture and true knots of the cord can, and do, cause fetal death and therefore merit being regarded as possible causes of abortion. A total of 28 such cases were found in Javert's series, and it would therefore appear that in only about 3% of his 1000 abortions could an abnormality of the cord be justifiably considered as a primary aetiological factor in abortion, a figure that I find perfectly acceptable.

A single umbilical artery is found more frequently in spontaneous abortions than in full-term live births; this anomaly is present in about 2.5% of aborted conceptuses (Thomas, 1962). In view of the known association between this abnormality and chromosomal disorders (Saller et al, 1990; Khong & George, 1992) this is a not unexpected finding, and there are certainly no grounds for assuming that the lack of one umbilical vessel is a cause of abortion.

Hathout (1964) and Monie (1965) have maintained that there is an association between abortion and velamentous or marginal insertion of the cord, but this has been specifically denied by Philippe et al (1968) and this interesting point remains to be settled.

Abnormalities of the placenta

It is rather unusual to have the opportunity to examine complete placentas from spontaneous abortions and, in general terms, macroscopic examination of such placentas commonly reveals little, if anything, that is helpful in elucidating the possible cause of the abortion. It is usually very difficult to say if placentas from first-trimester abortions are of normal shape or not, but I would agree with Scott's (1960) refutation of earlier claims (Hobbs & Rollins, 1934) of an excess of extrachorial placentation in abortion material.

Gaither and Sampson (1968) have suggested that perivillous fibrin deposition is an important feature of placentas from abortions whilst Salafia et al (1993) have noted a relatively high incidence of placental infarcts in first-trimester abortions. I would share the opinion of Bret et al (1967) that gross lesions, such as infarcts, intervillous thrombi and perivillous fibrin plaques, are not commonly seen in tissue from early pregnancy failures and occur no more frequently in placentas from spontaneous abortions than in placentas from induced therapeutic abortions of the same gestational age. Philippe et al (1968) found a high incidence of retroplacental haematomas in abortion material, but there must be considerable doubt as to whether the formation of such haematomas is a primary or a secondary change. Marginal placental haematomas have been noted in ultrasonographic studies of abortions (Mantoni, 1985) but these have received little pathological attention in first-trimester placentas.

Some authors have commented on the relatively frequent occurrence of a massive subchorial thrombosis (Breus's mole) in placentas from spontaneous abortions (Levy, 1956; Dydowicz & Pisarki, 1967; Abaci & Aterman, 1968; Bret & Grepinet, 1968; Philippe et al, 1968). This lesion (Figs 10.1 and 10.2) has been considered in more detail in Chapter 5, but it is worth reiterating here that both in Breus' (1892) original

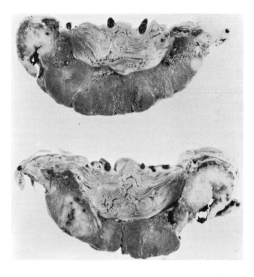

Figure 10.1. A massive laminated subchorial thrombus in an otherwise normal placenta from a chromosomally normal abortus.

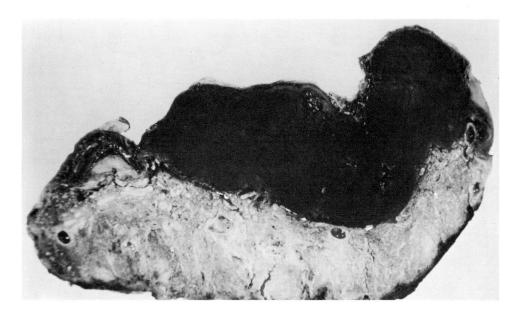

Figure 10.2. A massive subchorial thrombus in a placenta from a triploid abortus. The placenta shows focal microcystic change.

report, and in most subsequent descriptions, it has been assumed that the lesion is found only in abortion material and that it is either a cause or a result of fetal death. That this is an erroneous view has been shown by Shanklin and Scott's (1975) description of 10 massive subchorial thrombi, six of which were in placentas from pregnancies extending beyond the 30th week of gestation and seven of which were in placentas from live-born infants. Clearly, therefore, a massive subchorial thrombosis is not simply a *result* of fetal death nor is it specifically related to abortion: the lesion may be a cause of abortion but this remains to be proved.

A number, in my experience a very small number, of placentas from spontaneous abortions show maternal floor infarction (Rushton, 1988, 1995), a lesion discussed more fully in Chapter 5. Rushton considers this to be a post-mortem change and believes that maternal floor infarction increases the rigidity of the chorio-decidual attachment, reduces the maternal blood flow into the intervillous space and predisposes to a clean separation of the placenta from the uterus with minimal maternal blood loss.

Histological Abnormalities in the Placenta

About 40% of placentas from spontaneous abortions have villi that are fully normal for the length of the gestational period (Fig. 10.3), whilst a further 20–30% show only the changes that occur after fetal death, i.e. sclerosis and obliteration of fetal vessels and stromal fibrosis (Fig. 10.4). In between 20 and 40% of placentas from aborted fetuses, the villi show, either focally or diffusely, hydropic change, i.e. they appear swollen and oedematous, either hypovascular or, much more commonly, avascular and have an attenuated trophoblastic mantle (Figs 10.5 and 10.6). Hydropic change, sometimes wrongly and misleadingly classed as 'hydatidiform degeneration' of the villi, is not associated with the formation of central cisterns and is not apparent macroscopically as visible vesicles. It is worth noting that although hydropic change is usually considered to be due to villous oedema (Genest, 1994), a recent study has suggested that the villous swelling is due to an accumulation, within the villous stroma, of sulfated

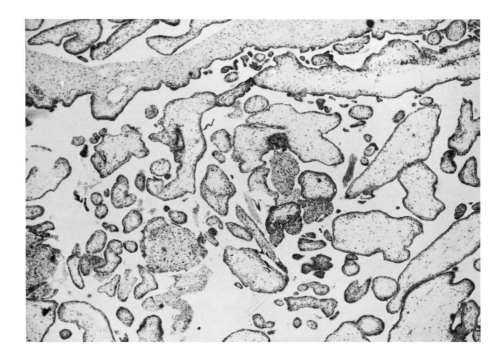

Figure 10.3. Normal histological appearances of the placental villi in a placenta aborted at the sixth week of gestation (H & E × 158).

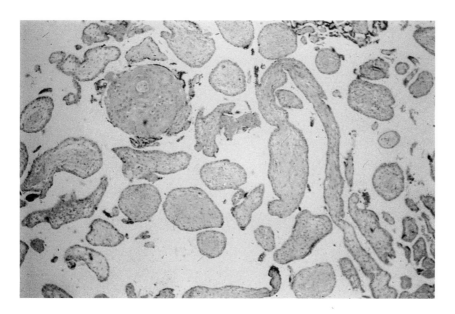

Figure 10.4. Placental tissue from a spontaneous abortion. The villi show only the changes that occur after fetal death.

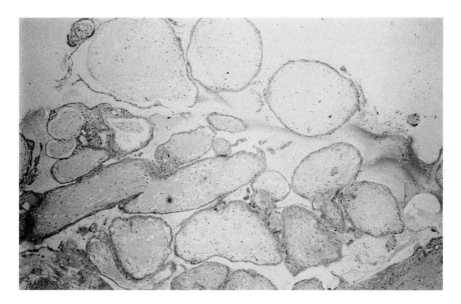

Figure 10.5. Hydropic change in the villi of a placenta from an aborted fetus (H & E ×55).

mucosubstances (Suster & Robinson, 1992), a finding that requires confirmation. A very unusual finding, reported only once, has been a massive chronic intervillositis occurring repetitively in placentas of a woman who suffered numerous spontaneous abortions (Doss et al, 1995).

In addition to these general findings there have been many claims that it is possible to correlate villous morphology in cases of early pregnancy failure either with specific chromosomal abnormalities or, less ambitiously, with an abnormal, as opposed to a normal, karotype (Bret & Grepinet, 1968; Philippe & Boué, 1969, 1970; Carr, 1971a,b; Cohen, 1972; Philippe, 1973, 1986; Honoré et al, 1976; Geisler & Kleinebrecht, 1978; Gocke et al, 1982, 1985; Canki et al, 1988; Muntefering et al, 1989; Rockelein et al, 1989; Horn et al, 1991). Those making these claims have stressed the

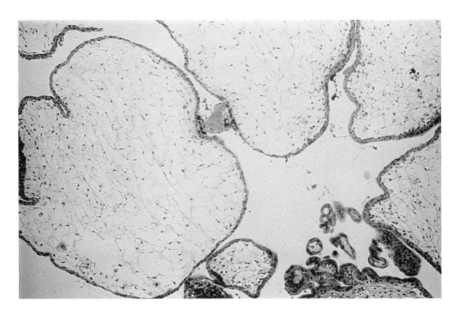

Figure 10.6. Higher power view of hydropic villi in a placenta of an abortus: there is no trophoblastic hyperplasia (H & E ×480).

diagnostic value of such features as vesicular change in the villi, irregular villous contours, the presence of trophoblastic pseudoinclusions, trophoblastic hyperplasia, the finding of abnormal stromal cells and, in the case of XO monosomy, villous fibrosis and hypoplasia.

It will be appreciated that many of these studies antedate the delineation of the partial hydatidiform mole and the recognition that this is the pathological hallmark of a diandrous fetal triploidy. Removal from many of these series of cases clearly seen to be, in retrospect, partial moles, dilutes considerably the significance of their findings. Further, some of these analyses have failed to take into account the changes that occur in the placental villi after fetal death.

Recent studies have cast considerable doubt on the ability of pathologists to identify villous changes that are characteristic of fetal karotypic abnormalities with, as ever, the exception of diandrous triploidy. First, it has been shown that the interobserver variation in the detection of histological features thought to be associated with fetal karotypic abnormalities is very considerable (van Lijnschoten et al, 1993a). Secondly, prospective studies have demonstrated, with some considerable clarity, that villous histology is an insensitive and inaccurate indicator of fetal chromosomal abnormalities (Novak et al, 1988; Minguillon et al, 1989; Rehder et al, 1989; Hustin & Jauniaux, 1992; van Lijnschoten et al, 1993b; Fukunaga et al, 1995; Genest et al, 1995), a view with which I would agree (Figs 10.7 and 10.8). Morphometric analysis of villous tissue has proved equally unrewarding in this respect (van Lijnschoten et al, 1993b), though it is only fair to say that this conclusion has been disputed by Rockelein and his colleagues who believe that karotypic abnormalities can be identified by morphomety and scanning electron microscopy of placental villi (Rockelein et al, 1990a,b). It is certainly possible that karotypic abnormalities alter villous growth in a rather subtle fashion; too subtle, however, to be detected on light microscopy but neither morphometry nor scanning electron microscopy is likely to have great appeal or value for histopathologists who have to deal with an abundance of tissue from early pregnancy failures.

It appears therefore that an accurate histological classification of placental villous morphology in spontaneous abortions, in terms of normal and abnormal karotypes, is not attainable. Is there then anything that can be gleaned from the histology of placentas from abortuses that gives any indication as to the cause of the pregnancy failure or affords any hint as to the prognosis of future pregnancies?

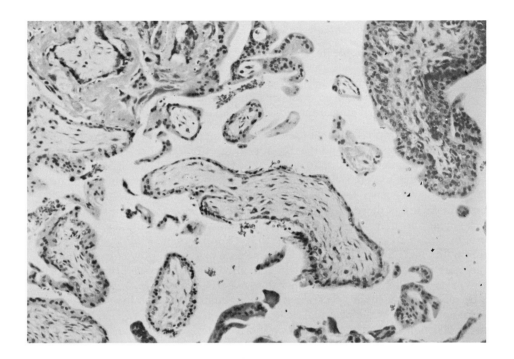

Figure 10.7. Villi in a placenta from an XO abortus; the appearances cannot be readily distinguished from those seen in a placenta showing post-mortem change (H & E ×400).

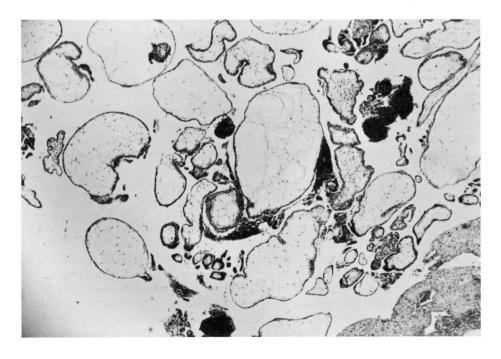

Figure 10.8. Villi in a placenta from a trisomic abortus; the appearances are simply those of a hydropic abortion (H & E ×158).

Rushton (1981, 1984, 1988, 1995) has codified the villous patterns seen in placental tissue from spontaneous abortions and has produced a morphological classification which, after excluding partial moles, may be paraphrased along the following lines:

Group 1. A considerable proportion of the villi show hydropic change.

Group 2. Some villi are hydropic but most show post-mortem change with stromal fibrosis.

Group 3. The villi show no evidence of hydropic or post-mortem change and are of normal appearance for the length of the gestational period.

Rushton has emphasized that each of these groups is, in terms of the aetiology of the abortion, heterogeneous and that the appearances reflect more the stage of gestation at which the pregnancy failed than any specific factor. Nevertheless it would be reasonable to assume that placentas from Group 1 are either from anembryonic pregnancies or from cases of very early fetal death. Under such circumstances the factor leading to pregnancy failure is more likely to be intrinsic to the fetus than to lie in the maternal environment and therefore a fetal karotypic abnormality is statistically the most likely cause. In Group 2 cases it is certain that, as in Group 1 cases, fetal death preceded the abortion, the fetus having been dead for some time before the pregnancy terminated. It is therefore probable, though not certain, that also in this group the primary factor leading to pregnancy failure was fetal rather than maternal. Finally, in Group 3 cases, which are usually from abortions occurring later in gestation than the other two groups, the normal appearance of the placental tissue indicates that the fetus was either alive at the time of abortion or had died only very shortly before the pregnancy terminated. It appears reasonable to postulate that in this group the pregnancy failed because of a fault in the maternal environment rather than because of any fetal abnormality.

The reasoning behind Rushton's approach is impeccable but how useful is this classification in practice? Any morphological classification of abortion material is probably only of real value in recurrent abortions and it is probable that most cases of repetitive pregnancy failure are due to maternal rather than fetal factors. A valid morphological classification of abortion material should therefore tend to identify those apparently sporadic cases of spontaneous abortion which are likely to recur and should reveal a different pattern in sporadic and repetitive pregnancy failures. Houwert-de Jong and his colleagues (Houwert-de Jong, 1989; Houwert-de Jong et al, 1990) have used Rushton's classification to examine placental material from both sporadic and recurrent abortions. They found that the pattern of placental changes was identical in these two groups and that, furthermore, they could not correlate the histopathological findings with the outcome of subsequent pregnancies. This does imply that current approaches to placental histological abnormalities in abortion material are unlikely to be of any great value in the study and management of cases of recurrent abortion.

In realistic terms, therefore, what is the value of histological examination of tissue from spontaneous abortions?

First, of course, to confirm that the patient has actually been pregnant, an aim achieved by the finding either of fetal tissue, villous tissue or of a placental site reaction in decidual tissue.

Secondly, to confirm that the pregnancy has been intrauterine, the only proof of which is the detection of a placental site reaction in decidual tissue (Fig. 10.9). The mere presence of placental villi in uterine curettings is not proof of an intrauterine gestation because these may be from a tubal pregnancy that has aborted into the uterus. Detection of a placental site reaction is usually a straightforward task but, in debateable cases, staining for cytokeratins or human placental lactogen (hPL) is of considerable help in identifying trophoblastic tissue (Khong et al, 1994).

Thirdly, to exclude gestational trophoblastic disease. It is in most cases relatively easy to exclude a complete hydatidiform mole though with complete moles increasingly being diagnosed by ultrasound at an early stage in their morphological evolution, this diagnosis is becoming somewhat more difficult (Paradinas, 1994). In theory the distinction between a hydropic abortus and a partial hydatidiform mole is straightforward

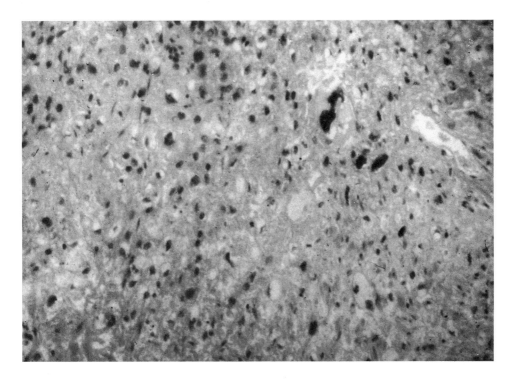

Figure 10.9. A placental site reaction in decidual tissue.

but in practice there is very considerable inter- and intra-observer error in making this differential diagnosis (Howat et al, 1993). It is often suggested that the distinction between these two forms of abortion rests upon the finding of villous trophoblastic hyperplasia in a partial mole but not in a hydropic abortus. This is a wrong approach because, in fact, there is no real trophoblastic hyperplasia in a partial hydatidiform mole and the differential diagnosis rests on the evidence of an abnormal pattern of trophoblastic growth in a partial mole, circumferential or multifocal trophoblastic growth being a feature of partial moles but never present in a non-molar pregnancy. In truly doubtful cases, flow or image cytometry may be of considerable diagnostic value in distinguishing triploid partial moles from diploid hydropic abortions (van Oven et al, 1989; Fukunaga et al, 1993; Lage & Popek, 1993; Topalovski et al, 1995) though it must be borne in mind that some hydropic non-molar abortions will be cases of digynic triploidies.

Fourthly, it may occasionally be necessary for medico-legal purposes to attempt to estimate the time of embryonic or fetal death. If the villi are hydropic and avascular and do not contain any erythrocytes it is reasonable to assume that embryonic death occurred before the 5th week of gestation, i.e. before vascularization of the villi. After this stage the ratio of nucleated to non-nucleated red cells in the fetal vessels may be of value as a chronological marker (Salafia et al, 1988; Szulman, 1991, 1995). Initially the red cells are of yolk sac origin and are nucleated but these are progressively replaced by non-nucleated red cells of fetal hepatic origin. Thus the ratio of nucleated to non-nucleated red cells is 9:1 at the 7th week of gestation and changes gradually to 1:9 at the 9th week of pregnancy, all the cells being non-nucleated by the 10th gestational week. After embryonic or fetal death the fetal red cells may persist in the collapsed villous vessels for several weeks and their nucleation status can provide a clue to the approximate date of fetal death.

These comments about the histological findings in spontaneous abortion refer principally to pregnancy failure in the first trimester or early second trimester. In the later stages of the second trimester, cases of abortion merge almost imperceptibly into cases that could almost be classed as very early premature onset of labour. In these cases chorioamnionitis becomes a relatively common and important finding (Gaillard et al, 1993).

A final point is that in 'iatrogenic spontaneous abortions', i.e. those following chorionic villus sampling, the placental tissue is usually fully normal for the length of the gestational period (McCormack et al, 1991).

INDUCED ABORTION

Currently, and until the value of antiprogesterone agents is more fully assessed, most pregnancy terminations are achieved by surgical means but a variety of well-established non-surgical techniques are still in use in some centres. The effects of these manoeuvres on the placenta have attracted attention, largely because of the widely held, though probably incorrect, belief that the production of placental damage is an important factor in the interruption of the pregnant state.

Intra-amniotic Injection of Hypertonic Saline

This has been a popular technique for inducing mid-pregnancy abortion. Stamm and de Watteville (1954) were the first to note that this procedure resulted in oedema and necrosis of the amnion, but they did not comment on lesions within the placental substance. Since then, however, a considerable number of observations have accumulated that give a clear picture of the changes that this technique of abortion induces in the cord, membranes and placenta, changes which, although variable in their extent and degree, are nevertheless remarkably consistent in pattern (Bengtsson & Stormby, 1962; Weingold et al, 1965; Christie et al, 1966; Gochberg & Reid, 1966; Pathak, 1968; Jakobovits et al, 1970; Berkowitz & Fuchs, 1971; Blaustein & Shenker, 1971; Gustavii & Brunk, 1972; Galen et al, 1974; Craig, 1975; Puri et al, 1976).

If the uterine contents are expelled shortly after the saline injection the placenta and membranes may appear macroscopically normal, but more commonly the placenta is pale, bulky and flabby and the membranes are oedematous, sometimes containing fluid-filled bullae. The chorionic vessels are congested and focal sub-amniotic haemorrhages are sometimes seen. Not uncommonly, thrombosis of the chorionic vessels is apparent: the cord is congested and oedematous. On slicing the placenta it can be seen that, whilst most of the placental substance appears normal, there is a very characteristic, thin, sharply demarcated subchorionic band which is solid and haemorrhagic. This band involves, at the most, between one-fifth and one-tenth of the full thickness of the placental tissue, and is usually no more than a few millimetres wide (Fig. 10.10).

Histological examination of the membranes confirms the presence of oedema, and reveals that the amniotic cells are patchy in distribution and have abnormalities ranging in nature from simple vacuolation to complete necrosis. Thrombosis of chorionic vessels is often seen and there may, on occasion, be a mild chorionic vasculitis. The cord is oedematous and thrombosis of funicular vessels is common. There may be an acute inflammatory cell infiltrate in Wharton's jelly. In the macroscopically abnormal subchorionic zone of the placental substance the intervillous space is occluded by a mixture of thrombus, fibrin and acute inflammatory cells, whilst the villi in this area show a variable degree of damage ranging from stromal oedema and trophoblastic vacuolation at one extreme to complete necrosis at the other. There is an abrupt transition from this grossly abnormal area of damaged or destroyed villi to normal placental tissue in which the intervillous space is free of obstruction and the villi are normal not only on light microscopy but also on electron microscopy (Wynn, 1965). Although the villi on the maternal side of the placenta are normal, there is a variable, but often extensive, degree of patchy necrosis of the decidual cells beneath Nitabuch's layer.

The distribution of the placental changes suggests that they are a direct result of

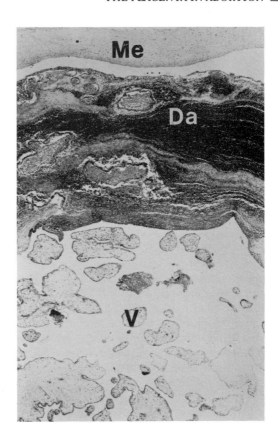

Figure 10.10. A placenta aborted after intra-amniotic injection of saline. Adjacent to the membranes (Me) there is a band of damaged tissue (Da) which is sharply demarcated from the more deeply situated normal intact villi (V) (H & E ×30).

chemical damage inflicted by the hypertonic saline in the amniotic fluid. It is difficult to attribute the decidual necrosis to a similar cause in view of the fact that the immediately adjacent villous tissue is completely normal, but as decidual changes of this type (and of similar degree) have also been noted in spontaneous mid-trimester abortions (Puri et al, 1976), they are very possibly not directly related to the intra-amniotic saline.

It has been considered that the placental damage produced by hypertonic saline is a direct cause of fetal death and subsequent abortion, but I find this difficult, indeed almost impossible, to accept, because the quantitative loss of villous tissue is modest and well within the compass of the functional reserve capacity of the placenta, particularly as the subchorionic zone is probably one of the less important sites of materno-fetal oxygen exchange within the placenta. A more sophisticated view suggests that placental damage leads to a fall in progesterone levels, with a consequent diminution of the adequacy of the myometrial progesterone block and subsequent onset of uterine contractions (Bengtsson & Csapo, 1962). Again, it is difficult to accept that the degree of placental damage could result in a significant fall in circulating progesterone levels, and Gustavii (1973) has pointed out that attempts to demonstrate reduced progesterone levels in saline-induced abortion or to show that the abortion can be delayed by administration of progestins have yielded conflicting and inconclusive results. Gustavii (1973) has postulated that the decidua is the target organ for hypertonic saline arguing that decidual cells have unusually labile lysosomes, which, under the influence of hypertonic saline, release enzymes capable of inducing local prostaglandin synthesis and secretion with consequent onset of uterine contractions. This is an attractive and quite persuasive hypothesis, but unfortunately it suffers from the defect that there is no proof that the noted decidual necrosis in these abortions is actually due to the saline, because similar changes of equivalent severity are, as already noted, not uncommonly found in spontaneous mid-pregnancy abortions. In abortion following intra-amniotic injection the fetus is nearly always born dead (Kovacs et al, 1970), and hence the view that the saline attacks principally the fetus to produce either acute desiccation or acute salt poisoning (Blaustein & Shenker, 1971; Galen et al, 1974) is, in my opinion, a reasonable and plausible explanation for its abortifacient effect.

Extra-amniotic Injection of Hypertonic Saline

This has been a less commonly used method of inducing abortion than intra-amniotic instillation and its effects have been less extensively studied. Oram et al (1963) found no lesions in placentas obtained by hysterotomy within 60 minutes of extra-amniotic injection, but this was probably too short a time interval to allow for the evolution of any pathological changes. Gustavii and Brunk (1972) noted changes in the membranes and placenta that were virtually identical to those found after intra-amniotic hypertonic saline injection; the sub-chorionic zone of damaged villi was, however, somewhat thinner than that seen with the intra-amniotic method (Fig. 10.11). Decidual necrosis was also apparent but was no more extensive or severe than that noted following intra-amniotic saline. These similarities between the effects of intra- and extra-amniotic injection of hypertonic saline are not altogether surprising, because it is known that extra-amniotic saline rapidly traverses the membranes to enter the amniotic fluid. The concentration attained within the liquor, however, is lower than that found following intra-amniotic instillation and this is presumably the reason why the subchorionic zone of villous necrosis is thinner. Extra-amniotic saline is presumed to induce abortion by a mechanism similar to that which occurs after intra-amniotic injection.

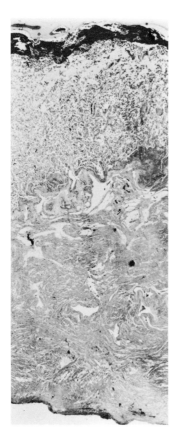

Figure 10.11. Section through the placenta and uterine wall. The tissue was obtained by hysterectomy 6 hours after extra-amniotic injection of saline. Only a very narrow zone of the placenta adjacent to the chorionic plate (above) shows any evidence of damage (H & E ×2.2)

Intra-amniotic Injection of Hypertonic Urea

Segal et al (1976) have observed that injection of hypertonic urea into the amniotic sac for abortifacient purposes produces placental and membranous lesions that are, in every way, identical to those seen after intra-amniotic instillation of hypertonic saline. It is of interest, however, that in this study no evidence was seen of decidual necrosis. It is assumed, though certainly not proved, that the mechanisms of both placental damage and abortion are similar to those that occur with intra-amniotic saline.

Intra-amniotic Injection of Glucose

This technique of pregnancy termination provides the best evidence that placental damage is not a necessary prerequisite for abortion when chemical substances are instilled into the amniotic sac, because reports of the abortifacient action of intra-amniotic glucose have made particular note of the absence of any resulting placental lesions (Brosset, 1958; Wood et al, 1962).

Intra-amniotic Injection of Prostaglandins

There have been few reports of the placental changes found with this technique of inducing abortion. Puri et al (1976) noted that after intra-amniotic injection of prostaglandin F_{ga2} the chorionic vessels showed marked thickening of their walls but were not thrombosed. The intervillous space in the immediately subchorionic area contained thrombus and fibrin, but the villi, both here and elsewhere in the placenta, were healthy and there was no evidence of trophoblastic damage. The membranes were not oedematous, but necrosis of the decidual cells beneath Nitabuch's layer was observed. Honoré (1976), in a similar study, reported that the most characteristic finding after intra-amniotic injection of prostaglandin F_{ga2} was extensive decidual haemorrhage with widespread necrosis of decidual cells and thrombosis of decidual vessels. He also described widespread degeneration of the placental villi, together with extensive perivillous thrombosis and fibrin deposition.

Extra-amniotic Injection of Prostaglandins

In a personally studied series of placentas obtained after induction of second-trimester abortion by the extra-amniotic injection of prostaglandins (Fox et al, 1978), no evidence was seen of damage to the villous tissue, the only reasonably consistent lesion being focal decidual haemorrhage.

Antiprogesterone Agents

Only preliminary information is available about the effects on the placenta of antiprogestational agents which are being used to induce early abortion, but villous degeneration and necrosis have been described (Xu et al, 1994; Liu et al, 1995).

Mechanical Induction of Abortion

The induction of second-trimester abortion by the intrauterine use of a rubber metreurynter after dilatation of the cervical canal by laminaria tents is not associated with the development of any placental lesions, at either the light or electron microscopic level (Manabe & Yoshida, 1973; Manabe et al, 1973).

REFERENCES

Abaci, F. and Aterman, K. (1968) Changes of the placenta and embryo in early spontaneous abortion. *American Journal of Obstetrics and Gynecology*, **102**, 252–263.

Alberman, E. (1988) The epidemiology of repeated abortion. In *Early Pregnancy Loss: Mechanisms and Treatment*, Beard, R.W. and Sharp, F. (Eds), pp. 9–17. London: Springer-Verlag.

Arnout, J., Spitz., Van Assche, A. and Vermylen, J. (1995) The antiphospholipid syndrome in pregnancy. *Hypertension in Pregnancy*, **14**, 147–178.

Baker, D.P. (1982) Trauma in the pregnant patient. *Surgical Clinics of North America*, **62**, 275–289.

Balen, A.H., Tan, S.L. and Jacobs, H.S. (1993a) Hypersecretion of luteinizing hormone: a significant cause of infertility and miscarriage. *British Journal of Obstetrics and Gynaecology*, **100**, 1082–1089.

Balen, A.H., Tan, S.L., MacDougall, J. and Jacobs, H.S. (1993b) Miscarriage rates following in-vitro fertilization are increased in women with polycystic ovaries and reduced by pituitary desensitization with buserelin. *Human Reproduction*, **8**, 959–964.

Bengtsson, L.P. and Csapo, A. (1962) Oxytocin response, withdrawal, and reinforcement of defence mechanism of the human uterus at midpregnancy. *American Journal of Obstetrics and Gynecology*, **83**, 1083–1093.

Bengtsson, L.P. and Stormby, N. (1962) The effect of intra-amniotic injection of hypertonic sodium chloride in human midpregnancy. *Acta Obstetricia et Gynecologica Scandinavica*, **41**, 115–123.

Bennett, M.J. (1987) Congenital abnormalities of the fundus. In *Spontaneous and Recurrent Abortion*, Bennett, M.J. and Edmonds, D.K. (Eds), pp. 109–129. Baltimore: Williams & Wilkins.

Berkowitz, R. and Fuchs, F. (1971) Hormonal and placental changes after intra-amniotic injection of hypertonic saline. *Clinical Obstetrics and Gynecology*, **14**, 179–191.

Berry, C.W., Brambati, B., Eskes, T.K.A.B. et al (1995) The Euro-team early pregnancy (ETEP) protocol for recurrent miscarriage. *Human Reproduction*, **10**, 1516–1520.

Blaustein, A. and Shenker, L. (1971) Pathologic findings after hypertonic saline installation in midtrimester abortion. *Clinical Obstetrics and Gynecology*, **14**, 192–203.

Boué, J., Boué, A. and Lazar, P. (1975) Retrospective and prospective epidemiological studies of 1500 karyotyped spontaneous human abortions. *Teratology*, **12**, 11–26.

Branch, D.W. (1994) Thoughts on the mechanism of pregnancy loss associated with the antiphospholipid syndrome. *Lupus*, **3**, 275–280.

Bret, J. and Grepinet, J. (1968) Etude comparative des éléments anatomo-cliniques dans une série d'avortements chromosomiques, dans une série témoin au cours de la mole de Breus. *Gynécologie et Obstétrique*, **67**, 313–328.

Bret, J., Lancret, P. and Bourel, M. (1967) Enquete anatomapathologique 'standard' sur le placenta dans 425 cas d'avortements. *Revue Francaise de Gynécologie et Obstétrique*, **62**, 409–412.

Brosset, A. (1958) The induction of therapeutic abortion by means of a hypertonic glucose solution injected into the amniotic sac. *Acta Obstetricia et Gynecologica Scandinavica*, **37**, 519–525.

Buttram, V.C. and Reiter, R.C. (1981) Uterine leiomyomata: etiology, symptomatology, and management. *Fertility and Sterility*, **32**, 40–46.

Byrne, J. and Warburton, D. (1986) Neural tube defects in spontaneous abortion. *American Journal of Medical Genetics*, **25**, 327–333.

Byrne, L.B.J. and Ward, K. (1994) Genetic factors in recurrent abortion. *Clinical Obstetrics and Gynecology*, **37**, 691–704.

Canki, N., Warburton, D. and Byrne, J. (1988) Morphological characteristics of monosomy X in spontaneous abortions. *Annales de Génétique*, **31**, 4–13.

Carr, D.H. (1971a) Chromosomes and abortion. In *Advances in Human Genetics*, Vol. 2, Harris, H. and Hirschorn, K.(Eds), pp. 201–257. New York and London: Plenum Press.

Carr, D.H. (1971b) The abortus. In *Symposium on the Functional Physiopathology of the Fetus and Neonate*, Abramson, H. (Ed.), pp. 94–109. St Louis: C V Mosby.

Chard, T. (1991) Frequency of implantation and early pregnancy loss in natural cycles. *Ballière's Clinical Obstetrics and Gynaecology*, **5**, 179–189.

Charles, D. and Larsen, B. (1990) Spontaneous abortion as a result of infection. In *Early Pregnancy Failure*, Huisjes, H.J. and Lind, T. (Eds), pp. 161–176. Edinburgh: Churchill Livingstone.

Christie, J.L., Anderson, A.B.M., Turnbull, A.C. and Beck, J.W. (1966) The human placenta and membranes: a histological and immunofluorescent study of the effects of intra-amniotic injection of hypertonic saline. *Journal of Obstetrics and Gynaecology of the British Commonwealth*, **73**, 399–409.

Clifford, K.A. and Regan, L. (1994) Recurrent pregnancy loss. In *Progress in Obstetrics & Gynaecology*, Vol. 11, Studd, J. (Ed.), pp. 97–110. Edinburgh: Churchill Livingstone.

Cohen, J. (1972) Intéret de l'examen du placenta dans les avortements spontanés du premier trimestre. *Revue Francaise de Gynécologie et d'Obstétrique*, **67**, 123–126.

Coulam, C.B. and Stern, J.J. (1994) Endocrine factors associated with recurrent spontaneous abortion. *Clinical Obstetrics and Gynecology*, **37**, 730–744.

Cowchock, F.S., Gibas, S. and Jackson, L.G. (1993) Chromosome errors as a cause of spontaneous abortion: the relative importance of maternal age and obstetric history. *Fertility and Sterility*, **59**, 1011–1014.

Craig, J.M. (1975) The pathology of birth control. *Archives of Pathology*, **99**, 233–236.

Creasy, R. (1988) The cytogenetics of spontaneous abortion in humans. In *Early Pregnancy Loss: Mechanisms and Treatment*, Beard, R.W. and Sharp, F. (Eds), pp. 293–304. London: Springer–Verlag.

Davison, E.V. and Burn, J. (1990) Genetic causes of early pregnancy loss. In *Early Pregnancy Failure*, Huisjes, H.J. and Lind, T. (Eds), pp. 55–78. Edinburgh: Churchill Livingstone.

Dawood, M.Y. (1994) Corpus luteal insufficiency. *Current Opinion in Obstetrics and Gynecology*, **6**, 121–127.

Daya, S. (1994) Issues in the etiology of recurrent spontaneous abortion. *Current Opinion in Obstetrics and Gynecology*, **6**, 153–159.

de Braekeleer, M. and Dao, T.N. (1990) Cytogenetic studies in couples experiencing repeated pregnancy losses. *Human Reproduction*, **5**, 519–528.

Donderwinkel, P.F., Dorr, J.P. and Willemsen, W.N. (1992) The unicornuate uterus: clinical implications. *European Journal of Obstetrics, Gynecology and Reproductive Biology*, **47**, 135–139.

Doss, B.J., Greene, M.F., Hill, J. et al (1995) Massive chronic intervillositis associated with recurrent abortions. *Human Pathology*, **26**, 1245–1251.

Dydowicz, M. and Pisarki, T. (1967) Estimation and classification of morphological changes in chorions on spontaneous abortions. *Bulletin Société des Amis des Science et des Lettres de Poznan*, **16**, 143–158.

Edmonds, D.K., Lindsay, K.S., Miller, J.F., Williamson, R. and Woods, P.J. (1982) Early embryonic mortality in women. *Fertility and Sterility*, **38**, 447–453.

Eiben, B., Bartels, I., Bahr-Porsch, S. et al (1990) Cytogenetic analysis of 750 spontaneous abortions with the direct-preparation method of chorionic villi and its implications for studying genetic causes of pregnancy wastage. *American Journal of Human Genetics*, **47**, 656–663.

Exalto, N. (1995) Early human nutrition. *European Journal of Obstetrics, Gynecology and Reproductive Biology*, **61**, 3–6.

Fantel, A.G., Shepard, T.H., Vadheim-Roth, C., Stephens, T.D. and Coleman, C. (1980) Embryonic and fetal phenotypes: prevalence and other associated factors in a large study of spontaneous abortion. In *Human Embryonic and Fetal Death*, Porter, I.H. and Hook, E.B. (Eds), pp. 71–87. New York: Academic Press.

Fedele, L., Dorta, M., Brioschi, D. et al (1989) Pregnancies in septate uteri: outcome in relation to site of uterine implantation as determined by sonography. *American Journal of Roentgenology*, **152**, 781–784.

Fox, H., Herd, M.E. and Harilal, K.R. (1978) Morphological changes in the placenta and decidua following extra-amniotic injection of prostaglandins. *Histopathology*, **2**, 145–150.

Fujikura, J., Froehlich, L.A. and Driscoll, S.G. (1966) A simplified anatomic classification of abortions. *American Journal of Obstetrics and Gynecology*, **95**, 902–905.

Fukunaga, M., Ushigome, S. and Fukunaga, M. (1993) Spontaneous abortions and DNA ploidy: an application of flow cytometric DNA analysis in detection of non-diploidy in early abortions. *Modern Pathology*, **6**, 619–624.

Fukunaga, M., Onda, T., Endo, Y. and Ushigome, S. (1995) Is there a correlation between histology and karotype in early spontaneous abortion? *International Journal of Surgical Pathology*, **2**, 295–300.

Gaillard, D.A., Paradis, P., Lallemand, A.V. et al (1993) Spontaneous abortions during the second trimester of gestation. *Archives of Pathology and Laboratory Medicine*, **117**, 1022–1026.

Gaither, D.B. and Sampson, C.C. (1968) Intervillous fibrin deposition associated with spontaneous abortion: analysis of 100 cases. *Journal of the National Medical Association*, **60**, 497–499.

Galen, R.S., Chauhan, P., Wietzner, H. and Navarro, C. (1974) Fetal pathology and mechanism of fetal death in saline-induced abortion: a study of 143 gestations and critical review of the literature. *American Journal of Obstetrics and Gynecology*, **120**, 347–355.

Garcia, C.R. and Tureck, R.W. (1984) Submucosal leiomyomas and infertility. *Fertility and Sterility*, **42**, 16–19.

Geisler, K. and Kleinebrecht, J. (1978) Cytogenetic and histologic analysis of spontaneous abortion. *Human Genetics*, **45**, 239–251.

Genest, D.R. (1994) The pathology of early pregnancy wastage. *Advances in Pathology and Laboratory Medicine*, **7**, 281–312.

Genest, D.R., Roberts, D., Boyd, D. and Bieber, F.R. (1995) Fetoplacental pathology as a predictor of karyotype: a controlled study of spontaneous first trimester abortions. *Human Pathology*, **26**, 201–209.

Geneva Conference (1966) Standardization of procedures for chromosome studies in abortions. *Cytogenetics* **5**, 361–393.

Gleicher, N., Pratt, D. and Dudkiewicz, A. (1993) What do we really know about autoantibody abnormalities and reproductive failure? a critical review. *Autoimmunity*, **16**, 115–140.

Gochberg, S.H. and Reid, D.E. (1966) Intra-amniotic injection of hypertonic saline for termination of pregnancy. *Obstetrics and Gynecology*, **27**, 648–654.

Gocke, H., Muradow, I. and Cremer, H. (1982) Morphologische und zytogenetische Befunde bei Fruhaborten. *Verhandlungen der Deutschen Gesellschichte für Pathologie*, **66**, 141–146.

Gocke, H., Schwanitz, G., Muradow, I. and Zerres, K. (1985) Pathomorphologie und Genetik in der Fruhschwangerschaft. *Pathologe*, **6**, 249–259.

Golan, A., Langer, R., Neuman, M. et al (1992) Obstetric outcome in women with congenital uterine malformations. *Journal of Reproductive Medicine*, **37**, 233–236.

Gustavii, B. (1973) Studies on the mode of action of intra-amniotically injected hypertonic saline in therapeutic abortion. *Acta Obstetricia et Gynecologica Scandinavica*, Supplement **25**, 1–22.

Gustavii, B. and Brunk, U. (1972) A histological study of the effect on the placenta of intra-amniotically and extra-amniotically injected hypertonic saline in therapeutic abortion. *Acta Obstetricia et Gynecologica Scandinavica*, **51**, 121–125.

Hassold, T.J., Chen, N., Funkhouser, J. et al (1980) A cytogenetic study of 1000 spontaneous abortions. *Annals of Human Genetics*, **44**, 151–178.

Hatasaka, H.H. (1994) Recurrent miscarriage: epidemiologic factors, definitions, and incidence. *Clinical Obstetrics and Gynecology*, **37**, 625–634.

Hathout, H. (1964) The vascular pattern and mode of insertion of the umbilical cord on abortion material. *Journal of Obstetrics and Gynaecology of the British Commonwealth*, **71**, 963–964.

Hertig, A.T. (1968) *Human Trophoblast*, Springfield, Illinois: Thomas.

Hertz, D.G. (1973) Rejection of motherhood: a psychosomatic appraisal of habitual abortion. *Psychosomatics*, **14**, 241–244.

Hobbs, J.E. and Rollins, P.R. (1934) Fetal death from placenta circumvallata. *American Journal of Obstetrics and Gynecology*, **28**, 78–83.

Honoré, L.H. (1976) Midtrimester prostaglandin-induced abortion: gross and light microscopic findings in the placenta. *Prostaglandins*, **11**, 1019–1032.

Honoré, L.H., Dill, F.J. and Poland, B.J. (1976) Placental morphology in spontaneous human abortuses with normal and abnormal karyotypes. *Teratology*, **14**, 151–166.

Horn, L.C., Rosenkranz, M. and Bilek, K. (1991) Wertigkeit der Plazentahistologie für die Erkennung genetisch bedingter Aborte. *Zeitschrift für Geburtshilfe und Perinatologie*, **195**, 47–53.

Houwert-de Jong, M.H. (1989) Habitual abortion; views and fact finding. *Thesis, University of Utrecht*.

Houwert-de Jong, M.H., Bruinse, H.W., Eskes, T.K.A.B. et al (1990) Early recurrent miscarriage: histology of conception products. *British Journal of Obstetrics and Gynaecology*, **97**, 533–535.

Howat, A.J., Beck, S., Fox, H. et al (1993) Can histopathologists reliably diagnose molar pregnancy? *Journal of Clinical Pathology*, **46**, 599–602.

Huisjes, H.J. (1990) Maternal disease and early pregnancy loss. In *Early Pregnancy Failure*, Huisjes, H.J. and Lind, T. (Eds), pp. 148–153. Edinburgh: Churchill Livingstone.

Hustin, J. and Jauniaux, E. (1992) Morphology and mechanisms of abortion. In *The First Twelve Weeks of Gestation*, Barnea, E.R., Hustin, J. and Jauniaux, E. (Eds), pp. 280–296. Berlin: Springer-Verlag.

Hustin, J. and Schaaps, J.P. (1987) Echographic and anatomic studies of the maternotrophoblastic border during the first trimester of pregnancy. *American Journal of Obstetrics and Gynecology*, **157**, 162–168.

Hustin, J., Jauniaux, E. and Schaaps, J.P. (1990) Histological study of the materno–embryonic interface in spontaneous abortion. *Placenta*, **11**, 477–486.

Infante-Rivard, C., David, M., Gauthier, R. and Rivard, G.E. (1991) Lupus anticoagulants, anticardiolipin antibodies, and fetal loss: a case control study. *New England Journal of Medicine*, **325**, 1063–1066.

Jakobovits, A., Traub, A., Farkas, M. and Morvay, J. (1970) The effect of intra-amniotic injections of hypertonic saline on the structure and endocrine function of the placenta. *International Journal of Gynaecology and Obstetrics*, **8**, 499–506.

Jauniaux, E., Zaidi, J., Jurcovic, D., Campbell, S. and Hustin, J. (1994) Comparison of colour Doppler features and pathological findings in complicated early pregnancy. *Human Reproduction*, **9**, 2432–2437.

Javert, C.T. (1957) *Spontaneous and Habitual Abortion*. New York: McGraw-Hill.

Javert, C.T. and Barton, B. (1952) Congenital and acquired lesions of the umbilical cord and spontaneous abortion. *American Journal of Obstetrics and Gynecology*, **63**, 1065–1077.

Kalousek, D.K. (1993) The effect of confined placental mosaicism on development of the human aneuploid conceptus. *Birth Defects: Original Article Series*, **29**, 39–51.

Kalousek, D.K. (1994) Current topic: confined placental mosaicism and intrauterine fetal development. *Placenta*, **15**, 219–230.

Kalousek, D.K., Barrett, I. and McGillivray, B.C. (1989). Placental mosaicism and intrauterine survival of trisomies 13 and 18. *American Journal of Human Genetics*, **44**, 338–343.

Kalousek, D.K., Fitch, N. and Paradice, B.A. (1990) *Pathology of the Human Embryo and Previable Fetus: An Atlas*. New York: Springer-Verlag.

Kalousek, D.K., Barrett, I.J. and Gartner, A.B. (1992) Spontaneous abortion and confined chromosomal mosaicism. *Human Genetics*, **88**, 642–646.

Kalousek, D.K., Pantzar, T., Tsai, M. and Paradice, B. (1993) Early spontaneous abortion: morphologic and karotypic findings in 3912 cases. *Birth Defects*, **29**, 53–61.

Keye, W. (1994) Psychologic relationships. *Clinical Obstetrics and Gynecology*, **37**, 671–680.

Khong, T.Y. and George, K. (1992) Chromosomal abnormalities associated with a single umbilical artery. *Prenatal Diagnosis*, **12**, 965–968.

Khong, T.Y., Liddell, H.S. and Robertson, W.B. (1987) Defective haemochorial placentation as a cause of miscarriage: a preliminary study. *British Journal of Obstetrics and Gynaecology*, **94**, 649–655.

Khong, T.Y., Stewart, C.J., Mott, C., Chambers, H.M. and Staples, A.J. (1994) The usefulness of human placental lactogen and keratin immunohistochemistry in the assessment of tissue from purported intrauterine pregnancies. *American Journal of Clinical Pathology*, **102**, 72–75.

Kline, J., Stein, Z. and Susser, W.D. (1985) Fever during pregnancy and spontaneous abortion. *American Journal of Epidemiology*, **121**, 832–842.

Kovacevic, M., Lusic, N. and Vukic, R. (1990) *Jugoslavenska Ginecologija Perinatologija*, **30**, 117–118.

Kovacs, L., Resch, B., Scollosi, J. and Herczeg, J. (1970) The role of fetal death in the process of therapeutic abortion induced by intra-amniotic injection of hypertonic saline. *Journal of Obstetrics and Gynaecology of the British Commonwealth*, **77**, 1132–1136.

Lage, J.M. and Popek, E.J. (1993) The role of DNA flow cytometry in evaluation of partial and complete hydatidiform moles and hydropic abortions. *Seminars in Diagnostic Pathology*, **10**, 267–274.

Laurini, R.N. (1990) Abortion from a morphological viewpoint. In: *Early Pregnancy Failure*, Huisjes, H.J. and Lind, T. (Eds), pp. 79–113. Edinburgh: Churchill Livingstone.

Lauritsen, J.G. (1976) Aetiology of spontaneous abortion: a cytogenetic and epidemiological study of 288 abortuses. *Acta Obstetricia et Gynecologica Scandinavica*, Supplement **52**, 1–29.

Levy, H. (1956) Mola de Breus – revisao des conceitos patogeneticos a proposito de nove casos proprios. *Gazeta Medica Portuguesa*, **9**, 341–363.

Liu, B., Sun, J. and Tao, W. (1995) The pathological investigations on termination of early pregnancy with mifepristone. *Chinese Journal of Obstetrics and Gynecology*, **30**, 7–9.

Ludmir, J., Samuels, P., Brooks, S. and Mennuti, M.T. (1990) Pregnancy outcome of patients with uncorrected uterine anomalies managed in a high-risk obstetric setting. *Obstetrics and Gynecology*, **75**, 906–910.

McCormack, M.J., Mackenzie, W.E., Rushton, D.I. and Newton, J.R. (1991) Clinical and pathological factors in spontaneous abortion following chorionic villus sampling. *Prenatal Diagnosis*, **11**, 841–846.

McFadden, D.E. and Kalousek, D. (1989) Survey of neural tube defects in spontaneously aborted embryos. *American Journal of Medical Genetics*, **32** 356–358.

Makino, T., Umeuchi, M., Nakada, K. et al (1992) Incidence of congenital uterine anomalies in repeated reproductive wastage and prognosis for pregnancy after metroplasty. *International Journal of Fertility*, **37**, 167–170.

Mall, F.P. and Meyer, A.W. (1921) Studies on abortuses: a survey of pathologic ova in the Carnegie embryological collection. *Contributions to Embryology. Carnegie Institution of Washington*, **12**, 1–364.

Manabe, Y. and Yoshida, Y. (1973) Light and electron microscopic studies of the placenta delivered by laminaria–metreurynter induced abortion in mid-pregnancy. *Endokrinologie*, **61**, 379–381.

Manabe, Y., Nakajima, A. and Griggs, J.F. (1973) Uterine contractility and placental histology in abortion by laminaria and metreurynter. *Obstetrics and Gynecology*, **41**, 753–759.

Manchesi, I., Manchesi, F., Parlato, F. et al (1989) Reproductive performance in women with uterus didelphys. *Acta Europaea Fertilitas*, **20**, 121–124.

Mantoni, M. (1985) Ultrasound signs in threatened abortion and their prognostic significance. *Obstetrics and Gynecology*, **65**, 471–475.

Melk, A., Mueller-Eckhardt, G., Polten, B., Lattermann, A., Heine, O. and Hoffmann, O. (1995) Diagnostic and prognostic significance of anticardiolipin antibodies in patients with recurrent spontaneous abortions. *American Journal of Reproductive Immunology*, **33**, 228–233.

Michalas, S.P. (1991) Outcome of pregnancy in women with uterine malformation: evaluation of 62 cases. *International Journal of Gynaecology and Obstetrics*, **35**, 557–559.

Michel, M.Z., Khong, T.Y., Clark, D.A. and Beard, R.W. (1990) A morphological and immunological study of human placental bed biopsies in miscarriage. *British Journal of Obstetrics and Gynaecology*, **97**, 984–988.

Michel-Wolfromm, H. (1967) Le facteur psychique dans l'avortement spontanés. *Revue Francaise de Gynécologie et d'Obstétrique*, **62**, 533–536.

Minguillon, C., Eiben, B., Bahr-Porsch, S., Vogel, M. and Hansmann, H. (1989) The predictive value of chorionic villus histology for identifying chromosomally normal and abnormal spontaneous abortions. *Human Genetics*, **82**, 373–376.

Monie, I.W. (1965) Velamentous insertion of the cord in early pregnancy. *American Journal of Obstetrics and Gynecology*, **93**, 276–281.

Moutos, D.H., Damewood, M.D., Schlaff, W.D. and Rock, J.A. (1992) A comparison of the reproductive outcome between women with a unicornuate uterus and women with a didelphic uterus. *Fertility and Sterility*, **58**, 88–93.

Muntefering, R., Dallenbach-Hellweg, G. and Ratscheck, M. (1989) Pathologische-anatomische Befunde bei der gestorten Fruhschwangerschaft. *Gynäkologie*, **21**, 262–272.

Novak, R.W., Agamonalis, D., Dasu, S. et al (1988) Histological analysis of placental tissue in first trimester abortions. *Pediatric Pathology*, **8**, 477–482.

Ohno, M., Meada, T. and Matsunobu, A. (1991) A cytogenetic study of spontaneous abortions with direct analysis of chorionic villi. *Obstetrics and Gynecology*, **77**, 394–398.

Oram, V., Svane, H. and Albrechtsen, O.K. (1963) Svangerskabsafbrydelse med saltvand. *Ugeskrift for Laeger*, **25**, 98–100.

Paradinas, F.J. (1994) The histological diagnosis of hydatidiform moles. *Current Diagnostic Pathology*, **1**, 24–31.

Pathak, U.N. (1968) Induction of labor by intraamniotic injection of saline: experience of 78 cases. *American Journal of Obstetrics and Gynecology*, **101**, 513–519.

Patton, P.E. (1994) Anatomic uterine defects. *Clinical Obstetrics and Gynecology*, **37**, 705–721.

Petri, M., Golbus, M., Anderson, R., Whiting-O'Keefe, Q., Corash, L. and Hellmann, D. (1987) Antinuclear antibody, lupus anticoagulant, and anticardiolopin antibody in women with idiopathic habitual abortion. *Arthritis and Rheumatism*, **30**, 601–606.

Philippe, E. (1973) Morphologie et morphometrie des placentas d'aberration chromosomique lethale. *Revue Francaise de Gynécologie et d'Obstétrique*, **68**, 645–653.

Philippe, E. (1986) *Pathologie Foeto-placentaire*. Paris: Masson.

Philippe, E. and Boué, J.G. (1969) Le placenta des aberations chromosomiques létales. *Annales d'Anatomie Pathologique*, **14**, 249–266.

Philippe, E. and Boué, J.G. (1970) Placenta et aberrations chromosomiques au cours des avortements spontanés. *Presse Médicale*, **78**, 641–646.

Philippe, E., Ritter, J., Dehalleux, J.M., Renaud, R. and Gandar, R. (1968) De la pathologie des avortements spontanés. *Gynécologie et Obstétrique*, **67**, 97–118.

Plouffe, L., White, E.W., Tho, S.P. et al (1992) Etiologic factors of recurrent abortion and subsequent reproductive performance of couples: have we made any progress in the past 10 years? *American Journal of Obstetrics and Gynecology*, **167**, 313–321.

Pratt, D., Novotny, M., Kaberlein, G., Dudkiewicz, A. and Gleicher, N. (1993) Antithyroid antibodies and the association with non-organ specific antibodies in recurrent pregnancy loss. *American Journal of Obstetrics and Gynecology*, **168**, 837–841.

Puri, S., Aleem, F. and Schulman, H. (1976) A histologic study of the placentas of patients with saline- and prostaglandin-induced abortion. *Obstetrics and Gynecology*, **48**, 216–220.

Quinn, M. (1993) Final report of the Medical Research Council/Royal College of Obstetricians and Gynaecologists multicentre randomised trial of cervical cerclage. *British Journal of Obstetrics and Gynaecology*, **100**, 1154–1155.

Quinn, P.A., Petric, M., Barkin, M. et al (1987) Prevalence of antibody to *Chlamydia trachomatis* in spontaneous abortion and infertility. *American Journal of Obstetrics and Gynecology*, **156**, 291–296.

Rae, R., Smith, I.W., Liston, W.A. and Kilpatrick, D.C. (1994) Chlamydial serologic studies and recurrent spontaneous abortion. *American Journal of Obstetrics and Gynecology*, **170**, 782–785.

Regan, L., Owen, E.J. and Jacobs, H.S. (1990) Hypersecretion of luteinizing hormone, infertility and miscarriage. *Lancet*, **336**, 1141–1144.

Rehder, H., Coerdt, W., Eggers, R., Klink, F. and Schwinger, E. (1989) Is there a correlation between morphological and cytogenetic findings in placental tissue from early missed abortions? *Human Genetics*, **82**, 377–385.

Roberts, C.J. and Lowe, C.R. (1975) Where have all the conceptions gone? *Lancet*, **i**, 498–499.

Rockelein, G., Schroder, J. and Ulmer, R. (1989) Korrelation von Karotype und Plazentamorphologie beim Fruhabort. *Pathologe*, **10**, 306–314.

Rockelein, G., Ulmer, R. and Schroder, J. (1990a) Karotype and placental structure of first trimester spontaneous abortions; a morphometrical study. *European Journal of Obstetrics & Gynecology and Reproductive Biology*, **38**, 25–32.

Rockelein, G., Ulmer, R. and Schwille, R. (1990b) Surface and branching of placental villi in early abortion: relationship to karyotype: scanning electron microscopic study. *Virchows Archives A Pathological Anatomy and Histopathology*, **417**, 151–158.

Rushton, D.I. (1981) Examination of products of conception from previable human pregnancies. *Journal of Clinical Pathology*, **34**, 819–835.

Rushton, D.I. (1984) The classification and mechanisms of spontaneous abortion. *Perspectives in Pediatric Pathology*, **8**, 269–287.

Rushton, D.I. (1988) Placental pathology in spontaneous miscarriage. In *Early Pregnancy Loss: Mechanisms and Treatment*, Beard, R.W. and Sharp, F. (Eds), pp. 149–157. London: Springer-Verlag.

Rushton, D.I. (1995) Pathology of abortion. In *Haines and Taylor: Obstetrical and Gynaecological Pathology*, 4th edn, Fox, H. (Ed.), pp. 1641–1675. Edinburgh: Churchill Livingstone.

Sagle, M., Bishop, K., Ridley, N. et al (1988) Recurrent early miscarriage and polycystic ovaries. *British Medical Journal*, **297**, 1027–1028.

Salafia, C.M., Weigl, C.A. and Foye, G.J. (1988) Correlation of placental erythrocyte morphology with gestational age. *Pediatric Pathology*, **8**, 495–502.

Salafia, C., Maier, D., Vogel, C., Burns, J. and Silberman, L. (1993) Placental and decidual histology in spontaneous abortion: detailed description and correlations with chromosome number. *Obstetrics and Gynecology*, **82**, 295–303.

Saller, D.N., Keene, C.L., Sun, C.-C.J. and Schwartz, S. (1990) The association of single umbilical artery with cytogenetically abnormal pregnancies. *American Journal of Obstetrics and Gynecology*, **163**, 922–925.

Scott, J.S. (1960) Placenta extrachorialis (placenta marginata and placenta circumvallata): a factor in antepartum haemorrhage. *Journal of Obstetrics and Gynaecology of the British Empire*, **67**, 904–918.

Segal, S., Ornoy, A., Bercovici, B., Antebi, S.O. and Polishuk, W.Z. (1976) Placental pathology in midtrimester pregnancies interrupted by intra-amniotic injection of hypertonic urea. *British Journal of Obstetrics and Gynecology*, **83**, 156–159.

Shanklin, D.R. and Scott, J.S. (1975) Massive subchorial thrombohaematoma (Breus' mole) *British Journal of Obstetrics and Gynaecology*, **82**, 476–487.

Silver, R.M. and Branch, D.W. (1994) Recurrent miscarriage: autoimmune considerations. *Clinical Obstetrics and Gynecology*, **37**, 745–760.

Silverman, M. (1970) Psychological aspects of habitual abortion. *Psychiatric Communications*, **13**, 35–40.

Simpson, J.L. (1992) The aetiology of pregnancy failure. In *Spontaneous Abortion: Diagnosis and Treatment*, Stabile, I., Grudzinskas, G. and Chard, T. (Eds), pp. 21–47. London: Springer-Verlag.

Simpson, J.L. and Bombard, A.T. (1987) Chromosomal abnormalities in spontaneous abortions: frequency, pathology and genetic counselling. In *Spontaneous Abortion*, Edmonds, K. and Bennet, M.J. (Eds), pp. 51–76. London: Blackwell.

Simpson, J.L., Elias, S. and Martin, A.O. (1981) Parental chromosomal rearrangements associated with repetitive spontaneous abortions. *Fertility and Sterility*, **36**, 584–590.

Sorensen, V.J., Bivins, B.A., Obeid, F.N. and Horst, H.M. (1986) Trauma in pregnancy. *Henry Ford Hospital Medical Journal*, **34**, 101–104.

Stagnaro-Green, A., Roman, S.H., Cobin, R.H., El-Harazy, E., Alvarez-Marfany, M. and Davies, T.F. (1990) Detection of at-risk pregnancy by means of highly sensitive assays for thyroid autoantibodies. *Journal of the American Medical Association*, **264**, 1422–1425.

Stamm, O. and de Watteville, H. (1954) Etude expérimentale sur le mécanisme d'avortement par hydramnios artificiel. *Gynécologie et Obstétrique*, **53**, 171–187.

Stein, A.L. and March, C.M. (1990) Pregnancy outcome in women with müllerian anomalies. *Journal of Reproductive Medicine*, **35**, 411–414.

Sthoeger, Z.M., Mozes, E. and Tartakovsky, B. (1993) Anti-cardiolipin antibodies induce pregnancy failure by impairing embryonic implantation. *Proceedings of the National Academy of Sciences USA*, **90**, 6474–6487.

Stirrat, G.M. (1990) Recurrent miscarriage. II. Clinical associations, causes and management. *Lancet*, **336**, 728–733.

Stirrat, G.M. (1992) Recurrent spontaneous abortion. In *Immunological Obstetrics*, Coulam, C.B., Faulk, W.P. and McIntyre, J.A. (Eds), pp. 357–376. New York: Norton.

Stray-Peterson, B., Eng, J. and Reikvam, T.M. (1978) Uterine T-mycoplasma colonization in reproductive failure. *American Journal of Obstetrics and Gynecology*, **130**, 307–311.

Summers, P.R. (1994) Microbiology relevant to recurrent miscarriage. *Clinical Obstetrics and Gynecology*, **37**, 722–729.

Suster, S. and Robinson, M.J. (1992) Placental intravillous accumulation of sulphated mucosubstances: a reevaluation of so-called hydropic degeneration of the villi. *Annales of Clinical and Laboratory Science*, **22**, 175–181.

Sweeney, A.M., Meyer, M.R., Aarons, J.H. et al (1988) Evaluation of methods for the prospective identification of early fetal losses in environmental epidemiology studies. *American Journal of Epidemiology*, **127**, 843–849.

Szulman, A.E. (1991) Examination of the early conceptus. *Archives of Pathology and Laboratory Medicine*, **115**, 696–700.

Szulman, A.E. (1995) Embryonic death: pathology and forensic implications. *Perspectives in Pediatric Pathology*, **19**, 43–58.

Thomas, J. (1962) Die Entwicklung von Fetus und Placenta bei Nabelgefssanomalien. *Archiv für Gynäkologie*, 198, 216–223.

Topalovski, M., Hankin, R.C., Michael, C. et al (1995) Ploidy analysis of products of conception by image and flow cytometry with cytogenetic correlation. *American Journal of Clinical Pathology* **103**, 409–414.

Treffers, P.E. (1990) Uterine causes of early pregnancy failure – a critical evaluation. In *Early Pregnancy Failure*, Huisjes, H.J. and Lind, T. (Eds), pp. 114–147. Edinburgh: Churchill Livingstone.

Triplett, D.A. (1992) Obstetrical complications associated with antiphospholipid antibodies. In *Immunological Obstetrics*, Coulam, C.B., Faulk, W.P. and McIntyre, J.A. (Eds), pp. 377–403. New York: Norton.

Tulppala, M., Stenman, U.-H., Cacciatore, B. and Ylikorkala, O. (1993) Polycystic ovaries and levels of gonadotrophins and androgens in recurrent miscarriage: prospective study in 50 women. *British Journal of Obstetrics and Gynaecology*, **100**, 348–352.

van Lijnschoten, G., Arends, J.W., De la Fuente, A.A., Schouten, H.J.A. and Geraedts, J.P.M. (1993a) Intra- and inter-observer variation in the interpretation of histological features suggesting chromosomal abnormality in early abortion specimens. *Histopathology* **22**, 25–29.

van Lijnschoten, G., Arends, J.W., Leffers, P. et al (1993b) The value of histomorphological features of chorionic villi in early spontaneous abortion for the prediction of karotype. *Histopathology*, **22**, 557–563.

van Oven, M.W., Schoots, C.J., Ossterhuis, J.W. et al (1989) The use of DNA flow cytometry in the diagnosis of triploidy in human abortions. *Human Pathology*, **20**, 238–242.

Wang, B.B.T., Rubin, C.H. and Williams, J. (1993) Mosaicism in chorionic villus sampling: an analysis of incidence and chromosomes involved in 2612 consecutive cases. *Prenatal Diagnosis*, **13**, 179–190.

Warburton, D., Stein, Z., Kline, J. and Susser, M. (1980) Chromosome abnormalities in spontaneous abortions: data from the New York City study. In *Human Embryonic and Fetal Death*, Porter, I.H. and Hook, E.B. (Eds), pp. 261–287. New York: Academic Press.

Watson, H., Kiddy, D.S., Hamilton-Fairley, D. et al (1993) Hypersecretion of luteinizing hormone and ovarian steroids in women with recurrent early miscarriage. *Human Reproduction*, **8**, 829–833.

Weingold, A.B., Seigal, S. and Stone, M.L. (1965) Intra-amniotic hypertonic solutions for induction of labor. *Obstetrics and Gynecology*, **26**, 622–627.

Wilcox, A.J., Weinberg, C.R., O'Connor, J.F. et al (1988) Incidence of early loss of pregnancy. *New England Journal of Medicine*, **319**, 189–194.

Witkin, S.S. and Ledger, W.J. (1992) Antibodies to *Chlamydia trachomatis* in sera of women with recurrent spontaneous abortions. *American Journal of Obstetrics and Gynecology*, **167**, 135–139.

Wood, C., Booth, R.T. and Pinkerton, J.H.M. (1962) Induction of labour by intra-amniotic injection of hypertonic glucose solution. *British Medical Journal*, **ii**, 706–709.

Wynn, R.M. (1965) Electron microscopic contributions to placental physiology. *Journal of Obstetrics and Gynaecology of the British Commonwealth*, **72**, 955–963.

Xu, M.F., Jin, Y.C. and Cen, H.X. (1994) Histopathology appearance of intrauterine residue after medical abortion by mifepristone and prostaglandin analogue. *Chinese Journal of Obstetrics and Gynecology*, **29**, 739–741.

11

INFECTIONS AND INFLAMMATORY LESIONS OF THE PLACENTA

In this chapter the term 'placenta' is used to include not only the placental parenchyma but also the cord and the membranes; similarly, the expression 'placentitis' is taken to indicate any inflammatory process in any of these sites.

ROUTES OF PLACENTAL INFECTION

The placenta and membranes may be infected by a variety of routes (Fig. 11.1):

1. By organisms ascending into the amniotic sac from the vagina or cervix or ascending via the decidua.
2. By organisms that reach the placenta in the maternal blood.
3. By direct spread of organisms from a focus of infection in the endometrium.
4. By organisms entering the uterine cavity through the Fallopian tube, either from an infection in the pelvis or from a focus of infection in the tube.
5. By the introduction of organisms into the amniotic sac from outside the mother's body during such procedures such as amniocentesis, intrauterine transfusion, percutaneous umbilical blood sampling or intra-amniotic injection of abortifacient substances.
6. By retrograde spread from the fetus following intrauterine fetal transfusion with infected blood.
7. As a result of fertilization of an ovum by an infected spermatozoon.

In practice, only the first two of these routes of infection are of real importance (Blanc, 1959, 1961; Benirschke, 1960). Infection of the placenta from a lesion in the endometrium is uncommon if only because an endometritis tends to mitigate against successful implantation. This is not an invariable rule, however, and there is certainly the possibility, known to exist in some animals, of a chronic viral infection of the endometrial glands which, without seriously diminishing fertility, may serve as a potential reservoir for placental infection.

Entry of organisms into the amniotic sac from the Fallopian tube is extremely rare, as is placentitis following intrauterine fetal transfusion with infected blood, the only well-documented example of this latter form of placental infection being due to *Acinetobacter calcoaceticus* (Scott & Henderson, 1972). Amniocentesis has been followed by both bacterial (MacVicar, 1970; Haag et al, 1974; Bastert et al, 1975) and monilial

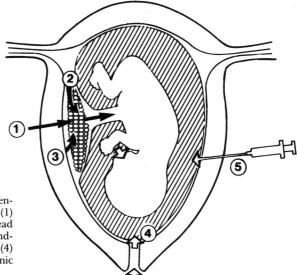

Figure 11.1. Pathways of feto-placental infection: haematogenous via (1) maternal bloodstream, (2) direct spread from endometrial infection, (3) via ascending decidual infection; ascending via (4) amniotic fluid infection or (5) iatrogenic amniotic fluid infection.

(Kérisit et al, 1973) infection of the amniotic sac whilst funipuncture has been complicated by fatal Group B streptococcal sepsis (McColgin et al, 1989); these are clearly preventable forms of placentitis.

Spermatozoa could, in theory, transmit organisms that were able to infect the ovum and hence also the developing trophoblast, but although the sperm nucleus could easily carry a provirus it has not yet been demonstrated that infection by this route actually occurs.

ASCENDING INFECTIONS

This term is applied to those infections of the placenta and membranes that are due to an entry of organisms into the amniotic sac from the maternal birth canal, this being by far the most common form of placentitis in humans. In this form of infection the brunt of the inflammatory process is borne by the membranes rather than by the placental tissue and the condition is usually classed as a 'chorioamnionitis' (or a 'chorionamnionitis'). It is currently thought that inflammation of the membranes is virtually always due to infection and that a chorioamnionitis is indicative of infection of the amniotic fluid. Nevertheless, infection of the amniotic fluid, as assessed by positive cultures, is not necessarily associated with histological evidence of chorioamnionitis and histologically proven chorioamnionitis occurs far more commonly than does clinically evident intra-amniotic infection.

Morphology of Ascending Infections

In most cases of chorioamnionitis the placenta and membranes appear macroscopically normal. In the relatively uncommon cases of severe and well-established bacterial infection, the membranes may be friable, oedematous, opaque, slimy and foul-smelling, whilst in infections of moderate severity there will be a variable degree of loss of the normal translucency of the membranes, which may have a slightly granular appearance. In the rare examples of chorioamnionitis caused by *Candida albicans* the membranes, and particularly the umbilical cord, may be studded with tiny yellow-white nodules or plaques which are usually of pin-point size.

Chorioamnionitis is, with rare exceptions which merit separate consideration, an acute inflammatory lesion and characteristically the first histological evidence of an ascending infection is a polymorphonuclear leucocytic infiltration of the extraplacental membranes (Fig. 11.2). The infiltrate appears first, and is subsequently most marked, at the lower pole of the amniotic sac. This is followed by an accumulation of polymorphonuclear leucocytes in the intervillous space immediately below the chorionic plate, which forms the roof of this space (Fig. 11.3). These cells are often enmeshed in fibrin, not because there is a fibrinous exudate but because the cells have infiltrated, and become embedded in, an already present layer of subchorionic fibrin. This aggregation of leucocytes is known accurately, but inelegantly, as a 'subchorial intervillositis'; inflammatory cells are rarely seen elsewhere in the intervillous space, whilst a villitis is rarely, with the possible exception of listeriosis, a feature of an ascending infection. The inflammatory cells in the roof of the intervillous space later extend upwards into the chorionic plate (Fig. 11.4) and it should be stressed that at this stage the inflammatory cellular response is purely maternal in origin, the leucocytes in the extraplacental membranes coming from maternal decidual vessels and those in the chorionic plate being derived from maternal blood in the intervillous space. Later, however, fetal leucocytes

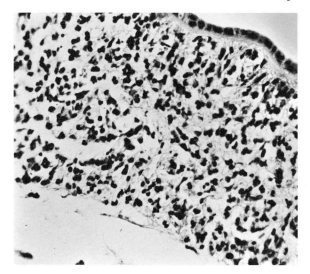

Figure 11.2. A polymorphonuclear leucocytic infiltration of the extraplacental membranes in an ascending infection. This is usually the first morphological hallmark of such an infection and the leucocytes are all maternal in origin (H & E ×950).

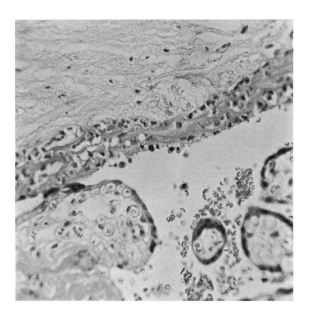

Figure 11.3. An accumulation of maternal polymorphonuclear leucocytes in the roof of the intervillous space ('intervillositis'); the leucocytes are infiltrating the subchorionic fibrin (H & E ×350).

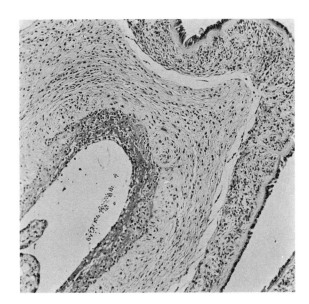

Figure 11.4. A polymorpho-nuclear leucocytic infiltration of the chorionic plate of a placenta involved in an ascending infection; an inter-villositis is also present and this is a later stage in the evolution of the inflammatory process than that which is shown in Fig. 11.3. Most, if not all, of these leucocytes are, how-ever, still of maternal origin (H & E ×90).

begin to migrate out from fetal vessels in the chorionic plate (Fig. 11.5), first from the veins and then later from the arteries, and subsequently an angiitis of the umbilical vessels is seen (Fig. 11.6) with eventual migration of fetal leucocytes into Wharton's jelly.

It is characteristic of ascending infections that the cellular migration from the fetal vessels is not concentric but is orientated towards the uterine cavity. Further, the vasculitis is limited to vessels in the chorionic plate and does not extend along their branches that run into the placental parenchyma. Similarly, any umbilical angiitis is confined to the vessels of the cord and stops short at the anterior abdominal wall of the fetus. The funiculitis is often very patchy and may be limited to an area of the cord that lay near to the cervical os, whilst occasionally an isolated funiculitis, unasso-ciated with a chorioamnionitis, is seen; nearly always when this occurs there has been a prolapse of the cord. The number of Hofbauer cells (i.e. placental macrophages) is often, but not invariably, moderately augmented in the inflamed membranes and

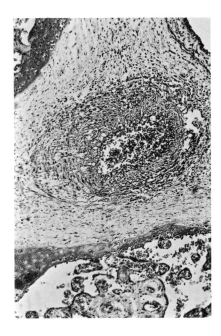

Figure 11.5. A vasculitis in a fetal vessel which is situated in the chorionic plate of a placenta involved in an ascending infection (H & E ×50).

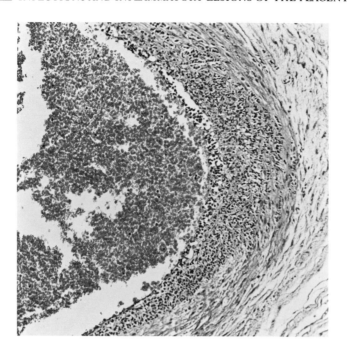

Figure 11.6. An umbilical angiitis found in association with a chorioamnionitis (H & E ×200).

there may be focal areas of necrosis; extensive necrosis of the membranes is, however, most uncommon.

In monilial chorioamnionitis the appearances may be identical to those found in a bacterial infection and the diagnosis may only become apparent if fungal elements are seen on microscopy (Fig. 11.7). More characteristically, however, small microabscesses are found, consisting of focal accumulations of leucocytes in areas of necrosis in which fungal structures may be scanty or numerous.

Several points about the histological changes in chorioamnionitis require emphasis. First, it will be appreciated that the inflammatory infiltrate is derived from both the mother and fetus and that therefore the fetally derived cells can only be present if the fetus is alive. If infection occurs after fetal death the maternal response is in no way diminished but the fetal component will be absent. Secondly, it has been indicated that

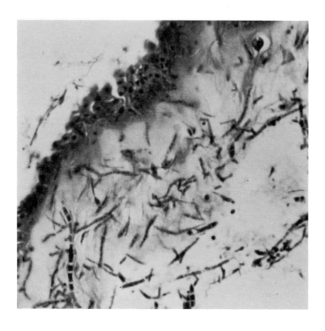

Figure 11.7. Fungal elements in the extraplacental membranes in a case of monilial chorioamnionitis (PAS ×1450).

in ascending infections the inflammatory process is largely confined to the membranes and chorionic plate and that the villous tissue of the placenta is not involved. However, if the infection is transmitted to the fetus and there is subsequently a fetal bacteraemia then the villi will show evidence of inflammation, simply because the placenta is a fetal organ. In such cases, which are not common, the original nature of the infection will still be apparent in the discrepancy between the severe cellular infiltration of the membranes and the mild villitis, a situation contrasting to that seen in haematogenous infections of the placenta, in which the inflammatory process is most marked in the villous tissue. Thirdly, it would be unwise to diagnose infection solely on the basis of an inflammatory infiltrate in the decidua and basal plate. Such an infiltrate can be considered as almost physiological, being present in 85% of normal pregnancies (Schneider, 1970). Fourthly, Naeye (1991, 1992) believes that there is a correlation between the length of time for which the membranes have been infected and the stage of evolution of the inflammatory picture, maintaining that in the first 48 hours of an infection there is simply a subchorial intervillositis and that only in the next few subsequent days do the polymorphonuclear leucocytes migrate into the chorionic plate. Whilst in general terms this is clearly true it is equally the case that not all infections progress at the same rate and, in my view, it would be imprudent to try to 'date' a chorioamnionitis with any degree of precision. Finally, it is often suggested that a chorioamnionitis should be graded and it is relatively easy to do this, using an admittedly subjective grading system such as 'mild', 'moderate' and 'severe'. However, there is no clear correlation between the intensity of the histological inflammatory process and the clinical severity of the amniotic sac infection, this being exemplified by infections by Group B streptococci in which there is often a marked disparity between a clinically serious infection and a minor degree of inflammatory infiltration of the membranes.

Aetiology of Chorioamnionitis

In the past the high incidence of negative cultures from inflamed membranes persuaded many that chorioamnionitis is of non-infective origin, being due to such factors as fetal hypoxia, changes in the pH of the amniotic fluid or the irritative effects of meconium. These theories have now been largely abandoned, partly because of the failure of experimental studies to confirm these contentions and partly because of the increased proportion of positive results obtained by modern microbiological techniques, and there is now a general acceptance of the infective nature of chorioamnionitis.

Chorioamnionitis commonly has a polymicrobiol aetiology and the organisms frequently isolated from inflamed membranes include enterococci, coagulase-positive staphylococci, anaerobic streptococci and *Escherichia coli*, all organisms normally found inhabiting the lower female genital tract during pregnancy (Rothbard et al, 1975). Fusobacteria are emerging as an important cause of amniotic infection (Altshuler & Hyde, 1985, 1988; Easterling & Garite, 1985) and, much less frequently, chorioamnionitis can be due to *Haemophilus influenzae* (Gibson & Williams, 1978; Campognone & Singer, 1986; Winn & Egley, 1987; Rusan et al, 1991; Ault et al, 1993; Shute & Kimber, 1994), *Neisseria gonorrhoeae* (Nickerson, 1973; Engebretsen, 1974; Rothbard et al, 1975; Smith et al, 1989) or *Streptococcus pneumoniae* (Duff & Gibbs, 1983). Occasional examples of chorioamnionitis due to relatively exotic organisms, such as *Streptobacillus moniliformis* (Faro et al, 1980), *Bacteroides fragilis* (Evaldson et al, 1982), *Pasteurella multocida* (Waldor et al, 1992; Wong et al, 1992), *Morganella morganii* (Carmona et al, 1992), *Kingella denitrificans* (Maccato et al, 1991) and *Capnocytophaga* sp. (Iralu et al, 1993) have been recorded.

Group B haemolytic streptococci, which intermittently colonize the genital tract, cause more perinatal morbidity and mortality than any other bacteria (Katz, 1993) and are an important cause of chorioamnionitis (Becroft et al, 1976; Vigorita & Parmley, 1979; Novak & Platt, 1985; Yancey et al, 1994). Nevertheless there is a rather poor correlation between neonatal streptococcal infection and the presence of a chorioamnionitis

(Altshuler, 1984), the organisms appearing to have the ability to pass rapidly through the membranes whilst only inducing a minimal inflammatory response.

In recent years there has been an increasing tendency to implicate *Chlamydia trachomatis*, *Ureaplasma* and the mycoplasmas as important factors in chorioamnionitis (Embree et al, 1980; Gibbs et al, 1982; Kundsin et al, 1984; Dong et al, 1987; Quinn et al, 1987; Hillier et al, 1988; Jacob-Cormier et al, 1989; Donders et al, 1991; Eschenbach, 1993; Smith & Taylor-Robinson, 1993) though it has to be admitted that the aetiological significance of these organisms, particularly that of *Chlamydia*, has been challenged (Romero et al, 1989c; Ismail et al, 1992).

The role played by *Gardnerella vaginalis* in the aetiology of chorioamnionitis is a complex one. This organism, by itself, does not appear to be pathogenic when present in the amniotic fluid (Gibbs et al, 1987) but the combination of *G. vaginalis* together with other organisms implicated in bacterial vaginosis, namely *M. hominis* and anaerobes, does appear to be quite an important cause of inflammation of the membranes (Silver et al, 1989; Gibbs, 1993).

Mycotic chorioamnionitis is uncommon and is nearly always due to *Candida albicans* (Benirschke & Raphael, 1958; Belter, 1959; Albarracin et al, 1967; Aterman, 1968; Lopez & Aterman, 1968; Hood et al, 1983; Bider et al, 1989; Donders et al, 1990; Schwartz & Reef, 1990; Mazor et al, 1993), though Sander et al (1983) described a case of ascending amniotic infection caused by *Torulopsis glabrata*; chorioamnionitis due to *C. parapsilosis* (Kellogg et al, 1974), *C. tropicalis* (Nichols et al, 1995) and *Aspergillus* (Bader, 1966) has also been reported. The relative rarity of monilial infection is surprising in view of the frequency with which this fungus is found in the vagina, and it has been suggested that this is because the pH of the amniotic fluid inhibits the growth of *Candida* (Galton & Benirschke, 1960).

The only virus that has been identified as a possible cause of chorioamnionitis is herpes simplex. Altshuler (1974) reported a necrotizing amnionitis, in which the infiltrate was primarily plasmacellular, in a case of congenital herpes infection whilst Benirschke and Kaufmann (1995) have described a similar case in which there was also subamniotic vesicle formation. Hyde and Giacoia (1993) noted focal, mild acute chorioamnionitis, necrosis of the amnion of the umbilical cord and a mild lymphoplasmacytic funisitis in a case of ascending herpes infection.

Incidence

In a prospective study of our own material at St Mary's Hospital in Manchester, which is a specialist obstetrical hospital with a large proportion of high-risk pregnancies, a thorough examination of 1000 consecutively delivered placentas showed that some degree of chorioamnionitis was present in 24.4%. An umbilical angiitis was, however, noted in only 6.6%, whilst a true funiculitis, with extension of leucocytes into Wharton's jelly, was seen in 3.7% (Fox & Langley, 1971). Somewhat similar figures have been quoted in other prospective, unselected studies from comparable obstetrical centres in the UK (Pryse-Davies et al, 1973; Zaaijma et al 1982). The frequency with which ascending infection is diagnosed in any particular centre is, however, influenced by several factors, these including:

1. Variations in the definition of inflammation. The criteria for recognizing that an inflammatory process is present vary from pathologist to pathologist. Some will consider that even an occasional leucocyte in the membranes is an indication of infection, whilst others will demand that a well-marked infiltrate be present before accepting that an infective lesion exists. This problem is perhaps most acute in the cord, where some will confidently diagnose infection solely on the basis of margination of leucocytes within the umbilical vessels, whilst others (including myself) would insist upon an angiitis being present.
2. Inclusion of decidual inflammation. As noted above, an inflammatory infiltrate in the decidua and basal plate is not, in itself, an indication of infection; nevertheless it is often taken as such.

3. The socio-economic status and ethnic constitution of the population at risk will influence the incidence of chorioamnionitis. Naeye and Blanc (1970) and Naeye et al (1971) have shown that, within a given population, this condition occurs with undue frequency in women of low socio-economic status. They also found that, in the USA, black women had a higher incidence of chorioamnionitis than white women, this ethnic bias being independent of socio-economic status.
4. The incidence of preterm deliveries in the hospital population. The incidence of chorioamnionitis is very high in placentas from pregnancies terminating before the 32nd week of gestation but then subsequently appears to decline, only to rise again in term deliveries.
5. Variations in obstetric practice from one centre to another, for example in Caesarean section rate, use of internal fetal monitoring or frequency of vaginal examination, will almost certainly influence the incidence of chorioamnionitis.

Defence Mechanisms against Ascending Infections

It may be thought that defence mechanisms against bacterial ascent are not a strict necessity, because in non-pregnant women organisms do not normally pass from the vagina into the uterine cavity. However, in pregnancy, and particularly during labour, the dilatation of the cervical canal, the possible suction action of uterine contractions, and the milking effect of rectal and vaginal examinations all predispose to an entry of organisms from the birth canal. Against this possibility are poised two principal defence mechanisms which protect the fetus and placenta against ascending infection, neither of which, unfortunately, can be considered as an absolute deterrent. These are:

1. The physical barrier offered to organisms by the intact membranes.
2. The antibacterial action of the amniotic fluid.

A further, probably equally important, but certainly less studied, defence is offered by the cervical mucus, which not only affords a physical block to bacterial ascent but also contains locally secreted antibodies of IgA type (Kutteh et al, 1993) and lysozyme (Chimura et al, 1993).

The Intact Membranes

The long-held belief that the intact membranes offer a virtually impregnable bar to the spread of bacteria has suffered considerable attrition in the last few decades. Recent *in vitro* studies have shown that the membranes have no inherent antibacterial activity (Talmi et al, 1991) and constitute only a weak barrier to bacterial penetration (Gyr et al, 1994) and it is now clear that, especially in preterm pregnancies, amniotic sac infection and chorioamnionitis can occur in the presence of intact membranes (Naeye & Peters, 1978; Miller et al, 1980; Bobitt et al, 1981; Royston & Geoghegan, 1985; Perkins et al, 1987; Guvenc et al, 1989; Romero et al, 1989c; Armer & Duff, 1991; Gaillard et al, 1993). It still remains true, however, that at term the fluid within an intact amniotic sac is usually sterile, a clear tribute to the role, albeit an imperfect one, played by the integrity of the membranes in protecting the bacteriological virginity of the fluid.

Whether the resistance offered by the membranes to bacterial spread is purely mechanical in nature is uncertain, but experimental studies Chany et al (1966) suggest that this is the case and have highlighted the importance, in this respect, of the inter-cellular matrix rather than that of the amniotic cells.

Antibacterial Activity of the Amniotic Fluid

Organisms entering the amniotic cavity come into contact with the amniotic fluid and their subsequent ability to produce a chorioamnionitis could be halted, or at least limited, if this fluid possessed any antibacterial activity. These is now clear evidence that the fluid does indeed contain substances inhibitory to bacterial growth (Larsen et al, 1974a,b; Larsen & Galask, 1975). Further, Schlievert et al (1975a,b) have demonstrated that the capacity of the fluid to inhibit bacterial growth is related to the length of the gestational period, being minimal or absent in fluids from pregnancies of less than 20 weeks' gestation and then progressively increasing to reach a peak between the 36th and 40th weeks.

The nature of the antibacterial factor in amniotic fluid has not been fully determined, but lysozyme, immunoglobulins, beta-lysin and a zinc-dependent low molecular weight polypeptide all appear to be important factors (Schlievert et al, 1976a; Scane & Hawkins, 1984; Hurley, 1988). It has been claimed that the phosphate concentration in the amniotic fluid determines the ability of the zinc-dependent polypeptide to exert its inhibitory effect on bacterial growth (Schlievert et al, 1976b, 1977) but studies of the zinc to phosphate ratio in relationship to the antibacterial activity of the fluid have yielded somewhat contradictory results (Hoskins et al, 1982).

Predisposing Obstetric Factors for Ascending Infections

Many cases of chorioamnionitis develop without any predisposing factor but in our own material there was a very significant relationship between prolonged rupture of the membranes and a high incidence of chorioamnionitis (Fox & Langley, 1971), the term 'prolonged' here being taken to mean a period of 24 hours or more. This association has been noted in every investigation of chorioamnionitis prior to, and since, our study but it is probable that membrane rupture for as relatively short a time as 6 hours is sufficient to lead to a marked increase in the incidence of amniotic infection (Blanc, 1961).

Prolonged labour is also a risk factor for chorioamnionitis (Soper et al, 1989) and this appears to be an independent factor rather than simply a surrogate for prolonged membrane rupture. The incidence of amniotic infection rises with an increasing number of vaginal examinations during labour (Newton et al, 1989; Soper et al, 1989) but the findings with regard to internal fetal monitoring have been conflicting, some finding this to have no influence on the incidence of chorioamnionitis (Zippel et al, 1975; Ledger, 1977) and others noting it to be associated with an increased incidence (Newton et al, 1989; Soper et al, 1989). There is a high incidence of chorioamnionitis in patients with cervical incompetence (Romero et al, 1992c).

Effects of Ascending Infection

Effects on the Fetus

There is now overwhelming evidence that an association exists between chorioamnionitis and preterm delivery, particularly when this occurs before the 35th week of gestation (Guzick & Winn, 1985; Perkins et al, 1987; Hillier et al, 1988, 1991; Martius, 1989; Romero et al, 1989c; Gibbs et al, 1992). The exact nature of this association is, however, not always clear for whilst it is almost certain that chorioamnionitis can both precipitate preterm labour and induce premature rupture of the membranes (Naeye & Peters, 1980; Romero et al, 1993) it is also possible that premature rupture of the membranes, due to non-infective factors, may be complicated by chorioamnionitis. Despite these uncertainties it is clear that chorioamnionitis is common in cases of early preterm labour, the incidence in various studies ranging from 19 to 74% (Chellam & Rushton, 1985; Guzick & Winn, 1985; Hillier et al, 1988; Mueller-Heubach et al, 1990; van der Elst et al, 1991).

It has been suggested that bacterial infection of the membranes may lead to their premature rupture because of the release of elastases and collagenases from the neutrophil polymorphonuclear leucocytes infiltrating the membranes (Naeye, 1987, 1991). Bacteria, by themselves, also diminish the tensile strength, elasticity and 'work to rupture' of the membranes by the release of proteolytic enzymes (McGregor et al, 1987) but the combination of some, but not all, bacteria and neutrophil polymorphonuclear leucocytes causes more damage to the membranes than either bacteria or acute inflammatory cells alone (Schoonmaker et al, 1989). The relationship between chorioamnionitis and premature onset of labour is more complex. Prostaglandins are thought to play a vital role in stimulating parturition and there is considerable evidence that infection is associated with a greatly increased production of prostaglandins by the amnion (Lopez-Bernal et al, 1987, 1989; Romero et al, 1987b; Bry & Hallman, 1989; van der Elst et al, 1991). It has been suggested that the high levels of prostaglandins are due to direct stimulation of their synthesis by bacterial products (Bennett et al, 1987; Romero et al, 1987a, 1988a,b; Lamont et al, 1990) but currently it is thought that cytokines play a predominant role, not only in stimulating the excess prostaglandin synthesis found in chorioamnionitis but also in evoking labour (Mitchell et al, 1993). The cytokines, produced by activated macrophages in response to infection, which have been particularly implicated in this respect are interleukin-1, interleukin-2, tumour necrosis factor, granulocyte colony-stimulating factor, interleukin-8 and interleukin-6. High levels of these cytokines are found in the amniotic fluid in cases of chorioamnionitis (Romero et al, 1989a,b, 1990, 1992a,b; Trautman et al, 1992; Greig et al, 1993; Hillier et al, 1993; Matsuzaki et al, 1993; Saito et al, 1993; Ohno et al, 1994; Steinborn et al, 1994), they can stimulate prostaglandin synthesis by the amnion and decidua (Romero et al, 1989b,d; Mitchell et al, 1991; Norwitz et al, 1992), inhibit progesterone synthesis (Ohno et al, 1994) and, under experimental conditions, directly elicit uterine contractility (Gibbs et al, 1992).

In our material we have not been able, after the confounding factor of prolonged membrane rupture has been taken into account, to establish any relationship between chorioamnionitis in term pregnancies and either fetal distress *in utero* or neonatal asphyxia. This negative finding is in accord with more recent studies which have shown that cord blood gas levels are usually normal in term neonates whose placentas show chorioamnionitis (Newton, 1993; Samueloff et al, 1994). There is, however, an excess incidence of neonatal asphyxia in those cases of chorioamnionitis associated with delivery before the 35th week of gestation. It is of course very difficult in these cases to distinguish between, and disentangle, the effects of a triad of factors, namely intra-amniotic infection, fetal or neonatal pneumonia and prematurity. Naeye (1987, 1991, 1992) has, however, maintained that chorioamnionitis stresses the fetus and that this results in villous oedema which compresses the fetal villous vessels with resulting diminished fetal oxygenation. It is of particular note that Naeye points out that the villous oedema, which he considers to be intracellular rather than extracellular, occurs most commonly before the 35th week of gestation and then diminishes progressively as the length of the gestational period increases. It is not fully clear to me why fetal stress should result in villous oedema and I believe it to be almost a physiological impossibility for oedema in a tissue to compress the vasculature of that tissue. I believe, and this view is clearly shared by others (Benirschke & Kaufmann, 1995), that many, possibly all, of the 'oedematous' villi noted by Naeye were, in fact, perfectly normal immature intermediate villi.

Salafia et al (1989) approached this problem in a rather convoluted fashion by showing that there was a relatively high incidence of chorioamnionitis and funisitis in cases in which there had been an abnormal fetal heart rate pattern; they suggested that there may be some factor in the infected amniotic fluid which has an effect on umbilical or chorionic vessels, a concept that has gained some experimental support (Hyde et al, 1989). It has to be said, however, that in the majority of cases of chorioamnionitis the fetal heart pattern is quite normal.

There is an association between chorioamnionitis and low birth weight but in many cases this is probably a reflection of the fact that the lower the weight of the fetus the longer, on average, is the time interval between membrane rupture and delivery (Lind & Hytten, 1969), possibly because the strength of the uterine contractions is related in some manner to the bulk of the uterine contents.

Chorioamnionitis is found in a moderate proportion of cases of intrauterine fetal death, but there is no convincing evidence that this form of infection can, in itself and in the absence of fetal infection, be held responsible for fetal demise. The frequent induction of labour and the consequently long period of membrane rupture observed in many cases of fetal death is probably responsible for many instances of this particular association.

A particular risk presented to the fetus by chorioamnionitis is clearly that of spread of infection to the fetus from the inflamed membranes. The fetus may inhale infected amniotic fluid and develop a 'congenital' pneumonia, whilst entry of the fluid into the upper respiratory tract can cause meningitis. The fetal skin or eyes can be infected by direct contact with organisms in the fluid, which is probably the aetiological mechanism in a proportion of cases of neonatal pyogenic dermatitis or ophthalmia. Swallowing of the fluid may be responsible for some cases of neonatal gastritis, enteritis or peritonitis. It should be stressed that all these unfortunate complications occur infrequently in chorioamnionitis; on the other hand they rarely occur in its absence (de Araujo et al, 1994).

Quite apart from the effects of direct contact with the infected amniotic fluid, the fetus may also be infected by organisms that enter the fetal circulation via the vessels on the inflamed surface of the placenta. The frequency with which this occurs is uncertain, but, in one representative study, positive cultures were obtained from the cord blood in only four out of 40 cases of chorioamnionitis, and only two of the infants with positive cultures showed any clinical evidence of infection (Engstrom & Ivemark, 1960). An incidence of bacteraemia in this range may appear quite alarming, but the available evidence suggests that in most instances such a bacteraemia is usually both transitory and without any clinical effects.

Chorioamnionitis is therefore, in most cases, a potential rather than an actual infective threat to the fetus and only infrequently is this threat realized. Nevertheless, most human fetal infections in late pregnancy are secondary to a chorioamnionitis, and eradication of this form of placentitis would radically reduce the incidence of 'congenital' or neonatal sepsis.

Effects on the Mother

Claims in some studies that chorioamnionitis is associated with an increased incidence of abruptio placentae (Darby et al, 1989) have been specifically refuted in others (Woods et al, 1986) and this correlation remains *sub judice* at the moment. It is certainly difficult see any reason why a chorioamnionitis in which the infection is confined to the membranes should be capable of causing placental abruption though Ando and Kanayama (1993) have suggested that decidual infiltration by acute inflammatory cells leads to the release of elastase from neutrophil polymorphonuclear leucocytes which inhibits decidual cell fibronectin receptor with resultant loss of cell cohesiveness.

In a quite high proportion of cases of chorioamnionitis the mother develops an intrapartum pyrexia together with tachycardia (Gibbs et al, 1992; Newton, 1993). This is not altogether surprising if it is borne in mind that the initial inflammatory response to infection of the membranes is maternal in origin. There is also an unduly high incidence of post-partum pelvic sepsis, uterine tenderness and maternal leucocytosis. The most serious risk presented to the mother by an amniotic infection is, however, the fortunately uncommon complication of endotoxic shock, this being confined to infections due to Gram-negative organisms.

Effects on the Placenta

Virtually nothing is actually known, as opposed to assumed, about the effects of ascending infections on placental function, though in general terms it would appear highly unlikely that an inflammatory process which neither involves the villi nor apparently interferes with the placental circulation would impair the functional efficiency of the organ.

HAEMATOGENOUS INFECTIONS

Many cases of placentitis are due to infective agents that reach the organ via the maternal circulatory system. It must, however, be admitted that a proportion of the placental infections to be considered in this section may well be secondary to an endometritis rather than to direct spread of organisms from the maternal blood. Nevertheless, the term 'haematogenous infection' serves as a useful portmanteau expression to cover all placental infections that are secondary to a systemic or pelvic infection of the mother and not due to an ascending infection from the birth canal. It will be apparent that haematogenous infection is always secondary to an overt or sub-clinical maternal infection by a pathogenic organism, this being in sharp contrast to ascending placental infections, in which the organisms are commonly normal inhabitants of the birth canal.

Morphology of Haematogenous Infections

Generally, haematogenous infections involve the placental parenchyma itself rather than the membranes; as the infection progresses it may extend to the membranes, but the inflammatory process is almost invariably less marked here than in the placental substance. The hallmark of a haematogenous infection is an inflammatory lesion within the villous substance (Fig. 11.8), this being known as a 'villositis' or 'villitis'. The villitis may be focal, with lesions present in random isolated villi, or diffuse, with extensive involvement of contiguous villi in many areas of the placenta. The focal form is the more common and very few villi may be involved, to the extent indeed that the lesions may be missed unless the placenta is extensively sampled.

Altshuler and Russell (1975) have segregated the villitides into various histological groups, which they have defined thus:

1. *Proliferative villitis*: inflammatory cells are present in the villi but there is no tissue necrosis.

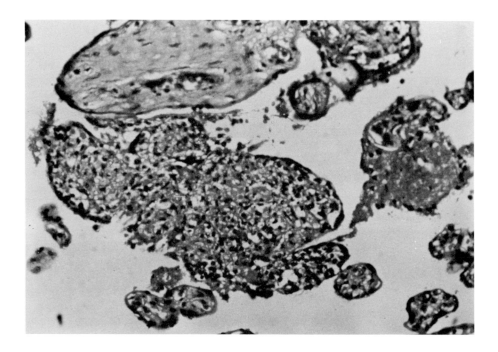

Figure 11.8. Villitis in a haematogenous infection of a placenta (H & E ×720).

2. *Necrotizing villitis*: inflammatory cells are present in the villi, and intravillous tissue necrosis is also present.
3. *Reparative villitis*: the inflammatory process within the villi is undergoing organization and repair, with granulation tissue formation and fibroblastic proliferation.
4. *Stromal fibrosis*: the villi are fibrotic, scarred and shrunken but show little or no evidence of any active inflammatory process.

It will be appreciated that this is a rather artificial classification which simply demarcates the progress of any inflammatory lesion. The placental findings in any particular infection will vary with, and depend upon, the stage reached in the evolution and repair of the inflammatory process at the time of delivery.

Villitides may be further subdivided in terms of both the topography of the inflammatory lesions and the type of inflammatory cells found in the villi (Russell, 1980). Thus a villitis may be basal, the inflamed villi being predominantly those adjacent to the basal plate, or non-basal, the inflamed villi being randomly distributed with no obvious relationship to the basal plate.

In an acute villitis, caused by infection with pyogenic organisms, the villi are infiltrated by polymorphonuclear leucocytes (Fig 11.9); indeed, in severe cases individual villi may be converted into microabscesses. A chronic villitis is, however, usually characterized by a mixed villous infiltrate of lymphocytes, plasma cells and histiocytic cells, though in a minority of cases the infiltrate is either purely lymphocytic or wholly histiocytic. A pure lymphocytic villitis is commonly basal in type and associated with little tissue destruction, while a histiocytic villitis is invariably randomly distributed and frequently associated with trophoblastic necrosis and villous destruction. It should perhaps be remarked that it is far from clear how one distinguishes, in simple morpholgical terms, between a purely histiocytic villitis and a villous lesion in which there is a proliferation of Hofbauer cells, a proliferation which may not be due to an infection. Granulomas of either histiocytic or tuberculoid type are occasionally seen in a villitis.

The lesions of villitis may be very scattered but all except a tiny minority of cases will be detected if four sections of placental tissue are examined. A villitis may be graded in very subjective terms into 'mild', 'moderate' or 'severe' or, still subjectively but less so, in the following manner:

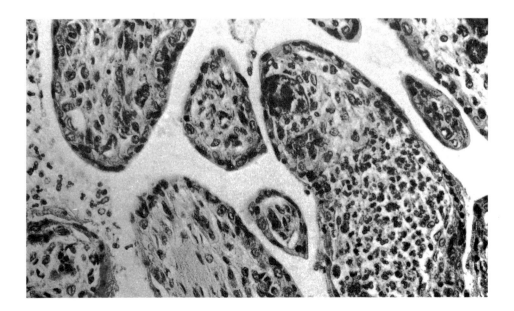

Figure 11.9. Acute suppurative villitis. There is a polymorphonuclear leucocytic infiltration of a villus on the right of the field (H & E ×450).

Grade 1: only one or two foci of villous inflammation in the entire four sections, and in each focus only a very few villi are involved.

Grade 2: up to six foci of villous inflammation in the four sections, each focus containing up to 20 villi.

Grade 3: multiple inflammatory foci, each occupying up to half a low-power microscopical field.

Grade 4: large areas of villous inflammation in most or all of the four sections.

Bacterial Infections

Pyogenic Organisms

Placental infection by organisms such as coagulase-positive staphylococci, haemolytic streptococci and pneumococci are uncommon simply because it is unusual for a bacteraemia or septicaemia caused by such organisms to complicate pregnancy. Staphylococcal and streptococcal infections of the placenta are usually due to an ascending infection. Nevertheless a haematogenous infection due to these organisms can occur and under these circumstances the placenta may show septic infarcts or septic intervillous thrombi. These do not differ macroscopically from the bland lesions of the type frequently found in non-infected placentas, but they are seen histologically to contain large numbers of neutrophil polymorph leucocytes. There is also often an acute intervillous thrombophlebitis and perivillous inflammation, whilst focal villous inflammation (Fig. 11.9) and necrosis are seen: sometimes villi are converted into minute abscesses.

Enteric and other Gram-negative Organisms

These usually reach the placenta from the birth canal and produce a chorioamnionitis. Haematogenous spread occasionally occurs from a septic focus in the pelvis and this will produce a histological picture similar to that seen with Gram-positive cocci.

Treponema pallidum

Hormann (1954) reviewed the many reports of placental syphilis that appeared during the earlier part of this century; more recent reports include those of Russell and Altshuler (1974), Walter et al (1982a), Horn et al (1992), Qureshi et al (1993), Samson et al (1994) and Schwartz et al (1994). The infected placenta is typically large and pale (Malan et al, 1990) and, as Russell (1995) has pointed out, usually presents a triad of histological appearances, none of which is specific but which when taken together are highly suggestive of syphilitic infection. First, there are changes that are secondary to infective haemolytic anaemia in the fetus, namely villous immaturity (Fig. 11.10) and the presence of nucleated erythrocytes in the fetal vessels. Secondly, there is an endarteritis and perivascultis of the villous stem vessels and, thirdly, there is a focal proliferative villitis which varies from lymphocytic to granulomatous but in which many plasma cells are characteristically present (Fig. 11.11); the number of Hofbauer cells tends to be increased. Qureshi et al (1993) have described examples of an acute villitis in placentas from mothers with syphilis but this seems an unlikely cellular response to a syphilitic infection and may be indicative of a superadded second infection.

A necrotizing funisitis (see later) may be found in syphilitic infections but claims that this is a specific lesion for, and diagnostic of, syphilis (Fojaco et al, 1989; Knowles & Frost, 1989) have been comprehensively refuted by Craver and Baldwin (1992). Schwartz et al (1994, 1995) examined the umbilical cords of placentas from 25 infants with confirmed congenital syphilis; 12 of the cords were histologically normal, in nine there was a necrotizing funisitis, in two there was an acute inflammatory infiltrate and there were single instances of mononuclear and plasma cell funisitis.

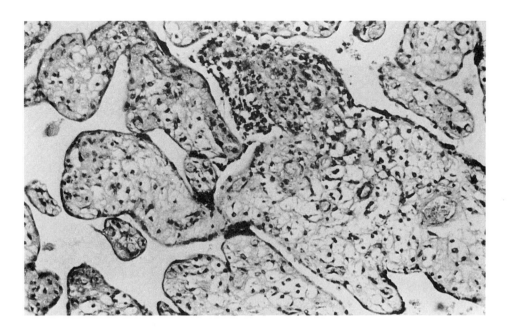

Figure 11.10. Placenta from a fetus with congenital syphilis. The villi are generally somewhat immature and oedematous and there is a focal villitis (H & E ×450).

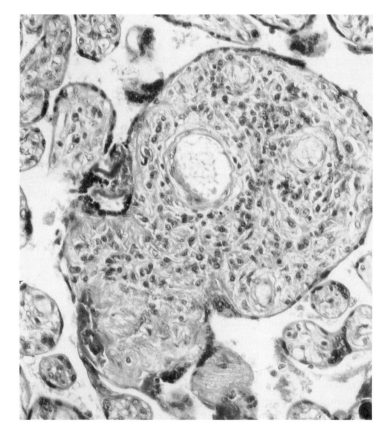

Figure 11.11. Congenital syphilis. A focal villitis showing an almost pure plasma cell infiltrate with only occasional lymphocytes (H & E ×440).

The spirochaetes may be identified in the placental tissues with a Warthin–Starry stain but the use of monoclonal antibodies, using either an immunofluorescent or an immunogold technique, is probably now the preferred technique for demonstration of the organisms (Schwartz et al, 1994, 1995). The umbilical cord appears to be the optimal site for detecting the presence of *Treponema pallidum*.

Samson et al (1994) have suggested that the villous abnormalities seen in syphilis are due to the local deposition, or formation, of immune complexes, a concept that merits further investigation.

Francisella tularensis

Tularaemia is an unusual complication of pregnancy, but Lide (1947) has described an example of placentitis caused by this disease. The placenta was grossly unremarkable, but histological examination revealed numerous granulomatous foci which were predominantly in the intervillous space. These were formed principally of polymorphs, histiocytes and lymphocytes enmeshed in fibrin, and usually showed a central area of necrosis. Many of these lesions were confluent and involved adjacent villi, whilst a proportion of the villi also showed mononuclear cell infiltration and patchy necrosis. Numerous organisms were demonstrated both in the granulomas and in the villi.

Listeria monocytogenes

This organism may reach the placenta by either the ascending or the haematogenous route; indeed, in most cases it is not possible to determine which of these routes has been involved because there are usually both lesions in the villous parenchyma and a chorioamnionitis (Yamazaki et al, 1977; Lallemand et al, 1992; Gersell, 1993). Infected placentas may be somewhat bulky but most are of normal size. There are usually seen within the parenchyma or on the placental surface (Figs 11.12 and 11.13) minute or small scattered whitish-yellow lesions which, histologically, are microabscesses consisting of foci of necrosis in which many polymorphonuclear leucocytes and organisms are present (Fig. 11.14). At the margin of these foci (Fig. 11.15) there is often a rim of palisaded histiocytic cells (Driscoll et al, 1962; Bret & Grepinet, 1967; Pageaut et al, 1967; Sarrut & Alison, 1967; Duval et al, 1976); much larger macroabscesses may also be present (Steele & Jacobs, 1979; Topalovski et al, 1993). Villi can be caught up and enmeshed in intervillous fibrin and inflammatory debris, whilst large masses of necrotic villi may be present, these often appearing to be contiguous with an inflamed and necrotic septum (Scott & Henderson, 1968). In addition to these gross lesions, a focal

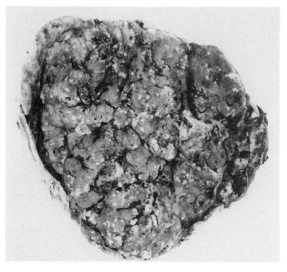

Figure 11.12. Placental listeriosis. Numerous whitish-yellow lesions are seen on the maternal surface of the placenta.

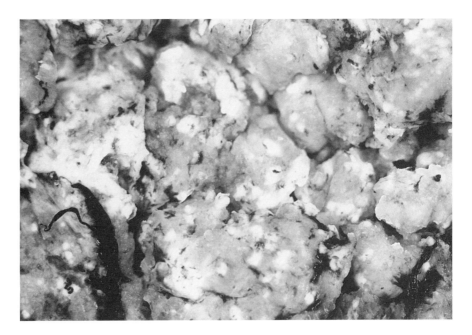

Figure 11.13. Higher-power view of the maternal surface lesions shown in Fig. 11.12.

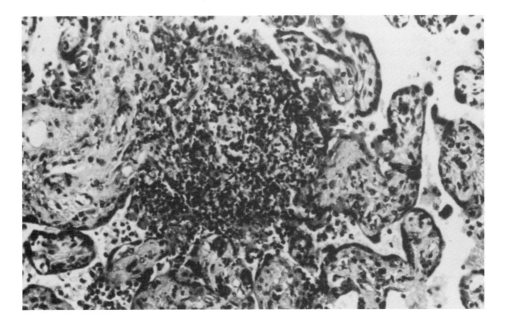

Figure 11.14. A microabscess in a case of placental listeriosis; the lesion consists of necrotic debris and polymorphonuclear leucocytes (H & E ×220).

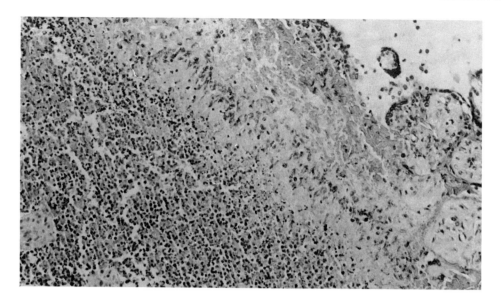

Figure 11.15. Placental listeriosis. The margin of a microabscess showing central polymorphonuclear leucocytes and peripherally palisaded histiocytes (H & E ×210).

villitis may also be present, in which, characteristically, localized collections of polymorphonuclear leucocytes are seen between the trophoblast and the villous stroma.

Bacillus Species

The genus *Bacillus* consists of saprophytic, aerobic, spore-forming, ubiquitous bacteria which are being increasingly recognized as pathogens. Workowski and Flaherty (1992) reported a case of placentitis caused by *Bacillus puma* in an intravenous drug abuser: there was a severe acute villitis and numerous Gram-positive bacilli were present in the placental tissues.

Chlamydia

Chlamydia trachomatis is a known cause of pelvic infections and may play a role in abortion and in the development of a chorioamnionitis. It was at one time postulated that this organism could be linked to villitis of unknown aetiology but proof of this has never been established (Russell, 1980).

Chlamydia psittaci is a well-documented cause of placentitis and abortion in sheep and Johnson et al (1985) reported an abortion in a woman who had contracted an infection with this organism after assisting with lambing. The placenta appeared macroscopically normal but histologically there were large numbers of acute inflammatory cells in the intervillous space together with an early perivasculitis of occasional fetal stem vessels (Wong et al, 1985). Basophilic inclusions were present in the villous syncytiotrophoblast which, using an immunoperoxidase technique, stained positively for *C. psittaci*.

Brucella

Organisms of the *Brucella* group are amongst the more important causes of placentitis in animals, but infection of the human placenta with *Brucella abortus* appears to be rare and the placental lesions that this organism may cause have been poorly documented. Trifonova (1959) described 'dystrophic and necrobiotic changes' in placentas from women with chronic brucellosis, whilst Poole et al (1972), reporting an example of abortion which was apparently due to *B. abortus*, limited their description of the placenta to the statement that it was necrotic. It is of interest that Sarram et al (1974), working in an area of endemic brucellosis in Iran, were able to culture *Brucella melitensis* from placental tissue in three second-trimester abortions; they did not, however, describe the pathology of the infected placentas.

Campylobacter fetus

Organisms of the genus *Campylobacter* were previously classified within the genus *Vibrio* and are a recognized cause of placental infection and abortion in sheep and cattle. The first description of human placental lesions caused by *Campylobacter* came from Vinzent (1949) and Vinzent et al (1950) who described large areas of necrobiosis with a peripheral margin of polymorphonuclear leucocytes. From the description given, I am far from sure that the lesions were not just simple infarcts. There is no doubt, however, about the placental lesions in the case reported by Gilbert et al (1981) and reviewed by Coid and Fox (1983) of an abortion in a woman with *Campylobacter fetus* subsp. *jejuni* septicaemia. There were extensive areas of massive perivillous fibrin deposition which were heavily infiltrated by polymorphonuclear leucocytes, the acute inflammatory cells often being concentrated around, and destructively infiltrating, entrapped villi and being focally aggregated to form microabscesses. In the villi not entrapped in fibrin there was a very widespread villitis with a variable appearance which appeared to reflect the evolution and later resolution of an acute inflammatory process within the villi.

Rickettsia

Rickettsia burneti have been isolated from the placentas of women with chronic Q fever but have not been shown to be capable of producing any inflammatory or necrotic changes in this organ (Robson & Shimmin, 1959).

Mycobacterium tuberculosis

This organism can infect the placenta; indeed, tuberculosis was one of the first placental infections to be described accurately (Schmorl & Kockel, 1894; Schmorl & Geipl, 1904; Warthin & Cowie, 1904). More recent reports have been those of Boesaart (1959) and Kaplan et al (1980). The lesions range from typical miliary tubercles (Fig. 11.16) to

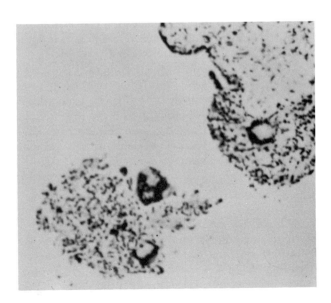

Figure 11.16. Placental tuberculosis. Two miliary tubercles are seen, one of which is in a villus whilst the other is in the intervillous space (H & E ×350).

large confluent caseous foci; the tubercles may be found within the villi or in perivillous fibrin. There is often a non-specific chronic deciduitis and granulomas may be seen at the junction of the decidua and the intervillous space.

Mycobacterium leprae

The placentas of infants born to women suffering from leprosy during pregnancy tend to be unduly small and the babies are often of low birth weight (Duncan, 1980). Nevertheless, evidence that leprosy actually involves the placenta is hard to come by. Sugai and Monobe (1913) examined 12 placentas from leprous women and found granulomatous lesion in the villous tissue of one; in more recent studies there has been a complete failure to detect any histological abnormality in the placentas of pregnant leprous women (King & Marks, 1958; Maurus, 1978; Duncan et al, 1984). Despite many claims in the past to have demonstrated acid-fast bacilli in placentas from leprous women by conventional histological techniques, Duncan et al (1984) could find no bacilli in the 81 placentas they examined. Homogenates from two of seven placentas from women with very active lepromatous leprosy did, however, contain acid-fast bacilli in very small numbers. Despite the apparent inability of *Mycobacterium leprae* to establish itself in placental tissue there is evidence that the disease can be transmitted across the placenta to the fetus (Melsom et al, 1981; Duncan et al, 1983).

Viral Infections

Rubella

The findings in rubella infection of the placenta have been described by Tondury and Smith (1966), Driscoll (1969), Ornoy et al (1973), Garcia et al (1985), Kaplan (1990, 1993), Horn and Becker (1992) and Horn et al (1993). In the acute stage of the infection there is a focal necrotizing villitis (Fig. 11.17) and a necrotizing endarteritis of the fetal villous vessels. The villitis is very variable: some involved villi show only focal necrosis of the trophoblast, whilst in others the trophoblast is totally necrotic with perivillous deposition of fibrin and polymorphs; small groups of villi are sometimes

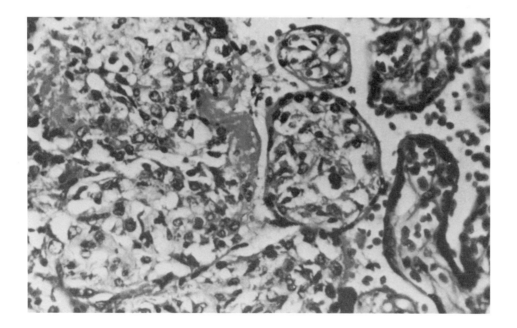

Figure 11.17. Placenta from a case of rubella. There is a focal necrotizing villitis involving the villi on the left of the field (H & E ×250).

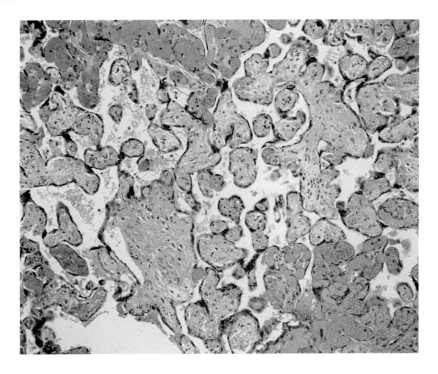

Figure 11.18. Placenta from a case of rubella. Villous inflammation has subsided leaving scarred avascular villi (H & E ×120).

agglutinated by fibrin. The villous stroma can be hypercellular or oedematous and often contains prominent Hofbauer cells, in the cytoplasm of which eosinophilic granules may be seen. The villous fetal vessels show, very characteristically, endothelial necrosis, whilst fragmented erythrocytes may be present in their lumina; there is sometimes also a well-marked perivasculitis. Eosinophilic inclusion bodies may be seen in the endothelial cells or, less frequently, in the villous trophoblast.

In placentas obtained after the acute stage of the disease has passed, there may be only scattered, avascular, shrunken fibrotic villi (Fig. 11.18), but in some both active and healed lesions are present simultaneously, which suggests continuing and progressive villous damage.

A not inconsiderable proportion of placentas from which rubella virus is isolated do not show any inflammatory lesions or morphological abnormality.

Vaccinia

Vaccinial infection of the placenta, which occurs as a rare complication of primary vaccination during pregnancy, is characterized by the presence of minute, pin-head sized, greyish-white scattered nodules, which are seen histologically to consist of foci of necrotic villi surrounded by fibrin and polymorphs (Wielenga et al, 1961; Entwistle et al, 1962; Hood & McKinnon, 1963); eosinophilic inclusion bodies may be seen.

Variola

Placental lesions caused by smallpox have not been described, but Garcia (1963) has documented the findings in two cases of placental involvement by variola minor (alastrim). Numerous tiny yellowish nodules with a creamy consistency were present both on the surface and within the parenchyma, and histological examination revealed multiple necrotizing tuberculoid granulomas together with patchy necrosis of villi and an intervillous accumulation of fibrin, polymorphs and inflammatory debris. Nuclear and cytoplasmic eosinophilic inclusion bodies were seen in decidual cells but not in villous tissue.

Varicella Zoster

Maternal varicella zoster infection in pregnancy can be transmitted to the fetus and can result in a 'varicella embryopathy'. Garcia (1963), Blanc (1978), Robertson and McKeever (1992) and Kaplan (1990, 1993) have described the pathological findings in placentas infected with varicella. The composite picture that emerges from these reports is of an acute necrotizing villitis in early and severe cases with a progression via a lymphocytic/granulomatous villitis in which histiocytic giant cells are present, to stromal fibrosis with obliteration of fetal vessels. Groups of agglutinated inflamed villi may be macroscopically visible and have been compared to 'rice seed'. Eosinophilic intranuclear inclusions may be present in decidual cells and within the histiocytic giant cells.

Herpes Simplex

In addition to its ability to produce a chorioamnionitis, this virus can infect the placenta by the haematogenous route, when it produces necrosis of the trophoblast of scattered villi and agglutination of groups of involved villi but, interestingly enough, often without provoking any significant inflammatory reaction (Witzleben & Driscoll, 1965) though there may be a mild lymphocytic villitis (Kaplan, 1993).

Epstein–Barr Virus

Ornoy et al (1982) studied five placentas from abortions induced because of maternal Epstein–Barr infection: a lymphoplasmacytic villitis, focal trophoblastic necrosis and necrosis of fetal endothelial cells were characteristic, though highly non-specific, features of these placentas.

Enteroviruses

The enteroviruses include coxsackievirus, echovirus, enterovirus and poliovirus. Poliovirus can cause an intrauterine fetal infection and has, under such circumstances, been isolated from the placenta (Schaeffer et al, 1954; Shelekov & Habel, 1956) but histological examination of placentas from such cases has not revealed any morphological abnormality (Baskin et al, 1950). Kilbrick and Benirschke (1958) studied a placenta from a fetus with intrauterine coxsackievirus B infection and could detect no histological abnormality.

In contrast to these disappointingly negative findings is the study of Garcia and her colleagues (Garcia et al, 1991). They examined 19 placentas from women with an enterovirus infection (16 with echovirus infection and three with coxsackievirus B infection); the outstanding findings were an extensive vasculitis of the fetal vessels of the placenta and a focal or extensive lymphocytic and histiocytic infiltration of the villous stroma with trophoblastic necrosis (Fig. 11.19).

In a case of coxsackievirus A infection of the placenta reported by Batcup et al (1985), examination of the placenta showed very extensive perivillous fibrin deposition and villous necrosis with a mononuclear cell infiltrate; just how specific these findings are is a matter for debate.

Mumps Virus

Herbst et al (1970) examined a placenta from a patient with epidemic parotitis; abnormalities, of a very non-specific nature, were seen only on electron microscopy.

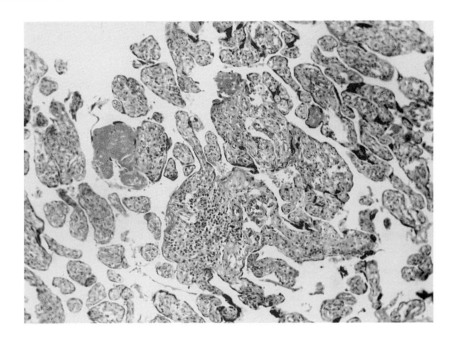

Figure 11.19. Echovirus infection of the placenta. There is a focal mononuclear villitis with trophoblastic necrosis (H & E ×70).

Garcia et al (1980) studied three placentas from pregnancies complicated by maternal mumps, one from a spontaneous abortion and two from induced abortions. In the placenta of the spontaneous abortion there was a widespread necrotizing villitis with an accumulation of necrotic material and mononuclear cells in the intervillous space; necrotizing granulomas containing giant cells and epithelioid cells were present in some villi (Fig. 11.20). There was a necrotizing endarteritis of the fetal villous vessels and inclusion bodies were seen in the cytoplasm of villous stromal cells and in decidual cells. In the two placentas from induced abortions, inclusion bodies were present in villous stromal cells and decidual cells but there were no inflammatory lesions.

Measles

Moroi et al (1991) reported the placental findings in a case of intrauterine fetal death associated with maternal measles. There was an intervillous mononuclear cell and fibrinous exudate with villous adhesions and villous syncytial necrosis. Measles virus antigen was demonstrated immunohistologically in villous syncytiotrophoblast.

Parvovirus

Parvovirus B-19 is a cause of fetal hydrops and death. Placentas infected by this virus tend to be large and may be oedematous. Histologically, the placental infection is characterized by the presence, within the fetal vessels, of a markedly increased number of nucleated red blood cells, some of which contain intranuclear inclusions consisting of a central clear or eosinophilic area with peripheral chromatin condensation (Kaplan, 1993). The diagnostic nuclear inclusions are not always found in the placenta, being present in only two of five placentas from fatal cases of fetal parvovirus infection studied by Rogers et al (1993). Patchy villous immaturity and oedema is common and although Kaplan (1993) maintained that a villitis is not seen in this infection, Morey et al (1992) noted that a vasculitis, affecting villous capillaries and occasionally stem arteries, is a common finding and is associated with a perivascular round cell inflammatory infiltrate.

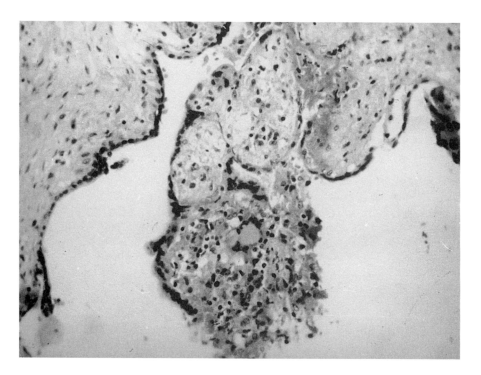

Figure 11.20. Placenta from a patient with mumps. A necrotizing granuloma is present in one villus (H & E ×250).

Cytomegalovirus

The placental changes induced by this virus have been documented quite extensively (Lepage & Schramm, 1958; Quan & Strauss, 1962; Cochard et al, 1963; Rosenstein & Navarrete-Reyna, 1964; Altshuler & McAdams, 1971; Benirschke et al, 1974; Mostoufi-Zadeh et al, 1984; Garcia et al, 1989). Grossly, the infected placenta is often unremarkable but is sometimes bulky and oedematous, whilst histologically there is characteristically a low-grade focal or diffuse lymphoplasmacytic villitis. The villi show, however, a spectrum of histological changes, ranging from, in the early stages, a focal necrotizing and proliferative villitis, sometimes with granulomatous features (Kaplan, 1993), to, in the later stages, atrophy and fibrosis. The brunt of the inflammatory damage is borne by the villous stroma rather than by the trophoblast, and whilst there is usually an infiltration of lymphocytes into the stroma, it is not uncommon to also find plasma cells (Fig. 11.21), these often being most numerous in the immediately perivascular areas. The lymphocytes appear to be all T-cells whilst the plasma cells may be IgM- or IgG-secreting (Schwartz et al, 1992). An increased number of Hofbauer cells may be present. Focal or generalized villous oedema is sometimes seen, and thrombosis of fetal vessels may occur. Deposition of haemosiderin pigment in the villi is often a particularly striking feature. Cytomegalovirus inclusion bodies can often be found in the infected placenta (Fig. 11.22) though they are usually few in number and are sometimes only detected after a prolonged search. They are usually seen in the endothelial cells of the fetal vessels but may occasionally be located in the stromal cells or in the trophoblast.

In many cases of documented intrauterine fetal cytomegalovirus infection the placenta appears normal on histological examination (Muhlemann et al, 1994) and it is known that cytomegalovirus can be isolated from such placentas (Davis et al, 1971; Hayes & Gibas, 1971; Strulovici et al, 1974). Furthermore, a villitis which is evoked by cytomegalovirus infection may show no specific features and can masquerade as a villitis of unknown aetiology. It is in cases such as these that

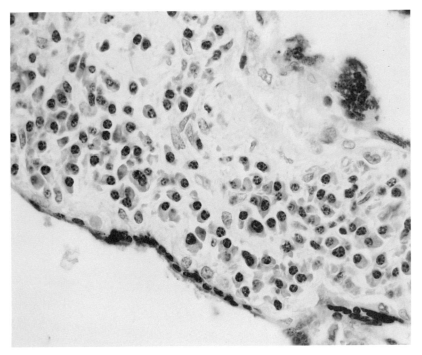

Figure 11.21. Cytomegalovirus infection of the placenta. There is a predominantly plasma cell infiltration of a villus (H & E ×480).

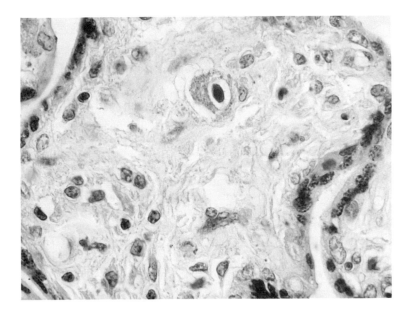

Figure 11.22. Cytomegalovirus infection of the placenta. A typical cytomegalic cell with an intranuclear inclusion is seen in a villus (H & E ×540).

immunofluorescence (Garcia et al, 1989), immunocytochemistry (Muhlemann et al, 1992, 1994; Sinzger et al, 1993), *in situ* hybridization (Borisch et al, 1988; Sachdev et al, 1990) and the polymerase chain reaction (Chehab et al, 1989; Nakamura et al, 1994) have proven to be of great value in demonstrating the presence of the virus in placental tissue.

Hepatitis Virus

Khudr and Benirschke (1972) studied two placentas from women with infective hepatitis and found that, although there was massive deposition of bilirubin in the macrophages of both the membranes and the villi, there was no evidence of any inflammatory lesion. Similar findings, but with the addition of focal syncytial necrosis without any inflammatory reaction, were noted by Benirschke and Kaufmann (1995) in a placenta from a woman who underwent therapeutic abortion for hepatitis B infection.

Lucifora et al (1988) have demonstrated, by immunocytochemistry, the presence of hepatitis B surface antigen in the villous Hofbauer cells and fetal villous vessel endothelial cells of asymptomatic HBsAg-carriers. They later (1990) showed that hepatitis B core antigen was also demonstrable in placentas from such carriers, the antigen being present not only in the Hofbauer and endothelial cells but also in the trophoblastic cell columns and in the infiltrating extravillous cytotrophoblast of the placental bed. The significance of this finding is debatable but it is impossible to accept the view of Lucifora et al (1990) that the infiltrating cells in the placental bed are actually Hofbauer cells and that these serve as a vehicle for transplacental infection of the fetus.

Influenza Virus

Yawn et al (1971) have documented a convincing example of transplacental transfer of influenza virus, in which the placenta was histologically normal. Melnikova et al (1987) reported 32 cases of placental involvement in influenza, describing trophoblastic necrosis, a lymphocytic infiltrate and necrosis of the endothelium of fetal stem vessels. Intracellular cytoplasmic inclusions were seen and an influenza virus was isolated from three of the placentas.

Human Immunodeficiency Virus

Vertical transplacental materno-fetal transmission of human immunodeficiency virus certainly occurs, though the virus does not reach the fetus in about 70% of pregnancies in seropositive mothers (Schwartz & Nahmias, 1991; Douglas & King, 1992; Ebbesen et al, 1994). The virus has been identified within placental tissue by electron microscopy (Jauniaux et al, 1988; Villegas-Castrejon et al, 1994), immunocytochemistry (Martin et al, 1992; Mattern et al, 1992; Backe et al, 1994), in situ hybridization (Lewis et al, 1990; Backe et al, 1992; Anderson et al, 1994), polymerase chain reaction and in situ polymerase chain reaction (Zevallos et al, 1994) and has been detected most frequently in the Hofbauer cells and less commonly in the trophoblast and fetal endothelial cells.

Placentas from women who are seropositive for human immunodeficiency virus usually appear macroscopically normal though in a few studies the placentas have been unduly heavy (Caretti et al, 1988; Jauniaux et al, 1988). Chorioamnionitis is unusually common (Jauniaux et al, 1988; Chandwani et al, 1991, 1992; Gichangi et al, 1993) but this is almost certainly because of a secondary opportunistic infection. Histologically there has been a widespread consensus that a villitis is not seen and that no specific abnormalities are present (Caretti et al, 1988; Jauniaux et al, 1988; Villegas-Castrejon et al, 1990; Chandwani et al, 1991, 1992; Schwartz et al, 1992; Backe et al, 1994). Anderson et al (1994) have described villous immaturity, villous oedema, focal trophoblastic necrosis, an excess of villous Hofbauer cells, necrosis of Hofbauer cells, excessive intravillous fibrin deposition and chorangiosis as features, albeit non-specific ones, of placentas exposed to possible infection by human immunodeficiency virus. They point out, however, that in their population these placentas are from women who are not only seropositive for the virus infection but who also tend to smoke cigarettes, are often addicted drug users and are subject to a wide range of opportunistic infections, all factors that may influence placental morphology.

C Virus

This virus (an endogenous retrovirus) has been detected in morphologically normal placentas from apparently healthy women (Kalter et al, 1973; Vernon et al, 1974; Johnson et al, 1990; Lyden et al, 1991) and is in fact probably present in all human placentas; strictly speaking, therefore, its presence does not denote a true infection or a pathological lesion. The function of this endogenous retrovirus, if any, is unknown but Lyden et al (1994) have argued that as the virus is expressed most strongly in the villous syncytiotrophoblast and as retroviruses cause cell fusion in cultures it is possible that it plays a role in the fusion of villous cytotrophoblastic cells to form syncytiotrophoblast. From a strictly practical point of view the significance of the presence of this virus is that it may be mistaken, on electron microscopy, for human immunodeficiency virus. Further, the endogenous retroviral proteins appear to have antigenic similarity with those of human immunodeficiency virus and may cross-react with antibodies to this latter virus (Lyden et al, 1994).

Fungal Infections

Coccidioides immitis

Examples of placental involvement in coccidioidomycosis have been described by Mendenhall et al (1948), Cohen (1951), Vaughan and Ramirez (1951), Baker (1955), Smale and Waechter (1970), VanBergen et al (1976) and McCaffree et al (1978). The spherules of *C. immitis* produce areas of placental necrosis with an acute inflammatory reaction and extensive fibrin deposition; areas of suppurative villitis may be present and tuberculoid granulomas are sometimes seen. Transplacental passage to the fetus does not appear to occur, partly because of the large size of the organisms and partly because of their entrapment in inflammatory exudate and fibrin (Spark, 1981).

Paracoccidioides brasiliensis

Examination of the placenta from a woman who was receiving treatment for juvenile-type paracoccidioimycosis showed numerous yeast forms in the intervillous space. These were enmeshed in a macrophage–histiocytic reaction and there was focal trophoblastic necrosis (Blotta et al, 1993).

Aspergillus

Ben-Rejeb et al (1993) described multiple large granulomas in the villi and intervillous space of a placenta from a woman with an *Aspergillus niger* infection.

Cryptococcus neoformans

Cryptococcal involvement of the placenta has been described in a patient with the acquired immunodeficiency syndrome (Kida et al, 1989) and in a woman with systemic lupus erythematosus (Molnar-Nasasdy et al, 1994). Multiple colonies of encapsulated budding yeasts were present in the intervillous space and these appeared to have elicited little or no inflammatory response; there was no involvement of villous tissue.

Candida albicans

This fungal organism is, as discussed earlier in this chapter, a cause of chorioamnionitis but Bittencourt et al (1984) described involvement of the villous tissue in a case of severe candidiasis of the membranes and fetus, the villous lesions being almost certainly due to haematogenous spread of the infection from the fetus. There was a striking infiltration of the intervillous space by polymorphonuclear leucocytes and a necrotizing villitis with infiltration of the villi by acute inflammatory cells: hyphae and spores were seen in the lumens of villous vessels.

Parasitic and Protozoal Infections

Toxoplasma gondii

Placentas infected by *Toxoplasma gondii* are often macroscopically normal, but a proportion are large, bulky and pale, thus resembling closely the hydropic placenta of severe materno-fetal rhesus incompatibility (Bain et al, 1956; Schubert, 1957). Histologically there is a low-grade smouldering chronic villitis which may involve single villi or groups of villi (Fig. 11.23); these show a mononuclear cell infiltration (predominantly lymphocytic but sometimes with a sprinkling of plasma cells), fibrosis, an excessive number of Hofbauer cells and, sometimes, necrosis (Elliot, 1970; Garcia et al, 1983; Abdel-Salam et al, 1990). Occasionally a granulomatous type of lesion may be seen in the villi (Elliott, 1970; Susani, 1981; Popek, 1992), whilst the fetal vessels often show an endarteritis (Sarrut, 1967). The intervillous space may contain nodular masses of histiocytes. Encysted and free forms of *Toxoplasma* may be seen, usually the former, and commonly in the chorionic plate or amnion (Fig. 11.24) rather than in the villi. The cysts are morphologically characteristic but can, if necessary, be specifically identified by a fluorescent antibody technique (Dallenbach & Piekarski, 1960; Foulon et al, 1990). The polymerase chain reaction is of considerable value for the recognition of toxoplasmosis if the diagnostic cysts are not present (Savva & Holliman, 1990).

In the hydropic form of placental toxoplasmosis the villi are oedematous, hypercellular and contain many Hofbauer cells (Altshuler, 1973a). The resemblance to the placenta of severe materno-fetal rhesus incompatibility may be further accentuated by the presence, because of fetal anaemia, of numerous nucleated red blood cells in the fetal

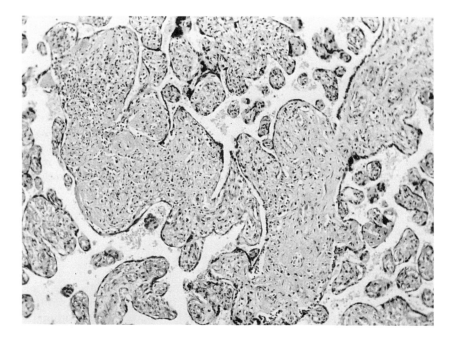

Figure 11.23. Placental toxoplasmosis. The villi are somewhat oedematous and there is a mononuclear cell villous infiltrate (H & E ×90).

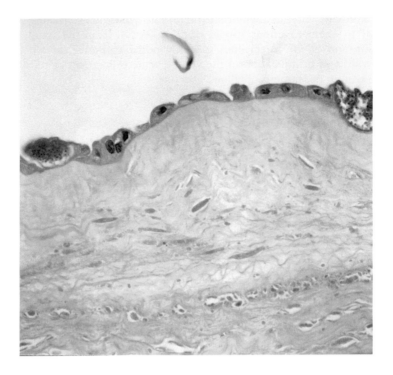

Figure 11.24. Toxoplasmosis. Encysted organisms in the amnion (H & E ×480).

vessels. The focal chronic villitis and the presence of encysted forms of the parasite allow for the differentiation of this form of placentitis from the placental changes of rhesus incompatibility.

Placentas have been described which contained numerous encysted forms of *Toxoplasma* but which did not show any morphological abnormality or evidence of inflammation (Werner et al, 1963; Glasser & Delta, 1965).

Schistosoma

Placental infestation with *Bilharzia* occurs in a relatively high proportion of women with the genital or urinary forms of this disease (Renaud et al, 1972). Ova may very occasionally be seen embedded in intervillous fibrin (Fig. 11.25), and although they usually elicit little or no inflammatory reaction there may be a granulomatous response (Bittencourt et al, 1980). Detection of the ova by conventional histological methods is dependent upon either good fortune or a massive infestation. Recognition of ova is, however, facilitated by digestion of placental segments in sodium hydroxide with subsequent light microscopy of the sediment (Sutherland et al, 1965).

Trypanosoma cruzi

Bittencourt and her colleagues have described placental involvement in Chagas' disease (Bittencourt, 1960, 1963, 1976; Bittencourt and Barbosa, 1972; Bittencourt et al, 1972). Characteristically there is an extensive necrotizing villitis which often has granulomatous features. The infecting organisms, transformed into amastigotes, can often, though not invariably, be seen with ease (Fig. 11.26), usually within Hofbauer cells but sometimes as a sub-syncytiotrophoblastic aggregate. Placental involvement is associated with a very high rate of transmission of the parasite to the fetus (Azogue & Darras, 1991).

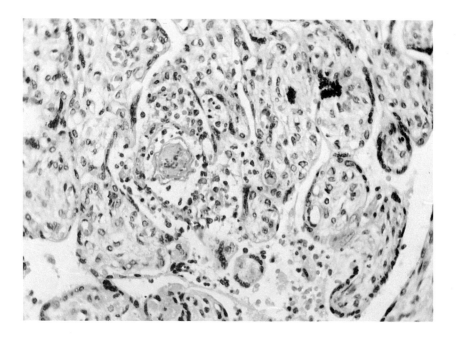

Figure 11.25. Schistosomiasis of the placenta. An ovum is seen in the intervillous space (H & E ×220).

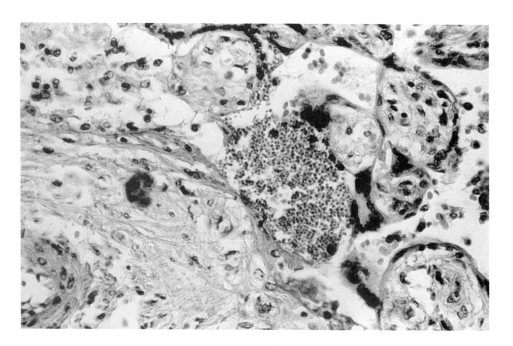

Figure 11.26. Chagas' disease involving the placenta. A large aggregate of the organisms is seen (H & E ×330).

Plasmodia

Malarial infection of the placenta is common in areas in which this disease is endemic. On histological examination (Wickramasuriya, 1935; Garnham, 1938; Covell, 1950; Galbraith et al, 1980a,b; Walter et al, 1982b; Philippe & Walter, 1985; Yamada et al, 1989; Bulmer et al, 1993a,b) parasites can often be seen in maternal red blood cells

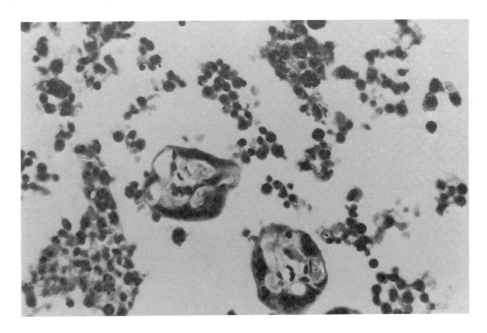

Figure 11.27. Placental malaria. There are large aggregates of maternal monocytic cells in the intervillous space (H & E ×150).

in the intervillous space and a variable amount of dark brown, coarse, granular malarial pigment is present. Much of the pigment appears within maternal monocytes in the intervillous space but it is sometimes apparent within villous Hofbauer cells. In some cases, free pigment is present within the villous syncytiotrophoblast and this is associated with focal syncytial necrosis. The pigment-bearing monocytes can form large aggregates within the intervillous space (Fig. 11.27) and these, together with parasitized erythrocytes, may be bound by intervillous fibrin to form an inflammatory-like mass. Within the villous tissue there may be some thickening of the trophoblastic basement membrane, an undue prominence of the villous cytotrophoblastic cells and an excess number of villi showing a variable degree of fibrinoid necrosis. It is noteworthy that parasitized maternal erythrocytes appear to be sequestrated in the intervillous space, to the extent that histological examination of the placenta is a more sensitive screening test for malaria than is a blood smear (Randrianjafisamindrakotroka et al, 1994).

Transmission of the malarial parasite to the fetus, presumably in transferred maternal red blood cells, is probably quite common (Marshall, 1983; Nnatu et al, 1987; Bachschmid et al, 1991) but in endemic areas congenital malaria is rare (Boukari et al, 1991; Hennequin & Bouree, 1991). Nevertheless, malaria in pregnancy is consistently associated with a significant reduction in birth weight (Jelliffe, 1967; McGregor et al, 1983; Kramer, 1987; Kaushik et al, 1992; Gazin et al, 1994; Morgan, 1994).

Villitis of Unknown Aetiology

Although it is clearly established that many infections reaching the placenta from either the maternal bloodstream or the endometrium result in a villitis, it remains true that in the vast majority of cases of villitis no specific infective organism can be identified. The incidence of villitis of unknown aetiology in large unselected series of third-trimester placentas in Western countries ranges from 6 to 14% (Altshuler & Russell, 1975; Russell, 1979, 1980; Knox & Fox, 1984). Both significantly higher (Garcia, 1982; Labarrere et al, 1982) and considerably lower (Rolschau, 1978) incidences of villitis have been recorded, but these were in relatively small series of highly selected placentas. Nakamura et al (1994) found a villitis in only just over 2% of placentas from a Japanese population but it is difficult to compare different populations because the incidence of villitis is influenced by ethnic, environmental and socio-economic factors (Loga et al, 1972). It should further be noted, when considering the cited incidence of villitis, that, although some cases of villitis of unknown origin are very extensive and easily recognized, many are detected only in extensively sampled and obsessively examined placentas. It is not uncommon for only 2–4% of the villous population to show an inflammatory infiltrate and lesions as scanty as these can easily be missed on routine histological examination. Furthermore, it can be very difficult to recognize a villitis, a point often not remarked upon in accounts of placental infections. There is, of course, no difficulty in recognizing those cases in which there is a dense inflammatory infiltrate and extensive villous necrosis but the distinction between minor degrees of cellular infiltration of the villi and mild villous stromal hypercellularity is often highly subjective. It is therefore hardly suprising that Khong et al (1993) found that even amongst experienced pathologists there is a significant degree of inter-observer variation in diagnosing villitis. The situation is further compounded by the fact that some authors feel that lesions very similar to those of a villitis of unknown aetiology can occur as a result of uteroplacental ischaemia (Naeye, 1992; Altshuler, 1993). This is a view with which I cannot concur and, after having examined carefully a photomicrograph purporting to show such a lesion (Altshuler, 1993), can see no way in which this differs from a conventional villitis.

Despite these codicils it is clear that villitis is a common finding and as infection can, and undoubtedly does, cause a villitis, the question arises as to whether a villitis is always due to infection. Altshuler (1973b) pointed out that focal villitis of unknown aetiology is usually histologically very similar to that seen in known cases of rubella infection of the placenta, and thought that most cases were due to an as yet unidentified viral agent. I have agreed with this view (Fox, 1993) and still do, and consider it almost certain that with the application of newer techniques for the diagnosis of viral infections the proportion of cases of villitis that are of 'unknown' origin will steadily decrease. Thus, Sachdev et al (1990), using *in situ* hybridization, found that three out of five cases of chronic villitis lacking the diagnostic features of cytomegalovirus infection reacted positively for cytomegalovirus DNA. Similarily, Nakamura et al (1994) found that with the aid of the polymerase chain reaction, cytomegalovirus genes were detectable in nearly 10% of cases of villitis of 'unknown' aetiology.

The view that villitis is a pathognomonic hallmark of infection has, however, been challenged by the suggestion that this lesion is the morphological expression of an immunological reaction within villous tissue. It has been argued that infection is one, but by no means the sole, cause of such an immune lesion, other possibilities being a maternal graft rejection or a graft-versus-host reaction (Labarrere et al, 1982, 1986; Althabe & Labarrere, 1985; Redline & Abramowsky, 1985; Hasegawa et al, 1990; Michaud et al, 1991; Redline, 1995). It has further been claimed that villitis should be defined in immunopathological rather than morphological terms, the characteristic, and specific, feature being the presence within the villi of macrophages that stain positively for class II (HLA-DR) antigens of the major histocompatibility complex (MHC) and also react positively with monoclonal antibodies to HLA-DP and HLA-DQ together with CD4 lymphocytes (Laberrere et al, 1989, 1990), a view confirmed by Altemani (1992). The problem with this definition is that villitis defined in terms of the presence of activated macrophages is present, to a greater or lesser degree, in virtually *all* placentas (Laberrere et al, 1989, 1990) and thus ceases to be a pathological process. Further, Khong (1995) has shown that there is no correlation between histological evidence of villitis and expression of MHC class II antigens; immunoreactivity may be absent in villi with a chronic inflammatory cell infiltrate and present in villi lacking any evidence of an inflammatory process.

The case for some instances of villitis being of non-infective origin is a seductive one, which is bolstered by the finding that fetal IgM levels are not elevated in cases of villitis of unknown aetiology (Mortimer et al, 1985; Altemani et al, 1989) and by the fact that maternal cells participate, and may even predominate, in the intravillous inflammatory infiltrate (Redline & Patterson, 1993; Labarrere & Faulk, 1995). It is, however, quite possible that in many cases an immune reaction is superimposed on, or is provoked by, an initial infectious insult (Gersell, 1993). Nevertheless, in our present state of knowledge it would still be prudent to regard a villitis of anything more than a trivial degree as being indicative of a possible infection.

The clinical significance of villitis of unknown origin is discussed later in this chapter.

The Placenta as a Barrier to Haematogenous Infection of the Fetus

The placenta is often considered as an obstacle to the free passage of organisms from the maternal circulation to the fetus. It must be conceded, however, that any barrier-like function of the placenta is not manifested with any great degree of consistency or success, because the variety of organisms known to be able to pass through the placenta and infect the fetus is legion. Indeed, it is doubtful if there is any infective agent that invariably fails to penetrate the defences of the placenta. It is true that there is both experimental and clinical evidence that cytomegalovirus may, on occasion, infect the placenta without involving the fetus (Johnson, 1969; Hayes & Gibas, 1971) but this is of little true significance, as it is well established that cytomegalovirus *can* cross the placenta to infect the fetus. This same comment also applies to other evidence often cited as proof of the placenta's barrier function, e.g., the fact that in maternal rubella the placenta is commonly affected, whilst spread to the fetus is relatively unusual (Mims, 1968).

The available evidence suggests, therefore, that the placenta can act only as a partial barrier to fetal infection: this partial resistance could be based on one, or more, of the following mechanisms:

1. The placenta may mount an immunological attack against infecting organisms.
2. The placenta could possess specific antibacterial or antiviral properties that enable it to resist infection.
3. Placental phagocytic activity.
4. The placenta may simply function as a non-specific physical barrier.

The first of these possibilities has little to recommend it because the placenta is a fetal organ and there is no convincing evidence that it possesses any immunological defence mechanism against infection that is either specific or differs significantly from that of other fetal tissues. Indeed, it has been argued that the reverse may be the case and that invading organisms could benefit coincidentally from the factor (or factors) that allows the placenta to resist maternal cell-mediated immune attack (Pearce & Lowrie, 1972).

There is evidence, however, that the placenta does possess specific non-immunologically mediated defence mechanisms against infection that are independent of those of the fetus. The placenta, specifically the villous syncytiotrophoblast, produces interferons when stimulated by viruses (Toth et al, 1990; Aboagye-Mathiesen et al, 1993) but whilst cell cultures of other fetal tissues produce higher levels of interferon when challenged by Sendai virus than when attacked by rubella virus, the reverse is true for cultured placental tissue (Banatvala et al, 1971). The autonomy of placental interferon synthesis is thus clearly apparent, and this is probably an important factor in limiting transplacental viral spread. This is emphasized by the fact that various strains of rubella virus have differing abilities to stimulate placental, but not fetal, interferon synthesis; their capacity in this respect is inversely proportional to their ability to cross the placenta (Banatvala et al, 1973).

Specific placental defence mechanisms against bacterial infection have not been defined and the bactericidal activity of placental tissue is similar to that of maternal and neonatal sera.

The Hofbauer cells of the placental villi have, as discussed in Chapter 1, all the characteristics of macrophages and are present in sufficient numbers for the placenta to be almost considered as a reticuloendothelial organ. This may be somewhat of an over-statement but it is nevertheless highly possible that the phagocytic capacity of the placenta is of considerable importance in limiting transplacental spread of infection (Vince & Johnson, 1996). This role has been emphasized by *in vitro* studies which have shown that when Hofbauer cells are infected with herpes simplex virus or echovirus the viruses are rapidly destroyed (Oliveira et al, 1992).

Despite these factors acting to prevent spread of infection to the fetus, the protection offered by the placenta as a simple physical barrier should not be underestimated. In most infections, however, the placenta appears only to delay the passage of organisms to the fetus, this delay being accounted for by the time taken for the organism to establish a focus of infection in the placental tissue from which the fetus is subsequently infected. In bacterial infections the organisms need only invade the placental tissue, but viruses must replicate in placental cells and, in theory, any virus unable to multiply in such cells would not pass through the placenta. In practice, however, most viruses appear to proliferate readily in placental tissue and are thus able to establish a focus from which the fetus is later involved. This is readily seen in rubella, in which the virus proliferates in the endothelium of fetal placental vessels, a site from which they can pass with ease into the fetal circulation.

The concept of the placenta as at least a partial barrier to fetal infection has, however, to be tempered by consideration of two other factors. First, the barrier function of the placenta may be modified by maternal factors. Thus, in experimental studies of *Brucella* infection in mice it has been clearly shown that maternal immunization with immune sera increased the placental barrier effect, insofar as fetal spread from heavily infected placentas was prevented (Bosseray & Plommet, 1988). How this restriction of spread from placenta to fetus is achieved, and whether this experimental model has any human counterpart, is a matter for conjecture, though it is worth noting that transplacental passage of malaria to the fetus occurs more commonly in non-immune populations than in immune populations.

Secondly, viewing the placenta as a protection against fetal infection may be, in some cases at least, a reversal of the true position. In many animal infections the placenta is a preferential site for localization of infecting organisms and many experimental infections can only be successfully induced if the animal is pregnant (Pearce & Lowrie, 1972). The increased susceptibility to infection of gravid animals appears, in many cases, to be due solely to the presence of placental tissue in which the organisms are able preferentially to proliferate. Nothing is currently known about facilitation of infections in humans by placental tissue but it would not be unreasonable to expect that a phenomenon which is so widespread in animal species may also be of relevance in some human infections.

Mechanisms of Placental Damage in Haematogenous Infections

Haematogenous infections could, in theory, cause placental damage by a variety of mechanisms, because the infecting organisms could:

1. Directly cause cell death and tissue damage.
2. Produce lesions in the uteroplacental vessels.
3. Produce a toxin which damages the placental tissue or vessels.
4. Provoke an immune response which is directed against placental tissue.

In infections of animal placentas there is often very extensive necrosis of the placental parenchyma, but in the human placenta a necrotizing inflammation rarely involves more than scattered individual villi or small groups of villi. It is true that in rare instances the necrosis may be very widespread with extensive villous destruction (Russell et al, 1980; Coid & Fox, 1983), but in the vast majority of cases the proportion of villi that is damaged is, in view of the considerable reserve capacity of the placenta, insufficient to compromise the functional ability of the placenta. Necrosis of villous tissue may, of course, be secondary to infective damage to the uteroplacental vasculature with widespread thrombosis; again, this occurs in a variety of animal infections, but is not, as far as is known, a feature of infection in humans.

Placental damage caused by bacterial toxins has been shown to occur under experimental conditions (Payne, 1958; McKay & Wong, 1964; Hall, 1974), but whether these laboratory models have any naturally occurring counterparts is unknown. Certainly it would be unwise to discount the possibility that toxic damage to trophoblast is more common than is usually recognized.

Corbel (1972) detected antiplacental antibodies in pregnant sheep infected with *Aspergillus fumigatus*; the titre of these reached a peak at the time of abortion. Both the significance of these antibodies and the relevance of this study to humans are highly dubious. It has been suggested that the finding of activated macrophages and T cells of the helper phenotype in the lesion of villitis is indicative of allogeneic recognition and a rejection reaction in the placenta (Labarrere & Faulk, 1992). The possibility that infection triggers off a cell-mediated immune attack on placental tissues can certainly not be excluded.

Effects and Clinical Significance of Haematogenous Infection

The most obvious consequence of haematogenous placental infection is that the establishment of an inflammatory lesion in the placental tissue serves as a focus from which the fetus is later infected.

It is an established fact that many cases of placental infection are associated with intrauterine fetal death or abortion, but, in most instances the demise of the fetus appears to be linked more to the direct effects of the infection on either the mother or the fetus than to placental damage. It has been shown experimentally that placental infection *per se*, without fetal infection or severe maternal illness, can be associated with a high incidence of fetal loss (Johnson, 1969), but there are no well-defined examples of this phenomenon in humans. Furthermore, the degree of tissue damage seen in most haematogenous placental infections in humans is such that its effects could be easily neutralized by the organ's considerable functional reserve.

The above remarks apply to those cases of villitis that are clearly due to a specific infection, such as rubella or syphilis. What, however, is the clinical significance of a villitis of unknown aetiology, which is presumed though not proven to be indicative of a haematogenous infection? There is an undoubted association between villitis of unknown aetiology and an increased incidence of intrauterine fetal growth retardation (Altshuler & Russell, 1975; Altshuler et al, 1975; Russell, 1979, 1980; Labarrere et al, 1982; Bjoro & Myhre, 1984; Knox & Fox, 1984; Althabe & Labarrere, 1985; Mortimer et al, 1985; Altemani et al, 1989; Nordenvall & Sandstedt, 1990; Salafia et al, 1992a,b; Redline & Patterson, 1994) though it must be stressed that in prospective studies the vast majority of neonates whose placentas show a villitis are of normal weight. Thus, in our own series only 6.8% of neonates from cases of villitis had a birth weight for gestational age that was below the 5th centile (Knox & Fox, 1984). A villitis of unknown aetiology can recur in successive pregnancies and it has been maintained that this recurrent form of villitis tends to be unusually extensive and shows a particularly strong association with fetal growth retardation (Russell et al, 1980; Redline & Abramowsky, 1985; Labarrere & Althabe, 1987). Such cases are very rare, however, and, of course, a pathologist examining a placenta usually does not know if any villitis that is present is recurrent or not.

The nature of the link between villitis of unknown aetiology and diminished fetal growth is far from being clear. Benirschke and Kaufmann (1995), whilst pointing out that there is no absolute relation between the severity of the villitis and the severity of growth retardation, consider nevertheless that the restriction of fetal growth is related to the elimination of a considerable amount of placental parenchyma from nutrient transfer. This may be true in occasional rare cases but is clearly not true in the vast majority of cases of villitis in which the inflammatory damage wreaked upon the placenta is far too limited in extent to dissipate the functional reserve of the organ. Hence some other cause must be sought. If, and it is admittedly quite a large 'if', a chronic villitis is commonly due to an unrecognized viral infection then it is perfectly possible that the virus passes through the inadequate barrier of the placenta to infect the fetus and restrict its growth, the inhibitory effect of viruses on fetal DNA synthesis being well established. It is true that neonates whose placentas show evidence of a villitis do not usually have any clinical evidence of an infection but the infection may have been relatively transitory and the growth restriction temporary. If, on the other hand, some cases of villitis are due to an immunological interaction between maternal and fetal tissues then this may be associated with abnormal placentation with consequent restriction of fetal growth, a point discussed more fully in Chapter 9.

Salafia et al (1991) have noted an association between villitis of unknown aetiology and preterm birth but this has not been our experience (Knox & Fox, 1984).

UNUSUAL INFLAMMATORY LESIONS OF THE PLACENTA

Chronic Chorioamnionitis

Chorioamnionitis is, as previously discussed, nearly always an acute inflammatory process but Gersell et al (1991) described 17 examples of a form of chorioamnionitis in which the membranes were infiltrated by chronic inflammatory cells. The inflammatory infiltrate in these cases consisted largely of mature lymphocytes but these were often admixed with smaller numbers of plasma cells and histiocytes; large lymphoid cells and immunocytes were occasionally seen. In six of the 17 cases the chronic inflammatory cell infiltrate was accompanied by a minor component of polymorphonuclear leucocytes which was in some cases distinct from the chronic inflammatory component and in others admixed with it. A chronic villitis was present in 11 of the 17 placentas.

Gersell et al (1991) pointed out that a chronic chorioamnionitis had been described, but not specifically commented on, in some cases of necrotizing funisitis and in occasional instances of proven viral and protozoal infections of the placenta. No specific infective agents could be identified in their cases but the combination of both a chorioamnionitis and a villitis does hint at the possibility of an unusual, modified response to a *Listeria* infection.

The clinical significance of a chronic chorioamnionitis is uncertain but there was a wide range of unrelated pregnancy complications in the cases described by Gersell and her colleagues. Premature rupture of the membranes occurred in two cases and there was prolonged rupture of the membranes in three patients. There was a high incidence of preterm labour.

Necrotizing Funisitis

The term 'necrotizing funisitis' was introduced by Navarro and Blanc (1974) to describe a form of chronic inflammation of the umbilical cord which is also sometimes classed as 'sclerosing funisitis' or 'constrictive sclerosis of the cord'. The cord may appear somewhat rigid and taut ('cooked macaroni' appearance) and on cross-section there are visible yellow-white or chalky bands surrounding thickened vessel walls (Fig. 11.28), an appearance likened to that seen in an Ouchterlony diffusion plate. Histologically there are concentric perivascular bands of necrotic Wharton's jelly containing acute and chronic inflammatory cells in various stages of degeneration (Fig. 11.29); calcification may occur in the necrotic areas. There is nearly always an associated chorioamnionitis.

Claims that this form of funisitis is a specific feature of, and is confined to, syphilis (Fojaco et al, 1989; Knowles & Frost, 1989) have not been confirmed, others finding that this lesion can be found in a wide range of infections (Craver & Baldwin, 1992; Jacques & Qureshi, 1992). There is, however, no doubt that it is a common finding in

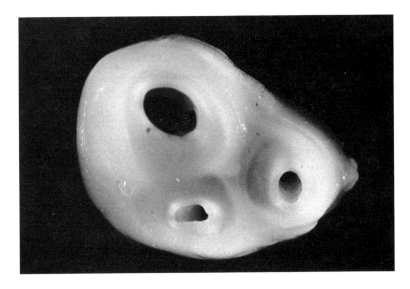

Figure 11.28. Necrotizing funisitis. Macroscopic appearances of a cross-section of the umbilical cord.

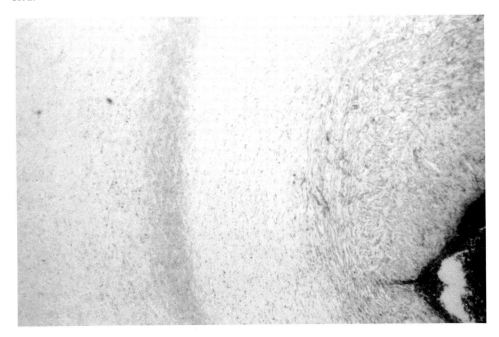

Figure 11.29. Necrotizing funisitis. Concentric bands of necrosis are seen in the wall of the cord (H & E ×60).

congenital syphilis, being present in about one-third of cases (Schwartz et al, 1995). Heifetz and Bauman (1994) considered that whilst no single pathogen causes necrotizing funisitis, there is nevertheless a strong association with latent herpes simplex infection of the endometrium.

It would appear that necrotizing funisitis is a non-specific lesion that results from long-standing chronic inflammation at a site from which inflammatory debris cannot be removed. Clinically there is an association between necrotizing funisitis and a high incidence of premature rupture of the membranes, pre-term labour, intrauterine growth retardation and intrauterine fetal death; the basis for these associations is not known.

Chronic Intervillositis

Labarrere and Mullen (1987) and Jacques and Qureshi (1993) have each described six placentas in which there was a massive histiocytic infiltration of the intervillous space. A concomitant villitis was present in four of the placentas described by Labarrere and Mullen but was found in only one of the placentas reported by Jacques and Qureshi. Fibrinoid change in the villi and atherosis in decidual vessels were quite frequently present whilst clinically there was a high incidence of fetal growth retardation. Doss et al (1995) have reported repetitive massive chronic intervillositis in placentas from a patient who suffered recurrent spontaneous abortions.

The nature of chronic intervillositis is unknown: no real evidence of an infective pathogenesis has been forthcoming and the concept that it indicates a maternal immune reaction to fetal tissues is largely speculative.

REFERENCES

Abdel-Salam, A.M., Eissa, M.H., Mangoud, A.M., Eissa, T.M. and Morsy, T.A. (1990) Pathologic examination of the placenta in human cases of toxoplasmosis. *Journal of the Egyptian Society of Parasitology*, **20**, 549–554.

Aboagye-Mathiesen, G., Toth, F.D., Petersen, P.M. et al (1993) Differential interferon production in human first and third trimester trophoblast cultures stimulated with viruses. *Placenta*, **14**, 225–234.

Albarracin, N.S., Patterson, W.S. and Haust, M.D. (1967) *Candida albicans* infection of the placenta and fetus: report of a case. *Obstetrics and Gynecology*, **30**, 838–841.

Altemani, A.M. (1992) Immunohistochemical study of the inflammatory infiltrate in villitis of unknown etiology: a qualitative and quantitative analysis. *Pathology Research and Practice*, **188**, 303–309.

Altemani, A.M., Fassoni, A. and Marba, S. (1989) Cord IgM levels in placentas with villitis of unknown etiology. *Journal of Perinatal Medicine*, **17**, 465–468.

Althabe, O. and Labarrere, C.A. (1985) Chronic villitis of unknown aetiology and intrauterine growth retarded infants of normal and low ponderal index. *Placenta*, **6**, 369–373.

Altshuler, G. (1973a) Toxoplasmosis as a cause of hydranencephaly. *American Journal of Diseases of Children*, **125**, 251–252.

Altshuler, G. (1973b) Placental villitis of unknown etiology: harbinger of serious disease. A four month experience of nine cases. *Journal of Reproductive Medicine*, **11**, 215–222.

Altshuler, G. (1974) Pathogenesis of congenital herpes virus infection: case report including a description of the placenta. *American Journal of Diseases of Children*, **127**, 427–429.

Altshuler, G. (1984) Placental infection and inflammation. In *Pathology of the Placenta*, Perrin, E.V.D.K. (Ed.), pp. 141–163. New York: Churchill Livingstone.

Altshuler, G. (1993) A conceptual approach to placental pathology and pregnancy outcome. *Seminars in Diagnostic Pathology*, **10**, 204–221.

Altshuler, G. and Hyde, S. (1985) Fusobacteria: an important cause of chorioamnionitis. *Archives of Pathology and Laboratory Medicine*, **109**, 739–743.

Altshuler, G. and Hyde, S. (1988) Clinicopathologic considerations of fusobacteria chorioamnionitis. *Acta Obstetricia et Gynecologica Scandinavica*, **67**, 513–517.

Altshuler, G. and McAdams, A.J. (1971) Cytomegalic inclusion disease of a nineteen-week fetus: case report including a study of the placenta. *American Journal of Obstetrics and Gynecology*, **111**, 295–298.

Altshuler, G. and Russell, P. (1975) The human placental villitides: a review of chronic intrauterine infection. *Current Topics in Pathology*, **60**, 64–112.

Altshuler, G., Russell, P. and Ermocilla, R. (1975) The placental pathology of small-for-gestational age infants. *American Journal of Obstetrics and Gynecology*, **121**, 351–359.

Anderson, V.M., Zevallos, E. and Gu, J. (1994) The HIV-exposed placenta: morphologic observations and interpretation. *Trophoblast Research*, **8**, 47–65.

Ando, K. and Kanayama, N. (1993) The study on mechanism of abruptio placentae caused by chorioamnionitis. *Acta Obstetricia et Gynaecologica Japonica* **45**, 1035–1041.

Armer, T.L. and Duff, P. (1991) Intraamniotic infection with intact membranes and preterm labor. *Obstetrical and Gynecological Survey*, **46**, 589–593.

Aterman, K. (1968) Pathology of *Candida* infection of the umbilical cord. *American Journal of Clinical Pathology*, **49**, 798–804.

Ault, K.A., Gabbs, S.G., O'Shaughnessy, R.W. and Ayers, L.W. (1993) Three cases of *Haemophilus influenzae* amnionitis. *American Journal of Perinatology*, **10**, 378–380.

Azogue, E. and Darras, C. (1991) Estudio prospectivo de la enfermedad de Chaga en recien nacidos con infection placentaria por *Trypanosoma cruzi* (Santa Cruz–Bolivia) *Revista da Sociedade Brasileira de Medicina Tropica*, **24**, 105–109.

Bachschmid, I., Soro, B., Coulibaly, A. et al (1991) Infection palustre a l'accouchement et issue de la grossesse a Becedi (Côte d'Ivoire) *Bulletin de la Société de Pathologie Exotique*, **84**, 257–265.

Backe, E., Jiminez, E., Unger, M., Schafer, A., Jauniaux, E. and Vogel, M. (1992) Demonstration of HIV-1 infected cells in human placenta by *in situ* hybridization and immunostaining. *Journal of Clinical Pathology*, **45**, 871–874.

Backe, E., Jiminez, E., Unger, M. et al (1994) Vertical human immunodeficiency virus transmission: a study of placental pathology in relation to maternal risk factors. *American Journal of Perinatology*, **11**, 326–330.

Bader, G. (1966) Beitrag zur Chorioamnionitis mycotica. *Archiv für Gynäkologie*, **203**, 251–255.

Bain, A.D., Bowie, J.H., Flint, W.F., Beverley, J.K.A. and Beattle, C.P. (1956) Congenital toxoplasmosis simulating haemolytic disease of the newborn. *Journal of Obstetrics and Gynaecology of the British Empire*, **63**, 826–832.

Baker, R.L. (1955) Pregnancy complicated by coccidioidomycosis: report of two cases. *American Journal of Obstetrics and Gynecology*, **70**, 1033–1038.

Banatvala, J.E., Potter, J.E. and Best, J.M. (1971) Interferon response to Sendai and rubella viruses in human foetal cultures. *Journal of General Virology*, **13**, 193–201.

Banatvala, J.E., Potter, J.E. and Webster, M.J. (1973) Foetal interferon responses induced by rubella virus. In *Intrauterine Infections CIBA Foundation Symposium 10*, pp. 77–99. Amsterdam: Associated Scientific Publishers.

Baskin, J.L., Soule, E.M. and Mill, D.S. (1950) Poliomyelitis of the newborn: pathologic changes in two cases. *American Journal of Diseases of Children*, **80**, 10–21.

Bastert, G., Rmer, E., Stein, W.W. and Schuhmann, R. (1975) Gefahr der Fruchtwasserinfektion bei Amniocentese. *Archiv für Gynäkologie*, **219**, 449–451.

Batcup, G., Holt, P., Hambling, M.H., Gerlis, L.M. and Glass, M.R. (1985) Placental and fetal pathology in coxsackie virus A9 infection: a case report. *Histopathology*, **9**, 1227–1235.

Becroft, D.M.C., Farmer, K., Mason, G.H., Morris, M.C. and Stewart, J.H. (1976) Perinatal infection by group B-haemolytic streptococci. *British Journal of Obstetrics and Gynaecology*, **83**, 960–966.

Belter, L.F. (1959) Thrush of the umbilical cord. *Obstetrics and Gynecology*, **14**, 796–798.

Benirschke, K. (1960) Routes and types of infection in the fetus and the newborn. *American Journal of Diseases of Children*, **99**, 714–721.

Benirschke, K. and Driscoll, S.G. (1967) *The Pathology of the Human Placenta*. Berlin, Heidelberg, New York: Springer Verlag.

Benirschke, K. and Kaufmann, P. (1995) *The Pathology of the Human Placenta*, 3rd edn. New York: Springer-Verlag.

Benirschke, K. and Raphael, S.I. (1958) *Candida albicans* infection of the amniotic sac. *American Journal of Obstetrics and Gynecology*, **75**, 200–202.

Benirschke, K., Mendoza, G.R. and Bazeley, P.L. (1974) Placental and fetal manifestations of cytomegalovirus infection. *Virchows Archiv Abteilung B Zell Pathologie*, **16**, 121–139.

Bennett, P.R., Rose, M.P. and Myatt, L. (1987) Preterm labor: stimulation of arachidonic acid metabolism in human amnion by bacterial products. *American Journal of Obstetrics and Gynecology*, **156**, 649–655.

Ben-Rejeb, A., Boubaker, S., Turki, I., Massaoudi, L., Chibani, M. and Khouja, H. (1993) L'aspergillose placentaire: mythe ou realite?. A propos d'une observation avec mort foetale in utero. *Journal de Gynécologie, Obstétrique at Biologie de la Reproduction*, **22**, 85–89.

Bider, D., Ben Rafael, Z., Barkai, G. and Mashiach, S. (1989) Intrauterine fetal death apparently due to *Candida* chorioamnionitis. *Archives of Gynecology and Obstetrics*, **244**, 175–177.

Bittencourt, A.L. (1960) Sobre a forma congenita da doenca de Chagas. *Revista do Instituto de Medicina Tropical de Sao Paulo*, **2**, 319–334.

Bittencourt, A.L. (1963) Placentite chagasica e transmissao congenita da doenca de Chagas. *Revista do Instituto de Medicina Tropical de Sao Paulo*, **5**, 62–67.

Bittencourt, A.L. (1976) Congenital Chagas disease. *American Journal of Diseases of Children*, **130**, 97–103.

Bittencourt, A.L. and Barbosa, H.S. (1972) Importancia do estodo do feto macerado para o diagnostico da forma congenita da doenca de Chagas. *Revista do Instituto de Medicina Tropical de Sao Paulo*, **14**, 260–263.

Bittencourt, A.L., Barbosa, H.S., Rocha, T., Sodre, I. and Sodre, A. (1972) Incidencia da transmissao congenita da doenca de Chagas em partos prematuros na maternidada tsylla balbino (Salvador, Bahia) *Revista do Instituto de Medicina Tropical de Sao Paulo*, **14**, 131–134.

Bittencourt, A.L., Cardoso de Almeida, M.A., Junes, M.A.F. and Casulari da Motta, L.D.C. (1980) Placental involvement in *Schistosomiasis mansoni*: report of four cases. *American Journal of Tropical Medicine and Hygiene*, **29**, 571–575.

Bittencourt, A.L., dos Santos, W.L.C. and de Oliveira, C.H. (1984) Placental and fetal candidiasis: presentation of a case of an abortus. *Mycopathologia*, **87**, 181–187.

Bjoro, K.J. and Myhre, E. (1984) The role of chronic non-specific inflammatory lesions of the placenta in intrauterine growth retardation. *Acta Pathologica, Microbiologica and Immunologica Scandinavica*, **92**, 133–137.

Blanc, W.A. (1959) Amniotic infection syndrome: pathogenesis, morphology and significance in circumnatal mortality. *Clinical Obstetrics and Gynecology*, **2**, 705–734.

Blanc, W.A. (1961) Pathways of fetal and early neonatal infection: viral placentitis, bacterial and fungal chorioamnionitis. *Journal of Pediatrics*, **59**, 473–496.

Blanc, W.A. (1978) Pathology of the placenta and cord in some viral infections. In *Viral Diseases of the Fetus and Newborn*, Hanshaw, J.B. and Dudgeon, J.A. (Eds), pp. 237–258. Philadelphia: Saunders.

Blotta, M.H., Altemani, A.M., Amaral, E., Silva, L.J. and Camargo, Z.P. (1993) Placental involvement in paracoccidioidomycosis. *Journal of Medical and Veterinary Mycology*, **31**, 249–257.

Bobitt, J.R., Hayslip, C.C. and Damato, J.D. (1981) Amniotic fluid infection as determined by trans-abdominal amniocentesis in patients with intact membranes in premature labor. *American Journal of Obstetrics and Gynecology*, **140**, 947–952.

Boesaart, J.W. (1959) Een geval van placenta-tuberculose. *Nederlands Tijdschrift voor Geneeskunde*, **103**, 1849–1852.

Borisch, B., Jahn, G., Scholl, B.C. et al (1988) Detection of human cytomegalovirus DNA and viral antigens in tissues of different manifestations of CMV infection. *Virchows Archiv B Cellular Pathology*, **55**, 93–99.

Bosseray, N. and Plommet, M. (1988) Serum- and cell-mediated immune protection of mouse placenta and fetus against *Brucella abortus* challenge: expression of barrier effect of fetus. *Placenta*, **9**, 65–79.

Boukari, B.S., Napo-Koura, G., Kampatibe, N., Kpodzro, K., Rabineau, D. and Vovar, M. (1991) Le paludisme congenital: considerations cliniques, parasitologiques et histologiques; à propos de 200 observations colligees au CHU de Lome et a l'Hopital de Kpalime. *Bulletin de la Société de Pathologie Exotique*, **84**, 448–457.

Bret, A.J. and Grepinet, J. (1967) Placentites et avortementes d'origine infectieuse: incidence des endometrites et de certains germes tels que le pyocyanique. *Revue Francaise de Gynécologie et d'Obstétrique*, **62**, 417–430.

Bry, K. and Hallman, M. (1989) Prostaglandins, inflammation and preterm labor. *Journal of Perinatology*, **9**, 60–65.

Bulmer, J.N., Rasheed, F.N., Francis, N., Morrison, L. and Greenwood, B.M. (1993a) Placental malaria. I. Pathological classification. *Histopathology*, **22**, 211–218.

Bulmer, J.N., Rasheed, F.N., Morrison, L., Francis, N. and Greenwood, B.M. (1993b) Placental malaria. II. A semi-quantitative investigation of the pathological features. *Histopathology*, **22**, 219–225.

Campognone, P. and Singer, D.B. (1986) Neonatal sepsis due to nontypable *Haemophilus influenzae*. *American Journal of Diseases of Children*, **140**, 117–121.

Caretti, N., Bertolin, A. and Dalla Pria, S. (1988) Placental alterations and fetal conditions in relation to the presence of anti-human immunodeficiency virus (HIV) in pregnant mothers. *Panminerva Medica*, **30**, 77–80.

Carmona, F., Fabregues, F., Alvarez, R., Vila, J. and Cararch, V. (1992) A rare case of chorioamnionitis by *Morganella morganii* complicated by septicemia and adult respiratory distress syndrome. *European Journal of Obstetrics, Gynecology and Reproductive Biology*, **45**, 67–70.

Chandwani, S., Greco, M.A., Mittal, K., Antoine, C., Krasinski, K. and Borkowsky, W. (1991) Pathology and human immunodeficiency virus expression in placentas of seropositive women. *Journal of Infectious Diseases*, **163**, 1134–1138.

Chandwani, S., Greco, M.A., Krasinski, K. and Borkowsky, W. (1992) Pathology of the placenta in HIV-1 infection. *Progress in AIDS Pathology*, **3**, 65–81.

Chany, C., Gresser, I., Venorely, C. and Robbe-Rossat, F. (1966) Persistent polioviral infection of the intact amniotic membrane. II. Existence of a mechanical barrier to viral infection. *Proceedings of the Society for Experimental Biology and Medicine*, **123**, 960–968.

Chehab, F.F., Xiao, X., Kan, Y.W. and Yen, T.S.B. (1989) Detection of cytomegalovirus infection in paraffin-embedded tissue specimens with the polymerase chain reaction. *Modern Pathology*, **2**, 75–78.

Chellam, V.G. and Rushton, D.I. (1985) Chorioamnionitis and funiculitis in the placentas of 200 births weighing less than 2.5 kg. *British Journal of Obstetrics and Gynaecology*, **92**, 808–814.

Chimura, T., Hirayama, T. and Takase, M. (1993) Lysozyme in cervical mucus of patients with chorioamnionitis. *Japanese Journal of Antibiotics* **46**, 726–729.

Cochard, A.M., Tan-Vinh, L. and Lelong, M. (1963) Le placenta dans la cytomegalie; étude anatomo-clinque de 3 observations personelles. *Archives Francaises de Pédiatrie*, **20**, 35–46.

Cohen R. (1951) Placental *Coccidioides*: proof that congenital *Coccidioides* is nonexistent. *Archives of Pediatrics*, **68**, 59–66.

Coid, C.R. and Fox, H. (1983) Campylobacters as placental pathogens. *Placenta*, **4**, 295–306.

Corbel, M.J. (1972) Production of antibodies to placental antigens by pregnant ewes experimentally infected with *Aspergillus fumigatus*. *British Veterinary Journal*, **128**, xliv–xlvi.

Covell, G. (1950) Congenital malaria. *Tropical Diseases Bulletin*, **47**, 1147–1167.

Craver, R.D. and Baldwin, V.J. (1992) Necrotizing funisitis. *Obstetrics and Gynecology*, **79**, 64–70.

Dallenbach, F. and Piekarski, G. (1960) Über den nachweis von *Toxoplasma gondii* im Gewebe mit Hilfe markierter fluorescierender Antikorpet (Methode nach Coons) *Virchows Archiv*, **333**, 607–618.

Darby, M.J., Caritis, S.N. and Shen–Schwartz, S. (1989) Placental abruption in the preterm gestation: an association with chorioamnionitis. *Obstetrics and Gynecology*, **74**, 88–92.

Davis, L.E., Tweed, G.V., Steward, J.A. et al (1971) Cytomegalovirus mononucleosis in a first trimester pregnant female with transmission to the fetus. *Pediatrics*, **48**, 200–206.

de Auraujo, M.C., Schultz, R., Vaz, F.A. et al (1994) A case-control study of histological chorioamnionitis and neonatal infection. *Early Human Development*, **40**, 51–58.

Donders, G.G.G., Moerman, P., Caudron, J. and Van Assche, F.A. (1990) Intrauterine *Candida* infection: a report of four infected fetuses from two mothers. *European Journal of Obstetrics, Gynecology and Reproductive Biology*, **38**, 233–238.

Donders, G.G.G., Moerman, P., de-Wet, G.H., Hooft, P. and Goubau, P. (1991) The association between *Chlamydia* cervicitis, chorioamnionitis and neonatal complications. *Archives of Gynecology and Obstetrics*, **249**, 79–85.

Dong, Y., St. Clair, P.J., Ramzy, I., Kagan-Hallet, S. and Gibbs, R.S. (1987) A morphologic and clinical study of placental inflammation at term. *Obstetrics and Gynecology*, **70**, 175–186.

Doss, B.J., Greene, M.F., Hill, J. et al (1995) Massive chronic intervillositis associated with recurrent abortions. *Human Pathology*, **26**, 1245–1251.

Douglas, G.C. and King, B.F. (1992) Maternal–fetal transmission of human immunodeficiency virus: a review of possible routes and cellular mechanisms of infection. *Clinical Infectious Disease*, **15**, 678–691.

Driscoll, S.G., (1969) Histopathology of gestational rubella. *American Journal of Diseases of Children*, **118**, 49–53.

Driscoll, S.G., Gorbach, A. and Feldman, D. (1962) Congenital listeriosis: diagnosis from placental studies. *Obstetrics and Gynecology*, **20**, 216–220.

Duff, P. and Gibbs, R.S. (1983) Acute intraamniotic infection due to *Streptococcus pneumoniae*. *Obstetrics and Gynecology*, **61**, 25S–27S.

Duncan, M.E. (1980) Babies of mothers with leprosy have small placentae, low birth weights and grow slowly. *British Journal of Obstetrics and Gynaecology*, **87**, 471–479.

Duncan, M.E., Melsom, R., Pearson, J.M.H. et al (1983) A clinical and immunological study of four babies of mothers with lepromatous leprosy, two of whom developed leprosy in infancy. *International Journal of Leprosy*, **51**, 7–17.

Duncan, M.E., Fox, H., Harkness, R.A. and Rees, R.J.W. (1984) The placenta in leprosy. *Placenta*, **5**, 189–198.

Duval, C., Sarrut, S., Henry-Suchet, J. et al (1976) La listériose de la femme enceinte: fréquence et moyens de diagnostic. *Journal de Gynécologie, Obstétrique et Biologie de la Reproduction*, **5**, 271–288.

Easterling, T.R. and Garite, T.J. (1985) Fusobacterium: anaerobic occult amnionitis and premature labor. *Obstetrics and Gynecology*, **66**, 825–828.

Ebbesen, P., Toth, F., Aboagye-Mathiesen, G. et al (1994) Vertical transmission of HIV: possible mechanisms and placental response. *Trophoblast Research*, **8**, 1–17.

Elliott, W.G. (1970) Placental toxoplasmosis. *American Journal of Clinical Pathology*, **53**, 413–417.

Embree, J.E., Krause, V.W., Embil, J.A. and Macdonald, S. (1980) Placental infection with *Mycoplasma hominis* and *Ureaplasma urealyticum*: clinical correlation. *Obstetrics and Gynecology*, **56**, 475–481.

Engebretsen, T. (1974) Gonoroisk chorioamnionitt. *Tidsskrift for den Norske Laegeforening*, **94**, 1903.

Engstrom, L. and Ivemark, B. (1960) Ascending infection in labour; its effect on mother and child. *Acta Obstetricia et Gynecologica Scandinavica*, **39**, 613–625.

Entwistle, D.M., Bray, P.T. and Laurence, K.M. (1962) Prenatal infection with vaccinia virus: report of a case. *British Medical Journal*, **ii**, 238–239.

Eschenbach, D.A. (1993) Ureaplasma urealyticum and premature birth. *Clinical Infectious Diseases*, **17**, Supplement 1, S100–S106.

Evaldson, G.R., Malmborg, A.S. and Nord, C.E. (1982) Premature rupture of the membranes and ascending infection. *British Journal of Obstetrics and Gynaecology*, **89**, 793–801.

Faro, S., Walker, C. and Pierson, R.L. (1980) Amnionitis with intact membranes involving *Streptobacillus moniliformis*. *Obstetrics and Gynecology*, **55**, 9S–11S.

Fojaco, R.M., Hensley, G.T. and Moskowitz, L. (1989) Congenital syphilis and necrotizing funisitis. *Journal of the American Medical Association*, **261**, 1788–1790.

Foulon, W., Naessens, A., de Catte, L. and Amy, J.-J. (1990) Detection of congenital toxoplasmosis by chorionic villus sampling and early amniocentesis. *American Journal of Obstetrics and Gynecology*, **163**, 1511–1513.

Fox, H. (1993) The placenta and infection. In *The Human Placenta*, Redman, C.W.G., Sargent, I.L. and Starkey, P.M. (Eds), pp. 313–333, Oxford: Blackwell.

Fox, H. and Langley, F.A. (1971) Leucocytic infiltration of the placenta and umbilical cord: a clinico-pathologic study. *Obstetrics and Gynecology*, **37**, 451–458.

Gaillard, D.A., Paradis, P., Lallemand, A.V. et al (1993) Spontaneous abortions during the second trimester of gestation. *Archives of Pathology and Laboratory Medicine*, **117**, 1022–1026.

Galbraith, R.M., Faulk, W.P., Galbraith, G.M.P., Holbrook, T.W. and Bray, R.S. (1980a) The human materno-fetal relationship in malaria. I. Identification of pigment and parasites in the placenta. *Transactions of the Royal Society of Tropical Medicine and Hygiene*, **74**, 52–60.

Galbraith, R.M., Fox, H., Hsi, B., Galbraith, G.M.P., Bray, R.S. and Faulk, W.P. (1980b) The human materno-fetal relationship in malaria. II. Histological, ultrastructural and immunopathological studies of the placenta. *Transactions of the Royal Society of Tropical Medicine and Hygiene*, **74**, 61–72.

Galton, M. and Benirschke, K. (1960) The implications of *Candida albicans* infection of the amniotic sac. *Journal of Obstetrics and Gynaecology of the British Empire*, **67**, 644–645.

Garcia, A.G.P. (1963) Fetal infection in chickenpox and alastrim, with histopathologic study of the placenta. *Pediatrics*, **32**, 895–901.

Garcia, A.G.P. (1982) Placental morphology of low-birth-weight infants born at term: gross and microscopic study of 50 cases. *Contributions to Gynecology and Obstetrics*, **9**, 100–112.

Garcia, A.G.P., Pereira, J.M.S., Vidigal, N., Lobato, Y.Y., Pegado, C.S. and Branco, J.P.C. (1980) Intrauterine infection with mumps virus. *Obstetrics and Gynecology*, **56**, 756–759.

Garcia, A.G.P., Coutinho, S.G., Amendoeira, M.R., Assumpacao, M.R. and Albano, M. (1983) Placental morphology of newborns at risk for congenital toxoplasmosis. *Journal of Tropical Pediatrics*, **29**, 95–103.

Garcia, A.G.P., Marques, R.L.S., Lobato, Y.Y., Fonseca, M.E.F. and Wigg, M.D. (1985) Placental pathology in congenital rubella. *Placenta*, **6**, 281–295.

Garcia, A.G.P., Fonseca, M.E.F., Marques, R.L.S. and Lobato, Y.Y. (1989) Placental morphology in cytomegalovirus infection. *Placenta*, **10**, 1–19.

Garcia, A.P.G., Basso, N.G.D., Fonseca, M.E.F., Zuardi, J.A.T. and Otanni, H.N. (1991) Enterovirus associated placental morphology: a light, virological, electron microscopic and immunohistologic study. *Placenta*, **12**, 533–547.

Garnham, P.C.C. (1938) The placenta in malaria with special reference to reticulo-endothelial immunity. *Transactions of the Royal Society of Tropical Medicine and Hygiene*, **32**, 13–34.

Gazin, P.P., Compaore, M.P., Hutin, Y. and Molez, J.F. (1994) Infection du placenta par les Plasmodium en zone d'endemie: les facteurs de risque. *Bulletin de la Société de Pathologie Exotique*, **87**, 97–100.

Gersell, D.J. (1993) Chronic villitis, chronic chorioamnionitis, and maternal floor infarction. *Seminars in Diagnostic Pathology*, **10**, 251–266.

Gersell, D.J., Phillips, N.J. and Beckerman, K. (1991) Chronic chorioamnionitis; a clinicopathologic study of 17 cases. *International Journal of Gynecological Pathology*, **10**, 217–229.

Gibbs, R.S. (1993) Chrioamnionitis and bacterial vaginosis. *Amrican Journal of Obstetrics and Gynecology*, **169**, 460–462.

Gibbs, R.S., Blanco, J.D., St. Clair, P.J. and Castaneda, Y.S. (1982) Quantitative bacteriology of amniotic fluid from women with intra-amniotic infection at term. *Journal of Infectious Diseases*, **145**, 1–8.

Gibbs, R.S., Weiner, M.H., Walmer, K. and St. Clair, P. (1987) Microbiologic and serologic studies of *Gardnerella vaginalis* in intra-amniotic infection. *Obstetrics and Gynecology*, **70**, 187–190.

Gibbs, R.S., Romero, R., Hillier, S.L., Eschenbach, D.A. and Sweet, R.L. (1992) A review of premature birth and subclinical infection. *American Journal of Obstetrics and Gynecology*, **166**, 1515–1528.

Gibson, M. and Williams, P.P. (1978) *Haemophilus influenzae* amnionitis associated with prematurity and premature membrane rupture. *Obstetrics and Gynecology*, **52**, 70S–72S.

Gichangi, P.B., Nyongo, A.O. and Temmerman, M. (1993) Pregnancy outcome and placental weights: their relationship to HIV-1 infection. *East African Medical Journal*, **70**, 85–89.

Gilbert, M.J., Davoren, R.A., Cole, M.E. and Radford, N.J. (1981) Midtrimester abortion associated with septicaemia caused by *Campylobacter jejuni*. *Medical Journal of Australia*, **1**, 585–586.

Glasser, L. and Delta, B.G. (1965) Congenital toxoplasmosis with placental infection in monozygotic twins. *Pediatrics*, **35**, 276–283.

Greig, P.C., Ernest, J.M., Teot, L., Erikson, M. and Talley, R. (1993) Amniotic fluid interleukin-6 levels correlate with histologic chorioamnionitis and amniotic fluid cultures in patients with premature labor with intact membranes. *American Journal of Obstetrics and Gynecology*, **169**, 1035–1044.

Guvenc, M., Guvenc, H., Cengiz, L., Cengiz, T. and Uslu, T. (1989) Subclinical amnionitis in patients with intact membranes in preterm labour. *Paediatric and Perinatal Epidemiology*, **3**, 367–374.

Guzick, D.S. and Winn, K. (1985) The association of chorioamnionitis with preterm delivery. *Obstetrics and Gynecology*, **65**, 11–16.

Gyr, T.N., Malek, A., Mathez-Loic, F. et al (1994) Permeation of human chorioamniotic membranes by *Escherichia coli* in vitro. *American Journal of Obstetrics and Gynecology*, **170**, 223–227.

Haag, B., Decker, K., Hinselmann, M. and Hirsh, H.A. (1974) Bakteriologische Befunde und Infektionsgefhrdung bei diagnostischer Fruchtwasserpunktion. *Gynäkologische Rundschau*, **14**, Supplement I, 59–60.

Hall, G.A. (1974) An investigation into the mechanism of placental damage in rats inoculated with *Salmonella dublin*. *American Journal of Pathology*, **77**, 299–312.

Hasegawa, I., Takakuwa, K., Adachi, S. and Kanazawa, K. (1990) Cytotoxic antibody against cytotrophoblast and lymphocytes present in pregnancy with intrauterine fetal growth retardation and its relation to anti-phospholipid antibody. *Journal of Reproductive Immunology*, **17**, 127–139.

Hayes, K. and Gibas, H. (1971) Placental cytomegalovirus infection without fetal involvement following primary infection in pregnancy. *Journal of Pediatrics*, **79**, 401–405.

Heifetz, S.A. and Bauman, M. (1994) Necrotizing funisitis and herpes simplex infection of placental and decidual tissues: study of four cases. *Human Pathology*, **25**, 715–722.

Hengst, P. and Budek, J. (1972) Untersuchungen zur Keim-aszension durch Amnioskopie. *Zentralblatt für Gynäkologie*, **94**, 842–848.

Hennequin, C. and Bouree, P. (1991) Paludisme de la femme gestante et du nouveau-ne. *Bulletin de la Société de Pathologie Exotique*, **84**, 465–470.

Herbst, R., Multier, A.M. and Jaluvka, V. (1970) Morphologische Untersuchungen der Plazenta einer an parotitis erkrankten Mütter. *Zeitschrift für Geburtshilfe und Perinatalogie*, **174**, 187–193.

Hillier, S.L., Martius, J., Krohn, M., Kiviat, N., Holmes, K.K. and Eschenbach, D.A. (1988) A case control study of chorioamnionic infection and histologic chorioamnionitis in prematurity. *New England Journal of Medicine*, **319**, 972–978.

Hillier, S.L., Krohn, M.A., Kiviat, N.B., Watts, D.H. and Eschenbach, D.A. (1991) Microbiologic causes and neonatal outcomes associated with chorioamnion infection. *American Journal of Obstetrics and Gynecology*, **165**, 955–961.

Hillier, S.L., Witkin, S.S., Krohn, M.A., Watts, D.H., Kiviat, N.B. and Eschenbach, D.A. (1993) The relationship of amniotic fluid cytokines and preterm delivery, amniotic fluid infection, histologic chorioamnionitis, and chorioamnion infection. *Obstetrics and Gynecology*, **81**, 941–948.

Hood, C.K. and McKinnon, G.E. (1963) Prenatal vaccinia. *American Journal of Obstetrics and Gynecology*, **85**, 238–240.

Hood, I.C., Desa, D.J. and Whyte, R.K. (1983) The inflammatory response in candidal chorioamnionitis. *Human Pathology*, **14**, 984–990.

Horn, L.C. and Becker, V. (1992) Morphologische Plazentabefunde bei klinisch-serologisch gesicherter und vermuteter Rotelninfektion in der zweiten Schwangerschaftshalfte. *Zeitschrift für Geburtshilfe und Perinatologie*, **196**, 199–204.

Horn, L.C., Emmrich, P. and Krugmann, J. (1992) Plazentabefunde bei Lues connata. *Pathologe*, **13**, 146–151.

Horn, L.C., Buttner, W. and Horn, E. (1993) Rotelnbedingte Plazentaveranderungen. *Perinatale Medizin*, **5**, 5–10.

Hoskins, I.A., Hemming, V.C., Johnson, T.R.B. and Winkel, C.A. (1982) Effects of alterations of zinc-to-phosphorus ratios and meconium content on Group B *Streptococcus* growth in human amniotic fluid *in vitro*. *American Journal of Obstetrics and Gynecology*, **157**, 770–773.

Hurley, R. (1988) Chorioamnionitis. *Journal of Obstetrics and Gynaecology*, **8**, 368–370.

Hyde, S.R. and Giacoia, G.P. (1993) Congenital herpes infection: placental and umbilical cord findings. *Obstetrics and Gynecology*, **81**, 852–855.

Hyde, S., Smotherman, J., Moore, J.I. and Altshuler, G. (1989) A model of bacterially induced umbilical vein spasm, relevant to fetal hypoperfusion. *Obstetrics and Gynecology*, **73**, 966–970.

Iralu, J.V., Roberts, D. and Kazanjian, P.H. (1993) Chorioamnionitis caused by *Capnocytophaga*: case report and review. *Clinical Infectious Diseases*, **17**, 457–461.

Ismail, M.A., Pridjian, G., Hibbard, J.U., Harth, C. and Moawad, A.A. (1992) Significance of positive cervical cultures for *Chlamydia trachomatis* in patients with preterm premature rupture of the membranes. *American Journal of Perinatology*, **9**, 368–370.

Jacob-Cormier, B., Petitjean, J., Asselin, D., Quibriac, M. and von Theobald, F. (1989) Ureaplasma urealyticum et chorioamniotite. *Revue Francaise de Gynécologie et d'Obstétrique*, **84**, 25–28.

Jacques, S.M. and Qureshi, F. (1992) Necrotizing funisitis: a study of 45 cases. *Human Pathology*, **23**, 1278–1283.

Jacques, S.M. and Qureshi, F. (1993) Chronic intervillositis of the placenta. *Archives of Pathology and Laboratory Medicine*, **117**, 1032–1035.

Jauniaux, E., Nessmann, C., Imbert, M.C., Meuris, S., Puissant, F. and Hustin, J. (1988) Morphological aspects of the placenta in HIV pregnancies. *Placenta*, **8**, 633–642.

Jelliffe, E.F.P. (1967) Placental malaria and foetal growth failure. In *Nutrition and Infection. CIBA Foundation Study Group No. 31*, Wolstenholme, G.E.W. and O'Connor, M. (Eds), pp. 18–35. London: J. & A. Churchill.

Johnson, K.P. (1969) Mouse cytomegalovirus: placental infection. *Journal of Infectious Diseases*, **120**, 445–450.

Johnson, F.W.A., Matheson, B.A., Williams, H. et al (1985) Abortion due to infection with *Chlamydia psittaci* in a sheep farmer's wife. *British Medical Journal*, **290**, 592–594.

Johnson, P.M., Lyden, T.W. and Mwenda, J.M. (1990) Endogenous retroviral expression in the human placenta. *American Journal of Reproductive Immunology*, **23**, 115–120.

Kalter, S.S., Helmke, R.J., Heberling, R.L. et al (1973) C-type particles in normal human placentas. *Journal of the National Cancer Institute*, **50**, 1081–1084.

Kaplan, C. (1990) The placenta and viral infections. *Clinical Obstetrics and Gynecology*, **33**, 232–241.

Kaplan, C. (1993) The placenta and viral infections. *Seminars in Diagnostic Pathology*, **10**, 232–250.

Kaplan, C., Benirschke, K. and Tarzy, B. (1980) Placental tuberculosis in early and late pregnancy. *American Journal of Obstetrics and Gynecology*, **137**, 858–860.

Katz, V.L. (1993) Management of group B streptococcal disease in pregnancy. *Clinical Obstetrics and Gynecology*, **36**, 832–842.

Kaushik, A., Sharma, V.K., Sadhana, B. and Kumar, R. (1992) Malarial placental infection and low birth weight babies. *Journal of Communicable Diseases*, **24**, 65–69.

Kellogg, S.G., Davis, C. and Benirschke, K. (1974) *Candida parapsilosis*: previously unknown cause of fetal infection: a report of two cases. *Journal of Reproductive Medicine*, **12**, 159–161.

Kérisit, J., de Villartay, A. and le Guilcher, P. (1973) Candidose placentaire; à propos d'une observation. *Ouest Médical*, **26**, 1478.

Kérisit, J., Herry, D., Ferrand, B., Denis, M.P. and Sénécal, J. (1975) Dépistace de l'infection néonatale par examen histopathologique extemporané du cordon umbilical. *Presse Médicale*, **4**, 2043–2044.

Khong, T.Y. (1995) Expression of MHC class II antigens by placental villi: no relationship with villitis of unknown origin. *Journal of Clinical Pathology*, **48**, 494–495.

Khong, T.Y., Staples, A., Moore, L. and Byard, R.W. (1993) Observer reliability in assessing villitis of unknown aetiology. *Journal of Clinical Pathology*, **46**, 208–210.

Khudr, G. and Benirschke, K. (1972) Placental lesion in viral hepatitis. *Obstetrics and Gynecology*, **40**, 381–384.

Kida, M., Abramowsky, C.R. and Santoscoy, C. (1989) Cryptococcosis of the placenta in a woman with acquired immunodeficiency syndrome. *Human Pathology*, **20**, 920–921.

Kilbrick, S. and Benirschke, K. (1958) Severe generalised disease (encephalohepato-myocarditis) occurring in the newborn period and due to infection with coxsackie virus group B: evidence of intrauterine infection with this organism. *Pediatrics*, **22**, 857–875.

King, J.A. and Marks, R.A. (1958) Pregnancy and leprosy: a review of 52 pregnancies in 26 patients with leprosy. *American Journal of Obstetrics and Gynecology*, **76**, 438–442.

Knowles, S. and Frost, T. (1989) Umbilical cord sclerosis as an indicator of congenital syphilis. *Journal of Clinical Pathology*, **42**, 1157–1159.

Knox, W.F. and Fox, H. (1984) Villitis of unknown aetiology: its incidence and significance in placentae from a British population. *Placenta*, **5**, 395–402.

Kramer, M.S. (1987) Determinants of low birth weight: methodological assessment and meta-analysis. *Bulletin of the World Health Organization*, **65**, 663–737.

Kundsin, R.B., Driscoll, S.G., Monson, R.R., Yeh, C., Biano, S.A. and Cochran, W.D. (1984) Association of *Ureaplasma urealyticum* in the placenta with perinatal morbidity and mortality. *New England Journal of Medicine*, **310**, 941–945.

Kutteh, W.H., Edwards, R.P., Menge, A.C. and Mestecky, J. (1993) IgA immunity in female reproductive tract secretions. In *Local Immunity in Reproductive Tract Tissues*, Griffin, P.D. and Johnson, P.M. (Eds), pp. 229–243. Delhi: Oxford University Press.

Labarrere, C.A. & Althabe, O. (1987) Chronic villitis of unknown aetiology in recurrent intrauterine fetal growth retardation. *Placenta*, **8**, 167–173.

Labarrere, C.A. and Faulk, W.P. (1992) Immunopathology of human extraembryonic tissues. In *Immunological Obstetrics*, Coulam, C.B., Faulk, W.P. and McIntyre, J.A. (Eds), pp. 439–463. New York: Norton.

Labarrere, C.A. and Faulk, W.P. (1995) Maternal cells in chorionic villi from placentae of normal and abnormal pregnancies. *American Journal of Reproductive Immunology*, **33**, 54–59.

Labarrere, C.A. and Mullen, E. (1987) Fibrinoid and trophoblastic necrosis with massive chronic inter-villositis: an extreme variant of villitis of unknown etiology. *American Journal of Reproductive Immunology and Microbiology*, **15**, 85–91.

Labarrere, C., Althabe, O. and Telenta, M. (1982) Chronic villitis of unknown aetiology in placentae of idiopathic small for gestational age infants. *Placenta*, **3**, 309–318.

Labarrere, C., Althabe, O., Calenti, E. and Musculo, D. (1986) Deficiency of blocking factors in intrauterine growth retardation and its relationship with chronic villitis. *American Journal of Reproductive Immunology and Microbiology*, **10**, 14–19.

Labarrere, C.A., Faulk, W.P. and McIntyre, J.A. (1989) Villitis in normal human term placentae: frequency of the lesion determined by monoclonal antibody to HLA-DR antigen. *Journal of Reproductive Immunology*, **16**, 127–135.

Labarrere, C.A., McIntyre, J.A. and Faulk, W.P. (1990) Immunohistologic evidence that villitis in human normal term placentas is an immunologic lesion. *American Journal of Obstetrics and Gynecology*, **162**, 515–522.

Lallemand, A.V., Gaillard, D.A., Paradis, P.H. and Chippaux, C.G. (1992) Fetal listeriosis during the second trimester of gestation. *Pediatric Pathology*, **12**, 665–671.

Lamont, R.F., Anthony, F., Myatt, L., Booth, L., Fürr, P.M. and Taylor-Robinson, D. (1990) Production of prostaglandin E_2 by human amnion *in vitro* in response to addition of media conditioned by microorganisms associated with chorioamnionitis and preterm labor. *American Journal of Obstetrics and Gynecology*, **162**, 819–825.

Larsen, B. and Galask, R.P. (1975) Host resistance to intraamniotic infection. *Obstetrical and Gynecological Survey*, **30**, 675–691.

Larsen, B., Snyder, I.S. and Galask, R.P. (1974a) Bacterial growth inhibition by amniotic fluid. I. *In vitro* evidence for bacterial growth inhibiting factor. *American Journal of Obstetrics and Gynecology*, **119**, 492–496.

Larsen, B., Snyder, I.S. and Galask, R.P. (1974b) Bacterial growth inhibition by amniotic fluid. II. Reversal of amniotic fluid growth inhibition by addition of a chemically defined medium. *American Journal of Obstetrics and Gynecology*, **119**, 497–501.

Ledger, W.J. (1977) Premature rupture of membranes and the influence of invasive monitoring techniques upon fetal and newborn infection. *Seminars in Perinatology*, **1**, 79–87.

Lepage, F. and Schramm, B. (1958) Aspects histologiques du placenta et des membranes dans la maladie des inclusions cytomégaliques. *Gynécologie et Obstétrique*, **57**, 273–279.

Lewis, S.H., Reynolds-Kohler, C., Fox, H.E. and Nelson, J. (1990) HIV-1 in trophoblastic and villous Hofbauer cells, and haematological precursors in eight-week fetuses. *Lancet*, **335**, 565–568.

Lide, T.N. (1947) Congenital tularemia. *Archives of Pathology*, **43**, 165–169.

Lind, T. and Hytten, F.E. (1969) Relation between birth weight and rupture-delivery interval. *Lancet*, **i**, 917–918.

Loga, E.M., Driscoll, S.G. and Munro, H.N. (1972) Comparison of placentae from two socio-economic groups. I. Morphometry. *Pediatrics*, **50**, 24–31.

Lopez, E. and Aterman, K. (1968) Intra-uterine infection by *Candida*. *American Journal of Diseases of Children*, **115**, 663–670.

Lopez-Bernal, A., Hansell, D.J., Canete Soler, R., Keeling, J.W. and Turnbull, A.C. (1987) Prostaglandins, chorioamnionitis and preterm labour. *British Journal of Obstetrics and Gynaecology*, **94**, 1156–1158.

Lopez-Bernal, A., Hansell, D.J., Khong, T.Y., Keeling, J.W. and Turnbull, A.C. (1989) Prostaglandin E production by the fetal membranes in unexplained preterm labour and labour associated with chorioamnionitis. *British Journal of Obstetrics and Gynaecology*, **96**, 1133–1139.

Lucifora, G., Calabro, S., Carroccio, G. and Brigandi, A. (1988) Immunocytochemical HBsAg evidence in placentas of asymptomatic carrier mothers. *American Journal of Obstetrics and Gynecology*, **159**, 839–842.

Lucifore, G., Martines, F., Calabro, S., Carroccio, G., Brigandi, A. and de Pasquale, (1990) HBcAg identification in the placental cytotypes of symptom-free HBsAg-carrier mothers: a study with the immunoperoxidase method. *American Journal of Obstetrics and Gynecology*, **163**, 235–239.

Lyden, T.W., Rote, N.S., Johnson, P.M. and Mwenda, J. (1991) Structural characterization of a placental endogenous retrovirus. *American Journal of Reproductive Immunology*, **25**, 66.

Lyden, T.W., Johnson, P.M., Mwenda, J. and Rote, N.S. (1994) Anti-HIV antibodies cross-react with normal human trophoblast. *Trophoblast Research*, **8**, 19–32.

McCaffree, M.A., Altshuler, G. and Benirschke, K. (1978) Placental coccidioidomycosis without fetal disease. *Archives of Pathology and Laboratory Medicine*, **102**, 513–514.

Maccato, M., McLean, W., Riddle, G. and Faro, S. (1991) Isolation of *Kingella denitrificans* from amniotic fluid in a woman with chorioamnionitis: a case report. *Journal of Reproductive Medicine*, **36**, 685–687.

McColgin, S.W., Hess, L.W., Martin, R.W., Martin, J.N. and Morrison, J.C. (1989) Group B streptococcal sepsis and death *in utero* following funipuncture. *Obstetrics and Gynecology*, **74**, 71–77.

McGregor, I.A., Wilson, M.E. and Billewicz, W.Z. (1983) Malaria infection of the placenta in The Gambia, West Africa: its incidence and relationship to stillbirth, birthweight and placental weight. *Transactions of the Royal Society of Tropical Medicine and Hygiene*, **77**, 232–244.

McGregor, J.A., French, J.I., Lawellin, D., Franco-Buff, A., Smith, C. and Todd, J.K. (1987) Bacterial protease-induced reduction of chorioamniotic membrane strength and elasticity. *Obstetrics and Gynecology*, **69**, 164–174.

McKay, D.G. and Wong, T.C. (1964) The effect of bacterial endotoxin on the placenta of the rat. *American Journal of Pathology*, **42**, 357–377.

MacVicar, J. (1970) Chorioamnionitis. *Clinical Obstetrics and Gynecology*, **13**, 272–290.

Malan, A.F., Woods, D.L., van der Elst, C.W. and Meyer, M.P. (1990) Relative placental weight in congenital syphilis. *Placenta*, **11**, 3–6.

Marshall, D.E. (1983) The transplacental passage of malaria parasites in the Solomon Islands. *Transactions of the Royal Society of Tropical Medicine and Hygiene*, **77**, 470–473.

Martin, A.W., Brady, K., Smith, S.I. et al (1992) Immunohistochemical localization of human immunodeficiency virus p24 antigen in placental tissue. *Human Pathology*, **23**, 411–414.

Martius, J. (1989) Die austeigende Infektion in der Schwangerschaft als eine Ursache de Fruhgeburt. *Zeitschrift für Geburtshilfe und Perinatologie*, **193**, 1–7.

Matsuzaki, N., Taniguchi, T., Shimoya, K. et al (1993) Placental interleukin-6 production is enhanced in intrauterine infection but not in labour. *American Journal of Obstetrics and Gynecology*, **168**, 94–97.

Mattern, C.F.T., Murray, K. and Jensen, A. (1992) Localization of human immunodeficiency virus core antigen in term human placentas. *Pediatrics*, **89**, 207–209.

Maurus, J.N. (1978) Hansen's disease in pregnancy. *Obstetrics and Gynecology*, **52**, 22–25.

Mazor, M., Chaim, W., Shinwell, E.S. and Glezerman, M. (1993) Asymptomatic amniotic fluid invasion with *Candida albicans* in preterm premature rupture of membranes: implications for obstetric and neonatal management. *Acta Obstetricia et Gynecologica Scandinavica*, **72**, 52–54.

Melnikova, V.F., Zinzerling, A.V., Aksenov, O.A., Vydumkina, S.P., Kalinina, N.A. and Mikhailova, L.E. (1987) Placental lesions in influenza. *Akusherstvo i Patologiya*, **49**, 19–25.

Melsom, R., Harboe, M., Duncan, M.E. and Bergsvik, H. (1981) IgA and IgM antibodies against *Mycobacterium leprae* in cord sera and in patients with leprosy: an indicator of intrauterine infection in leprosy. *Scandinavian Journal of Immunology*, **14**, 343–352.

Mendenhall, J.C., Black, W.C. and Potzz, G.E. (1948) Progressive (disseminated) coccidioidomycosis during pregnancy. *Rocky Mountain Medical Journal*, **45**, 472–476.

Michaud, P., Michenet, P., Lemaire, B., Maitre, F. and Tescher, M. (1991) La villité placentaire. *Revue Francaise de Gynécologie et d'Obstétrique*, **86**, 225–228.

Miller, J.M., Pupkin, M.J. and Hill, G.B. (1980) Bacterial colonization of amnionic fluid from intact fetal membranes. *American Journal of Obstetrics and Gynecology*, **136**, 796–804.

Mims, C.A. (1968) Pathogenesis of viral infections of the fetus. *Progress in Medical Virology*, **10**, 194–237.

Mitchell, M.D., Dudley, D.J., Edwin, S.S. and Lundin-Schiller, S. (1991) Interleukin-6 stimulates prostaglandin production by human amnion and decidual cells. *European Journal of Pharmacology*, **192**, 189–191.

Mitchell, M.D., Trautman, M.S. and Dudley, D.J. (1993) Cytokine networking in the placenta. *Placenta*, **14**, 249–275.

Molnar-Nasasdy, G., Haesly, I., Reed, J. and Altshuler, G. (1994) Placental cryptococcosis in a mother with systemic lupus erythematosus. *Archives of Pathology and Laboratory Medicine*, **118**, 757–759.

Morey, A.L., Keeling, J.W., Porter, H.J. and Fleming, K.A. (1992) Clinical and histopathological features of parvovirus B19 infection in the human fetus. *British Journal of Obstetrics and Gynaecology*, **99**, 566–574.

Morgan, H.G. (1994) Placental malaria and low birth weight neonates in urban Sierra Leone. *Annals of Tropical Medicine and Parasitology*, **88**, 575–580.

Moroi, K., Saito, S., Kurata, T., Sata, T. and Yanagida, M. (1991) Fetal death associated with measles virus infection of the placenta. *American Journal of Obstetrics and Gynecology*, **164**, 1107–1108.

Mortimer, G., MacDonald, D.J. and Smeeth, A. (1985) A pilot study of the frequency and significance of placental villitis. *British Journal of Obstetrics and Gynaecology*, **92**, 629–633.

Mostoufi-Zadeh, M., Driscoll, S.G., Biano, S.A. and Kundsin, R.B. (1984) Placental evidence of cytomegalovirus infection of the fetus and neonate. *Archives of Pathology and Laboratory Medicine*, **108**, 403–406.

Mueller-Heubach, E., Rubinstein, D.N. and Schwartz, S.S. (1990) Histologic chorioamnionitis and preterm delivery in different patient populations. *Obstetrics and Gynecology*, **75**, 622–626.

Muhlemann, K., Miller, R.K., Metlay, L. and Menegus, M.A. (1992) Cytomegalovirus infection of the human placenta: an immunocytochemical study. *Human Pathology*, **23**, 1234–1237.

Muhlemann, K., Miller, R.A., Metlay, L. and Menegus, M.A. (1994) Characterization of cytomegalovirus infection by immunocytochemistry. *Trophoblast Research*, **8**, 215–222.

Naeye, R.L. (1987) Functionally important disorders of the placenta, umbilical cord, and fetal membranes. *Human Pathology*, **18**, 680–691.

Naeye, R.L. (1991) Acute chorioamnionitis and the disorders that produce placental insufficiency. In *Pathology of Reproductive Failure*, Kraus, F.T., Damjanov, I. and Kaufman, N. (Eds), pp. 286–307. Baltimore: Williams & Wilkins.

Naeye, R.L. (1992) *Disorders of the Placenta, Fetus, and Neonate: Diagnosis and Clinical Significance*. St Louis: Mosby.

Naeye, R.L. and Blanc, W.A. (1970) Relation of poverty and race to antenatal infection. *New England Journal of Medicine*, **283**, 554–560.

Naeye, R.L. and Peters, E.C. (1978) Amniotic fluid infections with intact membranes leading to perinatal death: a prospective study. *Pediatrics*, **61**, 171–177.

Naeye, R.L. and Peters, E.C. (1980) Causes and consequences of premature rupture of fetal membranes. *Lancet*, **i**, 192–194.

Naeye, R.L., Dellinger, W.S. and Blanc, W.A. (1971) Fetal and maternal features of antenatal bacterial infections. *Journal of Pediatrics*, **79**, 733–739.

Nakamura, Y., Sakuma, S., Ohta, Y., Kawano, K. and Hashimoto, T. (1994) Detection of the human cytomegalovirus gene in placental chronic villitis by polymerase chain reaction. *Human Pathology*, **25**, 815–818.

Navarro, C. and Blanc, W.A. (1974) Subacute necrotizing funisitis: a variant of cord inflammation with a high rate of perinatal infection. *Journal of Pediatrics*, **85**, 689–697.

Newton, E.R. (1993) Chorioamnionitis and intraamniotic infection. *Clinical Obstetrics and Gynecology*, **36**, 795–808.

Newton, E.R., Prihoda, T.J. and Gibbs, R.S. (1989) Logistic regression analysis of risk factors for intraamniotic infection. *Obstetrics and Gynecology*, **73**, 571–575.

Nichols, A., Khong, T.Y. and Crowther, C.A. (1995) *Candida tropicalis* chorioamnionitis. *American Journal of Obstetrics and Gynecology*, **172**, 1045–1047.

Nickerson, C.W. (1973) Gonorrhea amnionitis. *Obstetrics and Gynecology*, **42**, 815–817.

Nnatu, S., Anyiwo, C.E. and Nwobu, R.U. (1987) Malaria parasitaemia at delivery in Nigerians. *East African Medical Journal*, **64**, 44–47.

Nordenvall, M. and Sandstedt, B. (1990) Placental villitis and intrauterine growth retardation in a Swedish population. *Acta Pathologica, Microbiologica and Immunologica Scandinavica*, **98**, 19–24.

Norwitz, E.R., Bernal, A.L. and Starkey, P.M. (1992) Tumor necrosis factor selectively stimulates prostaglandin F_2 production by macrophages in human term decidua. *American Journal of Obstetrics and Gynecology*, **167**, 815–820.

Novak, R.W. and Platt, M.S. (1985) Significance of placental findings in early-onset group B streptococcal neonatal sepsis. *Clinical Pediatrics*, **24**, 256–258.

Ohno, Y., Kasugi, M., Kurauchi, O., Mizutani, S. and Tomoda, Y. (1994) Effect of interleukin-2 on the production of progesterone and prostaglandin E2 in human fetal membranes and its consequence for preterm uterine contractions. *European Journal of Endocrinology*, **130**, 478–484.

Oliveira, L.H.S., Fonseca, M.E.F. and de Bonis, M. (1992) Placental phagocytic cells infected with herpes simplex type 2 and echovirus type 19: virological and ultrastructural aspects. *Placenta*, **13**, 405–416.

Ornoy, A., Segal, S., Nishmi, M., Simcha, A. and Polishuk, W.Z. (1973) Fetal and placental pathology in gestational rubella. *American Journal of Obstetrics and Gynecology*, **116**, 949–956.

Ornoy, A., Dudai, M. and Sadovsky, E. (1982) Placental and fetal pathology in infectious mononucleosis. *Diagnostic Gynecology and Obstetrics*, **4**, 11–16.

Pageaut, G., Oppermann, A., Eschbach, J., Percher, P. and Gauthier, C. (1967) La listériose placenta-foetale. *Annales d'Anatomie Pathologique*, **12**, 373–386.

Payne, J.M. (1958) Changes in the rat placenta and foetus following experimental infection with various species of bacteria. *Journal of Pathology and Bacteriology*, **75**, 367–385.

Pearce, J.H. and Lowrie, D.B. (1972) Tissue and host specificity in bacterial infection. In *Microbial Pathogenicity in Man and Animals*, 22nd Symposium of Society for General Microbiology, pp. 193–216. London: Cambridge University Press.

Perkins, R.P., Zhou, S.M., Butler, C. and Skipper, B.J. (1987) Histologic chorioamnionitis in pregnancies of various gestational ages: implications in preterm rupture of membranes. *Obstetrics and Gynecology*, **70**, 856–860.

Philippe, E. and Walter, P. (1985) Les lesions placentaires du paludisme. *Archives Francaise de Pediatrie*, **42**, Supplement 2, 921–923.

Poole, P.M., Whitehouse, D.B. and Gilchrist, M.M. (1972) A case of abortion consequent upon infection with *Brucella abortus* biotype 2. *Journal of Clinical Pathology*, **25**, 882–884.

Popek, E.J. (1992) Granulomatous villitis due to *Toxoplasma gondii*. *Pediatric Pathology*, **12**, 281–288.

Pryse-Davies, J., Beazley, J.M. and Leach, G. (1973) A study of placental size and chorio-amnionitis in a consecutive series of hospital deliveries. *Journal of Obstetrics and Gynaecology of the British Commonwealth*, **80**, 246–251.

Quan, A. and Strauss, L. (1962) Congenital cytomegalic inclusion disease: observations in a macerated fetus with a congenital defect, including a study of the placenta. *American Journal of Obstetrics and Gynecology*, **83**, 1240–1248.

Quinn, P.A., Butany, J., Taylor, J. and Hannah, W. (1987) Chorioamnionitis: its association with pregnancy outcome and microbial infection. *American Journal of Obstetrics and Gynecology*, **156**, 379–387.

Qureshi, F., Jacques, S.M. and Reyes, M.P. (1993) Placental histopathology in syphilis. *Human Pathology*, **24**, 779–784.

Randrianjafisamindrakotroka, N.S., Rakotomamonjy, J.C., Zafisaona, G. and Rakotoarimanana, D.R. (1994) Interet de l'examen anatomo-pathologique du placenta dans les zones d'endemie palustre et de faible niveau socio-culturel. *Journal de Gynécologie et d'Obstétrique et de Biologie de Reproduction*, **23**, 825–829.

Redline, R.W. (1995) Placental pathology: a neglected link between basic disease mechanisms and untoward pregnancy outcome. *Current Opinion in Obstetrics and Gynecology*, **7**, 10–15.

Redline, R.W. and Abramowsky, C.R. (1985) Clinical and pathologic aspects of recurrent placental villitis. *Human Pathology*, **16**, 727–731.

Redline, R.W. and Patterson, P. (1993) Villitis of unknown etiology is associated with major infiltration of fetal tissue by maternal inflammatory cells. *American Journal of Pathology*, **143**, 332–336.

Redline, R.W. and Patterson, P. (1994) Patterns of placental injury: correlations with gestational age, placental weight, and clinical diagnoses. *Archives of Pathology and Laboratory Medicine*, **118**, 698–701.

Renaud, R., Brettes, P., Castanier, C. and Loubiere, R. (1972) Placental bilharziasis. *International Journal of Gynaecology and Obstetrics*, **10**, 24–30.

Robertson, N.J. and McKeever, P.A. (1992) Fetal and placental pathology in two cases of maternal varicella infection. *Pediatric Pathology*, **12**, 545–550.

Robson, A.O. and Shimmin, C.D.G.L. (1959) Chronic Q fever. I. Clinical aspects of a patient with endocarditis. *British Medical Journal*, **ii**, 980–983.

Rogers, B.B., Mark, Y. and Oyer, C.E. (1993) Diagnosis and incidence of fetal parvovirus infection in an autopsy series. I. Histology. *Pediatric Pathology*, **13**, 371–379.

Rolschau, J. (1978) The significance of different forms of placentitis. *Acta Obstetricia et Gynecologica Scandinavica*, Supplement 72, 5.

Romero, R., Kadar, N., Hobbins, J.C. and Duff, G.W. (1987a) Infection and labor: the detection of endotoxin in amniotic fluid. *American Journal of Obstetrics and Gynecology*, **157**, 815–819.

Romero, R., Quintero, R., Emamian, M., Wan, M., Hobbins, J.C. and Mitchell, M.D. (1987b) Prostaglandin concentrations in amniotic fluid of women with intraamniotic infection and preterm labor. *American Journal of Obstetrics and Gynecology*, **157**, 1461–1467.

Romero, R., Hobbins, J.C. and Mitchell, M.D. (1988a) Endotoxin stimulates prostaglandin E_2 production by human amnion. *Obstetrics and Gynecology*, **71**, 227–228.

Romero, R., Roslansky, P., Oyarzun, E. et al (1988b) Infection and labor. II. Bacterial endotoxin in amniotic fluid and its relationship to the onset of preterm labor. *American Journal of Obstetrics and Gynecology*, **158**, 1044–1049.

Romero, R., Brody, D.T., Oyarzun, E. et al (1989a) Infection and labor. III. Interleukin-1: a signal for the onset of parturition. *American Journal of Obstetrics and Gynecology*, **160**, 1117–1123.

Romero, R., Manogue, K.R., Mitchell, M.D. et al (1989b) Infection and labor. IV. Cachectin-tumor necrosis factor in the amniotic fluid of women with intraamniotic infection and preterm labor. *American Journal of Obstetrics and Gynecology*, **161**, 336–341.

Romero, R., Sirtori, M., Oyarzun, E. et al (1989c) Infection and labor. V. Prevalence, microbiology and clinical significance of intraamniotic infection in women with preterm labor and intact membranes. *American Journal of Obstetrics and Gynecology*, **161**, 817–824.

Romero, R., Durum, S., Dinarello, C.A., Oyarzun, E., Hobbins, J.C. and Mitchell, M.D. (1989d) Interleukin-1 stimulates prostaglandin biosynthesis by human amnion. *Prostaglandins*, **37**, 13–22.

Romero, R., Avila, C., Santhanam, U. and Sehgal, P.B. (1990) Amniotic fluid interleukin-6 in preterm labor: association with infection. *Journal of Clinical Investigation*, **85**, 1392–1400.

Romero, R., Mazor, M., Sepulveda, W., Avila, C., Copeland, D. and Williams, J. (1992a) Tumor necrosis factor in preterm and term labor. *American Journal of Obstetrics and Gynecology*, **166**, 1576–1587.

Romero, R., Mazor, M., Brandt, F. et al (1992b) Interleukin-1 alpha and interleukin-1 beta in preterm and term human parturition. *American Journal of Reproductive Immunology*, **27**, 117–123.

Romero, R., Gonzalez, R., Sepulveda, W. et al (1992c) Infection and labor. VIII. Microbiol invasion of the amniotic cavity in patients with suspected cervical incompetence: prevalence and clinical significance. *American Journal of Obstetrics and Gynecology*, **167**, 1086–1091.

Romero, R., Nores, J., Mazor, M. et al (1993) Microbial invasion of the amniotic cavity during term labor: prevalence and clinical significance. *Journal of Reproductive Medicine*, **38**, 543–548.

Rosenstein, D.L. and Navarrete-Reyna, A. (1964) Cytomegalic inclusion disease: observation of the characteristic inclusion bodies in the placenta. *American Journal of Obstetrics and Gynecology*, **89**, 220–224.

Rothbard, M.J., Gregory, T. and Salerno, L.J. (1975) Intrapartum gonococcal amnionitis. *American Journal of Obstetrics and Gynecology*, **121**, 565–566.

Royston, D. and Geoghegan, F. (1985) Amniotic fluid infection with intact membranes in relation to stillborns. *Obstetrics and Gynecology*, **65**, 745–746.

Rusan, P., Adam, R.D., Petersen, P.A., Ryan, K.J., Sinclair, N.A. and Weinstein, I. (1991) *Haemophilus influenzae*: an important cause of maternal and neonatal infection. *Obstetrics and Gynecology*, **77**, 92–96.

Russell, P. (1979) Inflammatory lesions of the human placenta. II. Villitis of unknown etiology in perspective. *American Journal of Diagnostic Gynecology and Obstetrics*, **1**, 339–346.

Russell, P. (1980) Inflammatory lesions of the human placenta. III. The histopathology of villitis of unknown aetiology. *Placenta*, **1**, 227–244.

Russell, P. (1995) Infections of the placental villi (villitis) In *Haines and Taylor: Obstetrical and Gynaecological Pathology*, 4th edn, Fox, H. (Ed.), pp. 1541–1558. Edinburgh: Churchill Livingstone.

Russell, P. and Altshuler, G. (1974) The placental abnormalities of congenital syphilis. *American Journal of Diseases of Children*, **128**, 160–163.

Russell, P., Atkinson, K. and Krishnan, L. (1980) Recurrent reproductive failure due to severe placental villitis of unknown etiology. *Journal of Reproductive Medicine*, **24**, 93–98.

Sachdev, R., Nuovo, G.R., Kaplan, C. and Greco, M.A. (1990) In situ hybridization analysis for cytomegalovirus in chronic villitis. *Pediatric Pathology*, **10**, 909–917.

Saito, S., Kasahara, T., Kato, Y., Ishihara, Y. and Ichijo, M. (1993) Elevation of amniotic fluid interleukin-6 (IL6), IL8 and granulocyte colony stimulating factor (G-CSF) in term and preterm parturition. *Cytokine*, **5**, 81–88.

Salafia, C.M., Mangam, H.E., Weigl, C.A., Foye, G.J. and Silberman, L. (1989) Abnormal fetal heart rate patterns and placental inflammation. *American Journal of Obstetrics and Gynecology*, **160**, 140–147.

Salafia C.M., Vogel, C.A., Vintzileos, A.M., Bantham, K.F., Pezzullo, J. and Silberman, L. (1991) Placental pathologic findings in preterm birth. *American Journal of Obstetrics and Gynecology*, **165**, 934–938.

Salafia, C.M., Vintzileos, A.M., Silberman, L., Bantham, K.F. and Vogel, C.A. (1992a) Placental pathology of idiopathic intrauterine growth retardation at term. *American Journal of Perinatology*, **9**, 179–184.

Salafia, C.M., Vogel, C.A., Bantham, K.F., Vintzileos, A.M., Pezzullo, J. and Silberman, L. (1992b) Preterm delivery: correlations of fetal growth and placental pathology. *American Journal of Perinatology*, **9**, 190–193.

Samson, G.R., Meyer, M.P., Blake, D.R.B., Cohen, M.C. and Mouton, S.C.E. (1994) Syphilitic placentitis: an immunopathy. *Placenta*, **15**, 67–77.

Samueloff, A., Langer, O., Berkus, M.D., Field, N.Y., Xenakis, E.M. and Piper, J.M. (1994) The effect of clinical chorioamnionitis on cord blood gas at term. *European Journal of Obstetrics, Gynecology and Reproductive Biology*, **54**, 87–91.

Sander, C.H., Martin, J.N., Rogers, A.L., Barr, M., Jr and Heidelberger, K.P. (1983) Prenatal infection with *Torulopsis glabrata*: a case associated with maternal sickle cell anemia. *Obstetrics and Gynecology*, **61**, 21S–24S.

Sarram, M., Feiz, J., Foruzandeh, M. and Gazanfarpour, P. (1974) Intrauterine fetal infection with *Brucella melitensis* as a possible cause of second-trimester abortion. *American Journal of Obstetrics and Gynecology*, **119**, 657–661.

Sarrut, S. (1967) Renseignements fournis par l'étude histologique du placenta dans la toxoplasmose congénital. *Annales de Pédiatrie*, **14**, 2429–2435.

Sarrut, S. and Alison, F. (1967) Étude du placenta dans 21 cas de listériose congénitale. *Archives Francaises de Pédiatrie*, **24**, 285–302.

Savva, D. and Holliman, R.E. (1990) PCR to detect toxoplasma. *Lancet*, **336**, 1325.

Scane, T.M.N. and Hawkins, D.G. (1984) Antibacterial activity in human amniotic fluid: relationship to zinc and phosphate. *British Journal of Obstetrics and Gynaecology*, **91**, 342–348.

Schaeffer, M., Fox, M.J. and Li, C.P. (1954) Intrauterine poliomyelitis infection: report of a case. *Journal of the American Medical Association*, **155**, 248–250.

Schlievert, P., Larsen, B., Johnson, W. and Galask, R.P. (1975a) Bacterial growth inhibition by amniotic fluid. III. Demonstration of the variability of bacterial growth inhibition by amniotic fluid technique. *American Journal of Obstetrics and Gynecology*, **122**, 809–813.

Schlievert, P., Larsen, B., Johnson, W. and Galask, R.P. (1975b) Bacterial growth inhibition by amniotic fluid. IV. Studies on the nature of bacterial inhibition with the use of plate count determinations. *American Journal of Obstetrics and Gynecology*, **122**, 814–819.

Schlievert, P., Johnson, W. and Galask, R.P. (1976a) Bacterial growth inhibition by amniotic fluid. V. Phosphate-to-zinc ratio as a predictor of bacterial growth-inhibitory activity. *American Journal of Obstetrics and Gynecology*, **125**, 899–905.

Schlievert, P., Johnson, W. and Galask, R.P. (1976b) Bacterial growth inhibition by amniotic fluid. VI. Evidence of a zinc-peptide antibacterial system. *American Journal of Obstetrics and Gynecology*, **125**, 906–910.

Schlievert, P., Johnson, W. and Galask, R.P. (1977) Amniotic fluid antibacterial mechanisms: newer concepts. *Seminars in Perinatology*, **1**, 59–70.

Schmorl, G. and Geipl, L. (1904) Über die Tuberkulose der menschlichen Plazenta. *Münchener Medizinische Wochenschrift*, **51**, 1676–1679.

Schmorl, G. and Kockel, K.V. (1894) Die Tuberkulose der menschlichen Placenta und ihre Beziehung zue kongenitalen Infection mit Tuberkulose. *Beitrage zur pathologischen Anatomie und zur allgemeine Pathologie*, **16**, 313–339.

Schneider, L. (1970) Über Vorkommen und Bedeutung leukocytärer Infiltrate in Ablösingsvereich der spontan geborenen Placenta. *Archiv für Gynäkologie*, **208**, 247–254.

Schoonmaker, J.N., Lawellin, D.W., Lunt, B. and McGregor, J.A. (1989) Bacteria and inflammatory cells reduce chorioamniotic membranes' integrity and tensile strength. *Obstetrics and Gynecology*, **74**, 590–596

Schubert, W. (1957) Fruchttod und Hydrops universalis durch Toxoplasmose. *Virchows Archiv für pathologische Anatomie und Physiologie und für klinische Medizin*, **330**, 518–524.

Schwartz, D.A. and Nahmias, A.J. (1991) Human immunodeficiency virus and the placenta: current concepts of vertical transmission in relation to other viral agents. *Annals of Clinical and Laboratory Science*, **21**, 264–274.

Schwartz, D.A. and Reef, S. (1990) *Candida albicans* placentitis and funisitis: early diagnosis of congenital candidemia by histopathologic examination of umbilical cord vessel. *Pediatric Infectious Disease Journal*, **9**, 661–665.

Schwartz, D.A., Khan, R. and Stoll, B. (1992) Characterizaton of the fetal inflammatory response to cytomegalovirus placentitis. *Archives of Pathology and Laboratory Medicine*, **116**, 221–227.

Schwartz, D.A., Zhang, W., Larsen, S. and Rice, R.J. (1994) Placental pathology of congenital syphilis – immunohistochemical aspects. *Trophoblast Research*, **8**, 223–229.

Schwartz, D.A., Larsen, D.A., Beck-Sague, C., Fears, M. and Rice, R.J. (1995) Pathology of the umbilical cord in congenital syphilis: analysis of 25 cases. *Human Pathology*, **26**, 781–784.

Scott, J.M. and Henderson, A. (1968) A case of listeriosis of the newborn. *Journal of Medical Microbiology*, **1**, 97–103.

Scott, J.M. and Henderson, A. (1972) Acute villous inflammation in the placenta following intrauterine transfusion. *Journal of Clinical Pathology*, **25**, 872–875.

Shelokov, A. and Habel, K. (1956) Subclinical poliomyelitis in a newborn due to intrauterine infection. *Journal of the American Medical Association*, **160**, 465–466.

Shute, K.M. and Kimber, R.G. (1994) *Haemophilus influenzae* intra-amniotic infection with intact membranes. *Journal of the American Board of Family Practice*, **7**, 335–341.

Silver, H.M., Sperling, R.S., St. Clair, P.J. and Gibbs, R.S. (1989) Evidence relating bacterial vaginosis to intraamniotic infection. *American Journal of Obstetrics and Gynecology*, **161**, 808–812.

Sinzger, C., Muntefering, H., Loning, T., Stoss, H., Plachter, B. and Jahn, G. (1993) Cell types infected in human cytomegalovirus placentitis identified by immunohistochemical double staining. *Virchows Archiv A Pathological Anatomy and Histopathology*, **423**, 249–256.

Smale, M.E. and Waechter, K.G. (1970) Dissemination of coccidioidomycosis in pregnancy. *American Journal of Obstetrics and Gynecology*, **107**, 356–361.

Smith, J.R. and Taylor-Robinson, D. (1993) Infection due to *Chlamydia trachomatis* in pregnancy and the newborn. *Ballière's Clinics in Obstetrics and Gynaecology*, **7**, 237–255.

Smith, L.G., Jr. Summers, P.R., Miles, R.W., Biswas, M.K. and Pernoll, M.L. (1989) Gonococcal chorioamnionitis associated with sepsis: a case report. *American Journal of Obstetrics and Gynecology*, **160**, 574–577.

Soper, D.E., Mayhall, C.G. and Dalton, H.P. (1989) Risk factors for intraamniotic infection; a prospective epidemiologic study. *American Journal of Obstetrics and Gynecology*, **161**, 562–566.

Spark, R.P. (1981) Does transplacental spread of coccidioidomycosis occur? Report of a neonatal fatality and review of the literature. *Archives of Pathology and Laboratory Medicine*, **105**, 347–350.

Steele, P.E. and Jacobs, D.S. (1979) *Listeria monocytogenes* macroabscesses of placenta. *Obstetrics and Gynecology*, **53**, 124–127.

Steinborn, A., Gatje, R., Kramer, P., Kuhnert, M. and Halberstadt, E. (1994) Zytokine in der Diagnostik des Amnion-Infekt-Syndroms. *Zeitschrift für Geburtshilfe und Perinatologie*, **198**, 1–5.

Strulovici, D., Copelovici, Y., Bedivan, M., Maior, E. and Teodoru, G.C. (1974) Isolation of cytomegalic virus from the placenta in a case of inapparent human infection. *Revue Roumaine de Virologie*, **25**, 265–270.

Sugai, T. and Monobe, J. (1913) Uber histologische Befunde in der Placenta Tuberkolose- und Leprakranker. *Zentralblatt für Bakteriologie, Parasitenkunde, Infektionskrankheiten und Hygiene*, **13**, 262.

Susani, M. (1981) Granulomatous villitis in toxoplasmosis. *Wiener Klinische Wochenschrift*, **93**, 24–28.

Sutherland, J.C., Berry, A., Hynd, M. and Proctor, N.S.F. (1965) Placental bilharziasis – report of a case. *South African Journal of Obstetrics and Gynaecology*, **3**, 76–80.

Talmi, Y.P., Sigler, L., Inge, E., Finkelstein, Y. and Zohar, Y. (1991) Antibacterial properties of human amniotic membranes. *Placenta*, **12**, 285–288.

Tondury, G.T. and Smith, D.W. (1966) Fetal rubella pathology. *Journal of Pediatrics*, **68**, 867–879.

Topalovski, M., Yang, S.S. and Boonpasat, Y. (1993) Listeriosis of the placenta: clinicopathologic study of seven cases. *American Journal of Obstetrics and Gynecology*, **169**, 616–620.

Toth, F.D., Juhl, B.C., Norskov-Lauritsen, N., Aboagye-Mathiesen, G. and Ebbesen, P. (1990) Interferon production by cultured human trophoblasts and choriocarcinoma cell lines by Sendai virus. *Journal of General Virology*, **71**, 3067–3069.

Trautman, M.S., Dudley, D.J., Edwin, S.S., Collmer, D. and Mitchell, M.D. (1992) Amnion cell biosynthesis of interleukin-8: regulation by inflammatory cytokines. *Journal of Cell Physiology*, **153**, 38–43.

Trifonova, S.F. (1959) Pathomorphology of the placenta in brucellosis. *Akusherstvo i Ginekologiya*, **2**, 41–44.

VanBergen, W.S., Fleury, J.F. and Cheatle, E.L. (1976) Fatal maternal disseminated coccidioidomycosis in a nonendemic area. *American Journal of Obstetrics and Gynecology*, **124**, 661–663.

van der Elst, C.W., Lopez-Bernal, A. and Sinclair-Smith, C.C. (1991) The role of chorioamnionitis and prostaglandins in preterm labor. *Obstetrics and Gynecology*, **77**, 672–676.

Vaughan, J.E. and Ramirez, H. (1951) Coccidioidomycosis as a complication of pregnancy. *California Medicine*, **74**, 121–125.

Vernon, M.L., McMahon, J.M. and Hackett, J.J. (1974) Additional evidence of type-C particles in human placentas. *Journal of the National Cancer Institute*, **52**, 987–989.

Vigorita, V.J. and Parmley, T.H. (1979) Intramembranous localization of bacteria in β-hemolytic group B streptococcal chorioamnionitis. *Obstetrics and Gynecology*, **53**, 13S–15S.

Villegas-Castrejon, H., Reyes-Fuentes, A., Pinon-Lopez, M.J. and Arredondo-Garcia, J.L. (1990) Aspectos morfologicos de placenta, tejidos embrionarios y semen en infecciones por virus de inmuno-deficiencia humana. *Ginecologia y Obstetricia de Mexico*, **58**, 333–337.

Villegas-Castrejon, H., Carrillo-Farga, J., Paredes, Y., Barron, A. and Karchmer, S. (1994) Estudio ultra-estructural de placentas en mujeres serpositivas para el VIH. *Ginecologia y Obstetricia de Mexico*, **62**, 136–142.

Vince, G.S. and Johnson, P.M. (1996) Current topic: immunobiology of human uteroplacental macrophages – friend and foe? *Placenta*, **17**, 191–199.

Vinzent, R. (1949) Une affection mecomme de la grossesse: l'infection placentaire a *Vibrio fetus. Presse Médical*, **57**, 1230–1232.

Vinzent, R., de la Rue, J. and Herbert, H. (1950) L'infection placentaire a *Vibrio fetus. Annales de Médicine*, **51**, 23–68.

Waldor, M., Roberts, D. and Kazanjian, P. (1992) In utero infection due to *Pasteurella multocida* in the first trimester of pregnancy: case report and review. *Clinical Infectious Diseases*, **14**, 497–500.

Walter, P.R., Blot, P. and Inanoff, B (1982a) The placental lesions in congenital syphilis: a study of six cases. *Virchows Archiv A Pathological Anatomy and Histology*, **397**, 313–326.

Walter, P.R., Garin, Y. and Blot, P. (1982b) Placental pathologic changes in malaria: a histologic and ultrastructural study. *American Journal of Pathology*, **109**, 330–342.

Warthin, A.S. and Cowie, D.M. (1904) A contribution to the casuistry of placental and congenital tuber-culosis. *Journal of Infectious Diseases*, **1**, 140–169.

Werner, J., Schmidtke, L. and Thomascheck, G. (1963) *Toxoplasma* Infektion und Schwangerschaft, der histologische Nachweis des intrauterinen Infektionweges. *Klinische Wochenschrift*, **41**, 96–101.

Wickramasuriya, G.A.W. (1935) Some observations on malaria occurring in association with pregnancy. *Journal of Obstetrics and Gynaecology of the British Empire*, **42**, 816–834.

Wielenga, G., van Tongeren, H.A.E., Ferguson, A.H. and van Rijssel, T.G. (1961) Prenatal infection with vaccinia virus. *Lancet*, **i**, 258–260.

Winn, H.N. and Egley, C.C. (1987) Acute *Haemophilus influenzae* chorioamnionitis associated with intact amniotic membranes. *American Journal of Obstetrics and Gynecology*, **156**, 458–459.

Witzleben, C.L. and Driscoll, S.G. (1965) Possible transplacental transmission of herpes simplex infec-tion. *Pediatrics*, **36**, 192–199.

Wong, G.P., Cimolai, N., Dimmick, J.E. and Martin, T.R. (1992) *Pasteurella multocida* chorioamnionitis from vaginal transmission. *Acta Obstetricia et Gynecologica Scandinavica*, **71**, 384–387.

Wong, S.Y., Gray, E.S., Buxton, D., Finlayson, J. and Johnson, F.W.A. (1985) Acute placentitis and spon-taneous abortion caused by *Chlamydia psittaci* of sheep origin: a histological and ultrastructural study. *Journal of Clinical Pathology*, **38**, 707–711.

Woods, D.L., Edwards, J.N. and Sinclair-Smith, C.C. (1986) Amniotic fluid infection syndrome and abruptio placentae. *Pediatric Pathology*, **6**, 81–85.

Workowski, K.A. and Flaherty, J.P. (1992) Systemic *Bacillus* species infection mimicking listeriosis of pregnancy. *Clinical Infectious Diseases*, **14**, 694–696.

Yamada, M., Steketee, R. and Abramowsky, C. (1989) *Plasmodium falciparum* associated placental patho-logy: a light and electron microscopic and immunohistologic study. *American Journal of Tropical Medicine and Hygiene*, **41**, 161–168.

Yamazaki, K., Price, J.T. and Altshuler, G. (1977) A placental view of the diagnosis and pathogenesis of congenital listeriosis. *American Journal of Obstetrics and Gynecology*, **129**, 703–705.

Yancey, M.K., Duff, P., Clark, P., Kurtzer, T., Frentzen, B.H. and Kublis, P. (1994) Peripartum infection associated with vaginal group B streptococcal colonization. *Obstetrics and Gynecology*, **84**, 816–819.

Yawn, D.H., Pyeatte, J.C., Joseph, J.M., Eichler, S.L. and Garcia-Bunuel, R. (1971) Transplacental trans-fer of influenza virus. *Journal of the American Medical Association*, **212**, 1022–1023.

Zaaijma, J.T., Wilkinson, A.R., Keeling, J.W., Mitchell, R.G. and Turnbull, A.C. (1982) Spontaneous pre-mature rupture of the membranes: bacteriology, histology and neonatal outcome. *Journal of Obstetrics and Gynaecology*, **2**, 155–160.

Zevallos, E.A., Anderson, V.M., Bard, E. and Gu, J (1994) Detection of HIV-1 sequences in placentas of HIV infected mothers by in situ polymerase chain reaction. *Cell Vision*, **1**, 116–121.

Zippel, H.H., Citolor, P. and Zippel, C. (1975) Leukozytre Infiltration der Plazenta bei Intensivüberwachung in der Geburtshilfe. *Geburtshilfe und Frauenheilkunde*, **35**, 478–481.

12

IMMUNOPATHOLOGY
OF THE PLACENTA

It has long been believed, largely but not solely by immunologists, that immunopathological mechanisms probably play an important role in many of the problems that can beset a pregnancy, that the placenta may occupy a pivotal role both as a triggering mechanism of, and as a target organ for, such immune processes, and that immunopathological studies may help to unravel some of the complex problems of placental dysfunction.

It has to be remarked, however, that the high hopes held 20 years ago that immunological studies would solve many of the problems of placental pathology have not, in my opinion, been fulfilled and that the excitement felt at that time for immunopathology has now been replaced by a similar, indeed heightened, enthusiasm for molecular biological techniques (which may or may not fulfil their proponent's expectations). I was therefore tempted to discard this chapter from the present edition but have retained it, albeit in shortened form, because I still believe that immunological interactions between maternal and fetal tissues are of prime importance in both normal and abnormal pregnancies.

There is a vast body of work on placental immunobiology and immunopathology and only a brief summary of this can be outlined here. This summary will, of necessity, be highly selective and it has to be stressed that it represents a sifting of the available evidence by one who is, like many who have contributed to this field, not a professional immunologist.

THE PLACENTA AS A SEMI-ALLOGENEIC GRAFT

The placenta, being a fetal organ, contains paternal-type antigens that are alien to the mother, and is therefore an allograft, or transplant, which should be rejected. Quite patently, such a rejection does not usually occur and, just as Sherlock Holmes was intrigued by the dog that failed to bark, so immunologists have been fascinated by the failure of the maternal immune system to dispose of what has been aptly, though perhaps somewhat coyly, termed 'nature's transplant'.

Many possible explanations for this phenomenon have been proffered and many of these, such as the beliefs that the conceptus is not immunogenic, that maternal immune responses are non-specifically depressed during pregnancy, that the uterus is an immunologically privileged site and that the placenta acts as an immunological barrier separating mother from fetus, have failed to stand the tests of time and critical scrutiny (Jones et al, 1992; Sargent et al, 1993; Johnson, 1995). Currently it is thought that the survival of the placenta as a graft is not dependent upon any single factor but is the result of a complex interplay between trophoblastic antigenicity and specific maternal immune responsiveness. Because there is no alteration in systemic maternal immune responsiveness during pregnancy and because there is no real evidence for conventional antibody or cellular responses directed specifically against trophoblast in normal pregnancies (Bulmer & Johnson, 1995), interest in the maternal arm of this equation has been lately focused on local immune reactions in decidual tissue.

Trophoblast Immunobiology

HLA Antigens

It has now been clearly established that the stromal mesenchymal cells of the placental villi express conventional class I HLA antigens and that class II HLA antigens are expressed by the villous Hofbauer cells (Sunderland et al, 1981; Sutton et al, 1983, 1986; Bulmer et al, 1988a). By contrast, there is no detectable expression of classical class I or class II HLA antigens by villous trophoblast at any stage of gestation (Johnson, 1992). The failure of villous trophoblast to express class I HLA antigens appears to be at the transcriptional level because detectable amounts of HLA class I mRNA are low (Boucrat et al, 1993) and the failure of class I HLA expression is resistant to cytokine upregulation (Hunt et al, 1987). Whatever may be the mechanism for this remarkable non-expression of conventional HLA molecules by villous trophoblast, this phenomenon is clearly of central importance in protecting the tissue from both maternal immune recognition and maternal cytotoxic cell attack.

Extravillous cytotrophoblastic cells do, however, express a class I HLA antigen though this is not a classical HLA-A or HLA-B antigen (Hsi et al, 1984; Redman et al, 1984; Wells et al, 1984) and has now been identified as HLA-G (Ellis, 1990; Kovats et al, 1990). This a non-polymorphic antigen and it has been suggested that it may serve to protect the invasive trophoblast of the placental bed from maternal natural killer (NK) cell attack by acting as a passive non-polymorphic cell surface class I molecule (Chumbley et al, 1994).

Complement Regulatory Molecules

Early studies with polyclonal antisera raised against syncytiotrophoblast identified an antigen system that was shared by trophoblast and maternal immunocompetent cells and classified as the trophoblast–leucocyte common (TLX) antigen system (McIntyre & Faulk, 1982a,b). It was subsequently shown that these antigens were identical to several complement regulatory molecules (decay accelerating factor, membrane co-factor protein and membrane attack complex inhibitory factor) which protect cell surfaces from deposition of certain complement components (Holmes et al, 1990; Purcell et al, 1990; Hsi et al, 1991). Expression of these molecules by the trophoblast will therefore protect this tissue from any complement-mediated damage that could occur as a result of maternal antibody attack.

Immunobiology of Decidua

There is considerable evidence that decidual tissue exerts a local immunosuppressive effect (Starkey, 1993) though exactly how this is achieved is a matter for debate.

There is a population of T lymphocytes in the decidua and these are mostly CD8 suppressor cells (Bulmer & Sunderland, 1984; Bulmer et al, 1988b). However, the number of such cells is almost certainly too small for them to be able to exert any significant immunomodulatory effect. Decidual macrophages are quite abundant and it is probable that their main function is to act as scavengers (Bulmer, 1992). These macrophages may, however, also contribute substantially to decidual synthesis of prostaglandin, which is immunosuppressive (Lala et al, 1986; Parhar et al, 1988; Norwitz et al, 1991).

Large granulated lymphocytes are a major component of the leucocytic population of the decidua in early pregnancy, though their number diminishes as gestation progresses (Bulmer & Sunderland, 1984; Bulmer et al, 1991). These cells express many, but not all, markers of mature NK cells and their function is uncertain. However, it is possible that they play a role in the mediation of non-HLA-specific immunosuppression and thus act as natural suppressor cells (Maier et al, 1986; Bulmer, 1992).

Decidual stromal cells may also play a role in local immunosuppression, largely because of their ability to synthesize prostaglandins (Lala et al, 1986; Matthews & Searle, 1987). These cells also produce a soluble immunosuppressive factor which inhibits lymphoproliferative activity and interleukin 2 activity (Matsui et al, 1989).

Cytokines

Cytokines are produced in both decidua and placenta and clearly play an important role in normal pregnancy. It has been suggested that cytokines may contribute to local immunoregulation (Hunt, 1989) but, as Bulmer and Johnson (1995) have written, 'despite ever increasing localization of cytokines, their receptors and inhibitory molecules in uteroplacental tissues their in vivo role is unknown'.

Survival of the Placental Graft

It is clear that a full explanation of the ability of the placenta to survive as a semi-allogeneic graft has not yet been achieved. It is almost certain, however, that the lack of expression of HLA antigens by villous trophoblast is a pivotal factor. The effect of any immunosuppressive effect of the decidua is likely to be of only secondary importance because in tubal pregnancies placentation appears to occur normally despite the usual lack of a decidual reaction and despite the absence of large granulated lymphocytes (Bulmer et al, 1987). Suppressor T cells are commonly present in the tubal implantation site but not in the density with which they occur in uterine decidua (Earl et al, 1987).

The ability of the placenta to flourish as a graft does not necessarily mean, however, that in normal placental tissue there is no evidence of any immune interaction between maternal and fetal tissues. Early immunohistological studies demonstrated that the villous trophoblastic basement membrane stains focally for C3c, C3d and C9, positive staining for C1q and C9 is found in the walls of fetal stem vessels (McCormick et al, 1971; Faulk & Johnson, 1977) and C3 may be found in the uteroplacental vessels in normal pregnancies (Weir, 1981). How exactly one interprets these immunopathological findings is perhaps a matter of opinion but they do indicate that immunological reactions of some sort are occurring in placental tissues from normal pregnancies. More recently, villitis of unknown aetiology has, as discussed in Chapter 11, been regarded as a hallmark of materno-fetal immune reactivity within the placenta. In immunohistological terms, villitis is defined as the presence within villous tissue of activated macrophages together, usually, with T-cells of the helper phenotype and a few suppressor T cells but no B cells (Labarrere et al, 1990), these cells being predominantly of maternal origin (Labarrere & Faulk, 1995). If villitis is defined in these terms it is present, to a lesser or greater extent, in all placentas (Labarrere et al, 1989) and is regarded by Labarrere and Faulk (1992) as representing a consequence of allogeneic recognition and rejection reactions in the placenta. The validity or otherwise of this belief is currently a matter for debate but, if true, it would indicate that a reaction against the placenta as an allograft is merely damped down rather than totally inhibited. This is of considerable theoretical, but little practical, interest because in most discussions of the ability of the placenta to resist graft rejection there has been an underlying assumption that a maternal immune response is potentially harmful to the fetoplacental graft, and that mechanisms for suppressing or inhibiting such a response must be invoked to explain the continuing viability of the fetus. There is, however, much to suggest that, in some respects at least, the reverse of this concept is the case and that materno-fetal antigenic disparity has a beneficial effect upon fetal and placental growth, the greater the degree of such disparity the more marked being the benefit obtained.

Billington (1964) noted in mice that F_1 hybrid fetuses were larger and had heavier placentas than did homozygous fetuses in a mother of a given genetic strain, and he proposed that this 'hybrid vigour' was due, not to genetic differences, but to antigenic disparity. Others have confirmed the increased weight of the F_1 hybrid fetus and placenta, both in mice and other animals (James, 1965; McCarthy, 1965; Beer & Billingham, 1971; Beer, 1975; Beer et al, 1975a,b. However, the dependence of this phenomenon on an immunological reaction involving the disparity of histocompatibility antigens has been questioned by workers who have been unable to show that materno-paternal differences in the major H-2 or H-3 loci had any effect on placental weight in matings between otherwise congenic strains of mice (Finkel & Lilly, 1971; Hetherington, 1971, 1973).

Nevertheless, placental and fetal weights can be influenced by manipulation of the immune status of the mother. This was originally shown by James (1965, 1967), who demonstrated that female mice rendered specifically immune to an antigenically disparate strain, by skin grafting or injection of splenic cells, produced heavier fetuses and placentas when subsequently mated with a male of that strain than did similarly mated females who had not been previously sensitized. Conversely, mice rendered tolerant to the antigens of the male mate produced unduly light fetuses and placentas. These findings have not been reproduced by Clarke (1971) or McLaren (1975), but have won considerable support from the studies of Beer and his colleagues (Beer & Billingham, 1971, 1974; Beer, 1975; Beer et al, 1975a). These latter workers were not only able to alter placental weight in either direction by prior immunization or desensitization to paternal antigens, but also showed that the para-aortic lymph nodes of female rats were larger in pregnancies resulting from the mating of genetically disparate strains than in those due to the mating of genetically similar strains. They subsequently demonstrated that prior removal of either the para-aortic lymph nodes or the spleen from female rats before conception abolished the beneficial effect on placental weight that results from mating between genetically dissimilar strains, and that the injection into already pregnant rats of hyperimmune serum directed against paternal antigens in hybrid gestations produced a further increment in placental weight above that found in an allogeneic control group. These results suggest strongly that, in animals, maternal immune reactions against paternal antigens exert a beneficial effect upon placental and fetal growth, and that hybrid vigour is unlikely, despite the eloquent plea of McLaren (1975), to be due solely to genetic heterosis.

Whether the same can be said for humans is, at the present time, a matter for conjecture. Studies of the effects of materno-fetal ABO incompatibility on placental weight have yielded conflicting results (Jones, 1968; Seppala & Tolonen, 1970; Toivanen & Hirvonen, 1970), but Jenkins and Good (1972) have claimed that the greater the degree of reactivity in mixed cultures of maternal and paternal lymphocytes the heavier is the placenta. Clearly, much work remains to be done on this topic, but it must be at least possible that the immune response of the mother to disparate fetal antigens may well act as a double-edged weapon with complex effects on the placenta.

PRE-ECLAMPSIA

Pre-eclampsia is one of the most fascinatingly enigmatic of all diseases but the belief that it is, either wholly or in part, immunologically mediated has won considerable support over the years. The evidence for this concept tends, however, to be tantalizingly inconclusive, consisting largely of several unrelated observations that resemble the pieces of a jigsaw puzzle which fail to yield a complete picture.

Any consideration of the immunopathology of pre-eclampsia leads inexorably to the placenta, because the disease occurs only when trophoblastic tissue is present, can develop independently of the presence of a fetus (as in hydatidiform mole), and can be cured with certainty only by removal of the placenta. Furthermore, it is well established that there is a direct relationship between placental mass and pre-eclampsia, those pregnancies in which the placenta is unusually large, e.g., twin gestation, placental hydrops and hydatidiform mole, being complicated unduly frequently by pre-eclampsia (Scott, 1958; McFarlane & Scott, 1976). It may be remarked that this does not appear to hold for the usual case of pre-eclampsia, in which the placenta is, on average, slightly smaller than is the norm in uncomplicated gestations. Such an observation, however, is based on the examination of placentas that have usually been faced, for some time before delivery, with a restricted maternal blood supply, and it is of great interest that women who later develop pre-eclampsia have, as measured by their dehydroisoandrosterone sulphate clearance rate, a larger placental mass in the early stages of pregnancy than do those whose gestations are not destined to suffer this complication (Gant et al, 1971).

The placenta, or at least the trophoblast, is still further implicated by the observation that the amount of trophoblastic tissue entering the uterine veins is very much higher in women with pre-eclampsia than in those with uncomplicated pregnancies (Jaameri et al, 1965; Chua et al, 1991). It is not known whether this excessive vascular entry precedes the development, or occurs as a complication, of pre-eclampsia.

Consideration of these facts has led to the not unreasonable postulate that pre-eclampsia may be due to an immune attack on placental tissue and that the condition is predisposed to if the mother is presented with an excessive load of trophoblastic antigens. Evidence to support this hypothesis is, however, sparse. The placenta itself does not show any overt evidence of immune-mediated damage in pre-eclampsia, with the possible exception of excessive villous fibrinoid necrosis, and immunohistological studies have shown that whilst there is an increased staining for C1q, C3d and C9 in placentas from pre-eclamptic women, the distribution of such staining is the same as that found in placentas from healthy women (Sinha et al, 1984). It has been suggested that the morphological changes seen in the arteries in pre-eclampsia mimic closely those observed in the vessels of rejected renal transplants (Robertson et al, 1967, 1975) and this view is strengthened, to some extent, by the demonstration of complement components and immunoglobulin deposits in the walls of these vessels (Kitzmiller & Benirschke, 1973; Labarrere & Faulk, 1992). An even more striking analogy between graft rejection and pre-eclampsia was drawn by Feeney et al (1977), who, taking cognizance of the clinical and experimental observation that prior blood transfusion appears to protect a renal transplant from rejection, have shown that women receiving a blood transfusion before pregnancy have a lower incidence of pre-eclampsia than do non-transfused patients.

DIABETES MELLITUS

Immunohistological studies of placentas from diabetic women have yielded results strikingly similar to those found in placentas from patients with pre-eclampsia. Thus, whilst there is increased staining for C1q, C3d and C9, the distribution within the placenta of such positive staining is the same as that in placentas from non-diabetic women (Galbraith et al, 1984; Labarrere & Faulk, 1992). The significance of this finding is somewhat opaque but it is of interest that the immunohistological findings in placentas from women with gestational diabetes are the same as those in placentas from well-established diabetics.

SPONTANEOUS ABORTION

Of all the ills that can befall a pregnancy, the one that bears the closest superficial resemblance to a graft rejection phenomenon is spontaneous abortion. Kerr surveyed the evidence then available in 1968 to support this concept and was led to conclude that 'the material which has been reviewed is too fragmentary to summarize coherently', a comment that is almost equally valid today. It is certainly possible to induce abortion by immunological means under experimental conditions, because it is well established that pregnancy in a variety of animals can be interrupted by the administration of heterologous antisera directed against trophoblastic tissue-specific antigens (Behrman, 1971; Beer et al, 1972), human chorionic somatotrophin (Howe, 1975) or alpha-fetoprotein (Slade, 1973). In humans, however, no such clear-cut data have been forthcoming.

Rocklin et al (1976) raised the possibility that abortion, far from being the result of an immune-mediated attack on the conceptus, could be due to a lack of normal immunological protective mechanisms. They demonstrated the presence in multi-gravid women of an antibody that blocked the specific immune response of maternal lymphocytes to paternal antigens *in vitro* and showed that these blocking antibodies were absent from the sera of some women with a history of recurrent abortion. The blocking antibodies were of IgG type and specifically directed against a non-HLA paternal antigen and in this particular study a woman whose serum lacked this blocking antibody and suffered recurrent abortions later developed the antibody and had a successful pregnancy. It was later suggested that these blocking antibodies were directed against allotypic antigens shared by trophoblast and immunocompetent cells and that these antigens were in linkage disequilibrium with HLA antigens (Faulk & McIntyre, 1983).

Meanwhile several studies had appeared which showed that women who suffered repetitive abortion often had an unusual degree of sharing of HLA antigens (Komlos et al, 1977; Gerencer et al, 1979; Schacter et al, 1979; Beer et al, 1981) (this later being perceived as serving as a surrogate for sharing of specific allotypic trophoblastic antigens). It was suggested that in such cases the women did not, in immunological terms, recognize that they were pregnant and therefore did not mount an immune response to their conceptuses and failed to produce blocking antibodies (Faulk et al, 1978). It was therefore proposed that such women should be immunized with HLA incompatible (and thus trophoblastic antigen incompatible) leucocytes (Taylor & Faulk, 1981), a suggestion that triggered off a decade of enthusiasm for immunotherapy of recurrent abortion, using not only donor leucocytes for immunization but also paternal leucocytes (Beer et al, 1981), trophoblastic membranes (Johnson et al, 1988) and immunoglobulins (Mueller-Eckhardt et al, 1989). Initial reports of high success rates for these various immunotherapeutic techniques (Beer et al, 1985; Mowbray et al, 1985; McIntyre et al, 1986) gradually became muted as it progressively emerged that the pregnancy rates achieved were, in fact, no greater than those in control women (Hill, 1990; Cauchi et al, 1991; Ho et al, 1991; Fraser et al, 1993). Furthermore, the claims that recurrent abortion is associated with an undue degree of materno-paternal HLA antigen sharing have not been substantiated in more recent studies (Adinolfi, 1986; Balasch et al, 1989; Christiansen et al, 1989).

Interest in immunotherapy for recurrent abortion has therefore waned, in many centres almost to the point of extinction, and a current view would be that there is no real evidence that alloimmune factors play any role in early pregnancy loss (Berry et al, 1995). Furthermore, as discussed in Chapter 10, the evidence that autoimmune mechanisms play a role in spontaneous abortion is either disputed or flimsy.

It has to be concluded that immunological factors have not been proven to have any role in early pregnancy loss, a conclusion in accord with the lack of any morphological evidence in the placentas of abortuses to suggest, however remotely, that they have been the objects of an immune-mediated attack.

REFERENCES

Adinolfi, M. (1986) Recurrent habitual abortion: HLA sharing and deliberate immunization with partner's cells: a controversial topic. *Human Reproduction*, **1**, 45–48.

Balasch, J., Coll, O., Martorell, J. et al (1989) Further data against HLA sharing in couples with recurrent spontaneous abortion. *Gynecological Endocrinology*, **3**, 63–69.

Beer, A.E. (1975) Immunogenetic determinants of the size of the fetoplacental unit and their modus operandi. *European Journal of Obstetrics, Gynecology and Reproductive Biology*, **5**, 135–146.

Beer, A.E. and Billingham, R.E. (1971) Immunobiology of mammalian reproduction. *Advances in Immunology*, **14**, 1–84.

Beer, A.E. and Billingham, R.E. (1974) Host response to intrauterine tissue, cellular and fetal allografts. *Journal of Reproduction and Fertility*, **21** (Supplement), 559–588.

Beer, A.E., Billingham, R.E. and Yang, S.L. (1972) Further evidence concerning the auto-antigenic status of the trophoblast. *Journal of Experimental Medicine*, **135**, 1177–1184.

Beer, A.E., Billingham, R.E. and Scott, J.R. (1975a) Immunogenetic aspects of implantation, placentation and feto-placental growth rates. *Biology of Reproduction*, **12**, 176–189.

Beer, A.E., Scott, J.R. and Billingham, R.E. (1975b) Histoincompatibility and maternal immunological status as determinants of fetoplacental weight and litter size in rodents. *Journal of Experimental Medicine*, **142**, 180–196.

Beer, A.E., Quebbeman, J.F., Ayers, J.W.T. and Haines, R.F. (1981) Major histocompatibility complex antigens – maternal and paternal immunoresponse and chronic habitual abortion. *American Journal of Obstetrics and Gynecology*, **141**, 987–997.

Beer, A.E., Semprini, A.E., Xiaoyn, Z. and Quebbeman, J.F. (1985) Pregnancy outcome in human couples with recurrent spontaneous abortion: HLA antigen profiles, HLA antigen sharing, female serum MLR blocking factors and paternal leucocyte immunization. *Experimental and Clinical Immunogenetics*, **2**, 137–153.

Behrman, S.J. (1971) Implantation as an immunologic phenomenon. In *The Biology of the Blastocyst*, Blandau, R.J. (Ed.), pp. 479–494. Chicago: Chicago University Press.

Berry, C.W., Brambati, B., Eskes, T.K.A.B. et al (1995) The Euro-team early pregnancy (ETEP) protocol for recurrent miscarriage. *Human Reproduction*, **10**, 1516–1520.

Billington, W.D. (1964) Influence of immunological dissimilarity of mother and fetus on size of placenta in mice. *Nature*, **202**, 317–318.

Boucrat, J., Hawley, S., Robertson, K. et al (1993) Differential nuclear expression of enhancer A DNA-binding proteins in human first trimester trophoblast cells. *Journal of Immunology*, **150**, 3882–3894.

Bulmer, J.N. (1992) Immunology of the uterine decidual response. In *Immunological Obstetrics*, Coulam, C.B., Faulk, W.P. and McIntyre, J.A. (Eds), pp. 245–255. New York: Norton.

Bulmer, J.N. and Johnson, P.M. (1995) The immunopathology of pregnancy. In *Haines and Taylor: Obstetrical and Gynaecological Pathology*, 4th edn, Fox, H. (Ed.), pp. 1807–1835. Edinburgh: Churchill Livingstone.

Bulmer, J.N. and Sunderland, C.A. (1984) Immunohistological identification of lymphoid populations in the early human placental bed. *Immunology*, **52**, 349–357.

Bulmer, J.N., Ritson, A., Earl, U. and Hollings, D. (1987) Immunocompetent cells in human decidua. In *Reproductive Immunology: Materno-Fetal Relationship*, Chaouat, G. (Ed.), pp. 89–100. Paris: Inserm.

Bulmer, J.N., Morrison, L. and Smith, J.C. (1988a) Expression of Class II MHC gene products by macrophages in human uteroplacental tissues. *Immunology*, **63**, 707–714.

Bulmer, J.N., Smith, J., Morrison, L. and Wells, M. (1988b) Maternal and fetal cellular relationships in the human placental basal plate. *Placenta*, **9**, 237–246.

Bulmer, J.N., Morrison, L., Longfellow, M., Ritson, A. and Pace, D. (1991) Granulated lymphocytes in human endometrium: histochemical and immunohistochemical studies. *Human Reproduction*, **6**, 791–798.

Cauchi, M.N., Lim, D., Young, D.E., Kloss, M. and Pepperell, R.J. (1991) Treatment of recurrent aborters by immunization with paternal cells – a controlled trial. *American Journal of Reproductive Immunology*, **25**, 16–17.

Christiansen, O.B., Riisom, K., Lauritsen, J.G. and Grunnet, N. (1989) No increased histocompatibility antigen-sharing in couples with idiopathic habitual abortion. *Human Reproduction*, **4**, 160–162.

Chua, S., Wilkins, T., Sargent, I. and Redman, C.W.G. (1991) Trophoblast deportation in pre-eclamptic pregnancy. *British Journal of Obstetrics and Gynaecology*, **98**, 973–979.

Chumbley, G., King, A., Robertson, K., Holmes, N. and Loke, Y.W. (1994) Resistance of HLA-G and HLA-A2 transfectants to lysis by decidual NK cells. *Cellular Immunology*, **155**, 312–322.

Clarke, A.G. (1971) The effects of maternal pre-immunization on pregnancy in the mouse. *Journal of Reproduction and Fertility*, **24**, 369–375.

Earl, U., Lunny, D.P. and Bulmer, J.N. (1987) Leukocyte populations in ectopic tubal pregnancy. *Journal of Clinical Pathology*, **40**, 901–910.

Ellis, S. (1990) HLA-G: at the interface. *American Journal of Reproductive Immunology*, **23**, 84–86.

Faulk, W.P. and Johnson, P.M. (1977) Immunological studies of human placentae: identification and distribution of proteins in mature chorionic villi. *Clinical and Experimental Immunology*, **27**, 365–375.

Faulk, W.P. and McIntyre, J.A. (1983) Immunological studies of human trophoblast: markers, subsets and functions. *Immunological Reviews*, **75**, 139–175.

Faulk, W.P., Temple, A., Lovins, R. and Smith, N.C. (1978) Antigens of human trophoblast: a working hypothesis for their role in normal and abnormal pregnancies. *Proceedings of the National Academy of Sciences USA*, **75**, 1947–1957.

Feeney, J.G., Tovey, L.A.D. and Scott, J.S. (1977) Influence of previous blood transfusion on incidence of pre-eclampsia. *Lancet*, **i**, 874–875.

Finkel, S.I. and Lilly, F. (1971) Influence of histocompatibility between mother and foetus on placental size in mice. *Nature*, **234**, 102–103.

Fraser, E.J., Grimes, D.A. and Schultz, K. (1993) Immunization as a therapy for recurrent spontaneous abortion: a review and meta-analysis. *Obstetrics and Gynecology*, **82**, 854–859.

Galbraith, R.M., Sinha, D., Galbraith, G.M.P. and Faulk, W.P. (1984) Immunological study of placentae in insulin dependent diabetes mellitus. In *Carbohydrate Metabolism in Pregnancy*, Sutherland, H. and Stowers, J. (Eds), pp. 23–33. London: Churchill Livingstone.

Gant, N.F., Hutchinson, H.T., Siiteri, P.K. and MacDonald, P.C. (1971) Study of the metabolic clearance rate of dehydroisoandrosterone sulfate in pregnancy. *American Journal of Obstetrics and Gynecology*, **111**, 555–561.

Gerencer, M., Pfeifer, S., Singer, Z., Skalow, D. and Kastelan, A. (1979) HLA-A, -B, and -D compatibility in couples with recurrent pathologic pregnancies. *Periodicum Biologorum*, **81**, 407–409.

Hetherington, C.M. (1971) The decidual cell reaction, placental weight, foetal weight and placental morphology in the mouse. *Journal of Reproduction and Fertility*, **25**, 417–424.

Hetherington, C.M. (1973) The absence of any effect of materno-foetal incompatibility at the H-2 and H-3 loci on pregnancy in the mouse. *Journal of Reproduction and Fertility*, **33**, 135–139.

Hill, J.A. (1990) Immunologic mechanisms of pregnancy maintenance and failure: a critique of theories and therapy. *American Journal of Reproductive Immunology*, **22**, 33–42.

Ho, H.-N., Gill, T.J., Hsieh, H.-J. et al (1991) Immunotherapy for spontaneous abortions in a Chinese population. *American Journal of Reproductive Immunology*, **25**, 10–15.

Holmes, C.H., Simpson, K.L., Okada, H. et al (1990) Preferential expression of the complement regulatory protein decay accelerating factor at the fetomaternal interface during human pregnancy. *Journal of Immunology*, **144**, 3099–3105.

Howe, C.W.S. (1975) Lymphocyte physiology during pregnancy: in vivo and in vitro studies. In *Immunobiology of Trophoblast*, Edwards, R.G., Howe, C.W.S. and Johnson, M.H. (Eds), pp. 131–146. London: Cambridge University Press.

Hsi, B.-L., Yeh, C.-J.G. and Faulk, W.P. (1984) Class I antigens of the major histocompatibility complex on cytotrophoblast of human chorion laeve. *Immunology*, **52**, 621–629.

Hsi, B.-L., Hunt, J.S. and Atkinson, J.P. (1991) Differential expression of complement regulatory proteins on subpopulations of human trophoblast cells. *Journal of Reproductive Immunology*, **19**, 209–223.

Hunt, J.S. (1989) Cytokine networks in the uteroplacental unit: macrophages as pivotal regulatory cells. *Journal of Reproductive Immunology*, **16**, 1–17.

Hunt, J.S., Andrews, G.K. and Wood, G.W. (1987) Normal trophoblasts resist induction of class I HLA. *Journal of Immunology*, **138**, 2481–2487.

Jaameri, K.E., Koivuniemi, A.P. and Carpen, E.O. (1965) Occurrence of trophoblasts in the blood of toxaemic patients. *Gynaecologia*, **160**, 315–320.

James, D.A. (1965) Effects of antigenic dissimilarity between mother and foetus on placental size in mice. *Nature*, **205**, 613–614.

James, D.A. (1967) Some effects of immunological factors on gestation in mice. *Journal of Reproduction and Fertility*, **14**, 265–275.

Jenkins, D.M. and Good, S. (1972) Mixed lymphocyte reaction and placentation. *Nature New Biology*, **240**, 211–212.

Johnson, P.M. (1992) Immunology of human extraembryonic fetal membranes. In *Immunological Obstetrics*, Coulam, C.B., Faulk, W.P. and McIntyre, J.A. (Eds), pp. 177–188. New York: Norton.

Johnson, P.M. (1995) Immunology of pregnancy. In *Turnbull's Obstetrics*, 2nd edn, Chamberlain, G. (Ed.), pp. 143–159. Edinburgh: Churchill Livingstone.

Johnson, P.M., Chia, K.V., Hart, C.A., Griffith, H.B. and Francis, W.J.A. (1988) Trophoblast membrane infusion for unexplained recurrent miscarriage. *British Journal of Obstetrics and Gynaecology*, **95**, 342–347.

Jones, M.C., MacLeod, A.M., Dilon, D.M. and Catto, G.R. (1992) The maternal immune response. In *Immunological Obstetrics*, Coulam, C.B., Faulk, W.P. and McIntyre, J.A. (Eds), pp. 227–244. New York: Norton.

Jones, W.R. (1968) Immunological factors in human placentation. *Nature*, **218**, 480.

Kerr, M.G. (1968) Immunological rejection as a cause of abortion. *Journal of Reproduction and Fertility*, **3** (Supplement), 49–55.

Kitzmiller, J.L. and Benirschke, K. (1973) Immunofluorescent study of placental bed vessels in preeclampsia of pregnancy. *American Journal of Obstetrics and Gynecology*, **115**, 248–251.

Komlos, L., Zamir, R., Joshua, H. and Halbrecht, I. (1977) Common HLA antigens in couples with repeated abortions. *Clinical Immunology and Immunopathology*, **7**, 330–335.

Kovats, S., Main, E.K., Librach, C. et al (1990) A class I antigen, HLA-G, expressed in human trophoblasts. *Science*, **248**, 220–223.

Labarrere, C.A. and Faulk, W.P. (1992) Immunopathology of human extraembryonic tissues. In *Immunological Obstetrics*, Coulam, C.B., Faulk, W.P. and McIntyre, J.A. (Eds), pp. 439–463. New York: Norton.

Labarrere, C.A. and Faulk, W.P. (1995) Maternal cells in chorionic villi from placentae of normal and abnormal human pregnancies. *American Journal of Reproductive Immunology*, **33**, 54–59.

Labarrere, C.A., Faulk, W.P. and McIntyre, J.A. (1989) Villitis in normal human term placentae: frequency of the lesion determined by monoclonal antibody to HLA-DR antigen. *Journal of Reproductive Immunology*, **16**, 127–135.

Labarrere, C.A., McIntyre, J.A. and Faulk, W.P. (1990) Immunohistologic evidence that villitis in human normal term placentas is an immunologic lesion. *American Journal of Obstetrics and Gynecology*, **162**, 515–522.

Lala, P.K., Parhar, R.S., Kearns, M., Johnson, S. and Scodras, J.M (1986) Immunological aspects of the decidual response. In *Proceedings of the 3rd International Congress on Reproductive Immunology*, Clark, D.A. and Croy, B.A. (Eds), pp. 190–198. Amsterdam: Elsevier.

Maier, T., Holda, J.H. and Claman, H.N. (1986) Natural suppressor (NS) cells: members of the LGL regulatory family. *Immunology Today*, **7**, 312–315.

Matsui, S., Yoshimura, N. and Oka, T. (1989) Characterization and analysis of soluble suppressor factor from early human decidual cells. *Transplantation*, **47**, 678–683.

Matthews, C.J. and Searle, R.F. (1987) The role of prostaglandins in the immunosuppressive effects of supernatants from adherent cells of murine decidual tissue. *Journal of Reproductive Immunology*, **12**, 287–295.

McCarthy, J.C. (1965) Genetic and environmental control of foetal and placental growth in the mouse. *Animal Production*, **7**, 424–431.

McCormick, J.N., Faulk, W.P., Fox, H. and Fudenberg, H. (1971) Immunohistochemical and elution studies of the human placenta. *Journal of Experimental Medicine*, **133**, 1–18.

McFarlane, A. and Scott, J.S. (1976) Pre-eclampsia/eclampsia in twin pregnancies. *Journal of Medical Genetics*, **13**, 208–211.

McIntyre, J.A. and Faulk, W.P. (1982a) Allotypic trophoblast-lymphocyte cross reactive (TLX) cell surface antigens. *Human Immunology*, **4**, 27–36.

McIntyre, J.A. and Faulk, W.P. (1982b) Allotypic trophoblast–lymphocyte cross reactive (TLX) antigens. *Progress in Clinical and Biological Research*, **854**, 463–472.

McIntyre, J.A., Faulk, W.P., Nichols-Johnson, V.R. and Taylor, C.G. (1986) Immunologic testing and immunotherapy in recurrent spontaneous abortion. *Obstetrics and Gynecology*, **67**, 169–175.

McLaren, A. (1975) Antigenic disparity: does it affect placental size, implantation or population genetics. In *Immunobiology of Trophoblast*, Edwards, R.G., Howe, C.W.S. and Johnson, M.H. (Eds), pp. 255–273. London: Cambridge University Press.

Mowbray, J.F., Gibbings, C., Liddell, H. et al (1985) Controlled trial of treatment of recurrent spontaneous abortion by immunisation with paternal cells. *Lancet*, **i**, 941–943.

Mueller-Eckhardt, G., Heine, O., Neppert, J., Kunzel, W. and Mueller-Eckhardt, C. (1989) Prevention of recurrent spontaneous abortion by intravenous immunoglobulin. *Vox Sang*, **56**, 151–154.

Norwitz, E.R., Starkey, P.M., Lopez-Bernal, A. and Turnbull, A.C. (1991) Identification by flow cytometry of the prostaglandin-producing cell populations of term human decidua. *Journal of Endocrinology*, **31**, 327–334.

Parhar, R.S., Kennedy, T.G. and Lala, P.K. (1988) Suppression of lymphocyte alloreactivity by early gestational human decidua. I. Characterization of suppressor cells and suppressor molecules. *Cellular Immunology*, **116**, 392–410.

Purcell, D.F.J., McKenzie, I.F.C., Lublin, D.M. et al (1990) The human cell surface glycoproteins HuLym5, membrane co-factor protein (MCP) of the complement system, and trophoblast-leucocyte common (TLX) antigen, are CD46. *Immunology*, **70**, 155–161.

Redman, C.W.G., McMichael, A.J., Stirrat, G.M., Sutherland, C.A. and Ting, A. (1984) Class I MHC antigens on human extravillous cytotrophoblast. *Immunology*, **52**, 457–468.

Robertson, W.B., Brosens, I. and Dixon, H.G. (1967) The pathological response of the vessels of the placental bed to hypertensive pregnancy. *Journal of Pathology and Bacteriology*, **93**, 581–592.

Robertson, W.B., Brosens, I. and Dixon, H.G. (1975) Uteroplacental vascular pathology. *European Journal of Obstetrics, Gynecology and Reproductive Biology*, **5**, 47–65.

Rocklin, R.E., Kitzmiller, J.L., Carpenter, C.B., Garovoy, M.R. and David, J.R. (1976) Maternal-fetal relation: absence of an immunologic blocking factor from the serum of women with chronic abortions. *New England Journal of Medicine*, **295**, 1209–1213.

Sargent, I.L., Redman, C.W.G. and Starkey, P.M. (1993) The placenta as a graft. In *The Human Placenta*, Redman, C.W.G., Sargent, I.L. and Starkey, P.M. (Eds), pp. 334–361. Oxford: Blackwell.

Schacter, B., Gyves, M., Muir, A. and Tasin, M. (1979) HLA-A compatibility in parents of offspring with neural-tube defects or couples experiencing involuntary fetal wastage. *Lancet*, **i**, 796–798.

Scott, J.S. (1958) Pregnancy toxaemia associated with hydrops fetalis, hydatidiform mole and hydramnios. *Journal of Obstetrics and Gynaecology of the British Empire*, **65**, 689–701.

Seppala, M. and Tolonen, M. (1970) Histocompatibility and human placentation. *Nature*, **225**, 950–951.

Sinha, D., Wells, M. and Faulk, W.P. (1984) Immunological studies of human placentae: complement components in pre-eclamptic chorionic villi. *Clinical and Experimental Immunology*, **56**, 175–184.

Slade, B. (1973) Antibodies to alpha-fetoprotein cause foetal mortality in rats. *Nature*, **246**, 493–494.

Starkey, P.M. (1993) The decidua and factors controlling placentation. In *The Human Placenta*, Redman, C.W.G., Sargent, I.L. and Starkey, P.M. (Eds), pp. 334–413. Oxford: Blackwell.

Sunderland, C.A., Naiem, M., Mason, D.Y., Redman, C.W.G. and Stirrat, G.M. (1981) The expression of major histocompatibility antigens by human chorionic villi. *Journal of Reproductive Immunology*, **3**, 323–331.

Sutton, L., Mason, D.Y. and Redman, C.W.G. (1983) HLA-DR positive cells in the human placenta. *Immunology*, **49**, 103–113.

Sutton, L., Gadd, M., Mason, D.Y. and Redman, C.W.G. (1986) Cells bearing class II MHC antigens in the human placenta and amniochorion. *Immunology*, **58**, 23–29.

Taylor, C. and Faulk, W.P. (1981) Prevention of recurrent abortions with leucocyte transfusion. *Lancet*, **ii**, 68–70.

Toivanen, P. and Hirvonen, T. (1970) Placental weight in foetal-maternal incompatibility. *Clinical and Experimental Immunology*, **7**, 533–539.

Weir, P.E. (1981) Immunofluorescent studies of the uteroplacental arteries in normal pregnancy. *British Journal of Obstetrics and Gynaecology*, **88**, 301–307.

Wells, M., Hsi, B.-L. and Faulk, W.P. (1984) Class I antigens of the major histocompatibility complex on cytotrophoblast of the human placental basal plate. *American Journal of Reproductive Immunology*, **6**, 167–174.

13

NON-TROPHOBLASTIC TUMOURS OF THE PLACENTA

PRIMARY NEOPLASMS

In theory, tumours could arise from any of the non-trophoblastic elements of the placenta and it would not afford one any great astonishment if a placental fibroma or leiomyoma were to be described. The fact is, however, that convincing examples of such neoplasms have not been reported, and the only primary non-trophoblastic tumours of the placenta that are known to occur are the relatively common haemangioma (which is regarded by many as not being a true neoplasm), the very rare teratoma (the existence of which is doubted by some) and the hepatocellular adenoma, of which only one example has been recorded.

Placental Haemangioma

Haemangiomas of the placenta have long excited the interest of both pathologists and obstetricians, and have been the recurring subject of several reviews (Siddall, 1926; Marchetti, 1939; de Costa et al, 1956; Strakosch, 1956; Fox, 1967; Philippe et al, 1969; Lin et al, 1970; Wallenburg, 1971; Rendina and Patrono, 1975; Sieracki et al, 1975; Schramm et al, 1987; Sfar et al, 1991; Tan & Yeo, 1992). They masquerade in the literature, however, under at least 22 synonyms, the only ones of which that are histogenetically correct, useful and enjoy wide usage are 'chorangioma' and 'chorioangioma'. This nomenclatural plethora is a reflection of the variable and pleomorphic histological appearances of the haemangioma, and there are no histogenetic or histological reasons for dignifying such a lesion in the placenta with a name that is separate and distinct from that given to it when occurring in other organs.

Incidence

It used to be thought that these tumours were excessively rare, and in the older literature their incidence is variously quoted as being between one in 8000 and one in 50,000 placentas (Marchetti, 1939). Such figures only apply, however, to the distinctly uncommon large, and hence easily visible, haemangiomas and do not reflect their true frequency, because it has been the experience of nearly all workers who have made a careful and systematic study of sliced placentas that these tumours are found in approximately 1% (Table 13.1). The only observer failing to note this high incidence was

Table 13.1 Incidence of haemangiomata in systematic studies of placentae

Author	Number of placenta examined	Number of haemangiomata
Siddall (1926)	600	6
Zeek and Assali (1952)	562	4
Shaw-Dunn (1959)	500	7
Thomsen (1961)	660	7
van Assche, Brosens and Lauwerijns (1963)	100	4
Wentworth (1965)	620	8
Wilkin (1965)	376	3
Fox (1966)	500	5
Philippe et al (1969)	1000	7
Wallenburg (1971)	700	7
Nessmann-Emmanuelli, Breart and Kone-Pale (1978)	1200	4

Kuhnel (1933), who was unable to detect any haemangiomas in 500 carefully studied placentas. He did note, however, that 'round intraplacental apoplexy' was surprisingly common, which suggests that he was including within this rather strange category not only intervillous thrombi but also small haemangiomas, two lesions that can be very difficult to distinguish on macroscopic examination.

Pathology

Placental haemangiomas are usually single (Fig. 13.1) but occasionally multiple; the apparent record is in the placenta described by Fisher (1940), which contained 25 discrete tumours, each having its own pedicle. There have also been several instances in which a placenta has been diffusely infiltrated by haemangiomatous tissue (Fig. 13.2) (Szarthmary, 1934; Burger et al, 1952; Bret et al, 1953; Karnauchow, 1957; Gruenwald, 1963; Berge, 1966; Müller & Rieckert, 1967; Battaglia & Woolever, 1968; Du et al, 1968; Blom & Gevers, 1974; Jaffe et al, 1985; Glaser et al, 1988; Angelone et al, 1989), a condition often known as chorangiomatosis.

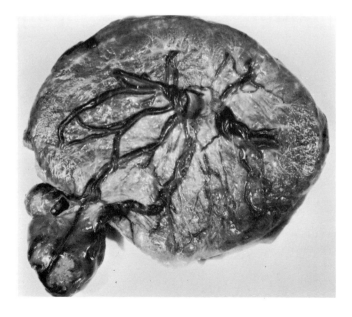

Figure 13.1. A large placental haemangioma; this is actually within the membranes and separate from the main placental mass, to which it is attached by a vascular pedicle.

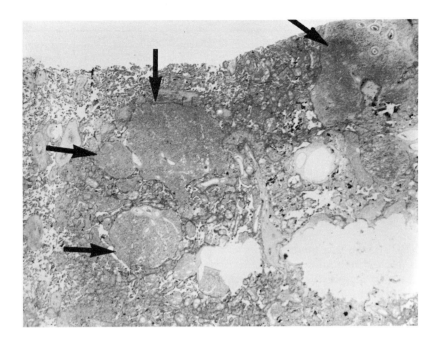

Figure 13.2. Multiple nodules of haemangiomatous tissue (arrowed) in the substance of a placenta (H & E ×2).

Large haemangiomas are seen most commonly as bulging protuberances on the fetal surface of the placenta, but a substantial minority occur on the maternal surface, where they may appear to replace the whole, or part, of a lobe (Fig. 13.3). Occasionally the tumour is situated entirely within the membranes, being attached to the placenta only by a vascular pedicle (Fig. 13.1). The vast majority of haemangiomas are, however, not visible on the external surface of the placenta; they are small and within the placental substance, and hence are unlikely to be noticed unless the placenta is systematically sliced. The tumours vary in size from a few millimetres in diameter (Fig. 13.4) to one

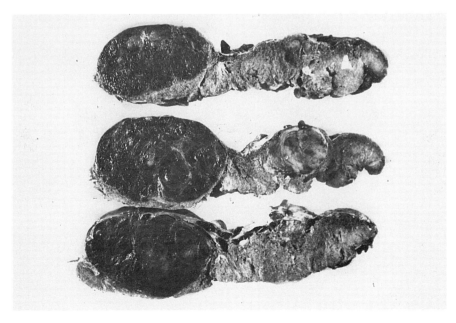

Figure 13.3. A large intraplacental haemangioma.

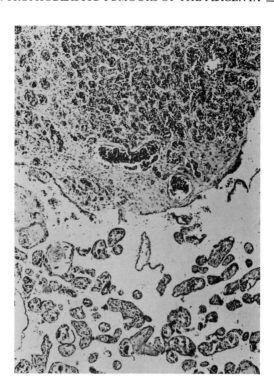

Figure 13.4. A small intraplacental haemangioma (above); this was only just visible to the naked eye (H & E ×40).

weighing 1500 g (Arodi et al, 1985). The large, externally visible haemangiomas usually have a purplish-red, glistening, encapsulated outer surface; they can be round, ovoid or reniform, are frequently bosselated, and sometimes deeply grooved by bands of fibrous tissue. The small intraplacental tumours are usually round and are demarcated from the surrounding normal villous tissue by an easily visible capsule. The cut surface of the tumour may be brown, yellow, tan, plum-coloured, red or white, and is usually smoother and firmer than normal placental tissue. The small haemangiomas may resemble intervillous thrombi, from which, however, they can be distinguished by the absence of lamination.

Placental haemangiomas show a very variable histological appearance, but usually fall into one of three microscopic types (Marchetti, 1939):

1. *Angiomatous*. Numerous blood vessels are set in a loose, inconspicuous stroma containing scanty fibrous tissue (Fig. 13.5); the vessels are usually small and of capillary size, but may be dilated to give a cavernous appearance.
2. *Cellular*. The tumour consists principally of loose, immature, cellular mesenchymal tissue containing only a few ill-formed vessels (Fig. 13.6).
3. *Degenerate*. The tumour shows myxoid change, hyalinization, necrosis or calcification; very rarely, fat may be present (Reddy et al, 1969).

This histological classification is useful for descriptive purposes but should not be taken as indicating any fundamental difference between the various subgroups; the cellular type is simply a less mature and less differentiated form of the angiomatous type. Indeed, many haemangiomas show a variable picture, being cellular in some areas and angiomatous in others (Figs 13.6 and 13.7), often with a gradual transition between the two histological patterns. The vast majority, however, do have an angiomatous pattern in at least one area and thus present no diagnostic challenge of any great severity, but the relatively uncommon tumours showing a cellular pattern throughout may give rise to difficulties, these sometimes being wrongly categorized as fibromas, myxomas or leiomyomas (Tapia et al, 1985).

Mitotic figures may occasionally be seen in a placental haemangioma and, very rarely, these are fairly numerous and associated with some degree of endothelial or

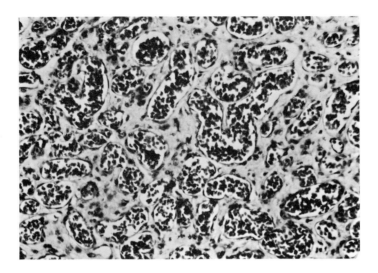

Figure 13.5. Histological appearance of a placental haemangioma; this has a typical 'angiomatous' pattern (H & E ×150).

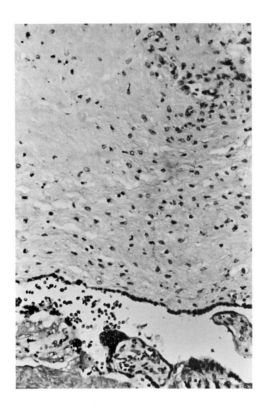

Figure 13.6. A placental haemangioma (above) which shows a 'cellular' pattern and is formed largely of loose, somewhat myxoid, mesenchymal tissue. Elsewhere there was a transition to a more characteristic, 'angiomatous' pattern (see Fig. 13.7) (H & E

stromal cell atypia. It has been suggested that tumours showing such features should be classified as 'atypical' haemangiomas (Majilessi et al, 1983) and although this is a fairly meaningless term, its use is certainly preferable to classifying these neoplasms as sarcomas (Cary, 1914; Ahrens, 1953) because there is no evidence that these tumours ever behave in a malignant fashion.

Electron microscopy has shown that the fine structure of the vessels in a placental haemangioma is very similar to that of normal capillaries, with apparently normal-looking endothelial cells resting on a basement membrane, outside of which are scattered pericytes (Kim et al, 1971; Cash & Powell, 1980).

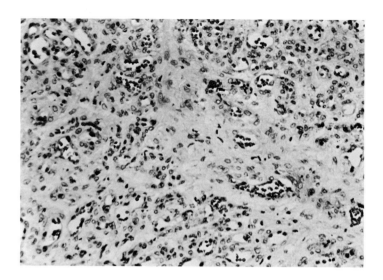

Figure 13.7. Another area of the same placental haemangioma that is illustrated in Fig. 13.6; here there is a transition from a 'cellular' to an 'angiomatous' pattern (H & E ×150).

Some workers have denied that haemangiomas are encapsulated, others have been able to trace a transition from normal villi to angiomatous tissue, whilst yet others have claimed that only a pseudo-capsule of compressed villi is present. In most cases, however, it is relatively easy to distinguish a well-delineated capsule of either fibrous tissue or syncytial epithelium (Fig. 13.8) together with, sometimes, cytotrophoblastic cells.

Two very unusual, and conceptually challenging, examples of a variant of a placental haemangioma, classed as a 'chorangiocarcinoma', have been described (Jauniaux et al, 1988; Trask et al, 1994). Both of these consisted of a typical haemangioma with a surrounding capsular mantle of atypical, proliferating trophoblast which closely

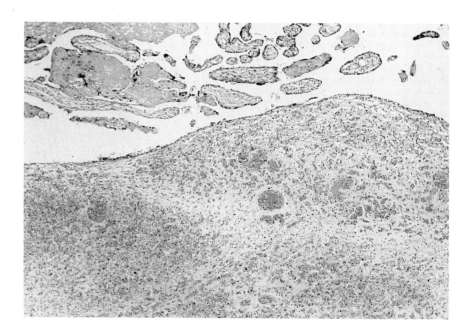

Figure 13.8. A placental haemangioma (on the right) is limited by a distinct capsule of attenuated syncytiotrophoblast.

resembled choriocarcinomatous tissue (Fig. 13.9). The nature, histogenetic status and significance of these extraordinary neoplasms are thoroughly obscure and the suggestion that they are intraplacental choriocarcinomas with associated tumour-stimulated angiogenesis (Trask et al, 1994) does not carry any conviction, if only because choriocarcinomas lack an intrinsic vasculature and do not appear to secrete angiogenic factors.

Chorangiomatosis, in which multiple nodules of haemangiomatous tissue are scattered throughout the placental substance, should be distinguished from 'chorangiosis' in which a proportion of the villi contain an excess of fetal vessels (Altshuler,

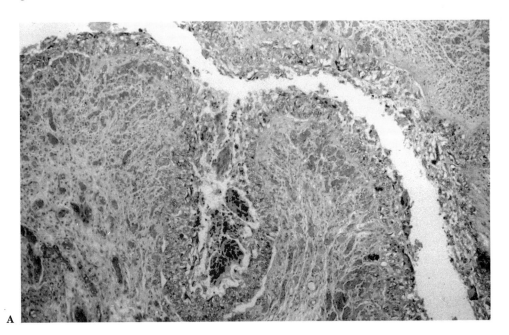

A

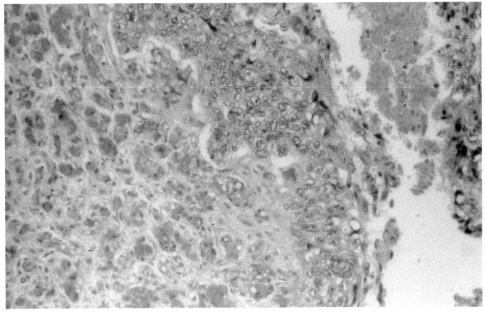

B

Figure 13.9. A placental chorangiocarcinoma. (**A**) General view showing a typical chorangioma with a surrounding mantle of atypical trophoblastic tissue which closely resembles a choriocarcinoma. (**B**) Higher-power view of covering mantle.

1984). In several reports in the literature, chorangiosis has been incorrectly used as a synonym for chorangiomatosis whilst it has sometimes been mooted that chorangiosis forms a link between normal villi and a haemangioma. However, there is no evidence that chorangiosis is an intermediate phase in the development, or a *form fruste*, of chorangiomatosis.

Associated Placental Features

The placenta containing a haemangioma is usually otherwise normal, but a small proportion are unduly heavy, sometimes weighing, after removal of the tumour, over a kilogram (Sen, 1970; Potashnik et al, 1973). It has been suggested that this bulkiness is due to vascular stasis within the placenta, as a result of compression of the umbilical veins by the tumour (Pensa, 1932), and although this is not a very plausible hypothesis it is nevertheless true that a few heavy placentas have been noted to be extremely oedematous (Earn & Penner, 1950; Lantéjoul & Heraux, 1951).

Occasional examples of haemangiomas occurring in circumvallate placentas have been reported, and it has been claimed that the abnormal shape of such placentas results from villous hyperplasia acting as a compensatory mechanism for the space occupied by the tumour (Eton, 1956). This is inherently unlikely (see Chapter 3) and the overall incidence of circumvallate forms in the reported cases of haemangiomas would not appear to be any higher than in a random series of placentas. Froehlich et al (1971) noted an association between haemangiomas and a single umbilical artery, a finding that has not, however, recieved any further confirmation.

A unique example has been described of a hydatidiform mole and a haemangioma occurring in the same placenta (Vermelin et al, 1957), a combination which is, bearing in mind the usual avascularity of a mole, rather curious. One placental haemangioma has been associated with bilateral ovarian theca-lutein cysts (King et al, 1991), a somewhat suprising finding because there is no evidence that placental haemangiomas secrete hCG.

Nature and Origin

Many of the early views on the histogenesis and nature of placental haemangiomas were highly speculative, often owing more to their proponents' imaginative powers than to their observational abilities; they include such hypotheses as those postulating the haemangioma to be due to villous hyperplasia, placental inflammation, villous fusion or organization of a thrombus, and that suggesting it to be an early stage in the evolution of a choriocarcinoma.

Today the haemangiomatous nature of these lesions is not disputed, but argument still persists as to whether they are true neoplasms or hamartomas; this argument is, of course, not confined to those haemangiomas that occur in the placenta. The occasional presence of mitotic figures and the frequent evidence of disproportionate growth between the angioma and the rest of the placenta have persuaded some that the placental haemangioma is a true neoplasm (Scott, 1924; Mugnai, 1938; Crainz, 1942; Davies, 1948; McInroy & Kelsey, 1954; Shaw-Dunn, 1959), but a majority opinion would incline towards its being a hamartoma which arises as a malformation of the primitive angioblastic tissue of the placenta, i.e. the chorionic mesenchyme. Indeed, the appearances of the cellular type of haemangioma mimic closely those seen in a primary villous stem during angiogenesis, which makes it probable that the tumour arises as a result of distorted angiogenesis in a single primary villous stem. This concept has been fully supported by an immunohistochemical study of the skeletal profile of five placental haemangiomas (Lifschitz-Mercer et al, 1989). This theory implies that the haemangioma arises during the earliest stages of placental development, and Snoeck and Wilkin (1952) have suggested that the malformation must occur at about the 16th day after fertilization. It is therefore a curious fact that there have been no reports of haemangiomas in placentas from first-trimester abortions.

Clinical Effects

The vast majority of placental haemangiomas are of no clinical importance, but a proportion are accompanied by a variety of complications that may affect the mother, the developing fetus or the neonate. It has usually been maintained that these complications are only found in association with tumours measuring more than 5 cm in diameter but in one study some haemangiomas of a smaller size were found to be clinically important (Mucitelli et al, 1990).

Complications during pregnancy

A high proportion of large haemangiomas are accompanied by polyhydramnios, the reported incidence of this association ranging from 16 to 33% (Fox, 1967). The only exception to this was in the series reported by Froehlich et al (1971), in which there was no excess incidence of this complication. This probably reflects the very low proportion of large tumours in this particular series because there seems little doubt that the presence of polyhydramnios is linked to the size of the haemangioma. Thus, Siddall (1924) found that if the tumour was 'larger than a hen's egg' the incidence of polyhydramnios was 48.7% whilst with smaller haemangiomas hydramnios occurred in only 11%. Kuhnel (1933) has disputed the implications of this observation, pointing out that many very large haemangiomas are not accompanied by polyhydramnios; this is perfectly correct, but it is equally true that it is usually only such tumours that are associated with polyhydramnios.

It has been maintained that the diagnosis of polyhydramnios is, in many cases of placental haemangioma, unfounded, being based only on the excessive size of the uterus, a sign that could be due solely to an unusually large placental mass. Nevertheless, the volume of liquor has been measured on several occasions, and figures such as 5, 6 or 10 litres (Merlino, 1939; Bury, 1954; de Costa et al, 1956; Bonneau et al, 1968) leave little doubt as to the authenticity of the hydramnios. Even so, it has been questioned whether a true causal relationship exists between the placental tumour and the polyhydramnios, it being pointed out that in some cases the accumulation of excess liquor is more likely to be due to an associated fetal abnormality such as spina bifida or anencephaly. Fox (1967) and Wallenburg (1971), however, in their reviews of placental haemangiomas, found that even after exclusion of all cases of fetal malformation, the incidence of polyhydramnios was still 14–22%, a figure too high to be dismissed as being purely coincidental.

The cause of the polyhydramnios is obscure; it has been suggested that liquor accumulates because of compression of the umbilical veins by the tumour (Klaften, 1929), but there is no evidence that those haemangiomas situated in close proximity to the cord are complicated unduly frequently by hydramnios (Wallenburg, 1971), whilst there have been several examples of tumours situated in the membranes, and thus totally incapable of compressing the cord, being associated with polyhydramnios (Fox, 1966). Kotz and Kaufman (1939) postulated that the fluid was a transudate from vascular channels on the fetal surface of the tumour, but this otherwise quite attractive hypothesis would clearly not account for those cases in which hydramnios complicates tumours situated entirely on the maternal surface of the placenta. McInroy and Kelsey (1954) proffered the ingenious view that the excess of liquor is the result of an increased secretion of fetal urine, the stimulus for which is the return to the fetus of waste products in the fetal blood that has passed through the physiologically useless tumour rather than through the placenta proper. Wallenburg (1971) has raised the possibility that fetal fluid imbalance caused by congestive cardiac failure, secondary to the haemangioma acting as a peripheral arterio-venous shunt, may be a factor in the development of the hydramnios. He points to those rare cases in which hydramnios appears to resolve spontaneously (MacIntosh & Osborn, 1968) and suggests that this could be due to thrombosis of the afferent vessels to the neoplasm, an event that would relieve the fetal cardiac embarrassment.

Which, if any, of these theories is correct is, at the moment, a matter for debate, though it is worth noting that a few haemangiomas are, for reasons even more cryptic, associated with oligohydramnios (Resnick, 1953; Engel et al, 1981; Wunsch & Furch, 1983).

There have been recurrent claims that an association exists between placental haemangiomas and pre-eclampsia (Heggtveit et al, 1965; Wentworth, 1965; Philippe et al, 1969; Froehlich et al, 1971; Sieracki et al, 1975), but this has not been everyone's experience (Asadourian & Taylor, 1968). If this association were proven, and I am far from convinced that it has been, no obvious explanation for it springs to mind. The suggestion of Wentworth (1965), that the pre-eclampsia is related to proliferation of cytotrophoblastic cells in the tumour capsule, is totally without appeal.

Antepartum bleeding may apparently complicate a placental haemangioma, but is usually caused by an unrelated accident of pregnancy. Very occasionally, however, haemorrhage may be secondary to retroplacental bleeding from a haemangioma (Sulman & Sulman, 1949) or to rupture of the vascular pedicle of a pedunculated tumour, a catastrophe that may lead to fetal exsanguination (Bukovinszky et al, 1960). It has been suggested that there may be a true, but rare, association between placental haemangiomas and abruptio placentae, it being postulated that the tumour alters the haemodynamics of the intervillous space in such a manner as to cause increased stress to an already fragile uteroplacental vessel (Kohler et al, 1976): this is an interesting view but one that remains to be proven.

It is often thought that placental haemangiomas predispose to premature onset of labour; indeed, in many series almost a third of pregnancies have terminated prematurely. However, this is nearly always due to labour being precipitated by polyhydramnios, and pregnancies uncomplicated by an excess accumulation of liquor usually proceed to term (Fox, 1967; Wallenburg, 1971).

It should be noted that placental haemangiomas, especially those large enough to be of possible clinical significance, can be readily diagnosed by ultrasound (Spirt et al, 1980; O'Malley et al, 1981; Liang et al, 1982; Wunsch & Furch, 1983; Scharl & Shlensker, 1987), even as early as the 19th week of gestation (Nahmanovici et al, 1982). Furthermore, a placental haemangioma may be associated with elevated levels of alpha-fetoprotein, either only in the maternal blood (Mann et al, 1983; Kapoor et al, 1989; Franca-Martins et al, 1990; Thomas & Blakemore, 1990) or in both maternal blood and amniotic fluid (Schnitger et al, 1980). Elevation of alpha-fetoprotein levels is, however, by no means a constant finding and is indeed present in only a minority of cases (Khong & George, 1994).

Complications during labour

Labour is usually normal in patients with a placental haemangioma, but there have been occasional instances in which a very large tumour has obstructed vaginal delivery (Emge, 1927). Rarely, the haemangioma may separate from the placenta during labour and be delivered per vaginum, either before delivery of the child or during the third stage before the placenta has separated (Shaw-Dunn, 1959; Bonneau et al, 1968). Exceptionally, the tumour may remain in the uterus after placental expulsion, an event that can lead to postpartum bleeding.

Complications affecting the fetus and neonate

The overall perinatal mortality in cases of placental haemangioma is only minimally increased (Fox, 1967). The very slight excess of deaths is in those rare cases in which either a large tumour, multiple tumours or a diffuse haemangiomatosis is present in the placenta. Fetal demise in these circumstances has been attributed to hypoxia because of shunting of fetal blood through the physiological dead space of the tumour, thus allowing it to bypass the functioning placental tissue and be returned to the fetus in an oxygen-depleted state (Shaw-Dunn, 1959). A similar explanation has been proffered for the exceptional instances in which large or multiple haemangiomas appear to be responsible for intrauterine fetal distress (Yule & O'Connor, 1964; Kamdom-Moyo et al, 1972; Ito et al, 1994). The view that fetal distress can be due to pressure of a large haemangioma on the normal placental tissue (Cardwell, 1988) has little to recommend it but fetal death can be due to cardiac failure as a consequence of the haemangioma acting as a peripheral arterio-venous shunt (Knoth et al, 1976; Hadi et al, 1993) or to compression of the cord by an unusually bulky tumour (Rodan & Bean, 1983).

The live-born infant whose placenta contains a haemangioma is usually normal, but a small proportion, particularly those with a placenta which is diffusely infiltrated by haemangiomatous tissue or which contains a very large tumour, are of low birth weight (Gruenwald, 1963; Vesanto et al, 1963; Müller & Rieckert, 1967; King & Lourien, 1978). In such circumstances it is again presumed that this is due to the shunting of blood through the tumour and its consequent return, in an unoxygenated and nutrient-poor state, to the fetus.

Skin angiomas have been noted in a few babies with a placental haemangioma (Ciulla, 1939; Bret & Duperrat, 1944; de Costa et al, 1956; Zawirska, 1964; Leblanc & Carrier, 1979), and were present in nine of the 74 cases reported by Froehlich et al (1971); these latter workers also noted cutaneous naevi in a further six infants. De Costa et al (1956) described a hepatic angioma in one of their infants with a placental haemangioma. There is some controversy as to whether there is otherwise an abnormally high incidence of congenital malformations in children with a placental haemangioma (Glaser et al, 1988). In the 344 cases that I reviewed (Fox, 1967) there were only eight malformed babies, a figure that did not particularly suggest a true association, especially in view of the tendency for such cases to be selectively and preferentially reported. This conclusion was, however, challenged by the findings of Froehlich et al (1971), who, in a prospective survey, encountered a high incidence of minor malformations; they included amongst these their examples of children with cutaneous angiomas or naevi and those with a single umbilical artery, but even after exclusion of such cases the incidence of malformation was still about 15%. It should be noted, however, that these were all of a relatively trivial nature, e.g., deformed ear or strabismus, and the findings of their survey do not suggest any real association between placental haemangiomas and major fetal malformation. Although one of the babies in the series of Froehlich et al (1971) was suffering from Down's syndrome, the combination of a placental haemangioma and a chromosomal abnormality has been reported in only one other instance (Wurster et al, 1969). Examples have been reported of placental haemangiomas occurring, almost certainly coincidentally, in association with the Beckwith–Wiedemann (Drut et al, 1992) and the Wolf–Hirschhorn (Verloes et al, 1991) syndromes.

The newborn infant whose placenta contains a large mass of haemangiomatous tissue is subject to several further complications, usually of a transitory nature, which are thought to be a direct consequence of the presence of the placental tumour (Table 13.2). Cardiomegaly may occur and has been attributed to the increased cardiac output required for shunting blood through the haemangioma which can, in haemodynamic terms, be considered as a peripheral arterio-venous shunt (Reiner & Fries, 1965). Neonatal oedema is uncommon and in some cases is a manifestation of cardiac failure (Nuttininen et al, 1988; Imakita et al, 1988; Eldar-Geva et al, 1988). In others, however, it has clearly been the result of fetal hypoalbuminaemia (Battaglia & Woolever, 1968; Jones et al, 1972; Sweet & Robertson, 1973; Sims et al, 1976), a deficiency thought to be due either to leakage of protein from the vessels of the haemangioma or to massive chronic feto-maternal bleeding. Du et al (1968) suggested that the rare instances of fetal anaemia could be due to sequestration of blood within the haemangioma, but this can also be due to a microangiopathic haemolytic anaemia resulting from injury inflicted on the red blood cells as they traverse the labyrinthine vascular channels of the tumour (Wallenburg, 1971; Bauer et al, 1978; Hirata et al, 1993). In some cases, however, the fetal anaemia has appeared to be due to a massive feto-maternal bleed, presumably from the tumour (Blom & Gevers, 1974; Sims et al, 1976; Stiller & Skafish, 1986; Santamaria et al, 1987; Franca-Martins et al, 1990). Neonatal thrombocytopenia is a rare complication of a placental vascular tumour; this may be due to platelet injury within the tumour vessels (Du et al, 1968) but can also be a manifestation of disseminated intravascular coagulation and a consumption coagulopathy which is triggered off by the release of a thromboplastic substance from the haemangioma (Jones et al, 1972; Ito

Table 13.2. Reported instances of transitory neonatal disorders ascribed to placental haemangiomas

Cardiomegaly	Burnard et al (1979)
Begg (1961)	Tonkin et al (1980)
Benson & Joseph (1961)	Green & Iams (1984)
Reiner & Fries (1965)	Stockhausen et al (1984)
Du et al (1968)	Imakita et al (1988)
Rauchenberg & Zeman (1971)	Hirata et al (1993)
Wallenburg (1971)	
Jones et al (1972)	*Anaemia*
Leonidas et al (1975)	Battaglia & Woolever (1968)
Leblanc & Carrier (1979)	Du et al (1968)
Tonkin et al (1980)	Mandelbaum et al (1969)
Green & Iams (1984)	Wurster et al (1969)
Eldar-Geva et al (1988)	Jones et al (1972)
Nuttininen et al (1988)	Sumathy et al (1973)
Koivu & Nuutinen (1990)	Blom & Gevers (1974)
Hirata et al (1993)	Sims et al (1976)
Ito et al (1994)	Bauer et al (1978)
	Wunsch & Furch (1983)
Oedema	Stockhausen et al (1984)
Phillip (1931)	Chazotte et al (1990)
Horn (1948)	Franca-Martins et al (1990)
Lantéjoul & Heraux (1951)	Lampe et al (1995)
Resnick (1953)	
Battaglia & Woolever (1968)	*Thrombocytopenia*
Monteforte (1968)	Froehlich et al (1971)
Mandelbaum et al (1969)	Jones et al (1972)
Jones et al (1972)	Sims et al (1976)
Sweet & Robertson (1973)	Bauer et al (1978)
Blom & Gevers (1974)	Lopez-Herce et al (1983)
Sims et al (1976)	Jaffe et al (1985)

et al, 1994). Neonatal thrombocytopenia resulting from a placental haemangioma has led to fatal intracerebral haemorrhage (Lopez-Herce et al, 1983).

Recurrence

Very little is known about the possibility of recurrence of placental haemangiomas in successive pregnancies, but Ludighausen and Sahiri (1983) described a case in which multiple large haemangiomas were present in the placenta of a woman's first and third pregnancies, both of which resulted in intrauterine fetal death. Chan and Leung (1988) have reported a not dissimilar patient who in successive pregnancies had a placenta containing multiple haemangiomas, these being associated in both gestations with intrauterine fetal demise.

Teratoma of Placenta

Placental teratomas are rare, less than 20 examples having been recorded (Table 13.3). The tumour always lies between the amnion and chorion, usually on the fetal surface of the placenta but sometimes in the membranes adjacent to the placental margin (Fig. 13.10). The teratoma described by Fujikura and Wellings (1964) was attached to the placenta by a short pedicle, but this is an unusual feature. The tumours are smooth, round or oval, and measure between 2.5 and 7.5 cm in diameter; they lack an umbilical cord and their arterial supply is usually from a branch of a fetal artery on the surface of the placenta, the only exception to this being the tumour of Fujikura and Wellings (1964), which was supplied by an arterial branch arising directly from an

Table 13.3. Reported cases of placental teratoma

Morville (1925)	Svanholm & Thordsen (1987)
Kuster (1928)	Reus & Geppert (1988)
Perez et al (1939)	Fernandez-Figueras et al (1989)
Fox & Butler-Manuel (1964)	Unger (1989)
Fujikura & Wellings (1964)	Block et al (1991)
Joseph & Vogt (1973)	Gayer et al (1994)
Kobos & Sporny (1982)	Sironi et al (1994)
Smith & Pounder (1982)	Williams & Williams (1994)
Nickell & Stocker (1987)	

umbilical artery. Histologically, these neoplasms have the usual appearances of a benign teratoma, and contain squamous epithelium, often with skin appendages, together with a mélange of fat, muscle, mesenchyme, neural tissue, gastrointestinal-type epithelium, cartilage and disorganized bone. In all the reported cases, the contained tissue elements have been fully mature and there has been no evidence of malignancy.

Placental teratomas are of no clinical significance, but that reported by Fox and Butler-Manuel (1964) was visible as a partially calcified intrauterine mass on radiological examination at the 33rd week of gestation. A placental teratoma may also be detectable on ultrasound examination (Williams & Williams, 1994).

Not everybody accepts that these tumours are teratomas and it has been argued that they are, in fact, wrongly diagnosed examples of fetus acardius amorphus (Benirschke & Driscoll, 1967; Smith & Pounder, 1982). It has been suggested that a distinction can be drawn between these two entities (Fox & Butler-Manuel, 1964) on the following grounds:

1. A fetus acardius amorphus has a separate umbilical cord which is attached either to the placenta of a normal (or relatively normal) twin or to a separate placenta; such a cord may be poorly developed or even rudimentary, but is, in many cases, almost fully developed and easily recognizable. A placental teratoma does not have an umbilical cord and receives its arterial blood from a major fetal vessel coursing over the surface of the placenta.

2. A fetus acardius amorphus is usually described as an amorphous mass of tissue that is completely lacking in organization. In fact, a complete failure of organization is most unusual, and in many examples it is possible to recognize cranial and caudal ends of the fetus, whilst, in most, the central skeleton is relatively well developed. The pattern of skeletal development is notably consistent, in that the vertebral column is partially or wholly present in an easily recognizable form; ribs, pelvis and base of skull can often be identified. This degree of organization is not seen in a teratoma, in which any bone present is usually totally disorganized.

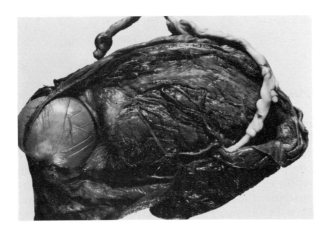

Figure 13.10. A placental teratoma which is situated in the membranes immediately adjacent to the main placental mass. The teratoma did not have an umbilical cord, showed no evidence of axial organization, and contained skin, neural tissue, fat, cartilage and bone.

These distinguishing criteria have, however, been criticized by Stephens et al (1989) who, in particular, claimed that lack of an umbilical cord does not help in the distinction between a teratoma and a fetus amorphus. These authors do allow that the extent of skeletal development is a reasonably valid criterion but nevertheless came to the conceptually nihilistic conclusion that distinction of a placental teratoma from a fetus amorphus is meaningless.

The histogenesis of a placental teratoma is a matter of considerable interest. There now seems little doubt that teratomas are derived from germ cells (Fox & Langley, 1976). These germ cells arise in the dorsal wall of the yolk sac (in the area that will eventually form the hind gut), migrate into the primitive gut wall, and then continue through the mesothelial coat and the root of the mesentery to the dorsal body wall and the genital folds. In the loose tissue at the base of the mesentery some of these cells may go astray and migrate to a more distant midline structure such as the pineal body or the mediastinum, where they can eventually give rise to a teratoma. During the first 3 months of gestation there is an evagination of primitive gut into the umbilical cord and, occasionally, well-formed intestinal epithelium is seen in the cord as late as the fourth month of pregnancy. It is possible that primordial germ cells may migrate out through the wall of this evaginated gut into the connective tissue of the cord. If they are arrested at this site they may give rise to a teratoma of the cord (see Chapter 15), but if they continue their migration they will pass into the loose connective tissue between the amnion and the fetal surface of the placenta and from there into the extraplacental membranes between chorion and amnion. It will be seen that the placental teratomas which have been described all lie along this proposed route of aberrant migration of germ cells.

McKay (cited by Joseph & Vogt, 1973) has suggested that, since the yolk sac and placental precursor are in such close geographic proximity during early development, it may not be necessary to invoke the histogenetic theory outlined above, because a nest of germ cells could easily be displaced to the developing placenta. This does not fully explain, however, why the teratomas should always lie between the amnion and chorion and not within the placental substance.

Hepatocellular Adenoma

A placental tumour of this type has been described by Chen et al (1986). This was an intraplacental tan-white mass that measured 7 cm in diameter and histologically resembled fetal liver. It is probable that this arose from heterotopic hepatic tissue, which can occur in the placenta, presumably developing from displaced yolk sac elements.

SECONDARY NEOPLASMS

Placental Metastases from Maternal Neoplasms

Malignant disease in a pregnant woman, although uncommon, is by no means exceptional, but in only a few cases have metastases to the placenta been noted. The documented examples, excluding instances of leukaemia or lymphoma, are detailed in Table 13.4.

Metastases to the placenta are invariably blood-borne and occur only in patients with widely disseminated malignant disease. It is probably not surprising, therefore, that malignant melanomas, which are prone both to develop in relatively young individuals and to undergo extensive vascular spread, figure so prominently amongst maternal neoplasms involving the placenta. Next in frequency are carcinomas of the breast and bronchus, this probably being a reflection not only of the high incidence of these neoplasms but also of their tendency to spread via the bloodstream at an early stage of their evolution. The infrequency with which gastrointestinal neoplasms metastasize to the placenta is worth noting, whilst reports of placental involvement by a cervical neoplasm are notable for their extreme rarity. This latter deficiency is particularly striking in view of the fact that cervical carcinomas are amongst the most common

Table 13.4. Placental metastases from maternal neoplasms

Author	Maternal disease	Placenta			
		Gross deposits	Tumour cells in intervillous space	Villous invasion	Spread to fetus
Walz (1906)	Myxosarcoma thigh	+	+	+	0
Markus (1910)	Malignant melanoma	+	+	+	0
Senge (1912)	Carcinoma stomach	+	+	+	0
Gray et al (1939)	Carcinoma adrenal	0	+	+	0
Holland (1949)	Malignant melanoma	+	+	+	+
Bender (1950)	Carcinoma ethmoid	0	+	0	0
Bender (1950)	Carcinoma stomach	0	+	0	0
Cross et al (1951)	Carcinoma breast	+	+	0	0
Barr (1953)	Carcinoma bronchus	0	+	0	0
Byrd & McGanity (1954)	Malignant melanoma	+	+	0	0
Reynolds (1955)	Malignant melanoma	0	+	0	0
Freedman & McMahon (1960)	Malignant melanoma	+	+	0	0
Horner (1960)	Carcinoma ovary	0	+	0	0
Moschella (1961)	Malignant melanoma	+	+	0	0
Hesketh (1962)	Carcinoma bronchus	0	+	0	0
Pisarki & Mrozewski (1964)	Carcinoma breast	+	+	+	0
Rosemond (1964)	Carcinoma breast	0	+	0	0
Brodsky et al (1965)	Malignant melanoma	+	+	+	+
Rewell & Whitehouse (1966)	Carcinoma breast	0	+	0	0
Jones (1969)	Carcinoma bronchus	0	+	0	0
Metler et al (1970)	Carcinoma breast	0	+	0	0
Stephenson et al (1971)	Malignant melanoma	+	+	+	0
Rothman et al (1973)	Carcinoma rectum	+	+	0	0
Angate et al (1975)	Carcinoma breast	0	+	0	0
Gillis et al (1976)	Malignant melanoma	+	+	0	0
Smythe et al (1976)	Carcinomatosis – primary site unknown	0	+	0	0
Smythe et al (1976)	Carcinoma pancreas	0	+	0	0
Smythe et al (1976)	Malignant melanoma	0	+	0	0
Sokol et al (1976)	Malignant melanoma	+	+	+	0
Frick et al (1977)	Vaginal angiosarcoma	+	+	0	0
Russell & Laverty (1977)	Malignant melanoma	+	+	+	0
Looi & Wang (1979)	Malignant melanoma	0	+	+	0
Cailliez et al (1981)	Squamous cell carcinoma of cervix	+	+	+	0
Read & Platzer (1981)	Carcinoma bronchus	+	+	0	0
Greenberg et al (1982)	Ewing's sarcoma of bone	+	+	+	0
Orr et al (1982)	Squamous cell carcinoma of neck	+	+	+	0
Sedgeley et al (1985)	Angiosarcoma of breast				
Suda et al (1986)	Adenocarcinoma of lung	0	+	0	0
Anderson et al (1989)	Malignant melanoma	0	+	+	0
Delerive et al (1989)	Bronchial carcinoma	0	+	0	0
Patsner et al (1989)	Carcinoma ovary	0	+	0	0
Schmidt et al (1989)	Adenoid cystic carcinoma of trachea	0	+	0	0
Pfuhl & Panitz (1991)	Carcinoma breast	0	+	+	0
Pollack et al (1993)	Medulloblastoma	0	+	0	0
Brossard et al (1994)	Malignant melanoma	0	+	0	0
Brossard et al (1994)	Medulloblastoma	0	+	0	0
O'Day et al (1994)	Orbital rhabdomyosarcoma	+	+	0	0
Salamon et al (1994)	Carcinoma breast	0	+	0	0

tumours to complicate the pregnant state, but one that is perhaps explicable by the tendency for these neoplasms to spread principally by lymphatic routes. Only a few examples of maternal sarcomas that have involved the placenta have been recorded.

Placentas involved by a malignant melanoma are often, though not invariably, macroscopically abnormal; sometimes tumour deposits are visible as black or brown nodules of varying size within the placental substance, whilst not uncommonly the placenta is generally rather firm and has a brownish or greyish tinge. Histologically, malignant melanotic cells are invariably seen in the intervillous space, either as clumps or sheets (Fig. 13.11). Central necrosis is not uncommon in large masses of tumour cells and it should be noted that, to the unwary eye, the neoplastic cells may be mistaken for proliferating trophoblast. Villous involvement by melanoma cells is an inconstant finding, the villi often being enveloped by tumour cells without any obvious tissue invasion (Fig. 13.12). Nevertheless, infiltration of the villous stroma, and sometimes the villous fetal vessels, by malignant cells has been noted in approximately half of the reported

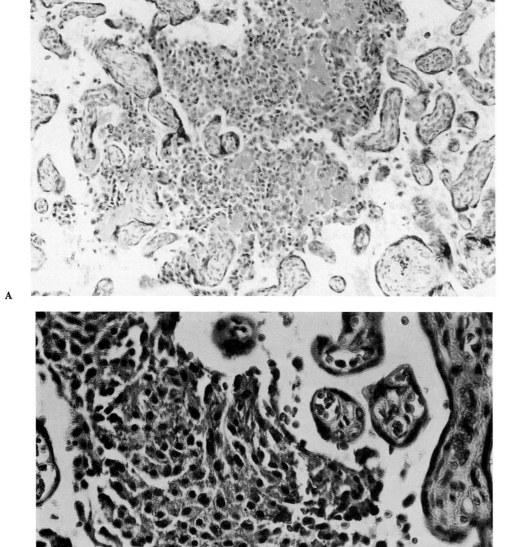

A

B

Figure 13.11. (A) A placental metastasis from a maternal malignant melanoma. The malignant cells are forming a sheet within the intervillous space and there is no infiltration of the villi (H & E ×80). **(B)** A higher-power view of a placental metastasis from a cutaneous malignant melanoma (H & E ×120).

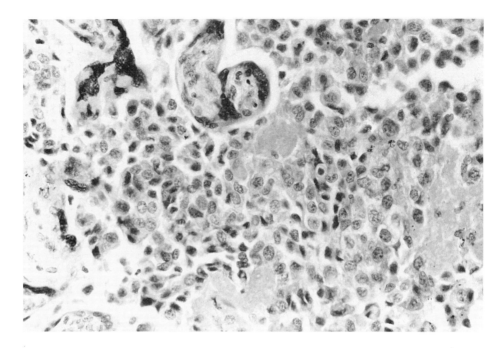

Figure 13.12. Metastatic malignant melanoma in the intervillous space. The neoplastic cells surround, but do not invade, a villus (H & E ×190).

cases. The villous Hofbauer cells often contain an abundance of melanin pigment, this being responsible for the generalized discoloration of the placenta; pigment deposition of this type occurs independently of villous invasion.

Placentas containing metastatic deposits of non-melanotic neoplasms usually appear normal to the naked eye because gross lesions, in the form of visible tumour deposits, are present in only just over a quarter of the reported cases; the deposits can be as large as 1–2 cm in diameter, but may be of only pin-head size. At the histological level, neoplastic cells are seen, as clumps or sheets, in the intervillous space with villous or fetal vascular invasion being rare (Fig. 13.13).

It should perhaps be stressed that, although the presence of malignant cells in the intervillous space is usually classed as a 'placental metastasis', the tumour cells are in fact still within the maternal vascular system and are not invading the placental tissue. This has led some workers to decry the use of the term 'metastasis' in this context and to propose that this is simply a sequestration phenomenon. Nevertheless, the large sheets of malignant cells found in the intervillous space in some instances suggest that tumour growth is occurring in this intravascular site. Further, the cells must have a point of contact with villous or extravillous trophoblast, either by direct implantation or by being bound down by fibrin, because the cells cannot simply float around unattached in the intervillous space. The fact that such an anchoring attachment has not been demonstrated is largely a reflection of the rather cursory examination to which most placentas containing malignant cells appear to have been subjected. The failure, in most cases, of maternal malignant cells to penetrate the villous tissue may be simply due to the trophoblast acting as a physical barrier, though the possibility that the fetal tissues of the placenta reject the maternal tumour cells by an immunological mechanism has often been mooted. The proponents of this latter view have, however, offered no proof for their suggestion, have not elaborated on the exact nature of the proposed immunological process involved, and have not remarked on the absence of immunocompetent cells in the villi that are resisting attack.

The placental barrier, whatever its nature, is not always inviolate and can be breached by malignant cells which pass over to the fetus; this occurs particularly, and indeed perhaps only, with malignant melanoma. Two instances have been fully

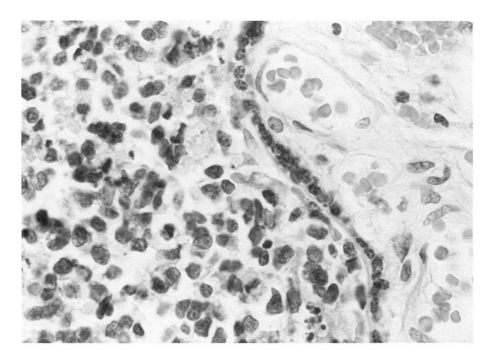

Figure 13.13. A metastatic deposit of Ewing's sarcoma in the intervillous space adjacent to an intact villus (H & E ×600).

documented: the child in Holland's (1949) case (which was also reported by Weber et al, 1930) died at 8 months of age, whilst the infant described by Brodsky et al (1965) died after 48 days of life. Widespread deposits of malignant melanoma were present in both children and it is of particular interest that in both these cases malignant cells had been seen within fetal villous vessels. The mere presence of malignant cells in the villous stroma or within fetal villous vessels should not, however, be taken as absolute proof of spread to the fetus, because in several cases in which this phenomenon has been noted, there has been no subsequent evidence of fetal involvement (see Table 13.3).

There have been only two well-documented examples of placental involvement by maternal malignant lymphoma, both being non-Hodgkin's lymphomas (Kurtin et al, 1992; Tsujimura et al, 1993), but there have been a few scattered reports of spread of leukaemic cells to the placenta in women suffering from acute or subacute leukaemia during pregnancy (Bierman et al, 1956; Rigby et al, 1964; Nummi et al, 1973; Honore & Brown, 1990). In each instance the leukaemic cells were confined to the intervillous space, where they appeared as sheets, clumps or groups (Fig. 13.14). Placental involvement in leukaemia is, however, possibly more common than the paucity of reported instances would suggest, because Diamandopoulos and Hertig (1963) noted that malignant cells were present in the intervillous space in 22 of 24 placentas from leukaemic women, whilst Gorbunova and Streneva (1967) found placental involvement in two of 14 women whose pregnancy had been complicated by this disease. There must, however, be some scepticism about the validity of the term 'placental involvement' in a proportion of the reported cases. Clearly, if the mother has an extremely high peripheral white blood count, many leukaemic cells will be seen in the maternal blood trapped in the intervillous space, and such a finding alone does not mean that the placenta is 'involved' in the malignant process; such an involvement should only be considered if large clumps or sheets of leukaemic cells are seen.

No instance of villous involvement by leukaemic cells has been reported. Some light has been shed on this deficiency by a study of a placenta from a woman with acute lymphoblastic leukaemia in which phagocytosis and destruction of neoplastic cells

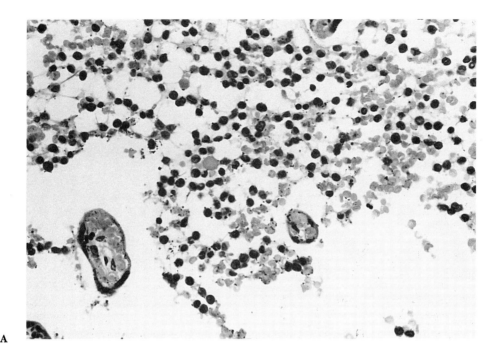

A

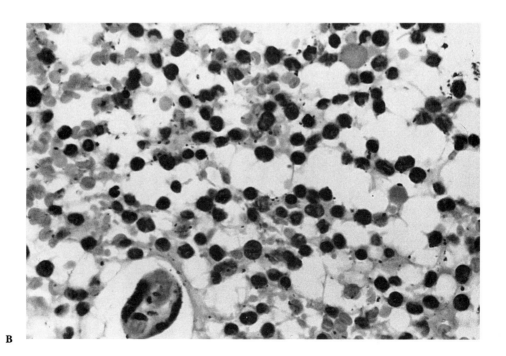

B

Figure 13.14. (A) Leukaemic cells in the intervillous space of a placenta from a woman suffering from acute leukaemia (H & E ×40). (B) Higher-power view of part of the field shown in Fig. 13.14A (H & E ×360).

within the villous trophoblastic cells was clearly demonstrable on electron microscopic examination (Wang et al, 1983).

Placental Metastases from Fetal Neoplasms

The dissemination of fetal malignant disease to involve the placenta is an event so uncommon as to rank almost as a curiosity. Nevertheless the apparent rarity of this phenomenon has probably been compounded by the fact that most congenital neoplasms are not apparent at birth and by the infrequency with which placentas are submitted to routine histological examination.

The tumour attracting most attention has been the neuroblastoma, and there are several well-documented examples of placental metastases from such a neoplasm (Strauss & Driscoll, 1964; Anders et al, 1970; Hustin & Chef, 1972; Jurkovik et al, 1973; Johnson & Halbert, 1974; Perkins et al, 1980; Stovring, 1980; van der Slikke & Balk, 1980; Smith et al, 1981; Mutz & Sterling, 1991). The descriptions given of the gross and microscopic features of the placentas in these cases have been strikingly uniform, as all were bulky, pale, oedematous and heavy (mostly weighing over 1000 g) and all bore a close resemblance to the hydropic placenta of severe erythroblastosis fetalis. In each case tumour deposits were not macroscopically visible, and the detection of neoplastic involvement was dependent on histological examination, which revealed plugging of the fetal villous vessels by nests and clumps of neuroblastomatous cells (Fig. 13.15). In some placentas the malignant cells were widely disseminated throughout the fetal vasculature and in one of Strauss and Driscoll's (1964) cases they were seen in every villus; this was perhaps an extreme example, but in all instances neoplastic cells have been seen in every low-power field. The tumour cells were usually confined to the fetal vessels and in only one case (Fig. 13.16) was invasion of the villous stroma seen (Perkins et al, 1980). The villi of the involved placentas have tended to be large, oedematous and rather immature with, sometimes, a proliferation of stromal mesenchymal cells. These abnormalities were present both in villi vascularized by tumour-infiltrated vessels and in those with vessels free of neoplastic cells.

It is not clear whether the failure of the neuroblastomatous cells to penetrate into the villous stroma is due to mechanical or immunological factors. Strauss and Driscoll (1964) tended to think that an immunological defence mechanism of some type was involved, basing this view on the general resemblance of these placentas to those seen in severe materno-fetal rhesus incompatibility, and on their finding, in one case, of nuclear debris in the perivascular villous stroma. The truth or otherwise of this concept is, at the moment, an imponderable, but the placental changes are certainly not due solely to the presence of neoplastic cells because Birner (1961) has described identical villous abnormalities in a placenta from a baby with a congenital neuroblastoma that had not spread to involve the placenta. This lends support to the view that the placental oedema and bulkiness is due simply to mechanical obstruction of venous return by a large intra-abdominal mass.

There have been single reports of placental metastases from a fetal hepatoblastoma (Robinson & Rolande, 1985) and from a fetal malignant melanoma which had arisen in a giant melanocytic naevus (Schneiderman et al, 1987). The placenta in this latter case was extremely bulky and melanoma cells were present both within the fetal villous vessels and in the stroma of the villi. Nests, or aggregates, of intravillous naevus cells have also been noted in placentas from fetuses with benign giant skin naevi (Holaday & Castrow, 1968; Werner, 1972; Demian et al, 1974; Sotelo-Avila et al, 1988; Jauniaux et al, 1993; Antaya et al, 1995) and these have usually been described as 'metastases'. It is, however, more probable that the naevus cell aggregates are due to aberrant migration of neural crest elements in early gestation.

No other solid fetal tumour has, to the best of my knowledge, been reported as having spread to the placenta, but a few instances of placental involvement in fetal leukaemia have been reported (Benirschke & Driscoll, 1967; Gray et al, 1986; Las Heras et al, 1986). The placentas in these cases have tended to be bulky and

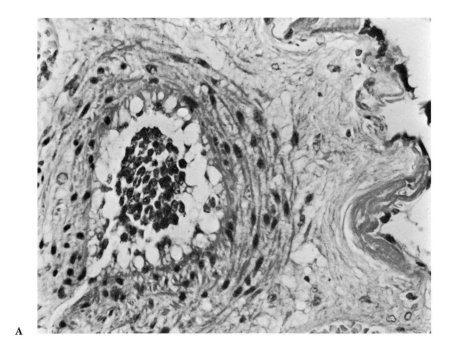

A

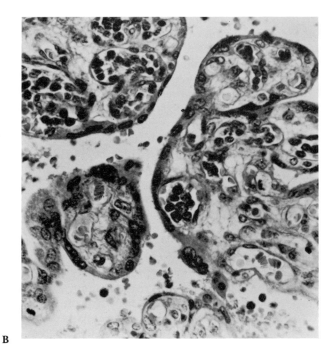

B

Figure 13.15. (**A**) A fetal stem artery in a placenta from a fetus with a widely metastasizing thoracic neuroblastoma. The arterial lumen is plugged by a clump of neuroblastomatous cells (H & E ×120). (**B**) Villi from the placenta illustrated in Fig. 13.15A. Many of the fetal villous vessels contain groups of malignant cells (H & E ×120).

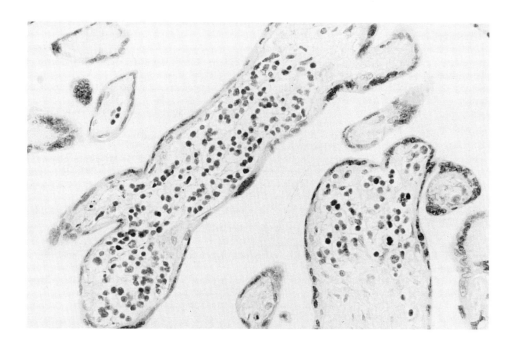

Figure 13.16. Villi in a placenta containing metastatic fetal neuroblastoma. The neoplastic cells have broken out from the fetal vessels and are infiltrating the villous stroma (H & E ×80).

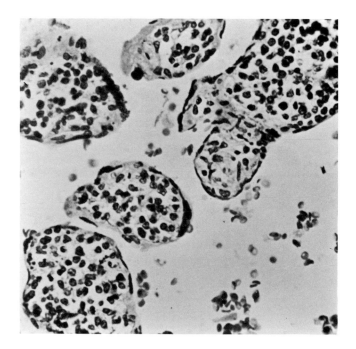

Figure 13.17. Villi in a placenta from a fetus with acute leukaemia. They are extensively infiltrated by leukaemic cells (H & E ×240).

oedematous and have contained large numbers of leukaemic cells both within the villous vessels and stroma, such cells being absent from the intervillous space. A further example of fetal leukaemia with placental villous involvement is shown in Fig. 13.17.

REFERENCES

Ahrens, C.A. (1953) Vier Falle von Plazentatumoren. *Zeitschrift für allgemeinen Pathologie und pathologische Anatomie*, **90**, 144.

Altshuler, G. (1984) Choriangiosis: an important placental sign of neonatal morbidity and mortality. *Archives of Pathology and Laboratory Medicine*, **108**, 71–74.

Anders, D., Frick, R. and Kindermann, G. (1970) Metastasierendes Neuroblastom des Feten mit Aussaat in die Plazenta. *Geburtshilfe und Frauenheilkunde*, **30**, 969–975.

Anderson, J.F., Kent, S. and Machin G.A. (1989) Maternal malignant melanoma with placental metastasis: a case report with literature review. *Pediatric Pathology*, **9**, 35–42.

Angate, A.Y., Loubiere R., Battesti, F., Coulibaly, A.O. and Fretillere, N. (1975) Métastase placentaire secondaire a un cancer du sein avec survie de trente et un mois de l'enfant. *Chirurgie*, **101**, 121–128.

Angelone, A., Caruso, A., Berghella, A., Sindici, G. and Bianchi, O. (1989) Sur un caso di emangioma diffuso della placenta. *Minerva Ginecologia*, **41**, 625–628.

Antaya, R.J., Keller, R.A. and Wilkerson, J.A. (1995) Placental nevus cells associated with giant congenital pigmented nevi. *Pediatric Dermatology*, **12**, 260–262.

Arodi, J., Auslender, R., Atad, J. and Abramovici, H. (1985) Case report: giant chorioangioma of the placenta. *Acta Obstetricia et Gynecologica Scandinavica*, **64**, 91–92.

Asadourian, L.A. and Taylor, H.B. (1968) Clinical significance of placental hemangiomas. *Obstetrics and Gynecology*, **31**, 551–555.

Barr, J.S. (1953) Placental metastases from a bronchial carcinoma. *Journal of Obstetrics and Gynaecology of the British Empire*, **60**, 895–897.

Battaglia, F.C. and Woolever, C.A. (1968) Fetal and neonatal complications associated with recurrent chorioangiomas. *Pediatrics*, **41**, 62–66.

Bauer, C.R., Fojaco, R.M., Bancalari, E. and Fernandez-Rocha, L. (1978) Microangiopathic hemolytic anemia and thrombocytopenia in a neonate associated with a large placental chorionangioma. *Pediatrics*, **62**, 574–577.

Begg, J.D.A. (1961) A further case of chorangioma. *Journal of Obstetrics and Gynaecology of the British Empire*, **68**, 229–231.

Bender, S. (1950) Placental metastases in malignant disease complicated by pregnancy; with a report of two cases. *British Medical Journal*, **i**, 980–981.

Benirschke, K. and Driscoll, S.G. (1967) *The Pathology of the Human Placenta*. Berlin, Heidelberg, New York: Springer-Verlag.

Benson, P.F. and Joseph, M.C. (1961) Cardiomegaly in a newborn due to a placental chorioangioma. *British Medical Journal*, **i**, 102–105.

Berge, T. (1966) Placental chorioangiomatosis. *Acta Pathologica et Microbiologica Scandinavica*, **66**, 465–470.

Bierman, H.R., Aggeler, P.M., Thelander, H., Kelly, K.H. and Cordes, F.L. (1956) Leukemia and pregnancy: a problem in transmission in man. *Journal of the American Medical Association*, **161**, 220–223.

Birner, W.F. (1961) Neuroblastoma as a cause of antenatal death. *American Journal of Obstetrics and Gynecology*, **82**, 1388–1391.

Block, D., Cruikshank, S., Kelly, K. and Stanley, M. (1991) Placental teratoma. *International Journal of Gynaecology and Obstetrics*, **34**, 377–380.

Blom, A.H. and Gevers, R.H. (1974) Een patiente met diffuse chorioangiomatosis placentae. *Nederlands Tijdschrift voor Geneeskunde*, **118**, 7–10.

Bonneau, H., Fouque, J.P., Varette, I., Blanc, B. and Danjoux, R. (1968) A propos de deux cas de chorioangiomes placentaires. *Bulletin de la Fédération des Sociétés de Gynécologie et d'Obstétrique de Langue Francaise*, **20**, 56–59.

Bret, J. and Duperrat, B. (1944) Angiome du placenta. *Gynécologie et Obstétrique*, **44**, 334.

Bret, A.J., Loewe-Lyon, Mme, Duperrat, B. and Gauthier, R. (1953) L'hémangiome racémeux du placenta. *Presse Médical*, **61**, 1193–1196.

Brodsky, I., Baren, M., Kahn, S.B., Lewis, G. Jr and Tellem, M. (1965) Metastatic malignant melanoma from mother to fetus. *Cancer*, **18**, 1048–1054.

Brossard, J., Abish, S., Bernstein, M.L., Baruchel, S., Kovacs, L. and Pollack, R. (1994) Maternal malignancy involving the products of conception: a report of malignant melanoma and medulloblastoma. *American Journal of Pediatric Hematology and Oncology*, **16**, 380–383.

Bukovinszky, L., Jakobovits, A. and Barna, J. (1960) Plazentatumor mit Gefässeruptur. *Zentralblatt für Gynäkologie*, **82**, 502–506.

Burger, P., Fruhling, L. and Wurch, T. (1952) Reticulo-hemangio-endotheliome diffus du placenta avec hydramnios et monstre coelosome porteur de malformations multiples. *Révue Francaise de Gynécologie et d'Obstétrique*, **47**, 45–54.

Burnard, N.J., Merino, W.T. and LiVolsi, V.A. (1979) Chorangiosis of the placenta and hydrops fetalis. *American Journal of Diagnostic Gynecology and Obstetrics*, **1**, 257–260.

Bury, R.D. (1954) A case of placental haemangioma. *Proceedings of the Royal Society of Medicine*, **47**, 911.

Byrd, B.F. and McGanity, W.J. (1954) The effect of pregnancy on the clinical course of malignant melanoma. *Southern Medical Journal*, **47**, 196–199.

Cailliez, D., Moirot, M.H., Fessaro, C., Hemet, J. and Philippe E. (1981) Localization placentaire d'un carcinoma du col uterin. *Journal de Gynécologie, Obstétrique et Biologie de la Reproduction*, **9**, 461–463.

Cardwell, M.S. (1988) Antenatal management of a large placental chorangioma: a case report. *Journal of Reproductive Medicine*, **33**, 68–70.

Cary, W.H. (1914) Report of a well authenticated case of sarcoma of the placenta. *American Journal of Obstetrics*, **69**, 658–664.

Cash, J.B. and Powell, D.E. (1980) Placental chorangioma: presentation of a case with electron-microscopic and immmunochemical studies. *American Journal of Surgical Pathology*, **4**, 87–92.

Chan, K.W. and Leung, C.Y. (1988) Recurrent multiple chorioangiomas and intrauterine death. *Pathology*, **20**, 77–78.

Chazotte, C., Girz, B., Koenigsberg, M. and Cohen, W.R. (1990) Spontaneous infarction of placental chorioangioma and associated regression of hydrops fetalis. *American Journal of Obstetrics and Gynecology*, **163**, 1180–1181.

Chen, K.T.K., Ma, C.K. and Kassel, S.H. (1986) Hepatocellular adenoma of the placenta. *American Journal of Surgical Pathology*, **10**, 436–440.

Ciulla, U. (1939) Angioma fetale associato angioma placentare. *Atti della Societa di Ostetricia e Ginecologia*, **35**, 48–53.

Crainz, F. (1942) L'angioma della placenta. *Monitore Ostetrico-Ginecologico di Endocrinologia e del Metabolismo*, **14**, 827–895.

Cross, R.G., O'Connor, M.H. and Holland, P.D.J. (1951) Placental metastasis of a breast carcinoma. *Journal of Obstetrics and Gynaecology of the British Empire*, **58**, 810–811.

Davies, D.V. (1948) A benign tumour of the placenta. *Journal of Obstetrics and Gynaecology of the British Empire*, **55**, 44–46.

de Costa, E.J., Gerbie, A.B., Andersen, R.H. and Gallanis, T.C. (1956) Placental tumors: hemangiomas with special reference to an associated clinical syndrome. *Obstetrics and Gynecology*, **7**, 249–259.

Delerive, C., Locquet, F., Mallat, A., Jamim, A. and Gosselin, B. (1989) Placental metastasis from maternal bronchial oat cell carcinoma. *Archives of Pathology and Laboratory Medicine*, **113**, 556–558.

Demian, S.D.E., Donnelly, W.H., Frias, J.L. and Monif, C.R.G. (1974) Placental lesions in congenital giant pigmented nevi. *American Journal of Clinical Pathology*, **61**, 438–442.

Diamandopoulos, G.T. and Hertig, A.T. (1963) Transmission of leukemia and allied diseases from mother to fetus. *Obstetrics and Gynecology*, **21**, 150–154.

Drut, R., Drut, R.M. and Toulouse J.G. (1992) Hepatic hemangioendotheliomas, placental chorioangiomas, and dysmorphic kidneys in Beckwith–Wiedemann syndrome. *Pediatric Pathology*, **12**, 197–203.

Du, J., Ko, C. and Lauchlan, S.C. (1968) Multiple chorangiomata of the placenta associated with fetal anemia. *Canadian Medical Association Journal*, **99**, 862–864.

Earn, A.A. and Penner, D.W. (1950) Five cases of chorangioma. *Journal of Obstetrics and Gynaecology of the British Empire*, **57**, 442–444.

Eldar-Geva, T., Hochner-Ceinikier, D., Ariel, I., Ron, M. and Yagel, S. (1988) Fetal high-output cardiac failure and acute hydramnios caused by large placental chorioangioma: a case report. *British Journal of Obstetrics and Gynaecology*, **95**, 1200–1203.

Emge, L.A. (1927) Dystocia caused by a hemangioma of the placenta. *American Journal of Obstetrics and Gynecology*, **14**, 35–40.

Engel, K., Hahn, T. and Kayschnia, R. (1981) Sonagraphische Diagnose eines Plazentatumors mit hochgradiger Mangelentwicklung, Aysbiloug einer Anhydramnios und nachfollen der Fruchttod. *Geburtshilfe und Frauenheilkunde*, **41**, 570–573.

Eton, B. (1956) A case of chorioangioma. *Journal of Obstetrics, Gynaecology of the British Empire*, **63**, 290–294.

Fernandez-Figueras, M.T., Vaz-Romero, M., Sancho-Poch, F.J. and Diaz-de-Losada, J.P. (1989) Teratoma of the placenta: a case report. *European Journal of Obstetrics, Gynecology and Reproductive Biology*, **32**, 160–172.

Fisher, J.H. (1940) Chorioangioma of the placenta. *American Journal of Obstetrics and Gynecology*, **40**, 493–498.

Fox, H. (1966) Haemangiomata of the placenta. *Journal of Clinical Pathology*, **19**, 133–137.

Fox, H. (1967) Vascular tumors of the placenta. *Obstetrical and Gynecological Survey*, **22**, 697–711.

Fox, H. and Butler-Manuel, R. (1964) A teratoma of the placenta. *Journal of Pathology and Bacteriology*, **88**, 137–140.

Fox, H. and Langley, F.A. (1976) *Tumours of the Ovary*. London: William Heinemann Medical Books.

Franca-Martins, A.M., Graubard, Z., Holloway, G.A. and Vander Merwe, F.J. (1990) Placental haemangioma associated with acute fetal anaemia in labour. *Acta Medica Portugesa*, **3**, 187–189.

Freedman, W.L. and McMahon, F.J. (1960) Placental metastasis: review of the literature and report of a case of metastatic melanoma. *Obstetrics and Gynecology*, **16**, 550–560.

Frick, R., Rummell, H.H., Heberling, D. and Schmidt, W.D. (1977) Placenta-Metastasen mutterlicher Neoplasien: angioblastische Sarkom der Vagina mit placentarer Aussatt. *Geburtshilfe und Frauenheilkunde*, **37**, 216–220.

Froehlich, L., Fujikura, T. and Fisher, P. (1971) Chorioangiomas and their clinical implications. *Obstetrics and Gynecology*, **37**, 51–59.

Fujikura, T. and Wellings, S.R. (1964) A teratoma-like mass on the placenta of a malformed infant. *American Journal of Obstetrics and Gynecology*, **89**, 824–825.

Gayer, N., Blumenthal, N. and Ruhen, L. (1994) Placental teratoma: simultaneous occurrence with ovarian teratoma complicating pregnancy. *British Journal of Obstetrics and Gynaecology*, **101**, 720–722.

Gillis, H., II, Hortel, R. and McGavran, M.H. (1976) Maternal malignant melanoma metastatic to the products of conception. *Gynecologic Oncology*, **4**, 38–42.

Glaser, G., Junemann, A., Tunte, W. (1988) Plazentares Chorangiom und kindliche Fehlbildungen. *Geburtshilfe und Frauenheilkunde*, **48**, 450–452.

Gorbunova, Z.V. and Streneva, T.N. (1967) Concerning the transplacental transmission of acute leukaemia. *Problemy Gematologii i Perelivaniya Krovi* (Moscow), **12**, 36–38.

Gray, E.S., Balch, N.J., Kohler, H.G., Thompson, W.D. and Simpson, J.G. (1986) Congenital leukaemia: an unusual cause of stillbirth. *Archives of Disease in Childhood*, **61**, 1001–1006.

Gray, J., Kenny, M. and Sharpey-Schafer, E.P. (1939) Metastasis of maternal tumour to products of gestation. *Journal of Obstetrics and Gynaecology of the British Empire*, **46**, 8–14.

Greenberg, P., Collins, J.D., Voet, R.L. and Jariwala, L. (1982) Ewing's sarcoma metastatic to placenta. *Placenta*, **3**, 191–197.

Green, E.E. and Iams, J.D. (1984) Chorioangioma: a case presentation. *American Journal of Obstetrics and Gynecology*, **148**, 1146–1148.

Gruenwald, P. (1963) Chronic fetal distress and placental insufficiency. *Biologia Neonatorum*, **5**, 215–265.

Hadi, H.A., Finley, J. and Strickland, D. (1993) Placental chorioangioma: prenatal diagnosis and clinical significance. *American Journal of Perinatology*, **10**, 146–149.

Heggtveit, H.A., de Carvalho, R. and Nuyens, A.J. (1965) Chorioangioma and toxemia of pregnancy. *American Journal of Obstetrics and Gynecology*, **91**, 291–292.

Hesketh (1962) A case of carcinoma of the lung with secondary deposits in the placenta. *Journal of Obstetrics and Gynaecology of the British Empire*, **69**, 514.

Hirata, G.I., Masaki, D.I., O'Toole, M., Medearis, A.L. and Platt, L.D. (1993) Color flow mapping and Doppler velocimetry in the diagnosis and management of a placental chorioangioma associated with nonimmune hydrops. *Obstetrics and Gynecology*, **81**, 850–852.

Holaday, W.J. and Castrow, F.F. (1968) Placental metastasis from fetal giant pigmented nevus. *Archives of Dermatology*, **98**, 486–488.

Holland, E. (1949) A case of transplacental metastasis of malignant melanoma of mother to foetus. *Journal of Obstetrics and Gynaecology of the British Empire*, **56**, 529–536.

Honore, L.H. and Brown, L.B. (1990) Intervillous placental metastasis with maternal myeloid leukaemia. *Archives of Pathology and Laboratory Medicine*, **114**, 450.

Horner, E.N. (1960) Placental metastases. Case report: maternal death from ovarian cancer. *Obstetrics and Gynecology*, **15**, 566–572.

Hustin, J. and Chef, R. (1972) Nephroblastome diffuse bilaterale: refléxions sur un nouveau cas. *Journal de Gynécologie, Obstétrique et Biologie de la Reproduction*, **1**, 373–384.

Imakita, M., Yutani, C., Ishibashi-Ueda, H., Murakami, M. and Chiba, Y. (1988) A case of hydrops fetalis due to placental chorangioma. *Acta Pathologica Japonica*, **38**, 941–945.

Ito, M., Kumamoto, T., Yamamoto, H. et al. (1994) A case report of placental hemangioma resulting in severe fetal distress. *Acta Paediatrica Japonica*, **36**, 207–211.

Jaffe, R., Seigal, A., Rat, L., Bernheim, J., Gruber, A. and Fejgin, M. (1985) Placental chorioangiomatosis: a high risk pregnancy. *Postgraduate Medical Journal*, **64**, 453–455.

Jauniaux, E., Zucker, M., Meuris, S., Verhesi, A., Wilkin, P. and Hustin, J. (1988) Chorangiocarcinoma: an unusual tumour of the placenta: the missing link? *Placenta*, **9**, 607–613.

Jauniaux, E., deMeeus, M.-C., Verellen, G., Lachapele, J.M. and Hustin, J. (1993) Giant congenital melanocytic nevus with placental involvement: long term follow up of a case and review of the literature. *Pediatric Pathology*, **13**, 717–721.

Ito, M., Kumamato, T., Yamamoto, H. et al (1994) A case report of placental hemangioma resulting in severe fetal distress. *Acta Pediatrica Japonica*, **36**, 207–211.

Johnson, A.T. and Halbert, D. (1974) Congenital neuroblastoma presenting as hydrops fetalis. *North Carolina Medical Journal*, **35**, 289–291.

Jones, C.E.M., Rivers, R.P.A. and Taghizadeh, A. (1972) Disseminated intravascular coagulation and fetal hydrops in a newborn infant in association with a chorangioma of placenta. *Pediatrics*, **50**, 901–907.

Jones, E.M. (1969) Placental metastases from bronchial carcinoma. *British Medical Journal*, **ii**, 491–492.

Joseph, T.J. and Vogt, P.J. (1973) Placental teratomas. *Obstetrics and Gynecology*, **41**, 574–578.

Jurkovic, I., Fric, I. and Boor, A. (1973) Placenta pri neuroblastome. *Ceskoslovenska Pediatrie*, **28**, 443–445.

Kamdom-Moyo, J., Hajeri, H., Winisdoerffer, C., Philippe, E., Beauvais, P. and Dreyfus, J. (1972) Souffrance foetal et chorioangiome: étude du rythme cardiaque foetal: à propos de 2 cas. *Journal de Gynécologie, Obstétrique et Biologie de la Reproduction*, **1**, 575–579.

Kapoor, R., Gupta, A.K., Sing, S., Sood, A. and Saha, M.M. (1989) Antenatal sonographic diagnosis of chorioangioma of the placenta. *Australasian Radiology*, **33**, 288–289.

Karnauchow, P.N. (1957) Chorioangiomatosis of the placenta. *Obstetrics and Gynecology*, **9**, 317–321.

Khong, T.Y. and George, K. (1994) Maternal serum alphafetoprotein levels in chorioangiomas. *American Journal of Perinatology*, **11**, 245–248.

Kim, C.G., Benirschke, L. and Connolly, K.S. (1971) Chorangioma of the placenta: chromosomal and electron microscopic studies. *Obstetrics and Gynecology*, **37**, 372–376.

King, C.R. and Lourien, E. (1978) Chorioangioma of the placenta and intrauterine growth failure. *Journal of Pediatrics*, **93**, 1027–1028.

King, P.A., Lopes, A., Tang, M.H., Lam, S.K. and Ma, H.K. (1991) Theca-lutein ovarian cysts associated with placental chorioangioma: case report. *British Journal of Obstetrics and Gynaecology*, **98**, 322–323.

Klaften, E. (1929) Chorionhaemangioma placentae. *Zeitschrift für Geburtshilfe und Gynäkologie*, **95**, 426–437.

Knoth, M., Rygaard, J. and Hesseldahl, H. (1976) Chorioangioma with hydramnios and intrauterine fetal death. *Acta Obstetricia et Gynecologica*, **55**, 279–281.

Kobos, J. and Sporny, S. (1982) Ein Teratom der Plazenta. *Zentralblatt für allgemeine Pathologie und pathologischen Anatomie*, **126**, 317–320.

Kohler, H.G., Iqbal, N. and Jenkins, D.M. (1976) Chorionic haemangiomata and abruptio placentae. *British Journal of Obstetrics and Gynaecology*, **83**, 667–670.

Koivu, M.K. and Nuutinen, E.N. (1990) Large placental chorioangioma as a cause of congestive heart failure in newborn infants. *Pediatric Cardiology*, **11**, 221–224.

Kotz, J. and Kaufman, M.S. (1939) Chorioangioma of the placenta. *Medical Annals of the District of Columbia*, **8**, 106–110.

Kuhnel, P. (1933) Placental chorangioma. *Acta Obstetricia et Gynecologica Scandinavica*, **13**, 143–149.

Kurtin, P.J., Gaffey, T.A. and Habermann T.M. (1992) Peripheral T-cell lymphoma involving the placenta. *Cancer*, **70**, 2963–2968.

Küster, J. (1928) Adultes Teratom ('Dermoid') der Placenta. *Archiv für Gynäkologie*, **133**, 93–99.

Lampe, S., Butterwegge, M. and Krech, R.H. (1995) Chorangiomatose de Plazenta: Diagnostik und geburtshliliches Management. *Zentralblatt für Gynäkologie*, **117**, 101–104.

Lantéjoul, P. and Heraux, A. (1951) Un cas de tumeur bénigne du placenta. *Presse Médical*, **5**, 1409.

Las Heras, J., Leal, G. and Haust, D.M. (1986) Congenital leukemia with placental involvement: report of a case with ultrastructural study. *Cancer*, **58**, 2278–2281.

Leblanc, A. and Carrier, C. (1979) Chorio-angiome placentaire, angiomes cutanes et cholestase neonatale. *Archives Francais de Pediatrie*, **36**, 484–486.

Leonidas, J.C., Beatty, E.C. and Hall, R.T. (1975) Chorangioma of the placenta: a cause of cardiomegaly and heart failure in the newborn. *American Journal of Roentgenology, Radium Therapy and Nuclear Medicine*, **23**, 703–707.

Liang, S.T., Wood, J.S.K. and Wong, V.C.W. (1982) Chorioangioma of the placenta: an ultrasonic study. *British Journal of Obstetrics and Gynaecology*, **89**, 480–482.

Lifschitz-Mercer, B., Fogel, M., Kushnir, I. and Czernobilsky B. (1987) Chorangioma: a cytoskeletal profile. *International Journal of Gynecological Pathology*, **8**, 349–356.

Lin, J.B., Misaka, N., Fukunaga, W. and Shimizu, S. (1970) Hemangioma of the placenta: case report and review of the literature. *Acta Obstetrica et Gynaecologica Japonica*, **17**, 107–114.

Looi, L.M. and Wang, F. (1979) Malignant melanoma metastases in chorionic villi: a case report. *Malaysian Journal of Pathology*, **2**, 73–75.

Lopez-Herce, C., Cid, J., Escriba Polo, R. and Escudero Loy, R. (1983) Corioangioma placentario y hemorraghia intracraneal neonatal. *Anales Espanoles de Pediatria*, **19**, 405–406.

Ludighausen, M.V. and Sahiri, I. (1983) Chorangiome der Plazenten als Ursache wiederhalter Totgeburten. *Geburtshilfe und Frauenheilkunde*, **43**, 233–235.

McInroy, R.A. and Kelsey, H.A. (1954) Chorio-angioma (haemangioma of placenta) associated with acute hydramnios. *Journal of Pathology and Bacteriology*, **68**, 519–523.

MacIntosh, A.M. and Osborn, R.A. (1968) Chorioangioma of the placenta: report of a case with spontaneous reabsorption of an acute hydramnios. *Medical Journal of Australia*, **2**, 313–314.

Majilessi, H.F., Wagner, K.M. and Brooks, J. (1983) Atypical cellular chorangioma of the placenta. *International Journal of Gynecological Pathology*, **1**, 403–408.

Mandelbaum, B., Ross, M. and Riddle, C.B. (1969) Hemangioma of the placenta associated with fetal anemia and edema: report of a case. *Obstetrics and Gynecology*, **34**, 335–338.

Mann, L., Alroomf, L. and Ferguson-Smith, M.A. (1983) Placental haemangioma; case report. *British Journal of Obstetrics and Gynaecology*, **90**, 983–984.

Marchetti, A.A. (1939) Consideration of certain types of benign tumors of the placenta. *Surgery, Gynecology and Obstetrics*, **68**, 733–743.

Markus, N. (1910) Gleichzeitige Entwicklung eines Melanosarcoma ovarii und Carcinoma hepatis in der Schwangerschaft. Eklampsie. Placentarmetastase. *Archiv für Gynäkologie*, **92**, 659–678.

Merlino, A. (1939) Contributo allo studio del corion-angioma. *Archivio di Ostetricia e Ginecologia*, **3**, 422–439.

Metler, S., Werner, B. and Meyer, J. (1970) Przerzuty raka sutka do lozyska. (Mammary cancer metastases to the placenta.) *Ginekologia Polska*, **41**, 301–307.

Monteforte, C. (1968) Osservagioni su due casi di corionangioma. *Archivio di Ostetricia e Ginecologia*, **73**, 329–344.

Morville, P. (1925) Une tératome placentaire. *Gynécologie et Obstétrique*, **11**, 29–32.

Moschella, S.L. (1961) A report of malignant melanoma of the skin in sisters. *Archives of Dermatology*, **84**, 1024–1025.

Mucitelli, D.R., Charles, E.Z. and Kraus, F.T. (1990) Chorioangiomas of intermediate size and intrauterine growth retardation. *Pathology Research and Practice*, **186**, 455–458.

Mugnai, U. (1938) Alcune considerazioni su un casi di 'angioma coriale'. *Monitore Ostetrico-Ginecologia di Endocrinologia e del Metabolizmo*, **10**, 261–290.

Müller, G. and Rieckert, H. (1967) Beitrag zur Frage Placentarinsuffizienz an Hand eines diffusen Chorangioms. *Archiv für Gynäkologie*, **204**, 78–88.

Mutz, I.D. and Sterling, R. (1991) Konnatales Neuroblastom und Plazentametastasen. *Monatsschrift für Kinderheilkunde*, **139**, 154–156.

Nahmanovici, C., Pancrazi, J. and Philippe, E (1982) Chorioangiome placentaire: diagnosie echographique de la 19 semaine. *Journal de Gynécologie, Obstétrique et Biologie de la Reproduction*, **11**, 593–597.

Nessmann-Emmanuelli, C., Breart, G. and Kone-Pale, B. (1978) Correlations entre la pathologie placentaire et les pathologies maternelles et neonatales. *Journal de Gynécologie, Obstétrique et Biologie de la Reproduction*, **7**, 933–944.

Nickell, K.A. and Stocker, J.T. (1988) Placental teratoma: a case report. *Pediatric Pathology*, **7**, 645–650.

Nummi, S., Koivisto, M. and Hakosalo, J. (1973) Acute leukaemia in pregnancy with placental involvement. *Annales Chirurgiae et Gynaecologiae Fenniae*, **62**, 394–398.

Nuttininen, E.M., Puistola, A., Herva, R. and Joivisto, M. (1988) Two cases of large placental chorioangioma with fetal and neonatal complications. *European Journal of Obstetrics, Gynaecology and Reproductive Biology*, **29**, 315–320.

O'Day, M.P., Nielsen, P., Al-Bozom, I. and Wilkins, I.A. (1994) Orbital rhabdomyosarcoma metastatic to the placenta. *American Journal of Obstetrics and Gynecology*, **171**, 1382–1383.

O'Malley, B.P., Toi, A., deSa, D.J. and Williams, G.L. (1981) Ultrasound appearances of placental chorioangioma. *Radiology*, **138**, 159–160.

Orr, J.W., Grizzle, W.E. and Huddleston, J.F. (1982) Squamous cell carcinoma metastatic to placenta and ovary. *Obstetrics and Gynecology*, **59**, 81s–83s.

Patsner, B., Mann, W.J., Jr and Chumas, J. (1989) Primary invasive ovarian adenocarcinoma with brain and placental metastases: a case report. *Gynecologic Oncology*, **33**, 112–115.

Pensa, A. (1932) Contributo allo studio del corioangiomi. *Monitore Ostetrico-Ginecologica di Endocrinologia e del Metabolismo*, **4**, 519–651.

Perez, M.L., Brachetto-Brian, D. and Ferrari, G.A. (1939) Sobre una observacion de teratoma de la placenta. *Archivos de la Sociedad Argentina de Anatomia Normal y Patologica*, **1**, 771–780.

Perkins, D.G., Kopp, C.M. and Haust, M.D. (1980) Placental infiltration in congenital neuroblastoma: a case study with ultrastructure. *Histopathology*, **4**, 383–389.

Pfuhl, J.P. and Panitz, H.G. (1991) Plazentametastasen maternaler maligner Tumoren. *Gynakologe*, **24**, 174–175.

Philippe, E., Muller, G., Dehalleux, J.M., de Mot, E., Lefakis, P. and Gandar, R. (1969) Le chorioangiome et ses complications foeto-maternelles. *Revue Francais de Gynécologie et d'Obstétrique*, **64**, 335–341.

Phillip, E. (1931) Choriohämangiom. *Zeitschrift für Geburtshilfe und Gynäkologie*, **99**, 599–604.

Pisarki, T. and Mrozewski, A. (1964) Przerzut raka sutka do lozyska. (The mammary gland cancer metastases to the placenta.) *Ginekologia Polska*, **35**, 277–286.

Pollack, N., Pollak, M. and Rochon, L. (1993) Pregnancy complicated by medulloblastoma with metastases to the placenta. *Obstetrics and Gynecology*, **81**, 858–859.

Potashnik, G., Ben Adereth, N. and Leventhal, H. (1973) Chorioangioma of the placenta: clinical and pathological implications. *Israel Journal of Medical Sciences*, **9**, 904–908.

Rauchenberg, M. and Zeman, V. (1971) Chorioangion placenty. *Casopis Lekaru Ceskych* (Prague), **110**, 727–733.

Read, E.J. and Platzer, P.B. (1981) Placental metastases from maternal carcinoma of the lung. *Obstetrics and Gynecology*, **58**, 387–391.

Reddy, C.R.R., Rao, A.V.N. and Sulochana, G. (1969) Haemangiolipoma of placenta. *Journal of Obstetrics and Gynaecology of India*, **19**, 653–655.

Reiner, L. and Fries, E. (1965) Chorangioma associated with arteriovenous aneurysm. *American Journal of Obstetrics and Gynecology*, **93**, 58–64.

Rendina, G.M. and Patrono, D. (1975) Il coriangioma nella patologia materno-fetale con particolare riferimento al parto pretermine. *Minerva Ginecologia*, **27**, 108–120.

Resnick, L. (1953) Chorangioma, with report of a case associated with oligohydramnios. *South African Medical Journal*, **27**, 57–60.

Reus, W.A. and Geppert, M. (1988) Teratom der Plazenta. *Geburtshilfe und Frauenheilkunde*, **48**, 459–461.

Rewell, R.E. and Whitehouse, W.L. (1966) Malignant metastasis to the placenta from carcinoma of the breast. *Journal of Pathology and Bacteriology*, **91**, 255–256.

Reynolds, A.G. (1955) Placental metastasis from a malignant melanoma. *Obstetrics and Gynecology*, **6**, 205–209.

Rigby, P.G., Hanson, T.A. and Smith, R.S. (1964) Passage of leukemic cells across the placenta. *New England Journal of Medicine*, **271**, 124–127.

Robinson, H.B., Jr and Rolande, R.P. (1985) Fetal hepatoblastoma with placental metastases. *Pediatric Pathology*, **4**, 163–167.

Rodan, B.A. and Bean, W.J. (1983) Chorioangioma of the placenta causing intrauterine fetal demise. *Journal of Ultrasound Medicine*, **2**, 95–97.

Rosemond, G.P. (1964) Management of patients with carcinoma of the breast in pregnancy. *Annals of the New York Academy of Sciences*, **114**, 851–856.

Rothman, L.A., Cohen, C.J. and Astarloa, J. (1973) Placental and fetal involvement by maternal malignancy: a report of rectal carcinoma and review of the literature. *American Journal of Obstetrics and Gynecology*, **115**, 1023–1034.

Russell, P. and Laverty, C.R. (1977) Malignant melanoma metastases in the placenta: a case report. *Pathology*, **9**, 251–255.

Salamon, M.A., Sherer, D.M., Saller, D.N., Jr, Metlay, L.A. and Sickel, J.Z. (1994) Placental metastases in a patient with recurrent breast carcinoma. *American Journal of Obstetrics and Gynecology*, **171**, 573–574.

Santamaria, M., Benirschke, K., Carpenter, P.M., Baldwin, V.J. and Pritchard, J.A. (1987) Transplacental hemorrhage associated with placental neoplasms. *Pediatric Pathology*, **7**, 601–615.

Scharl, A. and Schlensker, K.H. (1987) Chorioangiome – sonagraphische Diagnose und klinische Bedeutung. *Zeitschrift für Perinatologie*, **191**, 250–253.

Schmitt, F.C., Zelhandi-Felho, C., Bacchi, M., Castilho, E.D. and Bacchi, C.E. (1989) Adenoid cystic carcinoma of trachea metastatic to the placenta. *Human Pathology*, **20**, 193–195.

Schneiderman, H., Wu, A.Y., Campbell, W.A. et al (1987) Congenital melanoma with multiple prenatal metastases. *Cancer*, **60**, 1371–1377.

Schnitger, A., Lieogren, S., Radberg, C., Johansson, S.G.O. and Kjessler, B. (1980) Raised maternal serum and amniotic fluid alphafetoprotein levels associated with a placental haemangioma. *British Journal of Obstetrics and Gynaecology*, **87**, 824–826.

Schramm, T., Gruppe, B., Baltzer, J. and Zander, J. (1987) Plazentares Chorangiom – Kasuistik und Diskussion der moglichen Komplikationen. *Geburtshilfe und Frauenheilkunde* **47**, 422–424.

Scott, R.A. (1924) Benign tumors of the placenta: a review of the literature and report of a chorioangioma. *Surgery, Gynecology and Obstetrics*, **39**, 216–221.

Sedgely, M.G., Ostor, A.G. and Fortune, D.W. (1985) Angiosarcoma of the breast metastatic to breast and ovary. *Australian and New Zealand Journal of Obstetrics and Gynaecology*, **25**, 299–302.

Sen, D.K. (1970) Placental hypertrophy associated with chorioangioma. *American Journal of Obstetrics and Gynecology*, **107**, 652–654.

Senge, J. (1912) Sekundre Carcinosis der Placenta bei primarem Magenkarzinom. *Beitrage zur pathologischen Anatomie und zur allgemeinen Pathologie*, **53**, 532–549.

Sfar, E., Boubaker, S., Zitouna, M.M. and Kharouf, M. (1991) Les chorio-angiomes placentaires volumineux: a propos de deux observations. *Revue Francaise de Gynécologie et d'Obstétrique*, **86**, 115–118.

Shaw-Dunn, R.A. (1959) Haemangioma of placenta (chorioangioma) *Journal of Obstetrics and Gynaecology of the British Empire*, **66**, 51–61.

Siddall, R.S. (1924) Chorioangiofibroma (chorioangioma) *American Journal of Obstetrics and Gynecology*, **8**, 430–456.

Siddall, R.S. (1926) The occurrence of chorangiofibroma (chorioangioma) *Bulletin of the Johns Hopkins Hospital*, **38**, 355–364.

Sieracki, J.C., Panke, T.W., Horvat, B.L., Perrin, E.V. and Nanda, B. (1975) Chorioangiomas. *Obstetrics and Gynecology*, **46**, 155–159.

Sims, D.G., Barron, S.L., Wadhera, V. and Ellis, H.A. (1976) Massive chronic feto-maternal bleeding associated with placental chorioangiomas. *Acta Paediatrica Scandinavica*, **65**, 271–273.

Sironi, M., Declich, P., Isimbaldi, G., Monguzzi, A. and Poggi, G. (1994) Placental teratoma with three-germ layer differentiation. *Teratology*, **50**, 165–167.

Smith, C.R., Chan, H.S.L. and deSa, D.J. (1981) Placental involvement in congenital neuroblastoma. *Journal of Clinical Pathology*, **34**, 785–789.

Smith, L.A. and Pounder, D.J. (1982) A teratoma-like lesion of the placenta: a case report. *Pathology*, **14**, 85–87.

Smythe, A.R., Underwood, P.B. and Kreutner, A., Jr (1976) Metastatic placental tumors: report of three cases. *American Journal of Obstetrics and Gynecology*, **125**, 1149–1151.

Snoeck, J. and Wilkin, P. (1952) Le chorio-angiome: tumeur bénigne du placenta. *Bulletin de la Fédération des Sociétés de Gynécologie et d'Obstétrique de Langue Francaise*, **4**, 644–651.

Sokol, R.J., Hutchison, P., Cowan, D. and Reed, G.B. (1976) Amelanotic melanoma metastatic to the placenta. *American Journal of Obstetrics and Gynecology*, **124**, 431–432.

Sotelo-Avila, C., Graham, M., Hanby, D.E. and Rudolph, A.J. (1988) Nevus cell aggregates in the placenta: a histochemical and electron microscopic study. *American Journal of Clinical Pathology*, **89**, 395–400.

Spirt, B., Gordon, L., Cohen, W. and Martin, R. (1980) Antenatal diagnosis of chorioangioma of the placenta. *American Journal of Roentgenology*, **135**, 1273–1275.

Stephens, T.D., Spall, R., Urter, A.G. and Martin, R. (1989) Fetus amorphus or placental teratoma? *Teratology*, **40**, 1–10.

Stephenson, H.E., Jr, Terry, C.W., Lukens, J.N. et al (1971) Immunologic factors in human melanoma 'metastatic' to products of gestation (with exchange transfusion of infant to mother) *Surgery*, **69**, 515–522.

Stiller, A.C. and Skafish, P.R. (1986) Placental chorioangioma: a rare cause of feto-maternal transfusion with maternal hemorrhage and fetal distress. *Obstetrics and Gynecology*, **67**, 296–298.

Stockhausen, H.B., Hansen, H.G., Monkemeier, D. and Muhrer, A. (1984) Riesenhamangiome der Plazenta als Ursache einer lebensbedrohlichen Neugeborenanamie mit Hydrops congenitum. *Monatsschrift für Kinderheilkunde*, **132**, 182–185.

Stovring, S. (1980) Kongenit neuroblastom med metastaser til placenta. *Ugeskrift für Laeger*, **142**, 2977–2978.

Strakosch, W. (1956) Uber Chorionangiome. *Geburtshilfe und Frauenheilkunde*, **16**, 485–495.

Strauss, L. and Driscoll, S.G. (1964) Congenital neuroblastoma involving the placenta: reports of two cases. *Pediatrics*, **34**, 23–31.

Suda, R., Repke, J.T., Steer, R. and Niebyl, J.R. (1986) Metastatic adenocarcinoma of the lung complicating pregnancy: a case report. *Journal of Reproductive Medicine*, **31**, 1113–1116.

Sulman, F.G. and Sulman, E. (1949) Increased gonadotrophin production in a case of detachment of placenta due to placental haemangioma. *Journal of Obstetrics and Gynaecology of the British Empire*, **56**, 1033–1034.

Sumathy, V., Grimes, E.M. and Miller, G.L. (1973) Chorioangioma of placenta. *Missouri Medicine*, **70**, 647–649.

Svanholm, H. and Thordsen, C. (1987) Placental teratoma. *Acta Obstetricia et Gynecologica Scandinavica*, **66**, 179–180.

Sweet, L. and Robertson, N.R.C. (1973) Hydrops fetalis with chorioangioma of the placenta. *Journal of Pediatrics*, **82**, 91–94.

Szarthmary, Z. (1934) Ueber Geschwülste der Placenta. *Archiv für Gynäkologie*, **155**, 453–468.

Tan, S.A. and Yeo, S.H. (1992) Placental chorangioma: a case report and review. *Singapore Medical Journal*, **33**, 83–85.

Tapia, R.H., White, V.A. and Ruffolo, E.H. (1985) Leiomyoma of the placenta. *Southern Medical Journal*, **78**, 863–864.

Thomas, R.L. and Blakemore, K.J. (1990) Chorioangioma: a new inclusion in the prospective and retrospective evaluation of elevated maternal serum alpha-fetoprotein. *Prenatal Diagnosis*, **10**, 691–696.

Tonkin, I.L., Setzer, E.S. and Ermocilla, R. (1980) Placental chorangioma: a rare cause of congestive heart failure and hydrops fetalis in the newborn. *American Journal of Roentgenology*, **134**, 181–183.

Trask, C., Lage, J.M. and Roberts, D.J. (1994) A second case of 'chorangiocarcinoma' presenting in a term asymptomatic twin pregnancy: choriocarcinoma in situ with associated villous vascular proliferation. *International Journal of Gynecological Pathology*, **13**, 87–91.

Tsujimura, T., Matsumoto, K. and Aozasa, K. (1993) Placental involvement by maternal non-Hodgkin's lymphoma. *Archives of Pathology and Laboratory Medicine*, **117**, 325–327.

Unger, J.L. (1989) Placental teratoma. *American Journal of Clinical Pathology*, **92**, 371–373.

van der Slikke, J.W. and Balk, A.G. (1980) Hydramnios with hydrops fetalis and disseminated fetal neuroblastoma. *Obstetrics and Gynecology*, **55**, 250–253.

Verloes, A., Schaaps, J.P. and Herens, C. (1991) Prenatal diagnosis of cystic hygroma and chorioangioma in the Wolf–Hirschorn syndrome. *Prenatal Diagnosis*, **11**, 129–132.

Vermelin, H., Braye, M. and Colette, Cl. (1957) Association de chorio-angiome placentaire et de dégénérescence molaire. *Bulletin de la Fédération des Sociétés de Gynécologie et d'Obstétrique de Langue Francaise*, **9**, 225.

Vesanto, T., Jrvinen, P.A. and von Numers, C. (1963) Placentan hemangioomasta. *Duodecima*, **79**, 808–811.

Wallenburg, H.C.S. (1971) Chorioangioma of the placenta: thirteen new cases and a review of the literature from 1939 to 1970 with special reference to clinical complications. *Obstetrical and Gynecological Survey*, **26**, 411–425.

Walz, K. (1906) Ueber Placentartumoren. *Verhandlungen der Deutschen Gesellschaft für Pathologie*, **10**, 279–281.

Wang, T., Harman, W. and Hartge, R. (1983) Structural aspects of a placenta from a case of maternal acute lymphatic leukaemia. *Placenta*, **4**, 185–196.

Weber, F.P., Schwarz, K. and Hellenschied, R. (1930) Spontaneous inoculation of melanotic sarcoma from mother to foetus. *British Medical Journal*, **i**, 537–539.

Wentworth, P. (1965) The incidence and significance of haemangiomata of the placenta. *Journal of Obstetrics and Gynaecology of the British Commonwealth*, **72**, 81–88.

Werner, C. (1972) Melaninablagerungen in der Plazenta bei neurokutaner Melanophakomatose des Feten. *Geburtshilfe und Frauenheilkunde*, **32**, 891–894.

Williams, V.L. and Williams, R.A. (1994) Placental teratoma: prenatal ultrasonographic diagnosis. *Journal of Ultrasound in Medicine*, **13**, 587–589.

Wunsch, M. and Furch, W. (1983) Sonagraphische Diagnose eines grossen Plazentatumor in der Spatschwangerschaft: Falldarstellung und Uberlegungen zur Geburtsleitung. *Geburtshilfe und Frauenheilkunde*, **43**, 236–239.

Wurster, D.H., Hoefnagel, D., Benirschke, K. and Allen, F.H., Jr (1969) Placental chorangiomata and mental deficiency in a child with 2/15 translocation: 46, XX, t(2q;ms: 15q+) *Cytogenetics*, **8**, 389–399.

Yule, R. and O'Connor, D. (1964) Haemangioma of the placenta. *Medical Journal of Australia*, **1**, 157–158.

Zawirska, B. (1964) Naczyniaki lozyska. *Patologia Polska*, **15**, 89–94.

14

GESTATIONAL TROPHOBLASTIC DISEASE

The term 'gestational trophoblastic disease' could, in theory, be applied to any abnormality of the trophoblast but is, by convention, restricted to a small number of conditions, the classification of which is given in Table 14.1. This classification is based principally on morphology but, perhaps somewhat illogically, includes one non-morphological component, namely 'persistent trophoblastic disease'. This term is applied to a biochemical abnormality, i.e. an elevated level of human chorionic gonadotrophin (hCG) following a molar pregnancy, and this diagnosis not only lacks any specific morphological connotation but becomes invalid if a morphological diagnosis is achieved.

The term 'gestational trophoblastic neoplasia' has been used as an alternative to gestational trophoblastic disease and indeed many seem to feel, often at a subliminal level, that these various conditions represent a neoplastic spectrum, with moles at the benign end of this spectrum, choriocarcinoma at the malignant extreme and invasive hydatidiform mole being equivalent to a neoplasm of borderline malignancy. Even in current textbooks of gynaecological oncology, hydatidiform moles are discussed under the heading of 'benign gestational trophoblastic neoplasia' (Currie, 1996). This is a totally misleading approach because there is nothing to suggest that a hydatidiform mole, of any type, is a form of neoplasia; it is, without question, a specific form of abortion. A choriocarcinoma is usually considered to be neoplastic but, as will be discussed later, even this may be no more than an unusual type of abortus in some cases and the only undoubtedly neoplastic entity within this group of conditions is the placental site trophoblastic tumour.

HYDATIDIFORM MOLES

During the last few decades molar disease has been divided into complete and partial hydatidiform moles, the distinction between these two entities being based on their differing morphological and cytogenetic features (Vassilakos et al, 1977; Szulman & Surti, 1978a,b).

Epidemiology

There is a striking geographic variation in the incidence of molar disease with it generally being thought that the incidence of hydatidiform moles is much higher in Asia, Latin America and Africa than in Europe and North America (Elston, 1981; Grimes,

Table 14.1. Classification of gestational trophoblastic disease

Hydatidiform mole
Complete
Partial
Invasive hydatidiform mole
Persistent trophoblastic disease
Choriocarcinoma
Placental site trophoblastic tumour

1984; Bracken, 1987). The degree of this difference, however, is difficult to estimate because of the serious flaws that have characterized all but the most recent of epidemiological studies of molar pregnancies. Nevertheless it is now clear that molar gestations occur three to four times more frequently in Japan (Ishizuka, 1976; Fukunaga et al, 1995) and in the United Arab Emirates (Graham et al, 1990) than in the UK (Womack & Elston, 1985). The reasons for this geographic variation remain obscure. Molar disease tends to occur most frequently at the extremes of a woman's reproductive life (Hayashi et al, 1982; La Vecchia et al, 1984; Atrash et al, 1986; Bagshawe et al, 1986) and therefore populations in which pregnancy occurs at an early age and in which childbearing continues until late in life would be expected to have a higher incidence of molar disease than those in which pregnancies usually occur within a more restricted age range. This could explain some of the observed regional differences but certainly not all and attempts to define an ethnic, nutritional or socio-economic basis for this variability have not met with success (Bracken, 1987; Buckley, 1987).

Attempts to define risk factors within a single population for molar disease have, with the exception of pin-pointing maternal age as a key factor, not yielded consistent or convincing results though it has emerged that the woman most likely to suffer a molar pregnancy is one who has had a previous hydatidiform mole (Sand et al, 1984; La Vecchia et al, 1985).

Clinical Features

Traditionally, patients with a complete hydatidiform mole present with vaginal bleeding towards the end of the first trimester, occasionally with the passage of vesicular villi. Uterine enlargement to a size greater than would be expected for the length of the gestational period is often found and fetal heart sounds are, in the absence of a twin pregnancy, absent. Urinary and serum levels of beta-hCG are unduly elevated, sometimes to extremely high levels, and this over-production of gonadotrophins has, not totally convincingly, been held responsible for the development of ovarian theca-lutein cysts, hyperemesis and early-onset pre-eclampsia in a small proportion (probably about 10%) of cases. Occasional patients present with hyperthyroidism and in such cases it appears likely that the high hCG levels are responsible for the endocrinological syndrome (Yoshimura et al, 1994). The diagnosis of a complete mole is easily and accurately established by ultrasound (Hammond et al, 1979; Romero et al, 1985).

Women with partial hydatidiform moles most commonly also present with late first-trimester bleeding; fetal heart sounds are present in some cases and the uterus is usually either unduly small or of normal size for the length of the gestational period, only rarely being unusually large. Serum and urinary levels of beta-hCG are lower than those found in association with complete moles, not uncommonly being either normal or only slightly elevated. Nevertheless, occasional patients with a partial mole develop early onset pre-eclampsia (Cox & Klein, 1993; Slattery et al, 1993). The diagnosis of a partial mole by ultrasound is less accurate than is the case with complete moles (Naumoff et al, 1981).

Morphology

Complete Hydatidiform Mole

In its classical form a complete mole is characterized by diffuse vesicular change which involves, to a greater or lesser degree, the entire villous population, thus producing the classical 'bunch of grapes' appearance. The mass of villous tissue is markedly increased, to an extent that an *in situ* mole can fill or even distend the uterus (Fig. 14.1), no remnant of a normal placental shape is discernible and, traditionally, neither a fetus nor a gestational sac is present. Paradinas (1994) has, however, maintained that amniotic tissue is found in a small percentage of complete moles. Histological examination confirms that all the villi are swollen and oedematous, some very markedly so but others only minimally (Fig. 14.2); central cistern formation is common. The enlarged villi are generally rounded but collapsed villi may have an irregular outline. There is commonly a complete absence of stromal fetal vessels but residual vessels are seen in a small minority of cases and these may contain nucleated red cells (Paradinas, 1994; Paradinas et al, 1996). Paradinas and his colleagues (Paradinas, 1994; Paradinas et al, 1996) have stressed the diagnostic importance of stromal nuclear debris in the villi of complete moles, thus confirming the earlier observation of Szulman and Surti (1978b). It is usually maintained that trophoblastic hyperplasia is a characteristic feature of a complete mole and in some cases there is indeed a marked excess of villous trophoblastic tissue (Fig. 14.3). In many complete moles, however, the degree of trophoblastic proliferation is no greater, and sometimes less, than that seen in the normal first-trimester placenta (Fig. 14.4). It is the pattern, rather than the degree, of trophoblastic proliferation that is abnormal in a complete mole; whilst in a normal pregnancy trophoblast proliferates along one side or at one pole of a villus (Fig. 14.5), in a complete mole the villous trophoblastic proliferation is either circumferential or multifocal (see Fig. 14.4). A moderate degree of nuclear atypia is commonly present in molar trophoblast though this is often no more marked than that seen in the trophoblast of placentas from normal first-trimester pregnancies.

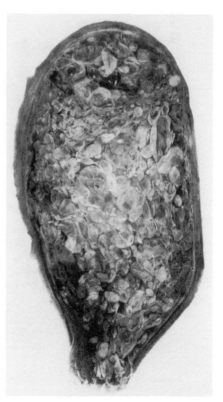

Figure 14.1. A uterus enlarged and distended by a complete hydatidiform mole. No normal placental tissue is present and all the villi show vesicular change.

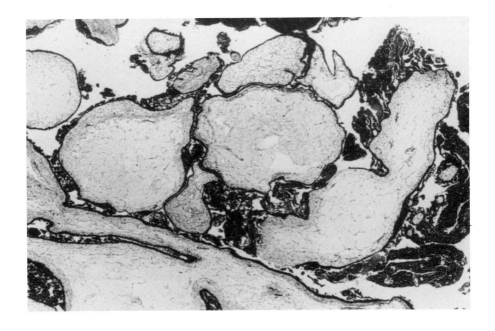

Figure 14.2. Complete hydatidiform mole. The villi are of abnormal appearance, are distended and show early central cistern formation: atypical trophoblastic proliferation is seen (H & E ×60).

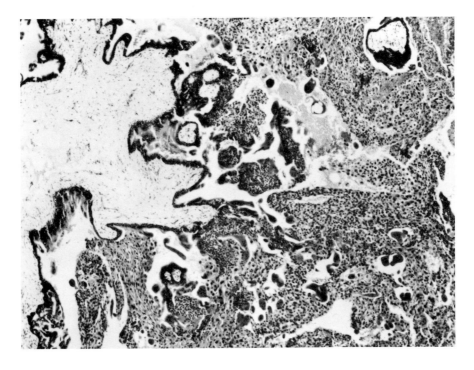

Figure 14.3. A complete hydatidiform mole showing marked trophoblastic proliferation (H & E ×50).

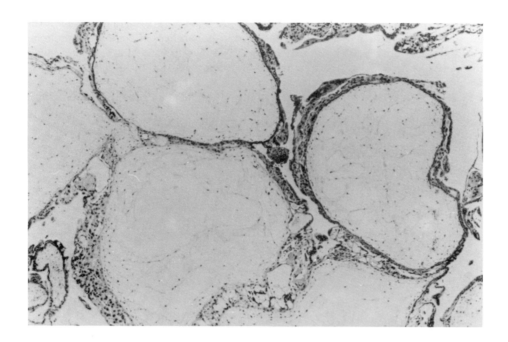

Figure 14.4. A complete hydatidiform mole in which there is only a slight degree of trophoblastic proliferation (H & E ×40).

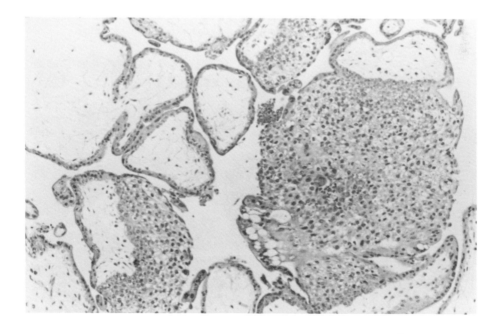

Figure 14.5. Placenta from a first-trimester termination of pregnancy. There is quite marked proliferation of trophoblast, though this has been exaggerated by tangential curetting. The trophoblastic proliferation is along one side or at one pole of a villus (H & E ×100).

This classical description of a complete mole is, however, based upon cases that have been diagnosed clinically. Because of the use of ultrasound, anembryonic gestations, and hence molar pregnancies, are now being diagnosed at an earlier stage of gestation than in the past. In these early lesions the typical gross appearances of a complete mole may not be apparent and vesicular villi may not be obvious to the naked eye. There may be, histologically, co-existing vesicular and non-vesicular villi and those villi that are not vesicular are often branching and have a polypoid or lobulated appearance (Figs 14.6 and 14.7): fetal vessels are present in most of the villi (Kajii et al, 1984; Paradinas, 1994).

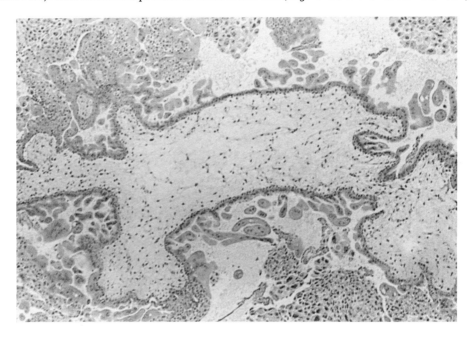

Figure 14.6. A polypoid villus from a very early complete hydatidiform mole.

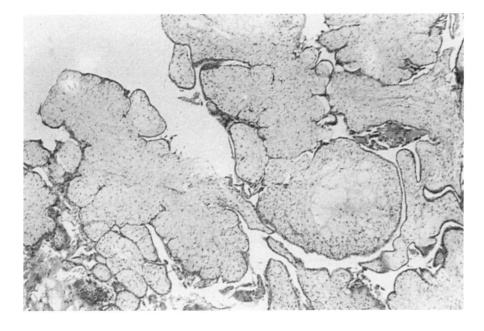

Figure 14.7. A very early complete hydatidiform mole: polypoid villi cut in cross-section have a lobulated appearance.

Partial Hydatidiform Mole

A partial mole differs in numerous respects from a complete mole: it tends to retain a placental shape, usually does not have an increased villous mass and is often associated with a fetus, though the quoted proportion of partial moles in which fetal tissue can be found has varied widely from 12% to 59% (Szulman et al, 1981; Conran et al, 1993; Heatley, 1994). Only a proportion of the villi show gross vesicular change, these being scattered within macroscopically normal placental tissue (Figs 14.8 and 14.9). Histologically the presence of both oedematous swollen villi and villi of normal size, albeit often with an unusually fibrotic or cellular stroma, is confirmed (Fig. 14.10). Fetal blood vessels containing erythrocytes are often present and in older partial moles an angiomatoid pattern is sometimes encountered. The vesicular villi may have large central cisternae and commonly have a very irregular, scalloped outline, this resulting in the 'Norwegian fjord' appearance (Fig. 14.11). Cutting of some of these deep indentations in cross-section results in the presence of so-called 'trophoblastic inclusions' within the villous stroma (Fig. 14.12). There is abnormal trophoblastic proliferation, this, as with complete moles, usually being either circumferential or multifocal; the degree of trophoblastic proliferation is usually not only less than that seen in complete moles but is sometimes less than that encountered in normal first-trimester placentas (see Figs 14.10 and 14.11). The villous trophoblast frequently has a somewhat vacuolated, or 'lacy', appearance. It is often maintained that partial moles are characterized by 'syncytiotrophoblastic hyperplasia' but it is, of course, quite impossible for the villous syncytiotrophoblast to be hyperplastic because this is a post-mitotic, terminally differentiated tissue which is incapable of DNA synthesis and cell division.

It should be noted that the use of the word 'partial' to describe a mole does not mean that one portion of the placenta is normal and another portion molar. This latter situation is encountered if a complete mole is part of a dizygotic twin pregnancy and associated with a normal twin (Miller et al, 1993; Steller et al, 1994a,b). In such pregnancies one placenta is molar and the other non-molar, whilst in a true partial mole there is an intermingling of molar and non-molar villi with the molar villi distributed throughout the entire placenta.

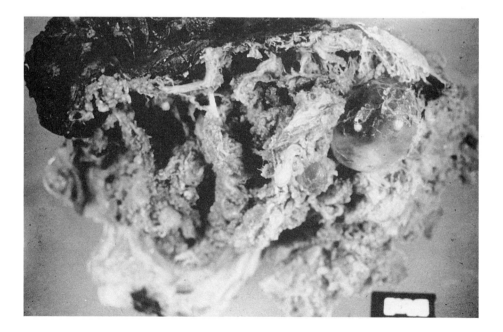

Figure 14.8. A partial hydatidiform mole. The normal placental shape is retained and whilst some of the villi are clearly vesicular, much of the villous tissue looks normal.

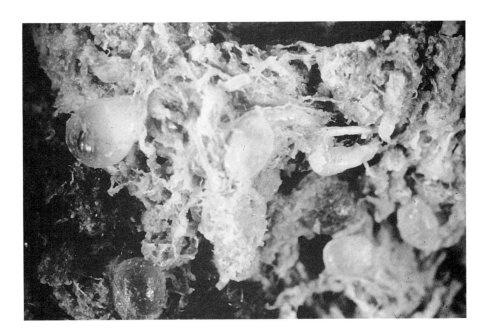

Figure 14.9. A close-up view of a partial hydatidiform mole: there is an admixture of normal and vesicular villi.

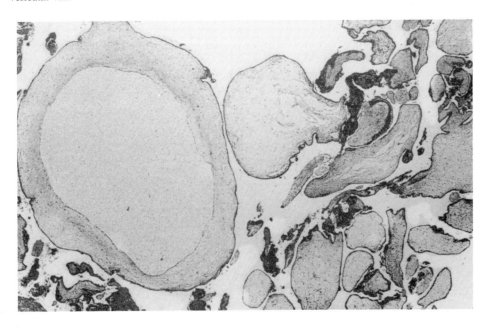

Figure 14.10. A partial hydatidiform mole. There is an admixture of large vesicular villi and small villi of normal configuration.

Cytogenetics

It has been recognized for some time that complete moles are androgenetic, i.e. all their nuclear DNA is paternally derived (Kajii & Ohama, 1977; Wake et al, 1978; Jacobs et al, 1980); furthermore approximately 85% of complete moles have a 46 XX chromosomal constitution, the remainder having a 46 XY karyotype (Kajii & Omaha, 1977;

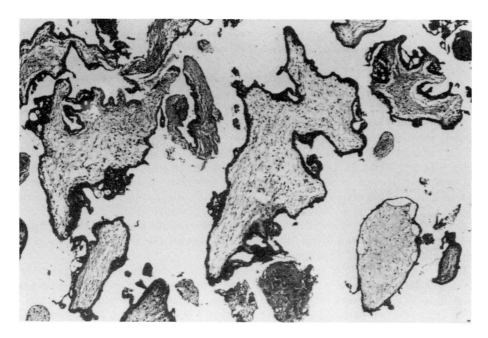

Figure 14.11. A partial hydatidiform mole. Many of the villi have a very irregular outline with the formation of 'fjords'.

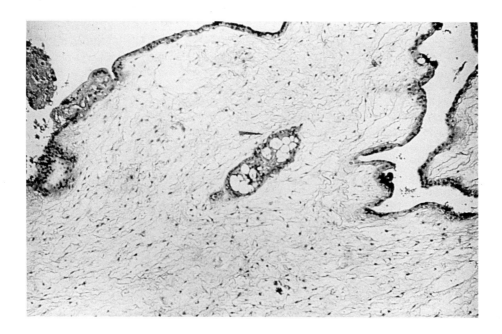

Figure 14.12. Villus in a partial hydatidiform mole. A deep surface indentation has been cut in cross-section to give the appearance of a 'trophoblastic inclusion'.

Szulman & Surti, 1978a; Jacobs et al, 1980). Banding studies have shown that the vast majority of 46 XX complete moles are derived from a single sperm (monospermic or homozygous moles) whilst all 46 XY moles and a small minority of 46 XX moles are derived from two sperms (dispermic or heterozygous moles). A hypothetical model has been proposed to explain these findings, namely that homozygous moles are due to fertilization of a 'dead' ovum (i.e. one containing no viable genomic material) by a single haploid sperm which then undergoes endoreduplication of its genetic material without cell division and that heterozygous moles result from entry into a 'dead' ovum of two haploid sperms which then fuse and replicate (Wake et al, 1978; Surti et al, 1979, 1982; Jacobs et al, 1980; Pattillo et al, 1981; Kajii et al, 1984; Lawler & Fisher, 1987; Sulti, 1987). It has to be stressed that this concept is purely theoretical and that the true nature of a 'dead' ovum has never been determined and, indeed, such an ovum has never been identified.

Partial moles contain both paternal and maternal genomic material and the vast majority are chromosomally triploid, usually 69 XXY but sometimes 69 XXX or 69 XYY (Szulman & Surti, 1978a; Szulman et al, 1981; Lawler et al, 1982; Surti, 1987; Lawler & Fisher, 1991). It is of course known that not all triploid gestations are associated with molar change in the placenta and it is now clear that if the extra chromosomal load is of paternal origin a partial mole will result, whilst if the extra chromosomal content is contributed from the mother a non-molar placenta will develop (Jacobs et al, 1982). It is thought that paternally derived triploidy is usually the result of two haploid sperms fertilizing a haploid ovum but that a few cases may be due to fertilization of a haploid ovum by a diploid 46 XX sperm.

This relatively simple subdivision into androgenetic diploid complete moles and biparentally derived triploid partial moles is not, however, the whole story. Cytogenetic studies have yielded a few instances of triploid and tetraploid complete moles and of diploid and tetraploid partial moles (Teng & Ballon, 1984; Surti et al, 1986; Verjeslev et al, 1987; Lage et al, 1989). To complicate the matter still further there have been very occasional instances of androgenetic partial moles and biparentally derived complete moles (Verjeslev et al, 1987), entities for which there is, at the moment, no very plausible explanation.

It should be noted that these anomalies have been detected in moles for which a rigorous morphological diagnosis had been made. Triploid complete moles may well be due to three haploid sperms entering a 'dead' ovum but many of the reported diploid partial moles have, in reality, been examples of a complete mole with an accompanying concomitant non-molar twin pregnancy. Nevertheless, a distinct entity of diploid partial mole does exist which, it has been suggested, merits consideration as a separate third type of molar pregnancy (Verjeslev et al, 1991), such cases possibly being a result of uniparental disomy.

The cytogenetic findings in molar pregnancy suggest strongly that paternal genes play a dominant role in placental development and growth and that maternal genes largely exert their influence on fetal development. This differential function of paternal and maternal genes has been confirmed by experimental animal studies (Barton et al, 1984; Kaufman et al, 1989) and it has been widely thought that moles are an excellent example of genomic imprinting. It has therefore come as somewhat of a surprising finding that maternally imprinted genes are expressed in complete moles (Ariel et al, 1994), this indicating a relaxation of imprinting.

Differential Diagnosis

Hydatidiform moles pose two diagnostic problems: first, the distinction between complete and partial moles and, secondly, the distinction between a hydatidiform mole and a hydropic abortion. In their classical fully established forms it is usually easy to distinguish, on morphological grounds alone, a complete from a partial mole but difficulties arise when an early complete hydatidiform mole is encountered. Under these circumstances neither the finding of villous fetal vessels containing erythrocytes nor an admixture of vesicular and non-vesicular villi is of any distinguishing value and greater stress has to be placed on the lobulated or polypoid appearance of the villi and the presence of stromal nuclear debris in complete moles (Paradinas, 1994; Paradinas et al, 1996).

Both flow and static cytometry have been used extensively to differentiate complete from partial moles (Fisher et al, 1987; Hemming et al, 1987; Lage et al, 1988, 1992; Conran et al, 1993; Fukunaga et al, 1993; Koenig et al, 1993; Lage & Popeck, 1993; van de Kaa et al, 1993; Cheville et al, 1995; Jeffers et al, 1995; Topalovski et al, 1995; Paradinas et al, 1996). Some of the technical problems in the interpretation of DNA histograms and the anomalies encountered in cytometric studies have been discussed by Lage and Bagg (1996) but the vast majority of partial moles are triploid and nearly all complete moles are diploid. The few exceptions to this general rule await elucidation but cytometry, either flow or image, has proved to be of considerable value in distinguishing between the two forms of molar disease and should probably now be considered as a routine diagnostic tool. Other techniques, such as interphase cytogenetics (van de Kaa et al, 1993), fluorescence *in situ* hybridization (Cheville et al, 1995) and the use of the polymerase chain reaction to detect Y chromosome-specific sequences (Azuma et al, 1990; Fisher & Newlands, 1993; Lane et al, 1993), whilst providing interesting results, are likely to remain the domain of the research laboratory for some considerable time.

Pathologists do encounter difficulties in distinguishing between partial hydatidiform moles and hydropic abortuses on purely morphological grounds (Messerli et al, 1987; Howat et al, 1993). In this situation cytometry is of less value because whilst diploidy does, to all intents and purposes, rule out a partial mole, the finding of triploidy does not necessarily indicate a diagnosis of a partial mole because a proportion of hydropic abortions, variously estimated as between 4% and 14% (Szulman et al, 1981; Lage et al, 1992; Paradinas et al, 1996), are triploid. Such cases are ones in which the extra chromosomal load is of maternal rather than paternal origin and it is possible, indeed probable, that it is just this group which causes most problems in morphological diagnosis. Attempts to distinguish partial moles from hydropic abortions by using the cell proliferation marker PCNA have yielded conflicting results (Suresh et al, 1993; Jeffers et al, 1994) and probably the most that can be said is that very careful analysis of the pattern of trophoblastic growth remains the best, but far from infallible and undoubtedly subjective, means of making this distinction.

An uncommon, but difficult, diagnostic problem may occur if curettage material is received from a twin pregnancy in which one twin has a normal placenta and the other is a complete hydatidiform mole, the difficulty being that the admixture of vesicular and non-vesicular villi may suggest a diagnosis of a partial mole. Under such circumstances it may be possible to discern that the vesicular villi have the features of a complete rather than a partial mole but an absolute diagnosis depends upon showing that all the villi are diploid and that whilst some are biparental others are androgenetic (van de Kaa et al, 1995).

Postmolar Disease

All women who have had a hydatidiform mole should be entered into a surveillance programme and monitored by regular assay of urinary or serum hCG levels. When the hCG levels return to normal, patients are advised not to become pregnant until hCG levels have remained normal for at least 6 months. Bagshawe et al (1986) found that if hCG levels fell to normal within 8 weeks of evacuation of a complete mole, follow-up could be safely limited to 6 months, but if the levels were still elevated after 8 weeks, follow-up should be continued for 2 years. The protocol for patients who have had a partial mole are less rigid and many feel that surveillance can be terminated as soon as hCG levels fall to normal. In very general terms treatment is not indicated if hCG levels are falling and the main indications for chemotherapy are a rising hCG level, high hCG levels 4 weeks after evacuation of the mole or prolonged uterine bleeding (Elston, 1995).

In the UK about 8% of patients who have had a complete mole will require chemotherapy for persistent trophoblastic disease (Womack & Elston, 1985; Bagshawe et al, 1986); the figure in the USA is rather higher, in the region of 20% (Currie, 1996), because of the use of different interventional criteria. The actual cause of persistent trophoblastic disease is generally unknown: there may have been incomplete removal of the mole but it is equally possible that many of these cases are invasive hydatidiform moles with residual invasive molar tissue within the myometrium or its vasculature; it is also possible that some are early cases of choriocarcinoma. It is thought that the risk of development of a clinically overt choriocarcinoma following a complete mole is in the region of 5%.

The incidence of persistent trophoblastic disease following a partial mole has been much disputed but there is now no doubt that it occurs, though the magnitude of the risk is very much lower than for complete moles (Mostoufi-Zadeh et al, 1987; Bagshawe et al, 1990; Rice et al, 1990; Lage et al, 1991; Goto et al, 1993). The eventual risk of choriocarcinoma in patients with partial moles is also unknown: choriocarcinomas have been reported following partial moles (Looi & Sivanesaratnam, 1981; Bagshawe et al, 1990; Gardner & Lage, 1992) but this, in itself, does not necessarily mean that this condition increases the risk of a choriocarcinoma as this can follow a normal pregnancy.

Prognostic Factors

As it is widely agreed that all women who have had a molar pregnancy should enter a follow-up surveillance programme, there is no practical point in attempting to define those cases at most risk of developing postmolar disease. Nevertheless, from a purely theoretical viewpoint it is of interest to consider if there are any features of a hydatidiform mole that indicate a high risk of postmolar complications. It was at one time considered that the risk of eventual postmolar disease was directly related to the degree of trophoblastic proliferation in the mole (Hertig & Sheldon, 1947) but this has proved not to be the case (Elston & Bagshawe, 1972a; Genest et al, 1991) and 'grading' of moles in terms of their degree of trophoblastic proliferation has now been abandoned. Attempts to forecast those cases at greatest risk for postmolar disease by the use of cell proliferation markers and flow cytometry (Hemming et al, 1988; Cheung et al, 1993) have failed but it has been maintained that heterozygous (dispermic) moles have a much higher risk of subsequent postmolar complications than do homozygous (monospermic) moles (Wake et al, 1987). Doubts have been cast upon this claim, however, by the failure to find any association between the presence of a Y chromosome, detected by the polymerase chain reaction, in a mole and an excess incidence of postmolar disease (Mutter et al, 1993).

INVASIVE HYDATIDIFORM MOLE

An invasive hydatidiform mole is one that penetrates into the myometrium or invades the uterine vasculature. The vast majority of moles that become invasive are of the complete type but a partial mole can also be invasive (Gabar et al, 1986).

A deeply invasive mole usually becomes clinically evident several weeks after apparently complete evacuation of a mole from the uterus, the patient usually presenting with haemorrhage. If a hysterectomy is performed at this stage the appearances range from, at one extreme, only a small haemorrhagic focus in the myometrium to, at the other end of the spectrum, a large deeply cavitating haemorrhagic lesion of the uterine wall (Fig. 14.13) which mimics a choriocarcinoma. Rarely, a mole penetrates the full thickness of the myometrium, leading either to uterine perforation or to extension of the mole into adjacent structures, such as the broad ligament. The histological distinction from a choriocarcinoma is dependent upon the finding of molar villi within the uterine wall, these more commonly being seen in the myometrial vascular channels than between the myometrial fibres (Fig. 14.14). The molar villi show a very variable degree of trophoblastic proliferation and sometimes this is far from being a conspicuous feature.

Invasive moles have, in the past, caused death from uterine bleeding or perforation but their mortality rate is now virtually zero because of the success achieved in

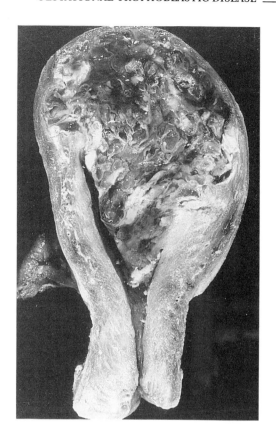

Figure 14.13. An invasive hydatidiform mole. The mole is invading deeply into the myometrium and at one point infiltrates almost to the serosa.

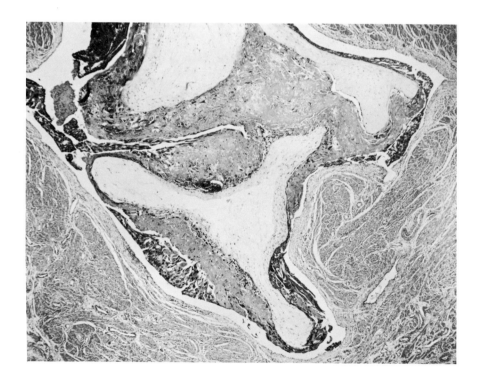

Figure 14.14. Invasive hydatidiform mole with molar villi lying within a dilated venous channel deep within the myometrium (H & E ×40).

their treatment by a limited course of chemotherapy. In fact the diagnosis of an invasive mole, which can only be made with certainty on a hysterectomy specimen, is now almost obsolete because nearly all invasive moles are subsumed into the category of persistent trophoblastic disease.

It has to be stressed that the invasive capacity of some moles is not an indication that they are neoplastic. Normal trophoblast has the ability to invade both the myometrium and the uterine vessels (Robertson et al, 1975; Pijnenborg et al, 1981) whilst villi from a normal placenta can invade deeply into, or even through, the uterine wall to give rise to a placenta increta or a placenta percreta (Fox, 1972), both of which are the exact non-molar equivalents of an invasive mole (Hertig, 1950).

Molar tissue can be transported via the bloodstream to extrauterine sites, particularly to the vagina and lungs. The transported molar trophoblast can then grow in these sites to form nodules that are either clinically or radiologically detectable. The development of 'metastatic' lesions implies that molar trophoblast has entered the uterine vessels (Fig. 14.15) and hence their presence is taken as *de facto* evidence of the presence of an invasive mole. The 'metastatic' nodules are not, however, usually associated with evidence of molar invasion of the myometrial tissues.

The 'metastatic' nodules usually appear several weeks after evacuation of a mole from the uterus but may occur concurrently with a mole or can be the presenting symptom of such a lesion. Vaginal lesions form haemorrhagic submucous nodules, the true nature of which only becomes apparent when microscopy reveals the presence of villous structures (Fig. 14.16), a finding which rules out a diagnosis of choriocarcinoma (Elston, 1976). Some vaginal nodules do not contain villi but consist solely of 'benign transported trophoblast' (Figs 14.17 and 14.18) lacking the features of a choriocarcinoma. Pulmonary lesions can cause haemoptysis but are usually an asymptomatic radiological finding: histological examination of these will also reveal their content of villi (Ring, 1972; Johnson et al, 1979). Reported, not always fully convincingly, rare sites of 'metastasis' include the paraspinal connective tissues (Delfs, 1957), spinal cord (Hsu et

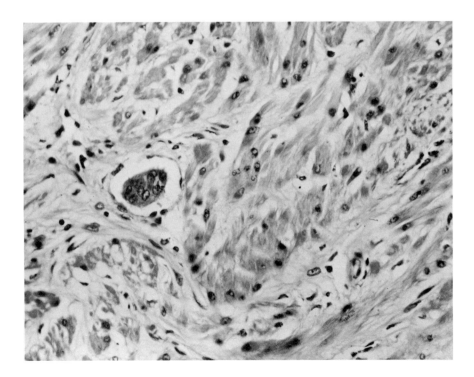

Figure 14.15. Small group of trophoblastic cells within a myometrial vessel: these were from a mole which showed only a very superficial villous invasion of the myometrium (H & E ×250).

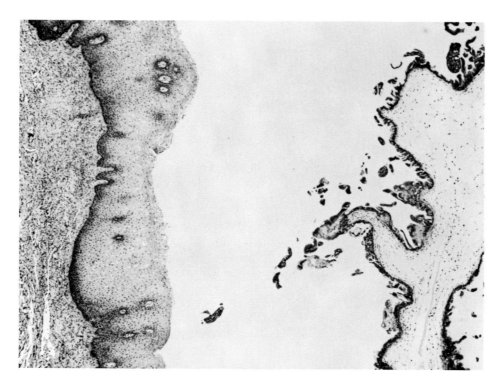

Figure 14.16. Molar villus with adjacent vaginal mucosa, obtained at biopsy of a vaginal nodule in a patient with a hydatidiform mole (H & E ×50).

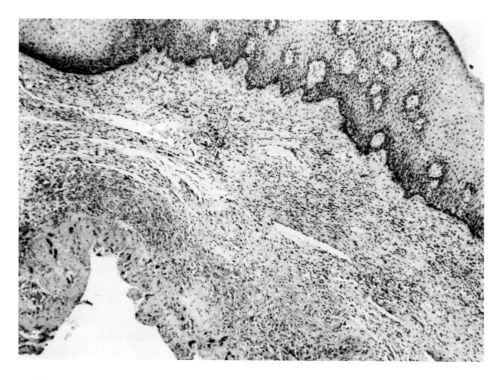

Figure 14.17. Biopsy of a vaginal nodule in a patient with a hydatidiform mole. The cavity at the bottom left is surrounded by inflammatory cells and occasional syncytiotrophoblast-like cells. The appearances are those of 'benign transported trophoblast' (H & E ×80).

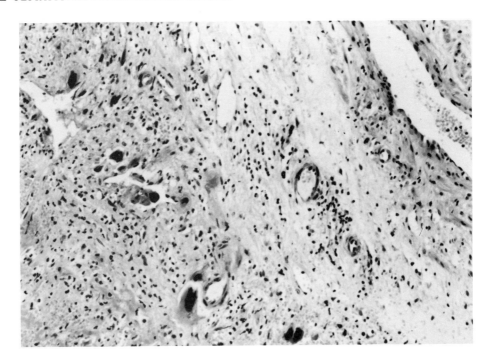

Figure 14.18. Higher magnification of nodule shown in Fig. 14.17. Syncytiotrophoblast-like cells are present: benign transported trophoblast (H & E ×160).

al, 1962) and brain (Ishizuka, 1967). These extrauterine lesions may resolve spontaneously but are commonly treated with limited chemotherapy, which achieves excellent results.

The fact that molar trophoblast is transported to extrauterine sites is not an indication of neoplastic behaviour. Trophoblast enters the maternal bloodstream in every normal pregnancy (Couone et al, 1984; Mueller et al, 1990) and is transported to sites such as the lung (Attwood & Park, 1961), this transported trophoblast only giving rise to detectable lesions if it is molar in nature.

There is no evidence that women with invasive moles are at increased risk of developing a choriocarcinoma and, indeed, the reverse may be the case (Chun & Braga, 1967).

CHORIOCARCINOMA

The variation in the incidence of choriocarcinoma is at least as great as is that for molar disease with those geographic areas having a high incidence of hydatidiform moles also having a high incidence of choriocarcinoma. Whether, however, the excess of choriocarcinoma in these regions is simply a reflection of the high incidence of moles or whether it indicates that the same factors which predispose to a molar gestation also predispose to choriocarcinoma is a moot point.

Approximately 50% of choriocarcinomas follow a molar pregnancy, 30% occur after an abortion and 20% follow an apparently normal gestation. The time interval between the antecedent pregnancy and the clinical presentation of a choriocarcinoma is very variable, ranging from a few weeks or months to 15 years. The most common symptom is vaginal bleeding but some women present with signs and symptoms due to metastatic disease, e.g., intracranial bleeding, haemoptysis, haematemesis or bluish nodules in the skin and mucous membranes. Occasional patients present with acute or subacute pulmonary hypertension caused by tumour growth in the pulmonary arteries (Bagshawe & Brooks, 1959; Seckl et al, 1991).

Morphology

Within the uterus a choriocarcinoma forms a single haemorrhagic mass (Fig. 14.19) or multiple haemorrhagic nodules which are often accompanied by local metastases to the cervix and vagina (Fig. 14.20). The neoplastic masses consist of a central area of haemorrhagic necrosis and, usually though not invariably, a peripheral rim of viable tumour tissue. The central, sometimes complete, necrosis of the neoplastic tissue is a reflection of the fact that a choriocarcinoma has no intrinsic blood supply, relying for its oxygenation on its ability to invade the uterine blood vessels. It is therefore only the growing edge of the tumour that is adequately oxygenated, the remainder undergoing ischaemic necrosis.

Histologically, a choriocarcinoma has a biphasic structure that recapitulates, often to a striking degree, that of the trophoblast of the normal implanting blastocyst, central sheets or cores of cytotrophoblast being 'capped' by a peripheral rim of syncytiotrophoblast (Fig. 14.21); occasional choriocarcinomas show a marked predominance of cytotrophoblast with minimal syncytiotrophoblast (Fig. 14.22). The cytotrophoblastic cells have large vesicular nuclei with prominent, sometimes multiple, nucleoli (Fig. 14.23) and clear or granular cytoplasm. The syncytial nuclei are smaller than those of the cytotrophoblastic cells and the cytoplasm of the syncytiotrophoblast is deeply eosinophilic. The trophoblastic cells in a choriocarcinoma may show no greater degree of atypia and mitotic activity than is seen in an implanting blastocyst but some show marked cytological atypia and contain many, sometimes abnormal, mitotic figures. Villi are never present in an extraplacental choriocarcinoma and, indeed, the presence of villous structures negates a diagnosis of choriocarcinoma.

Because of the need to obtain an oxygen supply, a choriocarcinoma is avariciously invasive of vascular channels in the myometrium, vessels which, it should be noted, are also invaded by trophoblast during the process of normal implantation. The tumour cells tend to form solid plugs within the myometrial vasculature (Fig. 14.24) and, although there is often extravascular extension, the malignant trophoblast tends to infiltrate between the muscle fibres with very little tissue destruction. The propensity

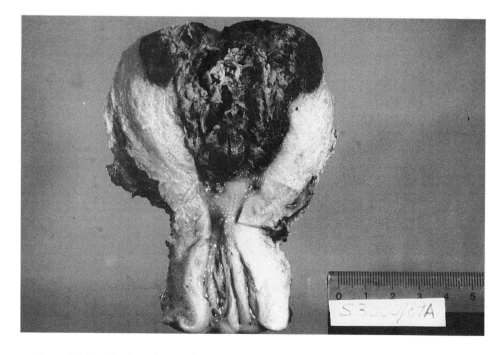

Figure 14.19. Choriocarcinoma. Section of a uterus containing a haemorrhagic mass of choriocarcinoma in the uterine body.

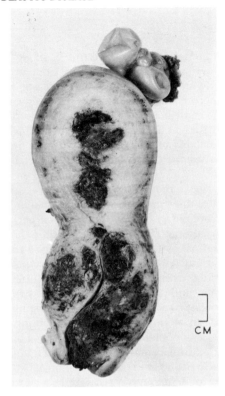

Figure 14.20. Hemisected uterus showing several haemorrhagic nodules of choriocarcinoma in the body and cervix.

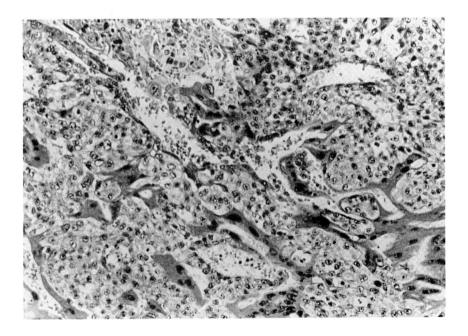

Figure 14.21. Choriocarcinoma composed of sheets of cytotrophoblast and syncytiotrophoblast (H & E ×100).

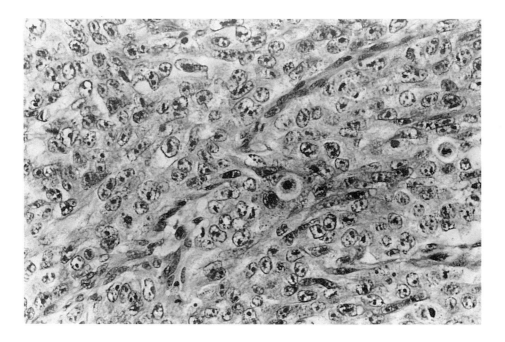

Figure 14.22. A choriocarcinoma in which there is a predominance of cytotrophoblast (H & E ×220).

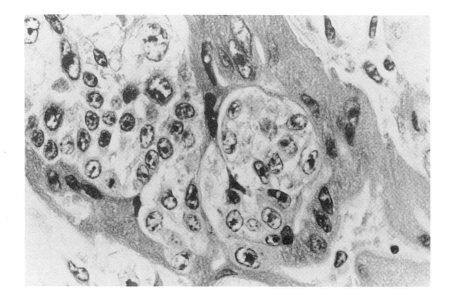

Figure 14.23. A choriocarcinoma showing central cores of cytotrophoblast surrounded by syncytiotrophoblast. The nucleoli are prominent, particularly in the cytotrophoblast (H & E ×520).

for vascular invasion is the basis for the predominantly haematogenous dissemination of a choriocarcinoma to sites such as the lungs, brain (Fig. 14.25), liver, kidney and gastrointestinal tract: large tumour emboli may impact within the pulmonary arteries. Lymph node deposits of a choriocarcinoma are usually tertiary metastases from a large extrauterine lesion.

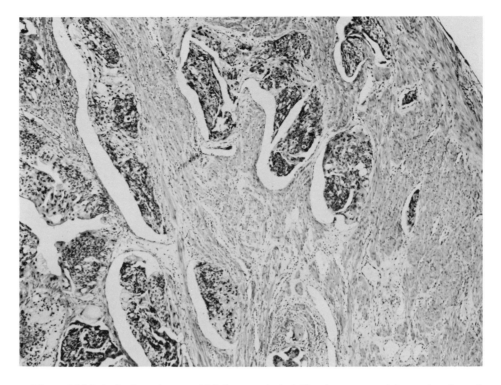

Figure 14.24. A choriocarcinoma which is extensively infiltrating myometrial vascular channels: the intervening myometrium is uninvolved (H & E ×50).

Histological Diagnosis of Choriocarcinoma in Curettage Material

Choriocarcinoma is often suspected if a woman complains of vaginal bleeding after either a normal pregnancy or a molar gestation. In a proportion of such cases, trophoblast will be present and Elston and Bagshawe (1972b) classified the type of trophoblastic tissue found under these circumstances into four groups:

1. Villous trophoblast
2. Simple trophoblast
3. Suspicious trophoblast
4. Trophoblast diagnostic of choriocarcinoma.

The term 'villous trophoblast' indicates that villi are present in the curettings. A diagnosis of 'simple trophoblast' is made if collections or clumps of monomorphous trophoblastic cells are present (Fig. 14.26) whilst if there are sheets of trophoblast showing a biphasic pattern of cytotrophoblast and syncytiotrophoblast (Figs 14.27 and 14.28) the diagnosis is 'suspicious trophoblast' if there is no evidence of endomyometrial invasion and 'trophoblast diagnostic of choriocarcinoma' if definite endomyometrial invasion is seen (Fig. 14.29).

The interpretation of these findings depends on the nature of the preceding pregnancy. If the preceding gestation was a hydatidiform mole then the finding of villous trophoblast, simple trophoblast or suspicious trophoblast in curettings indicates a diagnosis of persistent trophoblastic disease; under these circumstances choriocarcinoma should not be diagnosed and surveillance should be continued. Following a molar pregnancy a diagnosis of choriocarcinoma should only be made if invasive biophasic trophoblast (i.e. trophoblast diagnostic of choriocarcinoma) is seen. By contrast, if the preceding pregnancy was a normal pregnancy or a non-molar abortion, the pres-

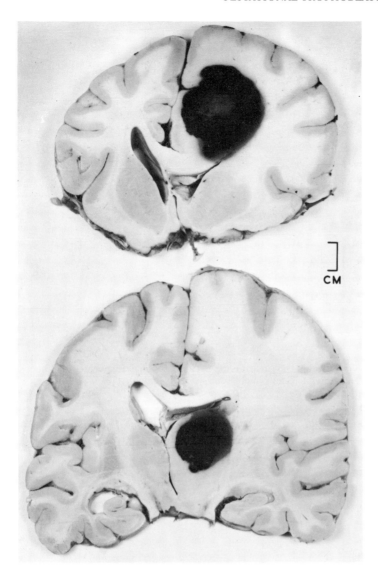

Figure 14.25. Cerebral metastases of a choriocarcinoma.

ence of villous trophoblast indicates the retention of placental tissue but the finding of non-villous trophoblast is an almost certain indication of a choriocarcinoma.

Origin

There are many puzzling aspects of choriocarcinomas such as their status as an allograft (which they must be because of their content of paternal antigens), their increased frequency in women of blood groups A with group O spouses and in group O women with group A spouses (Dawood et al, 1971; Bagshawe, 1973, 1976) and their rather strange, almost bizarre, epidemiological risk factors, which include dieting, a family history of dizygotic twins, more than one marriage and infrequent sexual intercourse (Buckley et al, 1988). By far the most perplexing problem they pose is their origin. As already remarked, choriocarcinomas may follow either a normal or a molar pregnancy, more commonly the latter, and there is a considerable gap in our knowledge as to the relationship between the previous pregnancy and the subsequent

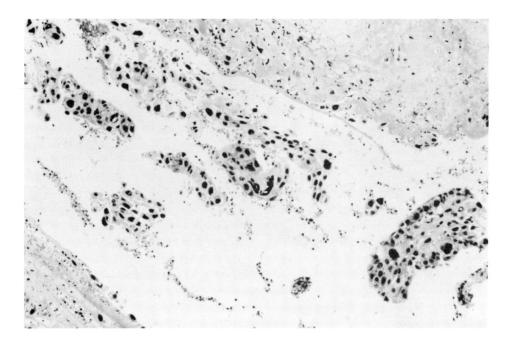

Figure 14.26. Simple trophoblast in a curetting. There are small fragments of pyknotic trophoblast with no clear differentiation into cytotrophoblast or syncytiotrophoblast (H & E ×120).

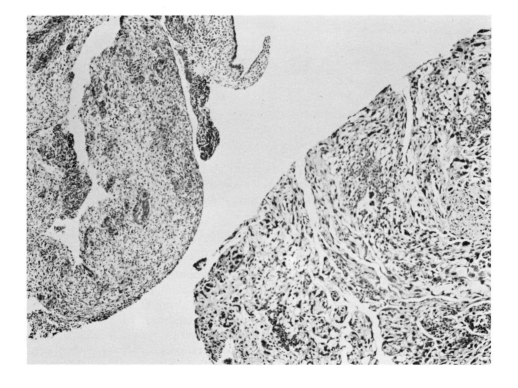

Figure 14.27. Suspicious trophoblast in a curetting. The fragment of trophoblast is to the right with decidual tissue to the left (H & E ×50).

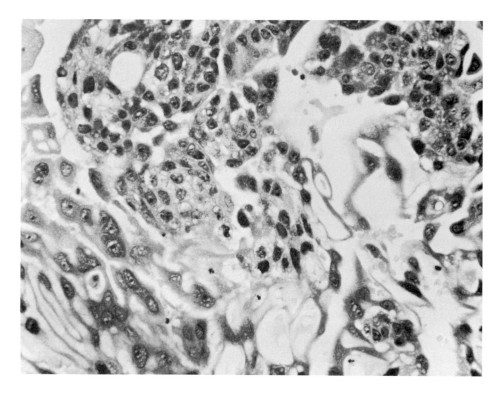

Figure 14.28. Higher magnification of the trophoblast shown in Fig. 14.27 showing cytotrophoblast and syncytiotrophoblast (H & E ×250).

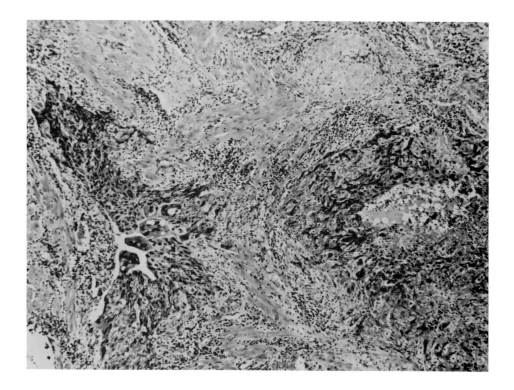

Figure 14.29. Invasive choriocarcinoma in a uterine curetting, the myometrium being infiltrated by choriocarcinoma (H & E ×70).

choriocarcinoma. Is the neoplasm actually derived from the trophoblast of the prior pregnancy and, if so, what has been happening to this trophoblast during the intervening months or years? The application of genetic techniques, such as the study of cytogenetic polymorphism (Chaganti et al, 1990), DNA restriction fragment-length polymorphism assays (Azuma et al, 1990; Osada et al, 1991; Fisher et al, 1992) or the study of tandem repeat regions amplified by the polymerase chain reaction (Suzuki et al, 1993; Fisher et al, 1995) has shown that some, but by no means all, choriocarcinomas are androgenetic. It has further been demonstrated that some of these androgenetic tumours were genetically identical to a previous molar gestation despite the fact that in two such cases there had been a full-term normal delivery intervening between the molar pregnancy and the development of the choriocarcinoma (Fisher et al, 1992, 1995; Suzuki et al, 1993). In one of these cases the time interval between the mole and the choriocarcinoma was 10 years (Fisher et al, 1992) and it is difficult to understand how tissue from the mole remained in the uterus for that length of time, and throughout a later normal pregnancy, to then subsequently undergo a neoplastic resurgence, this typifying the questions posed by this enigmatic lesion.

Some points are, however, becoming clearer; it is seeming increasingly probable that many, possibly most or even all, choriocarcinomas that follow an apparently normal pregnancy are, in reality, metastases from an undetected small intraplacental choriocarcinoma. Only a small number of intraplacental choriocarcinomas have been described (Driscoll, 1963; Brewer & Gerbie, 1966; Brewer & Mazur, 1981; Tsukamoto et al, 1981; Fox & Laurini, 1988; Hallam et al, 1990; Christopherson et al, 1992; Lage & Roberts, 1993) and in nearly all cases the choriocarcinoma was very small and easily overlooked unless the placenta was meticulously examined. In most cases the placenta had been subjected to such examination because metastases had developed in the mother during pregnancy and in only two cases had the tumour been detected in the absence of such complications (Driscoll, 1963; Fox & Laurini, 1988). One case (Hallam et al, 1990) is of particular interest insofar as a patient developed an apparently primary choriocarcinoma soon after a normal pregnancy; re-examination of the placenta at that time revealed a tiny intraplacental choriocarcinoma. Intraplacental choriocarcinomas are histologically identical to extraplacental choriocarcinomas (Fig. 14.30) but are often separated from the normal villous population by villi with a surrounding mantle of choriocarcinoma-like trophoblast which has replaced the normal trophoblast (Figs 14.31 and 14.32). This therefore confirms the long-held opinion, based largely on the ability of choriocarcinomas to secrete hCG, that a choriocarcinoma is a lesion of villous trophoblast despite the invariable absence of villi from extraplacental tumours.

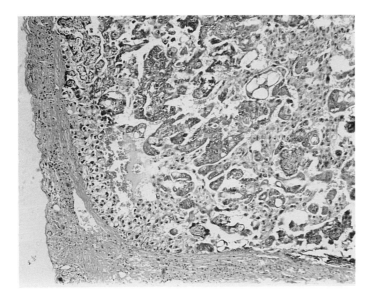

Figure 14.30. A focus of choriocarcinoma in a term placenta from an uncomplicated pregnancy.

If choriocarcinomas following a normal pregnancy are in reality metastases from an intraplacental choriocarcinoma, are those which follow a molar gestation similarly derived from an intramolar choriocarcinoma? This is certainly a possibility because one such lesion has been described (Heifetz & Csaja, 1992), though it was not associated with subsequent disease. The prolonged time interval in many cases between a molar pregnancy and the development of an overt choriocarcinoma does, however, suggest that by no means all postmolar choriocarcinomas are derived from intramolar lesions and though, as already discussed, some moles are genetically identical to prior moles,

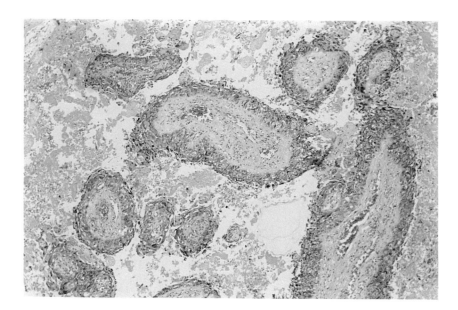

Figure 14.31. From the same case as Fig. 14.30. Between the normal villi and the focal choriocarcinoma were villi with a surrounding mantle of markedly abnormal trophoblast.

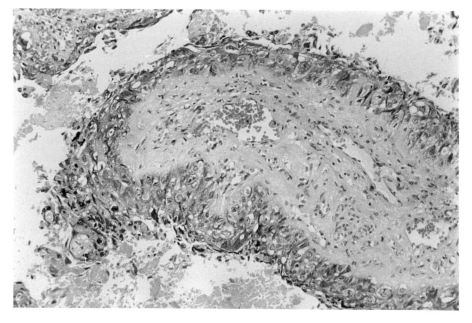

Figure 14.32. Higher magnification of the abnormal villous trophoblast shown in Fig. 14.31. The villous trophoblast closely resembles choriocarcinomatous tissue.

some postmolar choriocarcinomas are biparental. This raises the possibility that some choriocarcinomas are new pregnancies, the choriocarcinoma *ab initio* that has long been proposed (Acosta-Sison, 1955). There seems no good reason why a pregnancy, androgenetic or biparental, should not evolve directly into a choriocarcinoma and there is an excellent precedent for the belief that a pregnancy can appear to be neoplastic, namely the now generally agreed concept that a teratoma is a parthogenetic pregnancy (Fox, 1987). This raises the question, however, as to whether such pregnancies should be considered as truly neoplastic or simply as aberrant gestations. It is true that they invade vessels and spread to distant sites but so does normal trophoblast. They resemble acutely the trophoblast of the normal implanting blastocyst, and their response to methotrexate, whilst being quite different from that of virtually every other neoplasm, is not unlike that of a normal, but ectopic, early gestation. This is, of course, pure speculation but nevertheless the possibility that some choriocarcinomas are simply abnormal pregnancies should not be dismissed too lightly.

PLACENTAL SITE TROPHOBLASTIC TUMOUR

Clinical Features

This tumour is derived from the extravillous trophoblastic cells of the placental bed. It is a rare neoplasm though its true frequency is unknown: 77 cases had been reported in the English-language literature by 1995 (How et al, 1995) but there must be many cases that pass unrecorded.

In the majority of cases the neoplasm develops after a normal pregnancy; it is commonly stated that only 5% occur after a molar gestation (Lage & Young, 1993; Elston, 1995) but in their review How et al (1995) noted that the preceeding gestation was a molar pregnancy in 11 of 77 cases (14%). The age of women with this tumour has ranged from 19 to 53 years with a mean age of about 28 years. For obvious reasons the patients are usually in their reproductive era but there have been two instances in postmenopausal women (Eckstein et al, 1982; McLellan et al, 1991). Patients present at anything from a few weeks to several years after the antecedent pregnancy with a complaint of irregular vaginal bleeding or, perhaps more commonly, amenorrhoea. Occasional patients have been, for reasons that have not been satisfactorily explained, virilized (Nagelburg & Rosen, 1985; Nagamani et al, 1990) whilst a small proportion of patients develop a nephrotic syndrome which appears to be due to chronic intravascular coagulation initiated by factors released from the tumour (Young & Scully, 1984; Young et al, 1985). A patient described by How et al (1995) presented with only a history of anorexia, nausea and vomiting. Serum hCG levels are normal in approximately 23% of patients, slightly elevated in 46% and moderately elevated in 31% (Young et al, 1988; Lage & Young, 1993) this reflecting the fact that the principal secretory product of extravillous trophoblast is hPL rather than hCG.

Morphological Features

The uterus is commonly enlarged and the tumours tend to form tan, white or yellow masses either within the myometrium or protruding into the endometrial cavity in a polypoidal fashion (Fig. 14.33). Foci of haemorrhage and necrosis may be present but these are rarely a conspicuous feature and are not uncommonly completely absent.

Histologically, the neoplasm replicates, in an anarchic form, the appearances seen in the normal placental bed. The tumour is formed principally of mononuclear trophoblastic cells with an irregular and inconsistent admixture of multinucleated cells, the latter resembling the multinucleated cells of the placental bed rather than true syncytiotrophoblast. The polyhedral, rounded or spindle-shaped mononuclear tumour cells are arranged as cords, islands or sheets and infiltrate between, and dissect, the

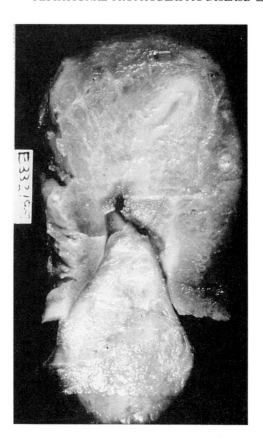

Figure 14.33. A placental site trophoblastic tumour: this is extensively infiltrating the myometrium and is also protruding
into the uterine cavity as a polypoid mass.

myometrial fibres with a striking absence of necrosis and haemorrhage (Figs 14.34 and
14.35). Invasion of vessels by tumour cells is common but the massive intravascular
growth that characterizes a choriocarcinoma is not seen and some vessels within the
tumour are surrounded, but not invaded, by neoplastic cells. Non-infiltrated vessels
often show fibrinoid necrosis of their wall, whilst a pseudodecidual change, and sometimes an Arias–Stella reaction, may be apparent in the adjacent endometrium. Mitotic
figures are almost invariably present and may range from sparse to abundant. There
may be an infiltrate, usually sparse, of chronic inflammatory cells, hyalinization is
occasionally seen whilst in rare instances there is an extensive deposition of fibrin-like
material (Lage & Young, 1993). The mononucleated tumour cells usually stain positively for hPL and cytokeratins but a small proportion stain positively for hCG, as do
the multinucleated cells (Kurman et al, 1984).

Differential Diagnosis

A placental site trophoblastic tumour has to be distinguished from an exaggerated
placental site reaction (Fig. 14.36), a distinction that is usually easy in a hysterectomy
specimen but difficult, indeed sometimes impossible, in curettage material. A useful,
but certainly not universally valid, criterion in making this differential diagnosis is the
time interval between the antecedent pregnancy and the curettage, because the longer
the time that has elapsed since the last gestation the more likely is it that infiltrating trophoblastic cells are neoplastic in nature. Villi have been noted in one slightly unusual
placental site trophoblastic tumour (Collins et al, 1990) but the presence of such structures normally indicates an exaggerated placental site reaction. An absence of mitotic
figures and a relative abundance of multinucleated trophoblastic cells (Fig. 14.37)
favour a diagnosis of exaggerated placental site reaction whilst, conversely, the presence

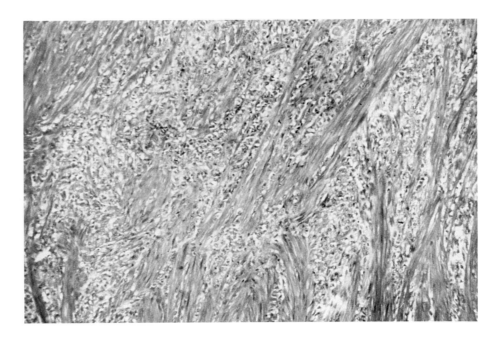

Figure 14.34. A placental site trophoblastic tumour. Cords of trophoblastic cells infiltrate between the smooth muscle fibres of the myometrium.

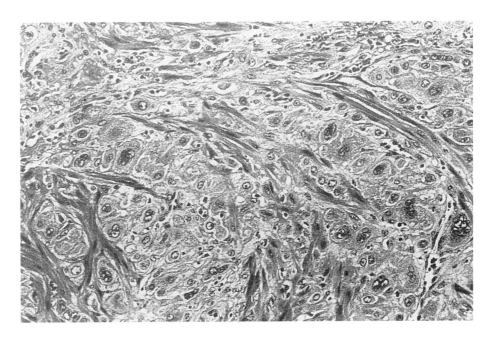

Figure 14.35. Higher-power view of the infiltrating trophoblast cells of a placental site trophoblastic tumour.

of mitotic figures, a paucity of multinucleated cells and the presence of sheets or conflu-ent masses of trophoblastic cells are indicative of a placental site trophoblastic tumour. If after taking into account all these considerations it is impossible to reach a firm con-clusion, it is usual to advise careful observation and repeat curettage within a month.

The trophoblast of the placental site can assume an aggregated pattern to form a placental site nodule which can persist for many years after a pregnancy (Young et al,

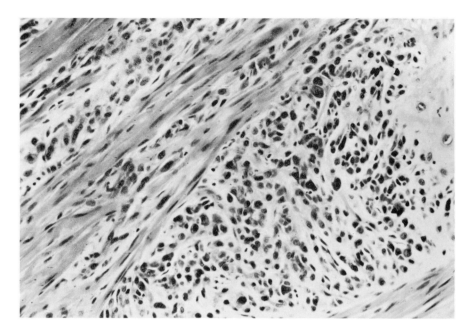

Figure 14.36. Exaggerated placental site reaction in myometrium: from a uterine curetting following a spontaneous abortion (H & E ×180).

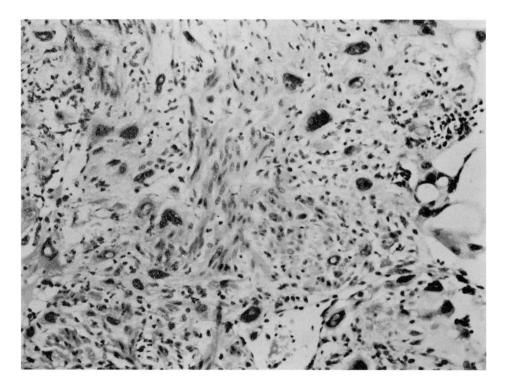

Figure 14.37. Higher magnification of an exaggerated placental site reaction; many typical multinucleated giant cells are present (H & E ×260).

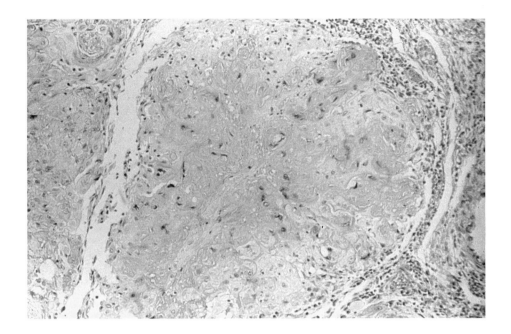

Figure 14.38. A sharply localized, hyalinized placental site nodule containing a few trophoblastic cells.

1990). These nodules, usually single but occasionally multiple, are well circumscribed, oval, elongated or rounded and are typically eosinophilic and extensively hyalinized (Fig. 14.38). Placental site nodules can be distinguished from a placental site trophoblastic tumour by their circumscribed, non-infiltrative nature, their lack of mitotic activity and their tendency to undergo hyalinization.

Occasional choriocarcinomas consist largely of cytotrophoblastic cells and these can be distinguished from a placental site trophoblastic tumour by their diffuse staining for hCG.

Prognosis

About 15–20% of placental site trophoblastic tumours behave in a malignant fashion (Young et al, 1988; Lage et al, 1993) and either recur locally or spread to such distant sites as the liver, lung, central nervous system, other abdominal viscera and vagina; lymph node metastases are uncommon. Assessment of the degree of malignancy of any individual neoplasm is, however, difficult because although those which have run a malignant course have usually had a mitotic count of above 4 per 10 high-power fields, this is not an invariable rule (Eckstein et al, 1982; Gloor et al, 1983; Finkler et al, 1988; Alvero et al, 1990; Fukunaga & Ushigome, 1993) and a low mitotic count should not necessarily engender a sense of security. By contrast, some tumours with very high mitotic counts appear to have pursued a benign course (Eckstein et al, 1982). Clinical stage is an obvious prognostic factor but tumour size, depth of myometrial invasion and vascular space invasion appear to be of no prognostic import (How et al, 1995).

It is of note that the placental site trophoblastic tumour responds very poorly to the cytotoxic drug therapy that is so successful in choriocarcinoma; indeed, the response to any form of chemotherapy is unsatisfactory and surgery is the basis of treatment, most patients requiring a hysterectomy (Finkler et al, 1988; Lathrop et al, 1988; Dessau et al, 1990).

Flow cytometry of placental site trophoblastic tumour has been performed only rarely but most of the tumours appear to be diploid; there has been one triploid neoplasm which, very suprisingly, followed a normal term pregnancy.

REFERENCES

Acosta-Sison, H. (1955) Can the implanting trophoblast of the fertilized ovum develop immediately into choriocarcinoma? *American Journal of Obstetrics and Gynecolology*, **69**, 442–444.

Alvero, R., Remmenga, S., O'Connor, D., Barnhill, D. and Park, R. (1990) Metastatic placental site trophoblastic tumor. *Gynecologic Oncology*, **37**, 445–449.

Ariel, I., Lustig, O., Oyer, C. et al. (1994) Relaxation of imprinting in trophoblastic disease. *Gynecologic Oncology*, **53**, 212–219.

Atrash, H.K., Hogue, C.J.R. and Grimes, D.A. (1986) Epidemiology of hydatidiform mole during early gestation. *American Journal of Obstetrics and Gynecology*, **154**, 906–909.

Attwood, H.D. and Park, W.W. (1961) Embolism to the lungs by trophoblast. *Journal of Obstetrics and Gynaecology of the British Commonwealth*, **68**, 611–617.

Azuma, C., Saji, F., Nobunaga, T. et al (1990) Studies of the pathogenesis of choriocarcinoma by analysis of restriction fragment length polymorphisms. *Cancer Research*, **50**, 488–491.

Bagshawe, K.D. (1973) Recent observations related to chemotherapy and immunology of gestational choriocarcinoma. *Advances in Cancer Research*, **18**, 231–263.

Bagshawe, K.D. (1976) Risk and prognostic factors in trophoblastic neoplasia. *Cancer*, **38**, 1373–1385.

Bagshawe, K.D. and Brooks, W.D.W. (1959) Subacute pulmonary hypertension due to chorionepithelioma. *Lancet*, **i**, 653–658.

Bagshawe, K.D., Dent, J. and Webb, J. (1986) Hydatidiform mole in England and Wales 1973–83. *Lancet*, **ii**, 673–677.

Bagshawe, K.D., Lawler, S.D., Paradinas, F., Dent, J., Brown, P. and Boxer, G.M. (1990) Gestational trophoblastic tumours following initial diagnosis of partial hydatidiform mole. *Lancet*, **335**, 1074–1076.

Barton, S.C., Surani, M.A.H. and Norris, M.L. (1984) Role of paternal and maternal genomes in mouse development. *Nature*, **311**, 374–376.

Bracken, M.B. (1987) Incidence and aetiology of hydatidiform mole: an epidemiological review. *British Journal of Obstetrics and Gynaecology*, **94**, 1123–1135.

Brewer, J.L. and Gerbie, A.B. (1966) Early development of choriocarcinoma. *American Journal of Obstetrics and Gynecology*, **94**, 692–710.

Brewer, J.L. and Mazur, M.T. (1981) Gestational choriocarcinoma: its origin in the placenta during seemingly normal pregnancy. *American Journal of Surgical Pathology*, **5**, 267–277.

Buckley, J. (1987) Epidemiology of gestational trophoblastic diseases. In *Gestational Trophoblastic Disease*, Szulman, A.E. and Buchsbaum, H.J. (Eds), pp. 8–26. New York: Springer-Verlag.

Buckley, J.D., Henderson, B.E., Morrow. C.P. et al (1988) Case-control study of gestational choriocarcinoma. *Cancer Research*, **48**, 1004–1010.

Chaganti, R.S.K., Koduru, P.R.K., Chakraborty, R. and Jones, W.B. (1990) Genetic origin of a trophoblastic choriocarcinoma. *Cancer Research*, **50**, 6330–6333.

Cheung, A.N., Ngan, H.Y., Chen, W.Z., Loke, S.L. and Collins, R.J. (1993) The significance of proliferating cell nuclear antigen in human trophoblastic disease: an immunohistochemical study. *Histopathology*, **22**, 565–568.

Cheville, J.C., Greiner, T., Robinson, R.A. and Benda, J.A. (1995) Ploidy analysis by flow cytometry and fluorescence *in situ* hybridization in hydropic placentas and gestational trophoblastic disease. *Human Pathology*, **26**, 753–757.

Christopherson, W.A., Kanbour, A. and Szulman, A.E. (1992) Choriocarcinoma in a term placenta with maternal metastases. *Gynecologic Oncology*, **46**, 239–245.

Chun, D. and Braga, C.A. (1967) Choriocarcinoma in Hong Kong. In *Proceedings of the 5th World Congess of Gynaecology and Obstetrics*, Wood, C. and Walters, W.A.W. (Eds), pp. 398–405. New South Wales: Butterworths.

Collins, R.J., Ngan, H.Y.S. and Wong, L.C. (1990) Placental site trophoblastic tumor with features between an exaggerated placental site reaction and a placental site trophoblastic tumor. *International Journal of Gynecological Pathology*, **9**, 170–177.

Conran, R.M., Hitchcock, C.L., Popek, E.J. et al (1993) Diagnostic considerations in molar gestations. *Human Pathology*, **24**, 41–48.

Couone, A.W., Multon, D., Johnson, P.M. and Adolfini, M. (1984) Trophoblast cells in peripheral blood from pregnant women. *Lancet*, **ii**, 841–843.

Cox, S.M. and Klein, V.R. (1993) Partial molar pregnancy associated with severe pregnancy-induced hypertension. *Journal of Perinatology*, **13**, 103–106.

Currie, J.L. (1996) Benign gestational trophoblastic neoplasia and overall surgical management. In *Gynecologic Oncology: Current Diagnosis and Treatment*, Shingleton, H.M., Fowler, W.C., Jr, Jordan, J.A. and Lawrence, W.D. (Eds), pp. 368–378. London: Saunders.

Dawood, M.Y., Teoh, E.S. and Ratnam, S.S. (1971) ABO blood group in trophoblastic neoplasia. *American Journal of Obstetrics and Gynecology*, **78**, 918–923.

Delfs, E. (1957) Quantitative chorionic gonadotrophin: prognostic value in hydatidiform mole and chorioepithelioma. *Obstetrics and Gynecology*, **9**, 1–24.

Dessau, R., Rustin, G.J.S., Dent, J., Paradinas, F.J. and Bagshawe, K.D. (1990) Surgery and chemotherapy in the management of placental site tumor. *Gynecologic Oncology*, **39**, 56–59.

Driscoll, S.G. (1963) Choriocarcinoma: an 'incidental finding' within a term placenta. *Obstetrics and Gynecology*, **21**, 96–102.

Eckstein, R.P., Paradinas, F.J. and Bagshawe, K.D. (1982) Placental site trophoblastic tumour (trophoblastic pseudotumour): a study of four cases requiring hysterectomy, including one fatal case. *Histopathology* **6**, 221–226.

Elston, C.W. (1976) The histopathology of trophoblastic tumours. *Journal of Clinical Pathology*, **29** (Supplement 10), 111–131.

Elston, C.W. (1981) Gestational tumours of trophoblast. In *Recent Advances in Histopathology*, Anthony, P.P. and McSween, R.N.M. (Eds), pp. 149–161.

Elston, C.W. (1995) Gestational trophoblastic disease. In *Haines and Taylor: Textbook of Obstetrical and Gynaecological Pathology*, 4th edn, Fox, H. (Ed.), pp. 1597–1639. New York: Churchill Livingstone.

Elston, C.W., and Bagshawe, K.D. (1972a) The value of histological grading in the management of hydatidiform mole. *Journal of Obstetrics and Gynaecology of the British Commonwealth*, **79**, 717–724.

Elston, C.W. and Bagshawe, K.D. (1972b) The diagnosis of trophoblastic tumours from uterine curettings. *Journal of Clinical Pathology*, **25**, 111–118.

Finkler, N.J., Berkowitz, R.S., Driscoll, S.G., Goldstein, D.P. and Bernstein, M.R. (1988) Clinical experience with placental site trophoblast tumors at the New England Trophoblast Disease Center. *Obstetrics and Gynecology*, **71**, 854–857.

Fisher, R.A. and Newlands, E.S. (1993) Rapid diagnosis and classification of hydatidiform moles with polymerase chain reaction. *American Journal of Obstetrics and Gynecology*, **168**, 563–569.

Fisher, R.A., Lawler, S.D., Ormerod, M.G., Imrie, P.R. and Povey, S. (1987) Flow cytometry used to distinguish between complete and partial hydatidiform moles. *Placenta*, **8**, 249–257.

Fisher, R.A., Newlands, E.S., Jeffreys, A.J. et al (1992) Gestational and non-gestational trophoblastic tumors distinguished by DNA analysis. *Cancer*, **69**, 839–845.

Fisher, R.A., Soteriou, B.A., Meredith, L., Paradinas, F.H. and Newlands, E.S. (1995) Previous hydatidiform mole identified as the causative pregnancy of choriocarcinoma following birth of normal twins. *International Journal of Gynecological Cancer*, **5**, 64–70.

Fox, H. (1972) Placenta accreta, 1945–1969. *Obstetrical and Gynecological Survey*, **27**, 475–490.

Fox, H. (1987) Biology of teratomas. In *Recent Advances in Histopathology 13*, Anthony, P.P. and MacSween, R.N.M. (Eds), pp. 33–43. Edinburgh: Churchill Livingstone.

Fox, H. and Laurini, R.N. (1988) Intraplacental choriocarcinoma: a report of two cases. *Journal of Clinical Pathology*, **41**, 1085–1088.

Fukunaga, M. and Ushigome, S. (1993) Metastasizing placental site trophoblastic tumor: an immunohistochemical and flow cytometric study of two cases. *American Journal of Surgical Pathology*, **17**, 1003–1010.

Fukunaga, M., Ushigome, S., Fukunaga, M. and Sugishita, M. (1993) Application of flow cytometry in diagnosis of hydatidiform moles. *Modern Pathology*, **6**, 353–359.

Fukunaga, M., Ushigome, S. and Endo, Y. (1995) Incidence of hydatidiform mole in a Tokyo hospital: a 5 year (1989 to 1993) prospective morphological and flow cytometric study. *Human Pathology*, **26**, 758–764.

Gabar, L.W., Redline, R.W., Mostoufi-Zadeh, M. and Driscoll, S.G. (1986) Invasive partial mole. *American Journal of Clinical Pathology*, **85**, 722–724.

Gardner, H.A.R. and Lage, J.M., (1992) Choriocarcinoma following a partial mole: a case report. *Human Pathology*, **23**, 468–471.

Genest, D.G., Laborde, O., Berkowitz, R.S., Goldstein, D.P., Bernstein, M.R. and Lage, J.M. (1991) A clinical-pathologic study of 153 cases of complete hydatidiform mole (1980–1990): histologic grade lacks prognostic significance. *Obstetrics and Gynecolology*, **77**, 111–115.

Gloor, E., Dialdas, J. and Hurlimann, J. (1983) Placental site trophoblastic tumor (trophoblast pseudotumor) of the uterus with metastases and fatal outcome: clinical and autopsy observations of a case. *American Journal of Surgical Pathology*, **7**, 483–486.

Goto, S., Yamada, A., Ishizuka, T. and Tomoda, Y. (1993) Development of postmolar trophoblastic disease after partial molar pregnancy. *Gynecologic Oncology*, **48**, 165–170.

Graham, I.H., Fajardo, A.M. and Richards, R.L. (1990) Epidemiological study of complete and partial hydatidiform moles in Abu Dhabi: influence of maternal age and ethnic group. *Journal of Clinical Pathology*, **43**, 661–664.

Grimes, D.A. (1984) Epidemiology of gestational trophoblastic disease. *American Journal of Obstetrics and Gynecology*, **150**, 309–318.

Hallam, L.A., McLaren, K.M., El-Jabbour, J.N., Helm, C.W. and Smart, G.E. (1990) Intraplacental choriocarcinoma: a case report. *Placenta*, **11**, 247–251.

Hammond, C.B., Haney, A.F. and Currie, J.L. (1979) The role of diagnostic tests in gestational trophoblastic disease. *American Journal of Diagnostic Obstetrics and Gynecology*, **1**, 319–330.

Hayashi, K., Bracken, M.B., Freeman, D.H., Jr and Hellenbrand, K. (1982) Hydatidiform mole in the United States (1970–1977): a statistical and theoretical analysis. *American Journal of Epidemiology*, **115**, 67–77.

Heatley, M. (1994) Fetal tissue as a diagnostic aid in hydatidiform mole. *British Journal of Obstetrics and Gynaecology*, **101**, 448–449.

Heifetz, S.A. and Csaja, J. (1992) In situ choriocarcinoma arising in partial hydatidiform mole: implications for risk of persistent trophoblastic disease. *Pediatric Pathology*, **12**, 601–611.

Hemming, J.D., Quirke, P., Womack, C., Wells, M. and Elston, C.W. (1987) Diagnosis of molar pregnancy and persistent trophoblastic disease by flow cytometry. *Journal of Clinical Pathology*, **40**, 615–620.

Hemming, J.D., Quirke, P., Womack, C., Wells, M., Elston, C.W. and Pennington, G.W. (1988) Flow cytometry in persistent trophoblastic disease. *Placenta*, **9**, 615–621.

Hertig, A.T. (1950) Hydatidiform mole and chorionepithelioma. In *Progress in Gynecology, Vol. 2*, Meigs, J.B. and Sturgis, S.H. (Eds), pp. 372–394. New York: Grune & Stratton.

Hertig, A.T. and Sheldon, W.H. (1947) Hydatidiform mole: a pathologico-clinical correlation of 200 cases. *American Journal of Obstetrics and Gynecology*, **53**, 1–36.

How, J., Scurry, J., Grant, P. et al (1995) Placental site trophoblastic tumor: report of three cases and review of the literature. *International Journal of Gynecological Cancer*, **5**, 241–249.

Howat, A.J., Beck, S., Fox, H. et al (1993) Can histopathologists reliably diagnose molar pregnancy? *Journal of Clinical Pathology*, **46**, 599–602.

Ishizuka, N. (1967) Chemotherapy of chorionic tumours. In *Chorioadenoma: Transactions of a Conference of the International Union against Cancer*, Holland, J.F. and Hreshchyshyn, M.M. (Eds), pp. 116–118. Berlin, Heidelberg, New York: Springer-Verlag.

Ishizuka, N. (1976) Studies of trophoblastic neoplasia. *Gann*, **18**, 203–216.

Jacobs, P.A., Wilson, C.M., Sprenkle, J.A., Rosenhein, N.B. and Migson, B.R. (1980) Mechanisms of origin of complete hydatidiform mole. *Nature*, **286**, 714–716.

Jacobs, P.A., Szulman, A.E., Funkmouska, J., Maatsura, J.S. and Wilson, C.C. (1982) Human triploidy: relationship between paternal origin of the additional haploid complement and development of partial hydatidiform mole. *Annals of Human Genetics*, **46**, 223–231.

Jeffers, M.D., Grehan, D. and Gillen. J.E. (1994) Comparison of villous trophoblast proliferation rate in hydatidiform mole and non-molar abortion by assessment of proliferating cell nuclear antigen expression. *Placenta*, **15**, 551–556.

Jeffers, M.D., Michie, B.A., Oakes, S.J. and Gillen, J.E. (1995) Comparison of ploidy analysis by flow cytometry and image analysis in hydatidiform mole and non-molar abortion. *Histopathology*, **27**, 415–421.

Johnson, T.R., Comstock, C.H. and Anderson, D.G. (1979) Benign gestational trophoblastic disease metastatic to pleura: unusual cause of hemothorax. *Obstetrics and Gynecology*, **53**, 509–511.

Kajii, T. and Ohama, K. (1977) Androgenetic origin of hydatidiform mole. *Nature*, **268**, 633–634.

Kajii, T., Kurashigo, H., Ohama, K. and Uchino, F.L. (1984) XY and XX complete moles: clinical and morphological correlations. *American Journal of Obstetrics and Gynecology*, **150**, 57–64.

Kaufman, M.H., Lee, K.K.H. and Speirs, S. (1989) Influence of diandric and digynic triploid genotypes on early mouse embryogenesis. *Development*, **105**, 137–145.

Koenig, C., Demopoulos, R.I., Vamvakas, E.C., Mittal, K.R., Feiner, H.D. and Espiritu, B. (1993) Flow cytometric DNA ploidy and quantitative histopathology in partial moles. *International Journal of Gynecological Pathology*, **12**, 235–240.

Kurman, R.J., Young, R.H., Norris, H.J., Lawrence, W.D. and Scully, R.E. (1984) Immunocytochemical localization of placental lactogen and chorionic gonadotrophin in the normal placenta and trophoblastic tumors with emphasis on intermediate trophoblast and the placental site trophoblastic tumor. *International Journal of Gynecological Pathology*, **3**, 101–121.

Lage, J.M. and Bagg, A. (1996) Hydatidiform moles: DNA flow cytometry, image analysis and selected topics in molecular biology. *Histopathology*, **28**, 379–382.

Lage, J.M. and Popek, E.J. (1993) The role of DNA flow cytometry in evaluation of partial and completely hydatidiform moles and hydropic abortions. *Seminars in Diagnostic Pathology*, **10**, 267–274.

Lage, J.M. and Roberts, D.J. (1993) Choriocarcinoma in a term placenta: pathologic diagnosis of tumor in an asymptomatic patient with metastatic disease. *International Journal of Gynecological Pathology*, **12**, 80–85.

Lage, J.M. and Young, R.H. (1993) Pathology of trophoblastic disease. In *Tumors and Tumorlike Lesions of the Uterine Corpus and Cervix*, Clement, P.B. and Young, R.H. (Eds), pp. 419–475. New York: Churchill Livingstone.

Lage, J.M., Driscoll, S.G., Yavner, D.L., Olivier, A.P., Mark, S.D. and Weinberg, D.S. (1988) Hydatidiform moles: application of flow cytometry in diagnosis. *American Journal of Clinical Pathology*, **89**, 596–600.

Lage, J.M., Weinberg, J.S., Yavner, D.L. et al (1989) Tetraploid partial hydatidiform moles: histopathology, cytogenetics, and flow cytometry. *Human Pathology*, **20**, 419–425.

Lage, J.M., Berkowitz, R.S., Rice, L.W., Goldstein, D.P., Bernstein, M.R. and Weinberg, D.S. (1991) Flow cytometric analysis of DNA content in partial hydatidiform moles with persistent gestational trophoblastic tumor. *Obstetrics and Gynecology*, **77**, 111–115.

Lage, J.M., Mark, S.D., Roberts, D.J., Goldstein, D.P., Bernstein, M.R. and Burkowitz, R.S. (1992) A flow cytometric study of 137 fresh hydropic placentas: correlation between types of hydatidiform moles and nuclear DNA ploidy. *Obstetrics and Gynecology*, **79**, 403–410.

Lane, S.A., Taylor, G.R., Ozols, B. and Quirke, P. (1993) Diagnosis of complete molar pregnancy by microsatellites in archival material. *Journal of Clinical Pathology*, **46**, 346–348.

Lathrop, J.C., Lauchlan, S., Nayak, R. and Ambler, M. (1988) Clinical characteristics of placental site trophoblastic tumor (PSTT) *Gynecologic Oncology*, **31**, 32–42.

La Vecchia, C.L., Parazzini, F., Decarli, A. et al (1984) Age of parents and risk of gestational trophoblastic disease. *Journal of the National Cancer Institute*, **73**, 639–642.

La Vecchia, C.L., Franceschi, S., Parazzini, F. et al (1985) Risk factors for gestational trophoblastic disease in Italy. *American Journal of Epidemiology*, **121**, 457–464.

Lawler, S.D. and Fisher, R.A. (1987) Genetic studies in hydatidiform mole with clinical correlations. *Placenta*, **8**, 77–88.

Lawler, S.D. and Fisher, R.A. (1991) A prospective genetic study of complete and partial hydatidiform moles. *American Journal of Obstetrics and Gynecology*, **164**, 1270–1277.

Lawler, S.D., Fisher, R.A., Pickhall, V.J., Povey, S. and Evans, M.W. (1982) Genetic studies on hydatidiform moles. I. The origin of partial moles. *Cancer Genetics and Cytogenetics*, **5**, 309–320.

Looi, L.M. and Sivanesaratnam, A. (1981) Malignant evolution with fatal outcome in a patient with partial hydatidiform mole. *Australian and New Zealand Journal of Obstetrics and Gynaecology*, **21**, 51–52.

McLellan, R., Buscema, J., Currie, J.L. and Woodruff, J.D. (1991) Placental site trophoblastic tumor in a postmenopausal woman. *American Journal of Clinical Pathology*, **95**, 670–675.

Messerli, M.L., Parmley, T.H., Woodruff, J.D. et al (1987) Inter- and intra-pathologist variability in the diagnosis of gestational trophoblastic neoplasia. *Obstetrics and Gynecology*, **69**, 622–626.

Miller, D., Jackson, R., Ehein, T. and McMurtrie, E. (1993) Complete hydatidiform mole coexistent with a twin live fetus: clinical course of four cases with complete cytogenetic analysis. *Gynecologic Oncology*, **50**, 119–123.

Mostoufi-Zadeh, M., Berkowitz, R.S. and Driscoll, S.G. (1987) Persistence of partial mole. *American Journal of Clinical Pathology*, **87**, 377–380.

Mueller, U.W., Hawes, C.S., Wright, A.E. et al (1990) Isolation of fetal trophoblast cells from peripheral blood of pregnant women. *Lancet*, **336**, 197–200.

Mutter, G.L., Pomponio, R.J., Berkowitz, R.S. and Genest, D.R. (1993) Sex chromosome composition of complete hydatidiform mole: relationship to metastasis. *American Journal of Obstetrics and Gynecology*, **168**, 1547–1551.

Nagamani, M., Kaspar, H., van Dinh, T., Hannigan, E.V. and Smith, E. (1990) Hyperthecosis of the ovaries in a woman with a placental site trophoblastic tumor. *Obstetrics and Gynecology*, **76**, 931–935.

Nagelberg, S.B. and Rosen, S.W. (1985) Clinical and laboratory investigation of a virilized woman with placental-site trophoblastic tumor. *Obstetrics and Gynecology*, **65**, 527–534.

Naumoff, P., Szulman, A.E., Weinstein, B., Mazer, J. and Surti, U. (1981) Ultrasonography of partial hydatidiform mole. *Radiology*, **140**, 467–470.

Osada, H., Kawata, M., Yamada, M., Okumura, K. and Takamizawa, H. (1991) Genetic identification of pregnancies responsible for choriocarcinoma after multiple pregnancies by restriction fragment length polymorphism analysis. *American Journal of Obstetrics and Gynecology*, **165**, 682–688.

Paradinas, F.J. (1994) The histological diagnosis of hydatidiform moles. *Current Diagnostic Pathology*, **1**, 24–31.

Paradinas, F.J., Browne, P., Fisher, R.A., Foskett, M., Bagshawe, K.D. and Newlands, E. (1996) A clinical, histological and flow cytometric study of 149 complete moles, 146 partial moles and 107 non-molar hydropic abortions. *Histopathology*, **28**, 101–109.

Pattillo, R.A., Sasaki, S., Katayama, K.T., Roesler, M. and Mattingley, R.F. (1981) Genesis of 46XY hydatidiform mole. *American Journal of Obstetrics and Gynecology*, **141**, 104–105.

Pijnenborg, R., Bland, J.M., Robertson, W.B., Dixon, H.G. and Brosens, I. (1981) The pattern of interstitial trophoblastic invasion of the myometrium in early human pregnancy. *Placenta*, **2**, 303–316.

Rice, L.W., Berkowitz, R.S., Lage, J.M., Goldstein, D.P. and Bernstein, M.R. (1990) Persistent gestational trophoblastic tumor after partial hydatidiform mole. *Gynecologic Oncology*, **36**, 358–362.

Ring, A.M. (1972) The concept of benign metastasizing hydatidiform moles. *American Journal of Clinical Pathology*, **58**, 111–117.

Robertson, W.B., Brosens, I. and Dixon, H.G. (1975) Uteroplacental vascular pathology. *European Journal of Obstetrics, Gynecology and Reproductive Biology*, **5**, 47–65.

Romero, R., Horgan, G., Kohorn, E.I. et al (1985) New criteria for the diagnosis of gestational trophoblastic disease. *Obstetrics and Gynecology*, **66**, 553–558.

Sand, P.K., Lurain, J.R. and Brewer, J.I. (1984) Repeat gestational trophoblastic disease. *Obstetrics and Gynecology*, **63**, 140–144.

Seckl, M.J., Rustin, G.J.S., Newlands, E.S., Gwyther, S.J. and Bomanji, J. (1991) Pulmonary embolism, pulmonary hypertension and choriocarcinoma. *Lancet*, **338**, 1313–1315.

Slattery, M.A., Khong, T.Y., Dawkins, R.R. et al (1993) Eclampsia in association with partial molar pregnancy and congenital abnormalities. *American Journal of Obstetrics and Gynecology*, **169**, 1625–1627.

Steller, M.A., Genest, D.R., Bernstein, M.R., Lage, J.M., Goldstein, D.P. and Berkowitz, R.S. (1994a) Natural history of twin pregnancy with complete hydatidiform mole and coexisting fetus. *Obstetrics and Gynecology*, **83**, 35–42.

Steller, M.A., Genest, D.R., Bernstein, M.R., Lage, J.M., Goldstein, D.P. and Berkowitz, R.S. (1994b) Clinical features of multiple conception with partial or complete molar pregnancy and coexisting fetuses. *Journal of Reproductive Medicine*, **39**, 147–154.

Suresh, U.R., Hale, R.J., Fox, H. and Buckley, C.H. (1993) Use of proliferation cell nuclear antigen immunoreactivity for distinguishing hydropic abortions from partial hydatidiform moles. *Journal of Clinical Pathology*, **46**, 48–50.

Surti, U. (1987) Genetic concepts and techniques. In *Gestational Trophoblastic Disease*, Szulman, A.E. and Buchsbaum, H.J. (Eds), pp. 111–121. New York: Springer-Verlag.

Surti, U., Szulman, A.E. and O'Brien, S. (1979) Complete (classic) hydatidiform mole with 46XY karyotype of paternal origin. *Human Genetics*, **51**, 153–155.

Surti, U., Szulman, A.E. and O'Brien, S. (1982) Dispermic origin and clinical outcome of three complete hydatidiform moles with 46 XY karyotype. *American Journal of Obstetrics and Gynecology*, **144**, 84–87.

Surti, U., Szulman, A.E., Wagner, K., Leppert, M. and O'Brien, S.J. (1986) Tetraploid partial hydatidiform moles: two cases with a triple paternal contribution and a 92 XXXY karyotype. *Human Genetics*, **72**, 15–21.

Suzuki, T., Goto, S., Nawa, A., Kurauchi, D., Saito, M. and Tomoda, Y. (1993) Identification of the pregnancy responsible for gestational trophoblastic disease by DNA analysis. *Obstetrics and Gynecology*, **82**, 629–634.

Szulman, A.E. and Surti, U. (1978a) The syndromes of hydatidiform mole. I. Cytogenetic and morphologic correlations. *American Journal of Obstetrics and Gynecology*, **131**, 665–671.

Szulman, A.E. and Surti, U. (1978b) The syndromes of hydatidiform mole. II. Morphologic evolution of the complete and partial mole. *American Journal of Obstetrics and Gynecology*, **132**, 20–27.

Szulman, A.E., Philippe, E., Boue, J.G. and Boue, A. (1981) Human triploidy; association with partial hydatidiform moles and nonmolar conceptuses. *Human Pathology*, **12**, 1016–1021.

Teng, N.N.H. and Ballon, S.C. (1984) Partial hydatidiform mole with diploid karyotype: report of three cases. *American Journal of Obstetrics and Gynecology*, **150**, 961–964.

Topalovski, M., Hankin, R.C., Hunter, M.C., Hunter, S.V., Edwards, A.M. and Chen, J.C. (1995) Ploidy analysis of products of conception by image and flow cytometry with cytogenetic correlation. *American Journal of Clinical Pathology*, **103**, 409–414.

Tsukamoto, N., Kashimura, Y., Sano, M., Salto, T., Kanda, T. and Taki, I. (1981) Choriocarcinoma occurring within the normal placenta with breast metastasis. *Gynecologic Oncology*, **11**, 348–363.

van de Kaa, C., Hanselaar, A.G.J.M., Hopman, A.H.N. et al (1993) DNA cytometric and interphase cytogenetic analyses of paraffin-embedded hydatidiform moles and hydropic abortions. *Journal of Pathology*, **170**, 229–238.

van de Kaa, C.A., Robben, J.C.M., Hopman, A.H.N., Hanselaar, A.G.J.M. and Vooijs, G.P. (1995) Complete hydatidiform mole in twin pregnancy: differentiation from partial mole with interphase cytogenetic and DNA cytometric analysis on paraffin embedded tissues. *Histopathology*, **26**, 123–129.

Vassilakos, P., Riotton, G. and Kajii, T. (1977) Hydatidiform mole: two entities: a morphologic and cytogenetic study with some clinical considerations. *American Journal of Obstetrics and Gynecolology*, **127**, 167–170.

Vejerslev, L.O., Fisher, R.A., Surti, U. and Walke, N. (1987) Hydatidiform mole: cytogenetically unusual cases and their implications for the present classification. *American Journal of Obstetrics and Gynecology*, **157**, 180–184.

Vejerslev, L.O., Sunde, L., Hansen, B.F., Larsen, J.K., Christensen, I.J. and Larsen, J. (1991) Hydatidiform mole and fetus with normal karyotype: support of a separate entity. *Obstetrics and Gynecology*, **77**, 868–874.

Wake, N., Takagi, N., and Sasaki, M. (1978) Androgenesis as a cause of hydatidiform mole. *Journal of the National Cancer Institute*, **60**, 51–53.

Wake, N., Fujino, T., Hoshi, S. et al (1987) The propensity to malignancy of dispermic heterozygous moles. *Placenta*, **8**, 318–326.

Womack, C. and Elston, C.W. (1985) Hydatidiform mole in Nottingham: a 12 year retrospective epidemiological and morphological study. *Placenta*, **6**, 95–105.

Yoshimura, M., Pekary, E., Pang, X.P. et al (1994) Thyrotropic activity of basic isoelectric forms of human chorionic gonadotropin extracted from hydatidiform mole tissues. *Journal of Clinical Endocrinology and Metabolism*, **78**, 862–866.

Young, R.H. and Scully, R.E. (1984) Placental site trophoblastic tumor: current status. *Clinical Obstetrics and Gynecology*, **27**, 248–258.

Young, R.H., Scully, R.E. and McCluskey, R.T. (1985) A distinctive glomerular lesion complicating placental site trophoblastic tumor: report of two cases. *Human Pathology*, **16**, 35–42.

Young, R.H., Kurman, R.J. and Scully, R.E. (1988) Proliferations and tumors of the placental site. *Seminars in Diagnostic Pathology*, **5**, 223–237.

Young, R.H., Kurman, R.J. and Scully, R.E. (1990) Placental site nodules and plaques: a clinicopathological analysis of 20 cases. *American Journal of Surgical Pathology*, **14**, 1001–1009.

15

PATHOLOGY OF THE UMBILICAL CORD

It is a cliché of obstetrical writing that the umbilical cord is the 'lifeline of the fetus'. Despite the obvious truth of this statement it is extraordinary how little attention was paid, until relatively recently, to lesions of the cord in the English-language literature. Indeed, until about 20 years ago, the student of obstetrical or perinatal pathology would have scoured in vain the pathological and obstetrical journals in search of information about this topic, and it will suffice to comment that in the 50-year period following the classical paper of Browne (1925) no detailed study of cord pathology was published in an English-language journal. It should in all fairness be added that this neglect appeared to be a purely Anglo-Saxon phenomenon because, during this time, the cord had received considerable attention in the German and French literature. Today the umbilical cord, the subject of a stream of publications, is now seen to be vitally important though possibly the pendulum has swung too far the other way with a tendency to overstress the clinical significance of even relatively minor abnormalities of the cord. These is no doubt that cord lesions can, and do, cause fetal demise but claims that such lesions are responsible for approximately 1 in 6 perinatal deaths (Wessell et al, 1992) seem somewhat exaggerated. The pathologist has to evaluate cord lesions very critically before concluding that they are functionally significant and a cause, rather than a result, of fetal death or damage. Even more caution is required before attributing fetal brain damage to cord lesions. It is true that under experimental conditions temporary occlusion of the cords of fetal lambs will produce neurological lesions (Clapp et al, 1988; Mallard et al, 1994), but direct extrapolation of these findings to human pregnancies is fraught with dangers.

DEVELOPMENTAL ABNORMALITIES

Congenital Absence of the Cord

Complete, or virtually complete, absence of the cord, also known as body stalk anomaly, is extremely uncommon and is usually only found in aborted fetuses who are grossly malformed. Browne (1925), however, referred to two infants who were born at term with achordia and further examples of this anomaly in relatively mature fetuses have since been described (Molz et al, 1980; Goldhofer & Merz, 1985; Lockwood et al, 1986; Giacoia, 1992; Gilbert-Barnes et al, 1993). Characteristically there is a large fetal anterior abdominal defect with most of the abdominal viscera lying in a sac which is directly attached to the placenta. It is thought that this anomaly, which is universally fatal, is a consequence of a fault in embryonic folding with failure of development of the body stalk (Lockwood et al, 1986). The abnormality is associated with a raised alpha-fetoprotein level (Giacoia, 1992) and can, and should, be distinguished from a severe short umbilical cord syndrome and from gastroschisis or omphalocele.

Abnormal Length of the Cord

The factors controlling cord length are still not fully understood but there is some evidence that cord length is related to the degree of fetal mobility, and hence to the tensile force placed upon the cord, particularly during the early stages of pregnancy. Thus, Miller et al (1981) found that conditions restricting fetal mobility, such as amniotic bands or oligohydramnios, were associated with unusually short cords and this finding is in accord with the fact that males, who are presumed to be more active, have slightly longer cords than females (Soernes & Bakke, 1986) and that infants with Down's syndrome, presumed though far from being definitely known to be less active, have relatively short cords (Moessinger et al, 1986). Clearly there must be other factors contributing to cord growth but tensile stress, despite some expressed scepticism based on finding relatively long cords in some cases of oligohydramnios (Fujinaga et al, 1990), does seem to play a role.

The average length of the normal umbilical cord is between 54 and 61 cm (Walker & Pye, 1960; Malpas, 1964; Purola, 1968); since Gardiner's (1922) calculation that the minimum cord length which would allow for a normal vertex delivery is 32 cm, it has been generally accepted that a cord of, or less than, this length should be considered as abnormally short. In most studies using this definition, the incidence of unduly short cords has been between 0.4 and 0.9% (di Terlizzi & Rossi, 1955; Giugni, 1967; Purola, 1968; Ragucci & Morandi, 1969) whilst Berg and Rayburn (1995) found that 2% of cords measured less than 35 cm in length. Many infants with an unduly short cord pass through delivery unscathed but it has been claimed that a significant proportion develop either intrauterine distress or neonatal asphyxia (Rosen, 1955; Bret & Coupez, 1956; Picinelli & Picinelli, 1968). Bain and Eliot (1976) described five examples of fetal distress during the first stage of labour which they believed to be due entirely to an abnormal cord brevity. It is usually thought that the cause of the fetal hypoxia in these circumstances is an excessive traction on the cord during descent of the fetus and that the resulting tension occludes the cord vessels. This has never actually been demonstrated to be the case and, indeed, umbilical blood pH and base deficit values are the same for neonates with short cords as they are for those with cords of normal length (Berg & Rayburn, 1995). A further, largely theoretical, risk of a very short cord is that it is unduly prone to either partial or complete rupture (Szecsi, 1955).

Quite apart from the complications that can occur during labour, Naeye (1985) has shown that there is a correlation between an unduly short cord and an increased frequency of subsequent childhood mental and motor impairment. He considered, quite correctly in my view, that the short cord was the result rather than the cause of the psychomotor abnormalities, these being associated with diminished fetal movement and hence with less stretching stress to the cord.

An abnormally long cord is thought to predispose to knotting, torsion and prolapse (Ottolenghi-Preti & Bailo, 1950), but it is rather difficult to define the limit that should be exceeded for the cord to be considered as unduly long. Purola (1968) considered that 100 cm was the maximum normal length, finding that only 0.5% of the cords in his series of 1713 cases exceeded this length, an incidence roughly similar to that previously noted by Earn (1951) and di Terlizzi and Rossi (1955). Berg and Rayburn (1995) defined an unusually long cord as being more than 80 cm in length and found that 3.7% of the 3019 cords they examined fell into this category.

Abnormal Coiling of the Cord

The umbilical vessels, and hence the cord, usually have a spiral or coiled, structure, the spirals predominantly running in a counterclockwise direction (Fletcher, 1993). Strong et al (1993) studied 894 cords and found a complete absence of spiralling in 4.3%; this abnormality was associated with an heightened incidence of fetal karotypic abnormalities and with an increased perinatal morbidity and mortality. The basis for this clinical significance of absent coiling is unknown but it was postulated that a primary developmental fault resulted in the cord being less able to resist external pressure forces. Subsequently Strong et al (1994) devised a 'coiling index' for the cord by dividing the number of complete coils by the length of the cord, this coming to a mean of 0.21. They found that fetuses whose cord coiling index was below 0.1 or above 0.3 had significantly increased rates of suboptimal perinatal outcome.

Vestigial Remnants

Remnants of the allantoic or omphalomesenteric ducts may be apparent on microscopic examination of the cord. Allantoic remnants were present in 14.5% of the 1000 cords examined by Jauniaux et al (1989a). They are usually seen between the two umbilical arteries and appear either as a solid cord or as a duct: in the latter case the lumen is lined by flattened epithelium and only very occasionally is transitional epithelium found. A unique case of an abscess in an allantoic duct remnant has been described in a 22-week-old fetus (Baill et al, 1989); this was thought to be secondary to a chorioamnionitis and funiculitis.

Remains of the omphalomesenteric duct (Fig. 15.1), found in 1.4% of cords by Jauniaux et al (1989a), are situated at the margin of the cord, are lined by a cuboidal or columnar epithelium, and may contain a little mucus. Very occasionally these remnants of the omphalomesenteric duct show differentiation into gastrointestinal-type structures (Fig. 15.2) with well-formed gastric or intestinal-type epithelium within, or on the surface of, the cord (Blanc & Allan, 1961; Harris & Wenzl, 1963; Lee & Aterman, 1968; Heifetz & Rueda-Pedraza, 1983a; Iwasaki et al, 1986; Dombrowski et al, 1987). The gastrointestinal epithelium may appear as a nodule or polyp and in one such case the presence of gastric-type mucosa appeared to be a causal factor in ulceration of an umbilical vein with massive fetal haemorrhage (Blanc & Allan, 1961). It is of interest to note that patent omphalomesenteric ducts are occasionally associated with focal atresia of the fetal small intestine (Dombrowski et al, 1987; Petrikovsky et al, 1988), possibly as a

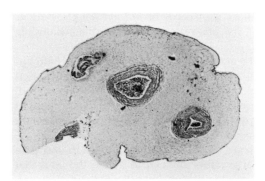

Figure 15.1A. Low-power view of umbilical cord containing a persistent remnant of the omphalomesenteric duct; this is seen above and to the left and is situated towards the margin of the cord (H & E ×8).

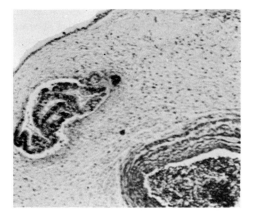

Figure 15.1B. Detail of Fig. 15.1A showing a remnant of omphalomesenteric duct above and to the left; this is lined by tall cuboidal epithelium (H & E ×38).

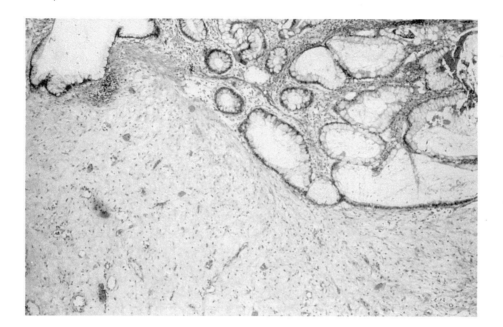

Figure 15.2. Large intestinal-type epithelium in the umbilical cord which was derived from a persistent remnant of the omphalomesenteric duct (H & E ×110).

result of strangulation of a loop of developing bowel by the persistent omphalomesenteric duct. Liver and biliary tissue described within the cord of a neonate (Cabrere et al, 1993) were probably not derived from omphalomesenteric duct remnants but were due to herniation.

These vestigial remnants may also give rise to cysts; these are discussed in a later section of this chapter.

Absence of Periarterial Wharton's Jelly

Labarrere et al (1985) described three examples of an extraordinary anomaly in which Wharton's jelly was completely absent around the umbilical cord arteries but was present around the umbilical vein. This abnormality, presumed to be a developmental error, was associated with perinatal death in all three cases.

ABNORMALITIES OF THE UMBILICAL VESSELS

Single Umbilical Artery

This anomaly was well recognized and fully described in the nineteenth century (Hyrtle, 1870), but subsequently fell into a neglect from which it was not rescued until Benirschke and Brown, in 1955, described a retrospective autopsy series of 55 cases and drew attention to its frequent association with fetal malformation. This paper stimulated both pathologists and obstetricians to examine the cord with somewhat greater care than had previously been the case, and this in turn provoked a flood of reports and studies of this abnormality which has only recently begun to subside. Despite this, and despite the comprehensive review of this topic by Heifetz (1984), there are still many aspects of the pathogenesis and significance of a single umbilical artery that remain controversial.

Incidence

In perinatal autopsy studies the incidence of a single umbilical artery has varied from 2.7 to 12% (Faierman, 1960; Seki and Strauss, 1964; Molz, 1965; Zeman, 1972; Heifetz, 1984; Saller & Neiger, 1994), whilst between 1.5 and 2.7% of spontaneous abortions show this anomaly (Thomas, 1961; Javert & Barton, 1952; Byrne & Blanc, 1985). These figures are, of course, highly selective and give little indication of the true frequency, which can only satisfactorily be established by prospective studies of a large number (i.e. at least 1000) of unselected consecutive deliveries. The results of such investigations are detailed in Table 15.1, and it can be seen that the reported incidence of single umbilical artery has ranged widely from 0.2 to 1.1%.

Some of the reasons for these discrepancies, but not all, can be pinpointed: the most important is that the frequency with which a single artery is noted varies considerably with the technique by which the cord is examined. If naked-eye examination of the fresh cord is relied upon as the sole means of diagnosis, a misleadingly low incidence will be obtained; the degree of error inherent in this method can be quite high, even in the hands of experienced workers searching specifically for the anomaly, and may be extreme if the results obtained by inexperienced or uninterested observers are relied upon. A considerably higher incidence of single umbilical artery is detected if inspection of the cord is delayed until after fixation in formalin or, preferably, glacial acetic acid. That these differences in technique are important is shown, for example, in Kristoffersen's (1969) study, in which the incidence of single umbilical artery in personally examined formalin-fixed cords was 1.15%, whilst that detected by the general obstetric staff looking at unfixed cords was only 0.37%. The highest, and presumably therefore the most accurate, yield of this abnormality is, however, found if the cord is subjected to histological examination. This was emphasized very clearly in Fujikura's (1964) series, in which an incidence of 0.5% was noted on naked-eye examination and one of 0.8% on microscopy, figures that leave little doubt that microscopy should be the definitive mode of diagnosis in all prospective studies.

One further point of technique should be emphasized, if only because it is so frequently neglected. As noted in Chapter 1, the two umbilical arteries may fuse at their lower end into a single trunk which subsequently divides into two rami (Szpakowski, 1974); if the cord is sectioned too closely to the chorionic plate (i.e. at a distance of less than 3 cm from the placental surface) this normal variation may be wrongly interpreted, and therefore a diagnosis of single umbilical artery should always be confirmed by a second section taken at a higher level.

A single umbilical artery can be detected ultrasonographically (Jassini et al, 1980; Tortora et al, 1984; Herrmann & Sidiropoulos, 1988; Sepulveda, 1991; Zienert et al, 1992; Jones et al, 1993) but this technique, whilst having a high specificity, has a rather poor sensitivity and will fail to diagnose about one-third of cases (Jones et al, 1993).

Many other factors, apart from the technique of examination, may influence the incidence of this abnormality in any particular series. In the USA it has been clearly shown that a single artery occurs at least twice as frequently in cords from white mothers than it does in those from black women (Peckham & Yerushalmy, 1965; Froehlich & Fujikura, 1966, 1973). The reasons for this ethnic bias, which may clearly influence the results in any particular series, are unknown, but it is of interest that it does not apply in India, where the incidence of single umbilical artery is at least as high as in Great Britain (Mital et al, 1969). It would be of considerable interest to know how frequently a single umbilical artery is found in Africa, but, to the best of my knowledge, no large series has been reported from that continent.

A considerable excess of single umbilical artery in association with maternal diabetes mellitus has been noted in some studies (Froehlich & Fujikura, 1966; Kristoffersen, 1969; Broussard et al, 1972) but was not confirmed by Bryan and Kohler (1974), whilst the occasional claims of an undue frequency in women of high parity or advanced age have not received support in most studies. The most controversial influence on the incidence is, however, that of twin pregnancy. Claims by some workers that the abnormality is found much more commonly in twin than in singleton pregnancies

Table 15.1. Reported incidence of single umbilical artery and of associated fetal malformation

Author	Number examined	Single umbilical artery[a]		Incidence of malformation in fetuses with single umbilical artery[a]	
Benirschke & Bourne (1960)	1500	15	(1)	7	(46.6)
Little (1961)	2800	21	(0.75)	10	(48)
Thomas (1961)	6970	27	(0.39)	5	(18.5)
Lenoski & Medovy (1962)	2500	5	(0.20)	1	(20)
Adler et al (1963)	2000	19	(0.95)	4	(22.2)
Soma (1963)	1200	9	(0.75)	5	(59)
Cairns & McKee (1964)	2000	20	(1)	2	(10)
Feingold et al (1964)	6080	32	(0.52)	15	(46)
Fujikura (1964)	5972	38	(0.6)	7	(18.4)
Gomori & Koller (1964)	1000	8	(0.8)	1	(12.5)
Gornicka et al (1965)	1620	14	(0.9)	2	(14.3)
Papadatos & Paschos (1965)	7886	32	(0.41)	10	(31.2)
Peckham & Yerushalmy (1965)	5848	51	(0.87)	12	(32.5)
Adrian (1966)	3688	25	(0.68)	5	(20)
Angiolillo & Picinelli (1966)	1000	2	(0.2)	2	(100)
Carrier et al (1966)	4138	33	(0.79)	5	(15.2)
Froehlich & Fujikura (1966)	26,539	203	(0.76)	58	(28.6)
Hnat (1967)	4590	38	(0.83)	6	(16)
Leissner (1967)	4000	26	(0.65)	6	(23)
Lewenthal et al (1967)	5135	50	(0.97)	12	(24)
Segovia (1967)	10,000	60	(0.6)	8	(13.3)
van Leeuwen et al (1967)	2000	6	(0.3)	2	(33.3)
Ainsworth & Davies (1969)	12,078	113	(0.94)	38	(33.6)
Jean et al (1969)	11,115	112	(1)	17	(15.1)
Kristoffersen (1969)	8751	41	(0.47)	11	(23.4)
Mital et al (1969)	4612	41	(0.89)	19	(46)
Müller et al (1969)	4600	27	(0.59)	2	(7.4)
Cederqvist (1970)	19,422	53	(0.27)	17	(32)
Broussard et al (1972)	9697	45	(0.46)	4	(8.8)
le Marec et al (1972)	5619	31	(0.53)	10	(33)
Vlietinck et al (1972)	2572	29	(1.1)	9	(31)
Froehlich & Fujikura (1973)	39,773	344	(0.9)	30	(8.7)
Johnsonbaugh (1973)	1152	9	(0.78)	1	(11)
Bryan & Kohler (1974)	20,000	143	(0.72)	25	(17.5)
Altshuler et al (1975)	4138	19	(0.45)	7	(39)
Eberst et al (1979)	22,293	137	(0.6)	24	(17.5)
Grall et al (1983)	42,815	194	(0.46)	44	(23)
Gnirs et al (1988)	15,388	78	(0.51)	29	(37)
Leung & Robson (1989)	56,919	159	(0.28)	71	(44.7)
Bourke et al (1993)	35,000	112	(0.32)		NS

[a] Figures in parentheses are the incidence expressed as a percentage.

(Benirschke & Bourne, 1960; Thomas, 1961; Benirschke, 1965; Mital et al, 1969; Giraud et al, 1971; Heifetz, 1984; Leung & Robson, 1989) have been specifically refuted by others (Papadatos & Paschos, 1965; Peckham and Yerushalmy, 1965; Lewenthal et al, 1967; Kristoffersen, 1969; Bryan & Kohler, 1974), an absolute disagreement for which there is no obvious explanation.

Associated Fetal Abnormalities

A single umbilical artery is often accompanied by fetal malformation, the reported frequency of this association varying considerably (Table 15.1) but being, in most studies, between 25 and 50%. Rather curiously, a recent report (Abuhamad et al, 1995) has suggested that complex fetal malformations are specifically associated with absence of the left umbilical artery, a finding which, to my mind at least, defies logical explanation. The malformations do not, despite occasional claims to the contrary, show a bias towards any particular organ or system; they are frequently multiple and often lethal. The vexed question of whether the incidence of malformation is higher than that which is clinically detectable at birth appeared to have been answered by Froehlich and Fujikura (1973). They followed up a very large series of infants with a single umbilical artery who survived the perinatal period, and found that, apart from an inexplicable tendency to develop an inguinal hernia, these developed normally and did not show any excess of congenital abnormalities. Later, however, Bryan and Kohler (1975) followed up 98 similar infants and found that previously occult malformations subsequently became manifest in 10, whilst Leung and Robson (1989) and Bourke et al (1993) have shown that there is a high incidence of clinically silent renal anomalies in infants with a single umbilical artery.

Infants with a single umbilical artery often have a low birth weight (Adler et al, 1963; Carrier et al, 1966; Froehlich & Fujikura, 1966; Gnirs et al, 1988; Herrmann & Sidiropoulos, 1988; Lilja, 1991). Seki and Strauss (1964) thought that the weight deficit was entirely due to congenital malformation and that the birth weight was usually normal for the gestational age when allowance was made for this factor, but Bryan and Kohler (1974) found the birth weight to be unduly low even in normally formed neonates.

The high incidence of serious malformation is the most important factor in the high perinatal mortality of infants with a single umbilical artery, one that is in the range of 15–50%. This is not, however, the sole cause of perinatal death, as there is an increased mortality rate even in normally formed infants (Little, 1961; Seki & Strauss, 1964; Peckham & Yerushalmy, 1965; Froehlich & Fujikura, 1966; Bryan & Kohler, 1974; Heifetz, 1984; Lilja, 1992). The reasons for this are far from being clear, though the trend towards a low birth weight may be of some importance in this respect.

Associated Placental Abnormalities

In many series a single umbilical artery has been associated frequently with circumvallate placentation, velamentous insertion of the cord and low placental weight (Benirschke, 1965; Dehalleux et al, 1966; Froehlich & Fujikura, 1966; Dellenbach et al, 1968; Kristoffersen, 1969; le Marec et al, 1972; Matheus and Sala, 1980), but this has not been everyone's experience (Peckham & Yerushalmy, 1965; Broussard et al, 1972) and, indeed, the placenta may sometimes be unduly bulky (Bret & Blanchier, 1968).

Note has been made of scattered groups of immature, oedematous villi in placentas supplied by a single umbilical artery (Seki & Strauss, 1964; Cipparone, 1966); however, this is a non-specific finding which is often seen in placentas from malformed infants, whether there be one or two umbilical arteries.

Aetiology and Pathogenesis

There has been considerable debate as to whether a single umbilical artery is due to a primary aplasia or to a secondary atrophy of the missing vessel. In favour of the primary aplasia concept is the well-documented occurrence of this anomaly in association with chromosomal abnormalities (German et al, 1962; Lewis, 1962; Miller et al, 1963; Gustavson, 1964; Uchida et al, 1968; Gnirs et al, 1988; Saller et al, 1990; Khong & George, 1992; Saller & Neiger, 1994), whilst the possibility of secondary atrophy has been suggested by the association of a missing vessel with maternal thalidomide administration (Russell & McKichan, 1962; Kajii et al, 1963). In fact it is almost certain that both of these mechanisms can be invoked because, whilst in some cases there is an absolute absence of a second artery in the cord, in others there is evidence of a previously present vessel, sometimes seen histologically as a small, shrivelled and involuted artery with an obliterated lumen but occasionally only recognizable by the presence of remnants of the muscular or elastic wall. Altshuler et al (1975) specifically investigated this point and found that in a series of 48 cases of single umbilical artery there appeared to be an aplasia in 29 and an atrophy in 19.

Where one artery is aplastic it has sometimes been thought that the single artery in the cord is a vitelline rather than an umbilical vessel (Gisel, 1938), but Monie and his colleagues (Monie, 1970; Monie & Khemmani, 1973) have argued, rather persuasively, that the single vessel represents the persistence of the normally transient single umbilical artery of early development. This is perhaps a rather academic point, as is also the question of whether a single umbilical artery is simply just one of a galaxy of congenital malformations or whether it can itself be a cause of congenital malformation. Those holding the latter view have maintained that the vascular anomaly acts as a teratogenic agent by increasing resistance to blood flow from fetus to placenta (Benirschke & Brown, 1955; Konstantinova, 1961) or by producing fetal tissue hypoxia. This view has not been generally accepted though it has been strongly supported by Chaurasia (1974), who demonstrated that the single umbilical artery often replaces the lower end of the abdominal aorta and argued that this could directly lead to a wide range of congenital malformations.

Supernumary Umbilical Vessels

Whilst the absence of one umbilical artery has provoked a profuse literature, the reverse anomaly, namely, an increased number of umbilical vessels, has attracted little attention. This is surprising because it is possibly more common than single umbilical artery and may be of equal significance. Meyer et al (1969) found an accessory fourth vessel in 16 of the 310 cords that they examined; this was usually small and they thought that it represented the persistence of either a vitelline or right umbilical vein. They could find no association between the presence of a fourth vessel and congenital malformation, but Karchmer et al (1966) noted four examples of supernumerary cord vessels in their study of 40 malformed infants; three of these had two arteries and two veins, whilst two had three arteries and one vein. Nadkarni (1969) found that in five of the cords from a consecutive series of 284 deliveries there were more than two umbilical arteries, but made no comment on the presence or otherwise of congenital malformation. It has to be remarked, however, that all these studies, with the exception of that of Meyer et al (1969), suffered from the fact that the possibility of the apparent extra vessel being artefactual, and due to vascular looping, was not rigidly excluded.

Gupta et al (1993) found more than three vascular profiles on cross-section in 40 (6%) of 644 cords from which samples at the fetal end, mid-portion and placental end were examined. The extra vascular profiles were seen most commonly in sections taken from the central portion of the cord and longitudinal dissection of the vessels showed that the appearances were due to branching rather than to looping or the presence of true supernumerary vessels. In this study an increased number of vascular profiles was found more commonly in cords from stillbirths than in those from live births and there was a clear association between this anomaly and a history of maternal cigarette smoking.

Miscellaneous Abnormalities of the Umbilical Arteries

Calcification of Umbilical Arteries

Calcification of umbilical cord vessels has been intermittently recorded (Rust, 1937; Walz, 1947; Perrin & Kahn-Vander Bel, 1965; Schiff et al, 1976) but the only detailed study of this lesion is that of Khong and Dilly (1989) who reported five cases. They considered that calcification of umbilical vessels took two forms, one characterized by complete obliteration of an umbilical artery and possibly an end stage of a thrombus and the other with calcification of the arterial wall (with or without involvement of Wharton's jelly) which was possibly related to infection. It is of note that only two of the five infants with calcified umbilical vessels were live births and that in both these cases there had been operative intervention for fetal distress. Calcification of the umbilical vessels is not associated with the syndrome of infantile arterial calcification and vice versa.

Segmental Thinning of Umbilical Vessels

Qureshi and Jacques (1994) noted marked segmental thinning of the umbilical cord vessels in 17 (1.5%) of 1100 consecutively examined placentas: in 13 cases the vein was affected whilst one or both arteries were involved in four cases. In each case the media was virtually absent in about a third of the vessel circumference in at least one level in the cord. In only half the cases was the deficient segment of the cord facing towards the cord surface. Congenital malformations were present in five of the 17 infants and there was a high incidence of fetal distress. The nature and origin of this rather strange lesion are completely unknown but it does appear to differ from the meconium-induced vascular lesions that have been described by Altshuler and his colleagues (see below).

Meconium-Induced Necrosis

Altshuler and his colleagues (Altshuler & Hyde, 1989; Altshuler et al, 1992) delineated a characteristic lesion of the umbilical arteries that appears to be induced by meconium and their description of this entity has been fully confirmed by Benirschke (1994). The lesion is always associated with prolonged passage of meconium and consists of segmental necrosis of the arterial wall, the vein usually not being involved: the necrotic segment of the artery always faces towards the cord surface and there are numerous meconium-laden macrophages within the Wharton's jelly. In long-standing cases there may be an accumulation of polymorphonuclear leucocytes within the necrotic segment of the vessel wall and in some instances there is also linear ulceration of the cord surface. Altshuler and Hyde (1989) showed that meconium produced vasoconstriction of isolated segments of umbilical veins *in vitro* and suggested that meconium-induced vasoconstriction could result in fetal cerebral damage. This is certainly a hypothesis that merits attention though the partially necrotic vessels seen after prolonged meconium passage would not be capable of contracting.

Aneurysm

Aneurysms of an umbilical artery are extremely rare. Fortune and Ostor (1978) described an arterial aneurysm arising in an otherwise normal cord that had extensively dissected and which, because of umbilical vascular compression, led to intrauterine fetal death. Siddiqi et al (1992) reported a fusiform aneurysm, measuring 13 cm in length and 5 cm in diameter, which developed in a single umbilical artery; this also led to fetal death, because of presumed umbilical vein compression.

ABNORMALITIES OF INSERTION (Fig. 15.3)

Eccentric and Marginal Insertion

Eccentric insertion of the cord can hardly be classed as an anomaly because in most studies it is found more commonly than a central insertion, its reported incidence ranging from 48 to 75% (Earn, 1951; Krone et al, 1964; Purola, 1968). In our own series of 1000 placentas, 620 were found to have an eccentric insertion of the cord (Uyanwah-Akpom & Fox, 1977). This feature appears to be of no clinical significance.

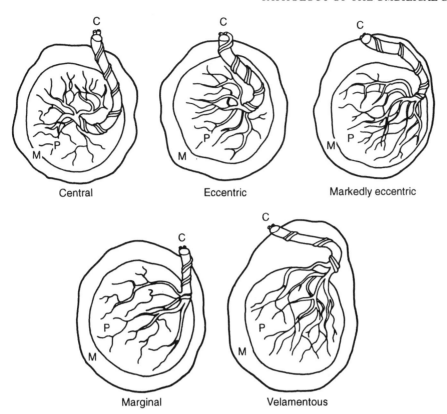

Figure 15.3. Diagrammatic representation of the various sites at which the cord may be inserted. C, cord; P, placenta; M, membranes.

Marginal insertion (the so-called 'battledore placenta') is less common than an eccentrically placed cord. Its reported incidence has varied widely (Table 15.2); this is probably because of differing interpretations of the rather subtle distinction between an 'extremely eccentric' and a marginal insertion. The significance of a marginal insertion is a matter for some debate. Hathout (1964) noted it was unduly common in abortion material, whilst Monie (1965) not only confirmed this finding but also described a greatly increased incidence of this form of insertion in the placentas of malformed infants, a finding subsequently specifically refuted by Robinson et al (1983). Raaflaub (1959) has claimed that babies whose cords are inserted in this fashion have a considerably increased incidence of neonatal asphyxia, whilst even more striking is Brody and Frenkel's (1953) finding that nearly 70% of placentas with a marginally inserted cord are from women who have gone

Table 15.2. Reported incidence of marginal insertion of the cord

Author	Number of placentas studied	Incidence of marginal insertion (%)
Earn (1951)	5412	15
Brody & Frenkel (1953)	512	6.2
Shanklin (1958)	514	1.9
Scott (1960)	3161	2
Krone et al (1964)	2868	7.9
Purola (1968)	1713	4.1
Foss & Vogel (1972)	684	7
Uyanwah-Akpom & Fox (1977)	1000	5.6
Robinson et al (1983)	44,677	8.5
Benirschke & Kaufmann (1995)	12,787	9.17

into premature labour. In our own series the incidence of marginal cord insertion was 5.6%, and this form of insertion was not associated with any excess incidence of abortion, premature labour, neonatal asphyxia or congenital malformation.

Velamentous Insertion

In this condition the cord is inserted, not into the placenta, but into the membranes, and hence the unprotected umbilical vessels run for some distance between the amnion and chorion before passing on to the placental surface. It is usually stated that velamentous insertion is found in about 1% of deliveries, but it will be seen from Table 15.3 that the reported frequency of this anomaly in singleton pregnancies varies quite strikingly; in our own series a velamentous insertion was found in 1.6% of 1000 placentas (Uyanwah-Akpom & Fox, 1977).

The incidence of velamentous insertion is considerably increased in multiple pregnancies (Benirschke & Kaufmann, 1995), but other proposed associations are more open to debate. Thus, for instance, although several workers have noted an increase of this abnormal form of insertion in extrachorial placentas (Thomas, 1962; Dellenbach et al, 1968), this was not found in the detailed study of Scott (1960). It has been claimed that there is an increased incidence of velamentous insertion in pregnancies following *in vitro* fertilization (Burton & Saunders, 1988) but the evidence for this is largely anecdotal. An association between velamentous insertion and a single umbilical artery has been noted (Thomas, 1962; Dellenbach et al, 1968; Foss & Vogel, 1972) and it has been claimed that a high proportion (up to 25%) of malformed infants have a cord that is velamentously inserted (Krone, 1961, 1962; Thomas, 1962; Stephan & Thomas, 1963; Krone et al, 1964; Monie, 1965). Robinson et al (1983) found that there was no excess

Table 15.3. Reported incidence of velamentous insertion of the cord

Author	Number of placentas examined	Incidence of velamentous insertion (%)
Lefevre (1896)	15,891	0.84
Slemens (1916)	600	0.17
Noldeke (1934)	10,000	1.1
Grieco (1936)	23,469	0.41
Zambelli (1942)	47,770	0.32
Rucker & Tureman (1945)	6421	0.24
Earn (1951)	5412	1.0
di Terlizzi & Rossi (1955)	15,416	0.09
Aguero (1957)	10,000	0.48
Shanklin (1958)	514	0.77
Raaflaub (1959)	500	13.6
Sauramo (1960)	5000	0.1
Scott (1960)	3161	1.5
Corkill (1961)	12,695	0.024
Thomas (1962)	18,316	1.3
Krone et al (1964)	2868	1.8
Dellenbach et al (1968)	4000	1.6
Leissner et al (1968)	2712	1.7
Purola (1968)	1713	0.9
Scheffel & Langanke (1970)	37,963	0.22
Foss & Vogel (1972)	684	1.5
Sirivongs (1974)	12,120	0.45
Uyanwah-Akpom & Fox (1977)	1000	1.6
Bjoro (1983)	14,050	2.17
Robinson et al (1983)	44,677	1.5
Tollison & Huang (1988)	25,558	0.02
Eddleman et al (1992)	16,210	0.5
Benirschke & Kaufmann (1995)	12,787	1.27

of true malformations in cases of velamentous insertion but that there was an increased incidence of deformations, i.e. an alteration in shape of a normally differentiated structure. It has further been maintained that a velamentous insertion is found in nearly a third of prematurely delivered babies (Noldeke, 1934), in 15% of abortions (Monie, 1965), in an unduly high proportion of abnormally adherent placentas (Krone et al, 1964), and in many cases of low birth weight (Busch, 1972). It is surprising that very little attempt has been made either to confirm or refute many of these claims, which, if true, could be of considerable significance. Philippe et al (1968) did, however, specifically deny that velamentous insertion was unduly common in abortions, whilst we have found that, although velamentous insertion was associated rather more commonly than would be expected with low birth weight, it was not associated unduly frequently with any other maternal or fetal complication. Eddleman et al (1992) have confirmed the correlation between velamentous insertion and a relatively high incidence of low-birth-weight infants and also noted an increased rate of intrapartum complications, such as variable decelerations in fetal heart rate, in cases with this form of cord insertion.

Neither the aetiology nor the pathogenesis of velamentous insertion is fully understood. The most popular theory of its pathogenesis has been that first proposed by von Franqué (1900) and later strongly supported by Ottow (1922, 1923). This is that the abdominal pedicle normally arises, and extends to the fetus, from that part of the chorion which is most richly vascularized, this usually being that in contact with the decidua basalis. Occasionally, however, the decidua capsularis may be the area of maximal vascularity during the first few days of pregnancy, and hence the abdominal pedicle will take its origin from the chorion in contact with this. As pregnancy progresses the vascularity of the decidua capsularis diminishes whilst that of the decidua basalis increases, and so the site of maximal vascularization will shift to that part of the chorion which is in contact with the decidua basalis and from which the definitive placenta will develop. Meanwhile, however, the abdominal pedicle retains its original position, and hence the cord will be inserted into the membranes.

Robinson et al (1983) and Benirschke and Kaufmann (1995) favour the concept of 'trophotropism', arguing that the cord is originally normally inserted but becomes stranded in the membranes by a process, during placental expansion, of central atrophy and unidirectional lateral growth of the chorion frondosum. They point out, with some validity, that this is the most logical explanation of the fact that a placenta bilobata usually has a cord that is velamentously inserted between the two lobes.

Monie (1965) has suggested that velamentous insertion results from an oblique implantation of the blastocyst, a view that appears to be supported by McLennan (1968), who, by using a rather complex mathematical theory, concluded that there must be an 'abnormal vector of implantation'.

There is no evidence that compels wholehearted adherence to any of these theories: possibly, they are all wrong; equally possibly, they may all be correct, insofar as there may be no single method of production of this anomaly.

Velamentous insertion of the cord is of serious import for the fetus because of the risk of damage to the exposed and unprotected fetal vessels during labour and delivery (Fig. 15.4). This danger is, of course, most prominent when the intramembranous vessels run across the internal os, a feature that can now be diagnosed before labour by transvaginal colour Doppler ultrasound (Nelson et al, 1990). The many reports of serious or fatal fetal bleeding from tearing of such a vessel (which produces the clinical picture of 'vasa praevia') have been reviewed most notably by Rucker and Tureman (1945), Torrey (1952), Naftolin and Mishell (1965), Paulino (1970) and Kouyoumdjian (1980), and most recently by VanDrie and Kammeraad (1981), Tollison and Huang (1988) and Cordero et al (1993), it being generally agreed that the fetal mortality rate resulting from this catastrophe is at least 60–70%. Although the bleeding is usually from fetal vessels in the region of the internal os, it is well established that haemorrhage can also occur from velamentous vessels in the upper uterine segment (Rucker & Tureman, 1945). This is less surprising than at first sight may appear because Scheuner (1965) has shown that the vessels in the chorion laeve are firmly bound

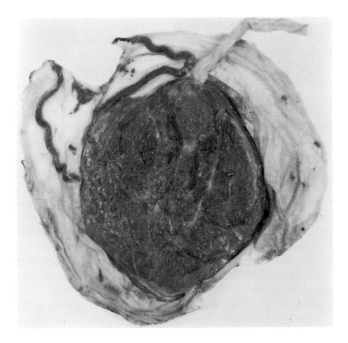

Figure 15.4. An example of velamentous cord insertion in which a fetal vessel running through the membranes has been torn (above and to the left) during delivery.

down by perivascular collagen, an anatomical arrangement that makes them particularly susceptible to damage during uterine contractions. It should not be thought, however, that the vessels of a velamentously inserted cord are only susceptible to damage during labour, because there have been several well-authenticated reports of bleeding from such vessels during the antepartum period (Bilek et al, 1962; Erb & Zeilinger, 1965).

Despite the obvious and dangerous possibility of bleeding from velamentous vessels, it has to be borne in mind that the vast majority of infants whose cords are velamentously inserted pass through labour and delivery without haemorrhage, it being estimated that this complication occurs in only 2% of such cases (Quek & Tan, 1972). The fetus is, however, at still further risk, as its life may be endangered by compression of the velamentous vessels against the wall of the pelvis during delivery; fetal distress under such circumstances is common and fetal demise by no means rare (Cordero et al, 1993).

Interposito Velamentosa

This is a very rare anomaly in which the cord appears to be inserted velamentously into the chorion laeve but the cord substance surrounds the fetal vessels until they reach the placenta (Ottow, 1922); its pathogenesis is unknown.

Insertion Funiculi Furcata (Furcate Insertion)

In this condition the site of cord insertion is normal but, prior to insertion, the vessels lose their protective covering of Wharton's jelly and branch before reaching the placental surface (Hyrtle, 1870; Ottow, 1923; Herberz, 1938). The exposed vessels are liable to damage and examples of fetal haemorrhage as a result of this anomaly have been described (Swanberg & Wiqvist, 1951; Kessler, 1960). The pathogenesis of this condition is uncertain: it may be a developmental error or may result from local degeneration and loss of the jelly.

MECHANICAL LESIONS

Knots

True knots can be formed in the umbilical cord (Fig. 15.5) and these are to be distinguished from 'false knots', which are either local dilatations of umbilical vessels or focal accumulations of Wharton's jelly. The literature on cord knots, which is not voluminous, has been reviewed by, amongst others, Browne (1925), Lundgren and Boice (1939), Hennessy (1944), Lucchetti (1965) and Mele (1968). Most of these authors agree that knots are found in between 0.3 and 0.5% of all deliveries, though in more recent prospective surveys the incidence has varied quite widely from 0.04% to 1.22% (Table 15.4). The incidence is notably high in monoamniotic twins and it is thought that a long cord, an excess of amniotic fluid and over-vigorous fetal movements all predispose to knot formation.

The functional significance of cord knotting was disputed in the past, and indeed still is to some extent, but Browne (1925) showed that under *in vitro* conditions a progressive tightening of a knot was accompanied by an increasing resistance to injection of fluid through the umbilical arteries. A pressure of 100–110 mmHg of mercury was required to overcome the resistance encountered in a tightly knotted cord with a 100 g weight suspended from it, this being a pressure exceeding that normally found in the umbilical arteries *in vivo*. It seems likely, therefore, that a tight knot can obstruct the fetal circulation through the cord, and it is not surprising that the presence of such knots is associated with a perinatal mortality rate in the region of 8–11% (di Terlizzi & Rossi, 1955; Scheffel & Langanke, 1970). In assessing the significance of a tight knot it should, however, be borne in mind that a previously loose knot may be suddenly tightened as the infant descends during delivery. Browne (1925) has pointed out that recently formed knots of this type can be distinguished from long-standing knots on the following grounds:

1. In an old knot there is marked and permanent grooving of the cord at the site of the knot.
2. At the site of a long-standing knot there is a loss of Wharton's jelly and a constriction of the umbilical vessels.
3. When an old knot is undone there is persistent curling of the cord at the site of the knot.

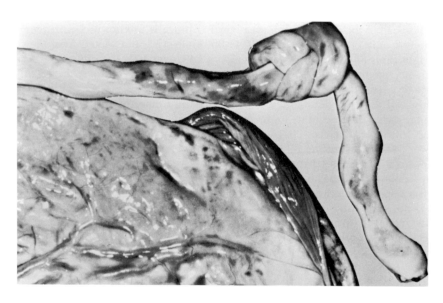

Figure 15.5. A knot in an umbilical cord.

Table 15.4. Reported incidence of umbilical cord knots in prospective surveys

Author	Number of cords studied	Number of knots[a]
Earn (1951)	5676	3 (0.05)
di Terlizzi & Rossi (1955)	15,416	48 (0.3)
Corkill (1961)	12,695	5 (0.04)
Ragucci & Morandi (1969)	8365	84 (1)
Scheffel & Langanke (1970)	61,810	115 (0.19)
Chasnoff & Fletcher (1977)	2000	7 (0.3)
Hartge (1979)	3400	33 (0.5)
Blickstein et al (1987)	4650	57 (1.22)
McLennan et al (1988)	1115	6 (0.5)

[a] Figures in parentheses are the incidence expressed as a percentage.

A knot formed during early labour will not usually show these features, but may nevertheless be responsible for intrapartum death, fetal distress or neonatal asphyxia. Examination of such a knot will, however, show oedema, congestion or thrombosis, and in the absence of these changes it would not be justifiable to attribute any functional significance to a knot. Failure to look carefully for such changes and lack of histological examination may be factors in those studies in which true knots have not been of any clinical importance (McLennan et al, 1988; Sopracordevole & Perissinotto, 1991).

Rupture

A rupture of the cord may be partial or complete. The term 'incomplete rupture' is usually taken to mean tearing of, or damage to, an umbilical vessel and thus represents one mechanism of cord haematoma formation (see section on vascular lesions). The extravasated blood is often confined to the cord but sometimes it ruptures into the amniotic sac (Itskovitz et al, 1980); such cases should be classed as 'rupture of an umbilical vessel' rather than as rupture of the cord, as should those cases in which rupture of velamentous vessels results in separation of the abnormally inserted cord from the placenta (Vestermark et al, 1990).

Complete rupture of the cord is extremely rare; Bahary et al (1965) could find only 12 recorded instances of this catastrophe in the literature and only a few further cases have been reported since their review (Leinzinger, 1972; Uher, 1975; Lurie et al, 1990). The actual incidence of complete cord rupture is unknown: Leinzinger (1972) encountered only one instance in over 41,000 deliveries, but Mateu-Aragones (1956) noted eight cases of cord rupture in a series of approximately the same size, though in his study he, like many others, does not make fully clear whether these are examples of complete or partial cord rupture.

The cord has considerable tensile strength and can withstand a severe degree of stretching, partly because of its high content of elastic tissue and partly because of the tortuous course that its vessels pursue. Nevertheless, Swanberg and Wiqvist (1951) quote work done during the nineteenth century which showed that a weight of 800 g will rupture a normal cord if allowed to fall through a height of 50 cm, whilst more recently Zink and Reinhardt (1969) have demonstrated that a weight of 3300 g falling through a height of 5 cm will cause complete rupture of 64% of cords. This being the case, it is not surprising that most ruptures of the cord complicate precipitate delivery, especially from the upright or squatting posture, and occur immediately after the birth of the child; the rupture is usually at the fetal end of the cord. Exceptionally, cord rupture may occur either during the early stages of labour or even before labour begins (Gallagher & Malone, 1956; Foldes, 1957; Rehn & Kinnunen, 1962). It is probable that in most such cases the cord rupture complicates a tight torsion, but it has been suggested that an unduly short cord, trauma or inflammation may also be of aetiological importance. One instance of complete rupture occurred as a result of focal 'maceration' of the cord for which no cause could be determined (Lurie et al, 1990). Separation of the cord from the placenta as an apparent result of implantation of a Lippes' loop at the funiculo–placental junction has been reported (Golden, 1973) but the pathogenetic role of the contraceptive device in this case has been disputed by Benirschke and Kaufmann (1995).

The effects of antepartum rupture are obviously catastrophic but some infants do survive rupture of the cord during the late stages of labour and delivery.

Torsion

The cord is, as previously remarked, normally twisted insofar as its vessels run a spiral course, but pathological torsion is usually readily distinguishable from the normal spiralling. The torsion may affect the whole cord, but is more commonly localized, and whilst a single lesion is usually found, there may occasionally be multiple twists. The characteristic site of torsion is at the fetal end of the cord (Fig. 15.6), but examples of torsion at the placental end have been recorded (Lucchetti, 1965).

The incidence of this complication is unknown because, whilst Corkill (1961) noted seven instances in a series of 12,696 deliveries, di Terlizzi and Rossi (1955) were unable to find a single example of cord torsion in 15,415 deliveries. Torsion is said, however, to be more common in multigravid pregnancies, supposedly because the laxity of the abdomen and the greater size of the uterus allow for greater freedom of fetal movement (Browne, 1925). Torsion also appears to occur predominantly with male infants as, it is suggested, these are stronger and more active than their female counterparts and hence more likely to twist their cords. It certainly seems that both cord stricture and an excessively long cord predispose to torsion whilst some authors have suggested that a focal deficiency of Wharton's jelly is an important aetiological factor (Marchesoni & Helfer, 1956). It may be, of course, that the loss of the jelly in such instances is secondary to the torsion rather than a provoking factor.

A tight cord torsion will clearly obstruct the umbilical vessels and can cause fetal death (Lange, 1968; Schultze, 1969); it has been argued that cord torsion is a postmortem event (Edmonds, 1954) and there is no doubt that excessive twisting of the

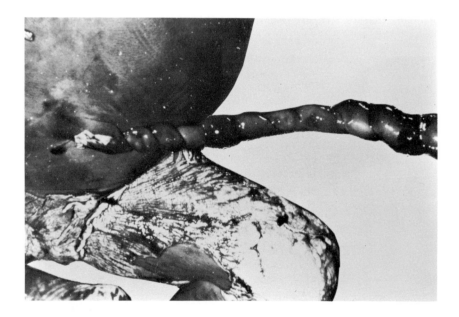

Figure 15.6. A tightly twisted cord in a macerated stillbirth. The torsion has occurred at the characteristic site, at the fetal end of the cord.

cord may occur after fetal death. An ante-mortem torsion can, however, be distinguished from post-mortem twisting by demonstrating that it remains permanently after separation of the fetus and placenta (Browne, 1925) and by histological examination, which will show congestion, oedema and, possibly, thrombosis at the site of torsion, all features absent from post-mortem twisting of the cord.

Stricture

A stricture of the cord is rare and is often, though by no means invariably, complicated by torsion; there is little doubt that the stricture is the precursor rather than the result of the torsion.

Browne (1925) and Weber (1963) have reviewed the cases of cord stricture that were reported during the nineteenth century and more recent examples have been described by Edmonds (1954), Piraux (1957), Quinlan (1965), Pal et al (1973), Gilbert and Zugibe (1974), Tavares-Fortuna and Lourdes-Pratas (1978), Virgilio and Spangler (1978), Robertson et al (1981), Ahrentsen and Andersen (1984), Glanfield and Watson (1986), and Kiley et al (1986). Javert and Barton (1952) found nine instances of cord stricture in their series of 297 spontaneous abortions, and this indication that the abnormality is possibly less uncommon than is usually supposed is further emphasized by Weber (1963), who found five cord strictures in a series of 1369 deliveries.

The stricture is usually well defined, short, single and at the fetal end of the cord (Fig. 15.7). Weber (1963), however, has described a cord with two discrete strictures and another in which the constriction was at the placental end. Javert and Barton (1952) emphasized the marked contraction of the umbilical vessels at the site of the stricture and hence employed the term 'coarctation' to describe the lesion; in Browne's (1925) case the umbilical vessels were obliterated in the constricted area. Most workers have, however, been less impressed by the vascular changes and have commented on the focal, and often extreme, deficiency of Wharton's jelly, this sometimes being accompanied by well-marked fibrosis.

Edmonds (1954) suggested that a cord stricture was a post-mortem artefact produced by maceration commencing at the fetal end of the cord. Weber (1963) has refuted this concept by pointing out that a stricture may be found in the cord of a live-born baby, that the stricture may develop at the placental end of the cord, and that

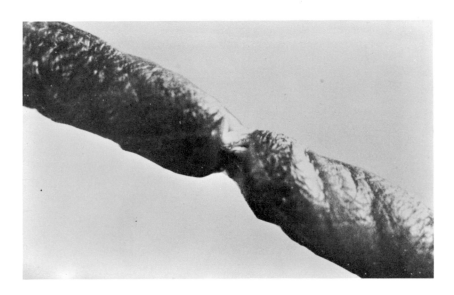

Figure 15.7. A sharply localized stricture in a cord from a stillborn infant.

most macerated fetuses do not have a cord stricture. Neither he nor any other students of this abnormality have, however, been able to provide a convincing pathogenetic theory, most suggesting only that there may be either a focal congenital lack, or a focal degeneration, of Wharton's jelly. One case has been attributed, not very convincingly, to damage caused by amniocentesis (Robertson et al, 1981). Benirschke (1994) feels that excessive fetal movement in the early months of gestation could be an important factor, though he does appear to be discussing a torsion rather than a primary stricture.

Although occasional babies with a cord stricture have been born alive, the vast majority have been stillbirths, and the evidence suggests strongly that cord stricture plays a role, possibly a very important one, in fetal demise in such cases.

VASCULAR LESIONS

Haematoma

Haematomas of the cord may be iatrogenic, complicating amniocentesis (Gassner & Paul, 1976; Morin et al, 1987), umbilical blood sampling (Jauniaux et al, 1989b; Chenard et al, 1990) or intrauterine intravascular blood transfusion (Keckstein et al, 1990).

This account is, however, concerned principally with spontaneous haematomas of the cord; these were described at length during the last century, but their importance was not fully realized until Dippel's review of this topic in 1940. Since then they have been the subject of a considerable number of reports and reviews, amongst which should be mentioned those of Bret and Bardiaux (1960), Overbeck (1960), Kretowicz (1961), Gardner and Trussell (1964), Hogg and Friesen (1964), Irani (1964), Bardiaux and Eliachar (1965), Slavov (1966), Ottolenghi-Preti et al (1972), Roberts-Thomson (1973), Clare et al (1979), Dillon and O'Leary (1981), Ruvinski et al (1981), Szabo and Esztergaly (1981), Virot et al (1981), Feldberg et al (1986) and Summerville et al (1987). Despite the critical attention that has been lavished upon this apparently simple lesion, it has to be admitted that its frequency is still undetermined, its pathogenesis awaits clarification and its clinical significance remains uncertain. The picture has been unduly confused by the tendency of some authors to limit their attention to those 80% of cord haematomas which are of the 'simple' variety, i.e. which are entirely intrafunicular. The findings in such studies will clearly contrast with those of workers who have also included within their remit the 20% of haematomas which rupture through the covering sheath into the amniotic cavity. Furthermore, the distinction between a ruptured haematoma and bleeding from a torn cord has not always been clearly drawn.

Dippel (1940) and Breen et al (1958) considered that 'simple' haematomas occurred only once in 5505 deliveries, but Bret and Bardiaux (1960) encountered 25 haematomas (of both simple and ruptured varieties) and maintained that their apparently low incidence was a tribute not so much to their rarity but to the infrequency with which the cord is adequately examined. Nevertheless, Corkill (1961) noted only one cord haematoma in 12,699 deliveries, whilst Schreier and Brown (1962) quoted an incidence of one per 5500 deliveries. More recently, Ottolenghi-Preti et al (1972) found an incidence of one in 8260 deliveries and Roberts-Thomson (1973) one in 6200 deliveries.

The haematomas, which consist of an extravasation of blood into Wharton's jelly, are usually single, though cords containing two separate and discrete haematomas have been noted on several occasions. They occur most commonly towards, or at, the fetal end of the cord, and present as a rounded or sausage-shaped turgid tumefaction which is usually reddish-purple or 'aubergine' coloured (Fig. 15.8). The haematomas vary considerably in size, and range from a diameter of just over 1 cm to a swelling 'the thickness of a child's arm'. They can be from 4 to 40 cm in length and Bret and Bardiaux (1960) have reported one example of a haematoma that ran the full length of the cord.

Very occasionally the source of a cord haematoma is due to extravasation of blood from a haemangioma (Dohmen & Bubenzer, 1978) whilst in a proportion of cases it is

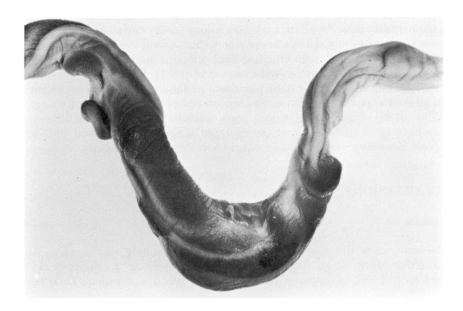

Figure 15.8. A small intrafunicular haematoma of the cord.

possible to demonstrate that the bleeding has come from a torn or ruptured umbilical vein (Clare et al, 1979): much less commonly the blood is clearly derived from a damaged umbilical artery. In many cases, however, no obvious large vessel lesion can be found and it has been suggested that in such circumstances the haemorrhage has been from persistent omphalomesenteric capillaries. This is a possible explanation for those haematomas that occur at the extreme fetal end of the cord, but will not suffice for that minority which develop at some distance from the umbilicus. Others have suggested that the blood may accumulate as a result of diapedesis of erythrocytes through weakened vessel walls, likening the whole process to a haemorrhagic pulmonary infarct. Bret and Bardiaux (1960) espouse this latter view with some enthusiasm and point to the occasional instance of a haematoma being associated with an umbilical vein thrombosis (Bertrand, 1962). They appear to place less emphasis on the fact that a vascular occlusion of this type is an exceptional finding in cord haematomas.

The aetiology of cord haematomas is as, if not more, obscure than their pathogenesis. Some examples of venous bleeding into the cord appear to have been clearly the result of rupture of a varix, whilst one example of bleeding due to a dissecting aneurysm of an umbilical vein has been noted (Lupovitch & McInerney, 1968). In some cases of arterial intrafunicular haemorrhage a localized deficiency of muscle and/or elastic tissue has been noted in the vessel wall at the site of rupture (Beckmann & Zimmer, 1929; Freisfeld, 1936; Schreier & Brown, 1962; Hogg & Friesen, 1963). In the vast majority of instances, however, no obvious lesion of this type is present, and amongst the suggested aetiological factors in such cases have been torsion, traction of an unduly short cord, trauma during delivery, non-specific inflammation of the cord, syphilis, prolapse of the cord, 'toxic' damage to the cord vessels, mucoid or fatty change in the umbilical vessels, a deficiency of Wharton's jelly, and a haemorrhagic diathesis in the infant. Benirschke (1994) considers excessive cord length and prolapse to be important aetiological factors though Dippel (1940), in his extensive review, showed clearly that most haematomas occurred in cords of normal length in which there had been no evidence of prolapse. Whilst it is conceivable that intrapartum trauma could cause bleeding in the cord, it is nevertheless true that many haematomas appear to develop before the onset of labour; indeed, these lesions have been noted in the cords of babies delivered by Caesarean section. I am aware of no evidence in favour of cord inflammation, syphilitic or otherwise, being of aetiological importance in haematoma formation, and I would regard many of the suggested arterial abnormalities as being totally imaginary in nature. Bret and Bardiaux (1960) cite occasional examples of cord haematomas being a manifestation of haemorrhagic disease of the neonate and this would seem perfectly reasonable; it would be less reasonable, however, to assume that this is a common aetiological precursor. It appears to me that one factor which has not been adequately evaluated is a deficiency of Wharton's jelly, because on reading case reports of cord haematomas it is apparent that a surprisingly high proportion occur in prolonged pregnancies, these being those, of course, in which there is often some loss of the jelly and hence a reduction in the support that it offers to the cord vasculature.

The perinatal mortality rate in infants whose cord contains a haematoma is in the region of 40–50%, but it is far from clear in many cases whether the haematoma is responsible for fetal demise or whether both the haematoma and fetal death are mutually dependent upon some common causal factor. It is possible for fetal exsanguination to occur because of bleeding into the amniotic sac from a ruptured haematoma (Ruvinski et al, 1981), but the bleeding is usually only slight and is insufficient to embarrass the fetus. It has also been postulated that the umbilical vessels may be occluded by a secondary thrombosis at the site of haematoma formation, but the inability, in most cases, to demonstrate such a thrombus argues against this concept. Many have thought that as the haematoma increases in size, it will compress the umbilical vessels and thus eventually produce a cessation of fetal blood flow. However, no clear-cut relationship exists between the size of the haematoma and the risk of fetal death, whilst Bret and Bardiaux (1960) have shown that in most fatal cases the vessels enveloped by the haematoma are, far from being compressed, widely patent and congested.

In our present state of knowledge, therefore, it would be unwise to attribute fetal death to a cord haematoma until all other possible causes of demise have been excluded.

Thrombosis of Umbilical Vessels

The far from abundant literature on this topic has been reviewed by Nayak (1967), Lednar et al (1970), Vous-Kristiansen and Thue-Nielsen (1985), Dieminger and Friebel (1986) and, most notably, Heifetz (1988). The condition is rare, being found in 1 in 1290 unselected deliveries and in 1 of 938 unselected perinatal autopsies by Heifetz (1988). A majority of cord thrombi appear to accompany, and are probably a complication of, cord compression, torsion, stricture or haematoma, whilst most of the remainder occur in association with obstetrical complications or fetal abnormalities. In the few remaining cases the pathogenesis of the thrombosis is obscure: Lerat et al (1969) reported two cases of umbilical venous thrombosis which they thought resulted from violent uterine contractions following administration of oxytocin and in occasional instances thrombosis has been attributed, not entirely convincingly, to an umbilical arteriopathy (Lednar et al, 1970).

The thrombi are usually (85%) in the umbilical vein, these occurring in isolation in about two-thirds of cases and being associated with thrombi in one or both arteries in about 20% of cases: only in a small proportion (11–15%) does an arterial thrombus occur alone. There is a theoretical risk, which is occasionally realized, of embolic spread from a cord thrombus to placental or fetal vessels (Heifetz, 1988; Cook et al, 1995).

A very high incidence of fetal death is found in association with an umbilical vessel thrombosis, but in most such cases it appears probable that fetal demise has been due principally to the condition of which the thrombotic episode is a complication, rather than to the thrombosis itself. There is no doubt that an infant can survive an umbilical vessel thrombosis, and this lesion is, in itself, likely to serve as a primary cause of fetal death in only a small minority of cases.

Oedema

Oedema of the cord had been reported occasionally (Walz, 1947; Javert & Barton, 1952; Howorka & Kapczynski, 1971) but had received little detailed attention until the meticulous study of Coulter et al (1975). These workers defined the condition as 'visible oedema in a cord with a minimal cross-sectional area of 1.3 cm^2', and they noted that the affected cord has a bloated, swollen appearance throughout, with a pale shiny surface (Fig. 15.9). On section, the oedematous cord has a loose, wet, jelly-like structure which is more translucent than normal Wharton's jelly.

Coulter and colleagues found that cord oedema was present in 10% of all deliveries but was seen unduly frequently in prematurely delivered babies, in infants delivered by Caesarean section, and in association with abruptio placentae, maternal diabetes, rhesus isoimmunization and macerated stillbirth. Babies whose cords were oedematous suffered no excess of fetal distress or neonatal asphyxia but did have a relatively high incidence of both respiratory distress syndrome and transient respiratory distress.

Coulter et al point out that the possible factors predisposing to cord oedema are a low fetal osmotic pressure, a raised hydrostatic pressure in the placenta and cord, and an increase in total water content in the fetoplacental unit. They suggest that low osmotic pressure may well be of aetiological importance in the development of cord oedema in pre-term infants, in those delivered by Caesarean section, and in rhesus isoimmunization.

Oedema of the cord must be differentiated from the gross swelling of the cord that may occur with a patent urachus (Chantler et al, 1969; Ente et al, 1970). In this condition the cord is thick, glistening, hydropic and tense but, when the cord stump falls off, urine is seen to be draining from the umbilicus.

ULCERATION

Bendon et al (1991) described three cases of linear ulceration of the umbilical cord associated with congenital intestinal atresia and Khong et al (1994) subsequently described a further example of this combination of lesions. The similarity of all these cases suggests that this association of cord and intestinal abnormalities is more than

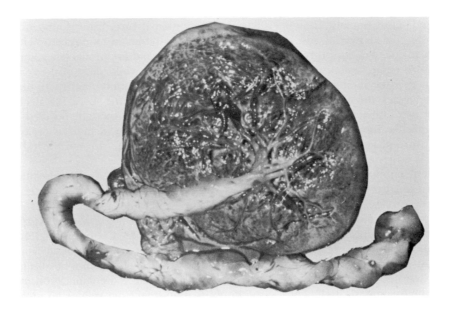

Figure 15.9. An oedematous umbilical cord.

coincidental and represents a true syndrome. In the neonate described by Khong et al (1994), there was an interstitial deletion of the long arm of chromosome 13 but whether this is a consistent karyotypic abnormality in this syndrome awaits further study. In three of the four cases there was severe haemorrhage from the ulcerated cord.

CYSTS

Umbilical cord cysts are of several varieties:

1. *Derived from vestigial remnants.* A cyst, usually situated near the fetal end of the cord, may develop from remnants of either the allantois or the omphalomesenteric duct. Those of allantoic origin are lined by cuboidal or flattened epithelium, which may, however, show a transitional epithelial pattern in some areas, whilst those arising from omphalomesenteric duct remnants are usually lined by epithelium of gastric or intestinal type, can have smooth muscle and nerve ganglia in their wall and are often surrounded by many small vessels which can appear almost angiomatoid (Kranzfeld, 1934; Palliez et al, 1956; Hoen, 1958; Suppi & Maschio, 1960; Heifetz & Rueda-Pedraza, 1983a). Cysts of this type are commonly small and of no clinical importance, but they may sometimes reach the size of a hen's egg, under which circumstances the theoretical possibility exists that they may compress the cord vessels.
2. *Derived from amniotic inclusions.* These are uncommon; they are usually small, and are lined by amniotic-type epithelium (Brown, 1925).
3. *Formed by degeneration of Wharton's jelly.* These are not true cysts but are cavitations which result from a mucoid degeneration of Wharton's jelly (Bergman et al, 1961); they lack an epithelial lining and contain clear mucoid material. Pseudocysts of this type have been described in cases of fetal trisomy 18 (Jauniaux et al, 1988) but whether this is a real, or even a frequent, association remains to be determined.
4. *Neoplastic cysts.* Cystic tumours are discussed in the next section.

INFLAMMATION

This topic, including the controversial entity of necrotizing funisitis, is discussed in Chapter 11.

TUMOURS

Tumours of the umbilical cord are rare, though possibly less so than their infrequent appearance in the obstetrical and pathological literature might suggest. The occurrence of a neoplasm in the cord appears to induce a state of diagnostic and nosological confusion in some pathologists, and the scanty literature on this topic is replete with such diagnoses as telangiectatic myxosarcoma, choriomyxoma and angiomyxoma. It is usually moderately clear that most, if not all, of the tumours that masquerade under these bizarre names are in fact haemangiomas, as are the few reported examples of arterio-venous malformations of the cord. The only other primary tumour that is known to occur in the cord is the teratoma.

Haemangiomas

Browne (1925) reviewed the five cases of cord haemangioma recorded during the previous 100 years; during the next 50 years only 10 further cases were reported (Schroderus, 1950; Barry et al, 1951; Benirschke & Dodds, 1967; Jakobovits & Herczec, 1970; Nieder & Link, 1970; Zeman & Rauchenberg, 1970; Dorste, 1973; Sikorski & Legiewski, 1974; Büttner & Gocke, 1975), bringing the total to a meagre 15 over a period of 150 years. It is almost certain that a greater awareness of the importance of cord pathology, rather than any true increase in the incidence of this lesion, has led to a recording of a further 28 cases of cord haemangioma during the last 20 years (Carvounis et al, 1978; Dohmen & Bubenzer, 1978; Barson et al, 1980; Fortune & Oster, 1980; Heifetz & Rueda-Pedraza, 1983b; Malaponte et al, 1985; Seifer et al, 1985; Dombrowski et al, 1987; Mishriki et al, 1987; Heep et al, 1988; Resta et al, 1988; Pollack & Bound, 1989; Yavner & Redline, 1989; Becmeur et al, 1990; Ghidini et al, 1990; Jauniaux et al, 1990; Gramellini et al, 1993; Weyerts et al, 1993; Armes & Billson, 1994; Bruhwiler et al, 1994; Carles et al, 1994; Sondergaard, 1994; Wilson et al, 1994; Richards et al, 1995). Nevertheless, despite this sudden plethora of reported cases, cord haemangiomas are apparently rare though it is worth noting that haemangiomas of the placenta, now considered as relatively common, were once regarded as exotic curiosities. Hence it is possible, indeed probable, that a systematic prospective study of umbilical cords would reveal an incidence of haemangiomas rather higher than that now considered to be the case.

The tumours tend to present as rounded or ovoid swellings in the cord, and those described have usually ranged from 3 to 17 cm in diameter, though one (Fig. 15.10) involved the entire length of the cord (Jauniaux et al, 1990): they are very variable in colour and consistency. In some cases attention had been drawn to the haemangioma by the presence of a cord haematoma, this presumably being due to local leakage from the neoplasm; in others the tumour has been found in an area of marked local oedema or 'pseudocyst' formation, the latter occasionally being very large (Yavner & Redline, 1989; Wilson et al, 1994). Histologically, the neoplasms have all had the appearances of either a capillary or cavernous haemangioma (Fig. 15.11), but the microscopic features have often been somewhat distorted by the loose, rather myxoid, stroma in which the tumour is set, and this has often resulted in the haemangioma being regarded as partially myxomatous in nature.

In some cases the haemangioma has clearly been supplied by one umbilical artery, in others it has apparently been connected with both an umbilical vein and an umbilical artery, and in yet others the tumour has been quite separate from the major vessels and appears to have arisen from capillaries in Wharton's jelly. It would appear highly

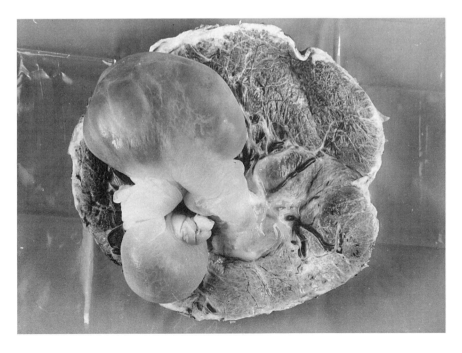

Figure 15.10. A haemangioma involving the entire length of the cord.

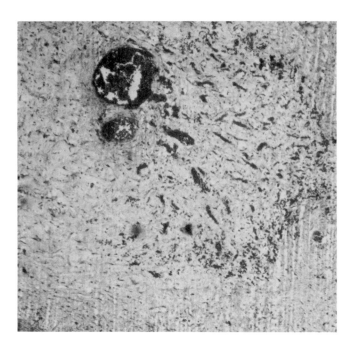

Figure 15.11. A small haemangioma of the cord. This was quite separate from any of the major umbilical vessels and was possibly derived from the omphalomesenteric vessels (H & E ×38).

probable that the haemangioma is a hamartoma rather than a true neoplasm and that it arises as a malformation of the primitive angiogenic mesenchyme of the developing cord.

Cord haemangiomas can be associated with an elevated maternal alpha-fetoprotein level; the elevation may be only slight but very high levels are sometimes attained (Barson et al, 1980; Resta et al, 1988; Yavner & Redline, 1989; Bruhwiler et al, 1994). An antenatal diagnosis can be achieved, in some but not all cases, by ultrasound examination (Pollack & Bound, 1989; Ghidini et al, 1990; Gramellini et al, 1993; Bruhwiler et al, 1994).

The cord haemangioma can thus be considered as very similar in origin and nature to the more common placental haemangioma, but whereas a whole range of complications have been recorded for the placental haemangioma (see Chapter 13), the clinical significance of cord haemangiomas is less well defined. An association with poly-hydramnios (Barry et al, 1951; Mishriki et al, 1987; Heep et al, 1988; Armes & Billson, 1994), fetal disseminated intravascular coagulation (Richards et al, 1995) and fetal hydrops (Seifer et al, 1985; Carles et al, 1994) has been described but such complications are inconsistent and of highly debatable pathogenesis. It is true that in a high proportion of the reported cases the fetus had died *in utero*, but this could be taken as indicating that the greater care with which the cord is examined under such circumstances may reveal a relatively high incidence of innocuous haemangiomas.

Teratoma

Budin, in 1887, described a partly solid and partly cystic mass in the umbilical cord of a live-born child; it measured 8 cm in diameter and was shown to contain epidermis, sebaceous glands, sweat glands, hair follicles, gastrointestinal-type epithelium, tubular and mucous glands, respiratory-type epithelium, fat, smooth muscle, cartilage and bone. The cord was incorporated in the border of this mass and contained the usual complement of vessels, none of which appeared to run into the tumour. Budin concluded, quite rightly in my opinion, that this was a teratoma of the cord.

Essentially similar cases have been recorded by Haendly (1922), Kreyberg (1958), Heckmann et al (1972), Bersch et al (1985), Calame and van der Harten (1985), Smith and Majmudar (1985), Nickell and Stocker (1987), Wagner et al (1993) and Kreczy et al (1994). Kreyberg did not exclude the possibility that the tumour he described was an acardiac twin whilst Calame and van der Harten, after some deliberation, finally concluded that their case was that of a fetus acardius. As discussed in Chapter 13, the distinction between these two entities can be difficult but most authors have agreed that the absence of any evidence of axial skeletal development and of a separate umbilical cord are features that distinguish a cord teratoma from an acardiac fetus. There is no doubt, however, that some pathologists have a conceptual difficulty in accepting that a teratoma can occur in the cord but this is parallelled by doubts in the minds of others as to whether an acardiac twin could be entirely intrafunicular. I share these latter doubts and can see no theoretical or practical reason why a teratoma should not occur in the cord.

As discussed more fully in Chapter 13, teratomas are derived from germ cells: these originally arise in the dorsal wall of the yolk sac, later migrate into the primitive gut wall, and then continue out through the root of the mesentery eventually to reach the genital folds. Not all germ cells complete this rather complicated journey and some may go astray to extragonadal sites, where they may eventually give rise to a teratoma. During the first few months of pregnancy there is an evagination of primitive gut into the umbilical cord, and it is possible that primordial germ cells may migrate out through the wall of this evaginated gut into the connective tissue of the cord, where they may then give rise to a teratoma.

Other Tumours

Banerjee (1962) has reported a myxoma of the cord; this did not contain any angiomatous areas and from the description and the illustration it appears clear that this was an area of localized oedema rather than a true neoplasm.

A case of metastasis of a fetal neuroblastoma to the cord has been recorded (Andersen & Hariri, 1983) in which neoplastic cells were blocking the umbilical vessels and were thought to be responsible for fetal death; interestingly, there was no metastatic tumour in the placenta.

REFERENCES

Abuhamad, A.Z., Shaffer, W., Mari, G., Copel, J.A., Hobbins, J.C. and Evans, A.T. (1995) Single umbilical artery: does it matter which artery is missing? *American Journal of Obstetrics and Gynecology*, **173**, 728–732.

Adler, J., Lewenthal, H. and Ben-Adereth, N. (1963) Absence of one umbilical artery and its relationship to congenital malformations. *Harefuah*, **65**, 286–288.

Adrian, K. (1966) Cited by Kristoffersen (1969).

Aguero, O. (1957) *Anomalias Morfologicas de la Placenta y su Significado Clinico*. Caracas, Venezuela: Artegrafia.

Ahrentsen, O.D. and Andersen, H.J. (1984) Intrauterin fosterdod forarsaget af navlesnorsstriktur og torsion. *Ugeskrift for Laeger*, **146**, 3374–3375; 137–142.

Ainsworth, P. and Davies, P.A. (1969) The single umbilical artery: a five year survey. *Developmental Medicine and Child Neurology*, **11**, 297–302.

Altshuler, G. and Hyde, S. (1989) Meconium-induced vasoconstriction: a potential cause of cerebral and other fetal hypoperfusion and of poor pregnancy outcome. *Journal of Childhood Neurology*, **4**, 137–142.

Altshuler, G., Tsang, R.C. and Ermocilla, R. (1975) Single umbilical artery: correlation of clinical status and umbilical cord histology. *American Journal of Diseases of Children*, **129**, 697–700.

Altshuler, G., Arizawa, M. and Molnar-Nadasdy, G. (1992) Meconium-induced umbilical cord vascular necrosis and ulceration: a potential link between the placenta and poor pregnancy outcome. *Obstetrics and Gynecology*, **79**, 760–766.

Andersen, H.J. and Hariri, J. (1983) Congenital neuroblastoma in a fetus with multiple malformations: metastasis in the umbilical cord as a cause of intrauterine death. *Virchows Archives A Pathological Anatomy and Histology*, **400**, 219–222.

Angiolillo, M. and Picinelli, M.L. (1966) Sui rapporti tra l'aplasia de una arteria del funicolo ombilicale e le malformazioni fetal congeneti. *Bollettino della Societa Italiana di Biologia Sperimentale*, **42**, 20–32.

Armes, J.E. and Billson, V.R. (1994) Umbilical cord haemangioma associated with polyhydramnios, congenital abnormalities and perinatal death in a twin pregnancy. *Pathology*, **26**, 218–220.

Bahary, C.M., Gabbai, M. and Eckerling, B. (1965) Rupture of the umbilical cord: report of a case. *Obstetrics and Gynecology*, **26**, 130–132.

Baill, I.C., Moore, G.W. and Hedrick, L.A. (1989) Abscess of allantoic duct remnant. *American Journal of Obstetrics and Gynecology*, **161**, 334–336.

Bain, C. and Eliot, B.W. (1976) Fetal distress in the first stage of labour associated with early fetal heart rate decelerations and a short umbilical cord. *Australian and New Zealand Journal of Obstetrics and Gynaecology*, **16**, 51–56.

Banerjee, D. (1962) A case of umbilical cord tumour. *Journal of Obstetrics and Gynaecology of India*, **12**, 649–650.

Bardiaux, M. and Eliachar, E. (1965) Hématome du cordon ombilical. *Archives Francaises de Pédiatrie*, **22**, 67–75.

Barry, F.E., McCoy, C.P. and Callahan, W.P. (1951) Hemangioma of the umbilical cord. *American Journal of Obstetrics and Gynecology*, **62**, 675–680.

Barson, A.J., Donnai, P., Ferguson, A., Donnai, D. and Reed, A.P. (1980) Haemangioma of the cord: further cause of raised alphafetoprotein. *British Medical Journal*, **281**, 1252.

Beckmann, S. and Zimmer, E. (1929) Ein Fall von isolierten Ruptur einer Nabelschnurarterie bei Spontangeburt. *Zentralblatt für Gynäkologie*, **52**, 3461–3465.

Becmeur, F., Geiss, S., Marcellin, L., Clavert, J.M. and Sauvage, P. (1990) L'angiome du cordon ombilical: à propos d'une observation. *Chirurgie Pédiatrique*, **31**, 60–62.

Bendon, R.W., Tyson, R.W., Baldwin, V.J., Cashner, K.A., Mimouni, F. and Miodovnik, M. (1991) Umbilical cord ulceration and intestinal atresia: a new association? *American Journal of Obstetrics and Gynecology*, **164**, 582–586.

Benirschke, K. (1965) Major pathologic features of the placenta, cord and membranes. *Birth Defects Original Article Series*, **1**, 52–63.

Benirschke, K. (1994) Obstetrically important lesions of the umbilical cord. *Journal of Reproductive Medicine*, **29**, 262–272.

Benirschke, K. and Bourne, G.L. (1960) The incidence and prognostic implication of congenital absence of one umbilical artery. *American Journal of Obstetrics and Gynecology*, **79**, 251–254.

Benirschke, K. and Brown, W.H. (1955) A vascular anomaly of the umbilical cord: the absence of one umbilical artery in the umbilical cords of normal and abnormal fetuses. *Obstetrics and Gynecology*, **6**, 399–404.

Benirschke, K. and Dodds, J.P. (1967) Angiomyxoma of the umbilical cord with atrophy of an umbilical artery. *Obstetrics and Gynecology*, **30**, 99–102.

Benirschke, K. and Kaufmann, P. (1995) *The Pathology of the Human Placenta*, 3rd edn. New York: Springer-Verlag.

Berg, T.G. and Rayburn, W.F. (1995) Umbilical cord length and acid-base balance at delivery. *Journal of Reproductive Medicine*, **40**, 9–12.

Bergman, P., Lundin, P. and Malmstrom, T. (1961) Mucoid degeneration of Wharton's jelly: an umbilical cord anomaly threatening foetal life. *Acta Obstetricia et Gynecologica Scandinavica*, **40**, 372–378.

Bersch, W., Mayer, M. and Dengler, H.M. (1985) Teratom der Nabelschnur: ein kasuistischer Beitrg. *Pathologe*, **6**, 38–40.

Bertrand, P. (1962) Thrombose des vaisseaux funiculaires. *Bulletin de la Fédération des Sociétés de Gynécologie et d'Obstétrique de Langue Francaise*, **14**, 420–421.

Bilek, K., Rothe, K. and Piskazeck, K. (1962) Insertio velamentosa – Blutung vor dem Blasensprung. *Zentralblatt für Gynäkologie*, **84**, 1536–1541.

Bjoro, K. (1983) Vascular anomalies of the umbilical cord. I. Obstetric implications. *Early Human Development*, **8**, 119–127.

Blanc, W.A. and Allan, G.W. (1961) Intrafunicular ulceration of persistent omphalomesenteric duct with intra-amniotic hemorrhage and fetal death. *American Journal of Obstetrics and Gynecology*, **82**, 1392–1396.

Blickstein, I., Shoham-Schwartz, Z. and Lancet, M. (1987) Predisposing factors in the formation of true knots of the umbilical cord – analysis of morphometric and perinatal data. *International Journal of Gynaecology and Obstetrics*, **25**, 395–398.

Bourke, W.G., Clarke, T.A., Mathews, T.G. O'Halpin, D. and Donoghue, V.B. (1993) Isolated single umbilical artery – the case for routine renal screening. *Archives of Disease in Childhood*, **68**, 600–601.

Breen, J.L., Riva, H.L. and Hatch, R.P. (1958) Hematoma of the umbilical cord: a case report. *American Journal of Obstetrics and Gynecology*, **76**, 1288–1290.

Bret, A.J. and Bardiaux, M. (1960) Hématome du cordon. *Revue Francaise de Gynécologie et d'Obstétrique*, **55**, 81–142.

Bret, A.J. and Blanchier, J. (1968) Artère ombilicale unique: valeur de l'examen systématique du placenta. *Revue Francaise de Gynécologie et d'Obstétrique*, **63**, 399–413.

Bret, A.J. and Coupez, F.J. (1956) De la brieveté du cordon. *Gynécologie et Obstétrique*, **55**, 240–249.

Brody, S. and Frenkel, D.A. (1953) Marginal insertion of the cord and premature labor. *American Journal of Obstetrics and Gynecology*, **65**, 1305–1312.

Broussard, P., Raudrant, D., Picaud, J.J., Bonglet, C. and Dumont, M. (1972) Artère ombilicale unique: étude de 45 cas. *Journal de Gynécologie, Obstétrique et Biologie de la Reproduction*, **1**, 551–558.

Browne, F.J. (1925) On the abnormalities of the umbilical cord which may cause antenatal death. *Journal of Obstetrics and Gynaecology of the British Empire*, **32**, 17–48.

Bruhwiler, H., Rabner, M. and Luscher, K.P. (1994) Pranatale Diagnose eines Nabelschnur-Hamangioms bei erhohtem Alphafetoprotein. *Ultraschall in der Medizin*, **15**, 140–142.

Bryan, E.M. and Kohler, H.G. (1974) The missing umbilical artery. I. Prospective study based on a maternity hospital. *Archives of Disease in Childhood*, **49**, 844–852.

Bryan, E.M. and Kohler, H.G. (1975) The missing umbilical artery. II. Paediatric follow-up. *Archives of Disease in Childhood*, **50**, 714–718.

Budin (1887) Cited by Browne, F.J. (1925).

Burton, G. and Saunders, D.M. (1988) Vasa praevia: another cause for concern in in vitro fertilization pregnancies. *Australian and New Zealand Journal of Obstetrics and Gynaecology*, **28**, 180–181.

Busch, W. (1972) Die placenta bei fetalen Mangelentwicklung: Makroskopie und Mikroskopie von 150 Placenten fetaler mangelentwicklungen. *Archiv für Gynäkologie*, **212**, 333–357.

Büttner, H.H. and Gocke, H. (1975) Kavernöses Hämangiom der Nabelschnur. *Zentralblatt für Gynäkologie*, **97**, 439–442.

Byrne, J. and Blanc, W.A. (1985) Malformations and chromosome anomalies in spontaneously aborted fetuses with single umbilical artery. *American Journal of Obstetrics and Gynecology*, **151**, 340–342.

Cabrere, R., Nunez, R. and Blesa, E. (1993) Hepatocolecistectomia neonatal por incarceracion en hernia de cordon. *Cirugia Pediatrica*, **6**, 204–205.

Cairns, J.D. and McKee, J. (1964) Single umbilical artery: a prospective study of 2000 consecutive deliveries. *Canadian Medical Association Journal*, **91**, 1071–1073.

Calame, J.J. and van der Harten, J.J. (1985) Placental teratoma or acrardius amorphus with amniotic band syndrome. *European Journal of Obstetrics, Gynecology and Reproductive Biology*, **20**, 265–273.

Carles, D., Maugey-Laulom, B., Roux, D., Jiminez, M., Saudubray, F. and Alberti, E.M. (1994) Anasarque foeto-placentaire letale secondaire à un hemangiome du cordon ombilical. *Annales de Pathologie*, **14**, 244–247.

Carrier, C., Matteau, P. and Jean, C. (1966) Aplasie d'une artère ombilicale. *Canadian Medical Association Journal*, **94**, 1001–1004.

Carvounis, E.E., Dimmick, J.E. and Wright, V.J. (1978) Angiomyxoma of umbilical cord. *Archives of Pathology and Laboratory Medicine*, **102**, 178–179.

Cederqvist, L. (1970) Die Bedeutung des Fehlens einer Arterie in der Nabelschnur: eine prospektive endemiologische Studie. *Acta Obstetricia et Gynecologica Scandinavica*, **49**, 113–117.

Chantler, C., Baum, J.D., Wigglesworth, J.S. and Scopes, J.W. (1969) Giant umbilical cord associated with a patent urachus and fused umbilical artery. *Journal of Obstetrics and Gynaecology of the British Commonwealth*, **76**, 273–274.

Chasnoff, I.J. and Fletcher, M.A. (1977) True knot of the umbilical cord. *American Journal of Obstetrics and Gynecology*, **117**, 425–427.

Chaurasia, B.D. (1974) Single umbilical artery with caudal defects in human fetuses. *Teratology*, **9**, 287–298.

Chenard, E., Bastide, A. and Fraser, W.D. (1990) Umbilical cord hematoma following diagnostic funipuncture. *Obstetrics and Gynecology*, **76**, 994–996.

Cipparone, J.R. (1966) Absence of one umbilical artery: analysis of 20 cases in a 5-year study. *American Journal of Clinical Pathology*, **45**, 247–251.

Clapp, J.F., Peress, N.S., Wesley, M. and Mann, L.I. (1988) Brain damage after intermittent partial cord occlusion in the chronically instrumented fetal lamb. *American Journal of Obstetrics and Gynecology*, **159**, 504–509.

Clare, N.M., Hayashi, R. and Khodr, G. (1979) Intrauterine death from umbilical cord hematoma. *Archives of Pathology and Laboratory Medicine*, **103**, 46–47.

Cook, V., Weeks, J., Brown, J. and Bendon, R. (1995) Umbilical artery obstruction and fetoplacental thromboembolism. *Obstetrics and Gynecology*, **85**, 870–872.

Cordero, D.R., Helfgott, A.W., Landy, H.J., Reik, R.F., Mendina, C. and O'Sullivan, M.J. (1993) A non-hemorrhagic manifestation of vasa previa: a clinicopathologic case report. *Obstetrics and Gynecology*, **82**, 698–700.

Corkill, T.F. (1961) The infant's vulnerable life-line. *Australian and New Zealand Journal of Obstetrics and Gynaecology*, **1**, 154–160.

Coulter, J.B.S., Scott, J.M. and Jordan, M.M. (1975) Oedema of the cord and respiratory distress in the newborn. *British Journal of Obstetrics and Gynaecology*, **82**, 453–459.

Dehalleux, J.M., Müller, G., L'Huillier, B., Philippe, E. and Gandar, R. (1966) Aplasia d'une artère ombilicale. *Gynécologie et Obstétrique*, **65**, 223–228.

Dellenbach, P., Leissner, P., Phillipe, E., Gillet, J.Y. and Muller, P. (1968) Artère ombilicale unique, insertion vélamenteuse du cordon ombilical et malformation foetale. *Revue Francaise de Gynécologie et d'Obstétrique*, **63**, 603–612.

Dieminger, H.J. and Friebel, L. (1986) Die Thrombose der Vena umbilicalis. *Zentralblatt für Gynäkologie*, **108**, 765–769.

Dillon, W.P. and O'Leary, L.A. (1981) Detection of fetal cord compromise secondary to umbilical cord hematoma with the nonstress test. *American Journal of Obstetrics and Gynecology*, **141**, 1102–1103.

Dippel, A.L. (1940) Hematomas of the umbilical cord. *Surgery, Gynecology and Obstetrics*, **70**, 51–57.

di Terlizzi, G. and Rossi, G.F. (1955) Studio clinico-statistico sulle anomalie del funicolo. *Annali di Ostetricia e Ginecologia*, **77**, 459–474.

Dohmen, W. and Bubenzer, J. (1978) Hamatom als Komplikation eines kavernös Hämangioms der Nabelschnur. *Zeitschrift für Geburtshilfe und Perinatologie*, **182**, 312–315.

Dombrowski, M.P., Budev, H., Wolfe, H.M., Sokol, R.J. and Perrin, E.V.D.K. (1987) Fetal hemorrhage from umbilical cord hematoma. *Obstetrics and Gynecology*, **70**, 439–442.

Dorste, P. (1973) Hämangiom der Nabelschnur. *Zentralblatt für Gynäkologie*, **95**, 1492–1496.

Earn, A.A. (1951) The effect of congenital abnormalities of the umbilical cord and placenta on the newborn and mother: a survey of 5676 consecutive deliveries. *Journal of Obstetrics and Gynaecology of the British Empire*, **58**, 456–459.

Eberst, B., Boog, G., Harzolf, G., Ritter, J. and Gander, R. (1979) L'artère ombilicale unique. *Revue Francaise de Gynécologie et d'Obstétrique*, **74**, 37–40.

Eddleman, K.A., Lockwood, C.J., Berkowitz, G.S., Lapinski, R.H. and Berkowitz, R.L. (1992) Clinical significance and sonographic diagnosis of velamentous umbilical cord insertion. *American Journal of Perinatology*, **9**, 123–126.

Edmonds, H.W. (1954) The spiral twist of the normal umbilical cord in twins and in singletons. *American Journal of Obstetrics and Gynecology*, **67**, 102–120.

Ente, G., Penzer, P.H. and Kenigsberg, K. (1970) Giant umbilical cord associated with patent urachus: an external clue to internal anomaly. *American Journal of Diseases of Children*, **120**, 82–83.

Erb, H. and Zeilinger, I. (1965) Spontane Gefassruptur bei Insertio velamentosa und intakter Fruchtblase. *Gynaecologia*, **159**, 25–32.

Faierman, E. (1960) The significance of one umbilical artery. *Archives of Disease in Childhood*, **35**, 285–288.

Feingold, M., Fine, R.N. and Ingall, D. (1964) Intravenous pyelography in infants with single umbilical artery. *New England Journal of Medicine*, **270**, 1178–1180.

Feldberg, D., Ben-David, M., Dicker, D., Samuel, N. and Goldman, J. (1986) Hematoma of the umbilical cord with acute antepartum fetal distress: a case report. *Journal of Reproductive Medicine*, **31**, 65–66.

Fletcher, S. (1993) Chirality in the umbilical cord. *British Journal of Obstetrics and Gynaecology*, **100**, 234–236.

Foldes, J.J. (1957) Spontaneous intra-uterine rupture of the umbilical cord. *Obstetrics and Gynecology*, **9**, 608–609.

Fortune, D.W. and Ostor, A.G. (1978) Umbilical cord aneurysm. *American Journal of Obstetrics and Gynecology*, **131**, 339–340.

Fortune, D.W. and Oster, A.G. (1980) Angiomyxomas of the umbilical cord. *Obstetrics and Gynecology*, **55**, 375–378.

Foss, I. and Vogel, M. (1972) Über Bezichungen zwischen Implantationsschäden der Plazenta und Plazentationsstorungen. *Zeitschrift für Geburtshilfe und Perinatologie*, **176**, 36–44.

Freisfeld, R. (1936) Ueber einen Fall von Nabelschnurhaematom. *Zentralblatt für Gynäkologie*, **60**, 1699–1701.

Froehlich, L.A. and Fujikura, T. (1966) Significance of a single umbilical artery: report from the collaborative study of cerebral palsy. *American Journal of Obstetrics and Gynecology*, **94**, 274–279.

Froehlich, L.A. and Fujikura, T. (1973) Follow-up of infants with single umbilical artery. *Pediatrics*, **52**, 22–29.

Fujikura, T. (1964) Single umbilical artery and congenital malformations. *American Journal of Obstetrics and Gynecology*, **88**, 829–830.

Fujinaga, M., Chinn, A. and Shepard, T.H. (1990) Umbilical cord growth in human and rat fetuses: evidence against the 'stretch hypothesis'. *Teratology*, **41**, 333–339.

Gallagher, J.P. and Malone, R.G.S. (1956) Intra-uterine rupture of the umbilical cord. *Journal of Obstetrics and Gynaecology of the British Empire*, **63**, 287–289.

Gardiner, J.P. (1922) The umbilical cord: normal length: length in cord complications: etiology and frequency of coiling. *Surgery, Gynecology and Obstetrics*, **34**, 252–256.

Gardner, R.F.R. and Trussell, R.R. (1964) Ruptured hematoma of the umbilical cord. *Obstetrics and Gynecology*, **24**, 791–793.

Gassner, C.B. and Paul, R.H. (1976) Laceration of umbilical cord vessels secondary to amniocentesis. *Obstetrics and Gynecology*, **48**, 627–630.

German, J.L., Rankin, J.K., Harrison, P.A., Donovan, D.J., Hogan, W.J. and Bearn, A.G. (1962) Autosomal trisomy of a group 16–18 chromosome. *Journal of Pediatrics*, **60**, 503–512.

Ghidini, A., Romero, R., Eisen, R.N., Smith, G.J. and Hobbins, J.C. (1990) Umbilical cord hemangioma: prenatal identification and review of the literature. *Journal of Ultrasound in Medicine*, **9**, 297–300.

Giacoia, G.P. (1992) Body stalk anomaly: congenital absence of the umbilical cord. *Obstetrics and Gynecology*, **80**, 527–529.

Gilbert, E.F. and Zugibe, F.T. (1974) Torsion and constriction of the umbilical cord: a cause of fetal death. *Archives of Pathology*, **97**, 58–59.

Gilbert-Barnes, E., Drut, R.M., Drut, R., Grange, D.K. and Opitz, J.M. (1993) Developmental abnormalities resulting in short umbilical cord. *Birth Defects: Original Article Series*, **29**, 113–140.

Giraud, J.R., Allal, A., Payard, J., Payen, J. and de Tourris, H. (1971) Artère ombilicale unique et pathologie périnatale. *Gynécologie et Obstétrique*, **70**, 433–446.

Gisel, A. (1938) Persistenz der Arteria omphalomesaraica und Fehlen der Nabel arterien bei einer Neugeborenen. *Zeitschrift für Anatomie und Entwicklungsgeschichte*, **108**, 686–694.

Giugni, A.J.M. (1967) Significacion clinica de la patologia del cordon umbilical. *Revista de Obstetricia y Ginecologia de Venezuela*, **27**, 459–481.

Glanfield, P.A. and Watson, R. (1986) Intrauterine death due to umbilical cord torsion. *Archives of Pathology and Laboratory Medicine*, **110**, 357–358.

Gnirs, J., Hendrik, J., Heberling, D. and Schmidt, W. (1988) Gafassanomalien der Nabelschnur – Incidenz, Bedeuting und Moglichkeit der pranatalen ultrasonographischen Erfassung. *Geburtshilfe und Frauenheilkunde*, **48**, 355–360.

Golden, A.S. (1973) Umbilical cord – placental separation a complication of IUD failure. *Journal of Reproductive Medicine*, **11**, 79–80.

Goldhofer, W. and Merz, E. (1985) Das Syndrom der fehlenden Nabelschnur im ultraschall. *Zeitschrift für Geburtshilfe und Perinatologie*, **189**, 241–243.

Gomori, A. and Koller, T. (1964) Über das Fehlen einer Arterie in der Nabelschnur. *Gynaecologia*, **157**, 177–190.

Gornicka, Z., Matusiak, J. and Teczinska, T. (1965) Znaczenie braky jednej tetnicy w sznurze pepowinowym w wykrywaniu wad wrodzonwych. *Ginekologia Polska*, **36**, 1261–1266.

Grall, J.Y., Coudrais, C., Jovan, H., Priov, G., Aras, P.L. and Kerisit, J. (1983) L'artère ombilicale unique: à propos de 194 observations. *Annals d'Anatomie et Cytologie Pathologiques*, **31**, 111–114.

Gramellini, D., Pedrazzoli, G., Sacchini, C., Montalto, M. and Piantelli, G. (1993) Color Doppler ultrasound in prenatal diagnosis of umbilical cord angiomyxoma: case report. *Clinical and Experimental Obstetrics and Gynecology*, **20**, 241–244.

Grieco, A. (1936) Rilievi clinico-statistici sulla inserzione velamentosa ed a racchetta del cordone ombellicale. *Monitore Ostetrico-Ginecologico di Endocrinologia e Metabolismo*, **8**, 89–102.

Gupta, I., Hillier, V.F. and Edwards, J.M. (1993) Vascular branching in the umbilical cord: an indication of maternal smoking habits and intrauterine distress. *Placenta*, **14**, 117–123.

Gustavson, K.H. (1964) *Down's Syndrome: A Clinical and Cytogenetical Investigation*. Uppsala: Almquist and Wiksells.

Haendly, P. (1922) Teratom der Nabelschnur. *Archiv für Gynäkologie*, **116**, 578–588.

Harris, L.E. and Wenzl, J.E. (1963) Heterotopic pancreatic tissue and intestinal mucosa in the umbilical cord. *New England Journal of Medicine*, **268**, 721–722.

Hartge, R. (1979) Über das Vorkommen von Nabelschnurknoten. *Geburtshilfe und Frauenheilkunde*, **39**, 976–980.

Hathout, H. (1964) The vascular pattern and mode of insertion of the umbilical cord in abortion material. *Journal of Obstetrics and Gynaecology of the British Commonwealth*, **71**, 963–964.

Heckmann, U., Cornelius, H.V. and Freudenberg, V. (1972) Das Teratom der Nabelschnur. Ein kasuistischer Beitrag zu den echten Tumoren der Nabelschnur. *Geburtshilfe und Frauenheilkunde*, **32**, 605–607.

Heep, J., Weidenkopf, K.L. and Tschahargane, C. (1988) Kapillares Hämangiom der Nabelschnur als Ursache eines Polyhydramnions. *Geburtshilfe and Frauenheilkunde*, **48**, 819–821.

Heifetz, S.A. (1984) Single umbilical artery: a statistical analysis of 237 autopsy cases and review of the literature. *Perspectives in Pediatric Pathology*, **8**, 345–378.

Heifetz, S.A. (1988) Thrombosis of the umbilical cord; analysis of 52 cases and literature review. *Pediatric Pathology*, **8**, 37–54.

Heifetz, S.A. and Rueda-Pedraza, E. (1983a) Omphalomesenteric duct cysts of the umbilical cord. *Pediatric Pathology*, **1**, 325–335.

Heifetz, S.A. and Rueda-Pedraza, E. (1983b) Hemangiomas of the umbilical cord. *Pediatric Pathology*, **1**, 385–398.

Hennessy, J.P. (1944) True knots of the umbilical cord. *American Journal of Obstetrics and Gynecology*, **48**, 528–536.

Herberz, O. (1938) Über die Insertio furcata funiculi umbilicalis. *Acta Obstetricia et Gynecologica Scandinavica*, **18**, 336–354.

Herrmann, U.J. and Sidiropoulos, D. (1988) Single umbilical artery: prenatal findings. *Prenatal Diagnosis*, **8**, 275–280.

Hnat, R.F. (1967) The practical importance of the single artery umbilical cord. *Journal of Reproduction and Fertility*, **14**, 195–201.

Hoen, E. (1958) Über Fehlbildungen im Bereich der Nabelschnur und des Nabels. *Kinderarztliche Praxis*, **26**, 494–497.

Hogg, G.R. and Friesen, R. (1964) Abnormal umbilical cord with fetal arterial haemorrhage. *American Journal of Obstetrics and Gynecology*, **83**, 1251–1252.

Howorka, E. and Kapczynski, W. (1971) Abnormal thickness of the fetal end of the umbilical cord. *Journal of Obstetrics and Gynaecology of the British Commonwealth*, **78**, 283.

Hyrtle, J. (1870) *Die Blutgefasse der menschlichen Nachgeburt in normalen und abnormalen Verhaltnissen*. Vienna: Braumüller.

Irani, P.K. (1964) Haematoma of the umbilical cord. *British Medical Journal*, **ii**, 1436–1437.

Itskovitz, J., Friedman, M., Peretz, B.A. and Brandes, J.M. (1980) Intrauterine rupture of the umbilical cord during delivery. *European Journal of Obstetrics, Gynecology and Reproductive Biology*, **10**, 35–40.

Iwasaki, I, Yu, T.J., Itahashi, K., Nito, A., Yamaguchi, H. and Onoki, J. (1986) Isolated well formed intestinal tissue in the umbilical cord: a variant of cyst of the omphalomesenteric duct. *Acta Pathologica Japonica*, **36**, 656–659.

Jakobovits, A. and Herczeg, J. (1970) Haemangioma of the umbilical cord. *Annales Chirurgiae et Gynaecologiae Fenniae*, **59**, 159–161.

Jassini, M.N., Brennan, J.N. and Merkatz, I.R. (1980) Prenatal diagnosis of single umbilical artery. *Journal of Clinical Ultrasound*, **8**, 447–448.

Jauniaux, E., Donner, C., Thomas, C., Francotte, J., Rodesch, F. and Avni, F.E. (1988) Umbilical cord pseudocyst in trisomy 18. *Prenatal Diagnosis*, **8**, 274–275.

Jauniaux, E., De Munter, C., Vanesse, M., Wilkin, P. and Hustin, J. (1989a) Embryonic remnants of the umbilical cord: morphologic and clinical aspects. *Human Pathology*, **20**, 458–462.

Jauniaux, E., Donner, C., Simon, P., Vanesse, M., Hustin, J. and Rodesch, F. (1989b) Pathological aspects of the umbilical cord after percutaneous umbilical blood sampling. *Obstetrics and Gynecology*, **73**, 215–218.

Jauniaux, E., Moscoso, G., Chitty, L., Gibb, D., Driver, M. and Campbell, S. (1990) An angiomyxoma involving the whole length of the umbilical cord: prenatal diagnosis by ultrasonography. *Journal of Ultrasound in Medicine*, **9**, 419–422.

Javert, C.T. and Barton, B. (1952) Congenital and acquired lesions of the umbilical cord and spontaneous abortion. *American Journal of Obstetrics and Gynecology*, **63**, 1065–1077.

Jean, C., Dupré, A. and Carrier, C. (1969) L'artère ombilicale unique: étude de 112 observations. *Canadian Medical Association Journal*, **100**, 1088–1091.

Johnsonbaugh, R.E. (1973) Unilateral short lower extremity and single umbilical artery: absence of a relationship. *American Journal of Diseases of Children*, **126**, 186–187.

Jones, T.B., Sorokin, Y., Bhatia, R., Zador, I.E. and Bottoms, S.F. (1993) Single umbilical artery: accurate diagnosis? *American Journal of Obstetrics and Gynecology*, **169**, 538–540.

Kajii, T., Shinohara, M., Kikuchi, K., Dohmen, S. and Akichika, M. (1963) Thalidomide and the umbilical artery. *Lancet*, **ii**, 889.

Karchmer, S.K., Medrano, P.G., MacGregor, C. and Dominguez, A.A. (1966) Anomalias del cordon umbilical y coexistencia de malformaciones congenitas. *Ginecologia y Obstetricia de México*, **21**, 831–837.

Keckstein, G., Tschurtz, S., Schneider, V., Hutter, W., Terinde, R. and Jonatha, W.D. (1990) Umbilical cord haematoma as a complication of intrauterine intravascular blood transfusion. *Prenatal Diagnosis*, **10**, 59–65.

Kessler, A. (1960) Blutungen aus Nabelschnurgefassen in der Schwangerschaft. *Gynaecologia*, **150**, 353–365.

Khong, T.Y. and Dilly, S.A. (1989) Calcification of umbilical artery: two distinct lesions. *Journal of Clinical Pathology*, **42**, 931–934.

Khong, T.Y. and George, K. (1992) Chromosomal abnormalities associated with a single umbilical artery. *Prenatal Diagnosis*, **12**, 965–968.

Khong, T.Y., Ford, W.D. and Haan, E.A. (1994) Umbilical cord ulceration in association with intestinal atresia in a child with deletion 13q and Hirschsprung's disease. *Archives of Disease in Childhood*, **71**, 212–213.

Kiley, K.C., Perkins, C.S. and Penney, L.L. (1986) Umbilical cord stricture associated with intrauterine fetal demise. *Journal of Reproductive Medicine*, **31**, 154–156.

Konstantinova, B.P. (1961) Zur Frage der Zustammenhanges zwischen der Fehlentwicklung der Nabelgefässe und der Entwicklung angeborener Missbildungen. *Zentralblatt für allgemeine Pathologie und pathologische Anatomie*, **103**, 62–66.

Kouyoumdjian, A. (1980) Velamentous insertion of the umbilical cord. *Obstetrics and Gynecology*, **56**, 737–742.

Kranzfeld, J. (1934) Zur Histologie kleinster Nabelschnurneubildunge. *Helvetica Medica Acta*, **1**, 302–305.

Kreczy, A., Alge, A., Menardi, G., Gassner, I., Geschhwendtner, A. and Mikuz, G. (1994) Teratoma of the umbilical cord: case report with review of the literature. *Archives of Pathology and Laboratory Medicine*, **118**, 934–937.

Kretowicz, J. (1961) Krwiak pepowiny jako przyczyna obumarcia plodu. (Case of haematoma of the umbilical cord, causing the death of the fetus.) *Ginekologia Polska*, **32**, 455–461.

Kreyberg, L. (1958) A teratoma-like swelling in the umbilical cord possibly of acardius nature. *Journal of Pathology and Bacteriology*, **75**, 109–112.

Kristoffersen, K. (1969) The significance of absence of one umbilical artery. *Acta Obstetricia et Gynecologica Scandinavica*, **48**, 195–214.

Krone, H.A. (1961) *Die Bedeutung der Eibettstrungen für die Entstehung menschlicher Missbildungen*. Stuttgart: Fischer.

Krone, H.A. (1962) Pathologische Fruchtentwicklung bei Placentaanomalien. *Archiv für Gynäkologie*, **198**, 224–227.

Krone, H.A., Jopp, H. and Schellerer, W. (1964) Die Bedeutung anamnestischer Befunde für die verschiedenen Formen des Nabelschnursatzes. *Zeitschrift für Geburtshilfe und Gynäkologie*, **163**, 205–213.

Labarrere, C., Sebastiani, M., Siminovich, M., Torassa, E. and Althabe, O. (1985) Absence of Wharton's jelly around the umbilical arteries: an unusual cause of perinatal mortality. *Placenta*, **6**, 555–559.

Lange, R. (1968) Ein Beitrag zum intrauterinen Fruchttod und Torsion der Nabelschnur. *Zentralblatt für Gynäkologie*, **90**, 1541–1542.

Lednar, A., Arfwedson, H. and Havu, N. (1970) Die Thrombose der Umbilikalgefasse. *Zentralblatt für Gynäkologie*, **92**, 435–442.

Lee, M.C.L. and Aterman, K. (1968) An intestinal polyp of the umbilical cord. *American Journal of Diseases of Children*, **116**, 320–323.

Lefevre, G. (1896) *De l'insertion vélamenteuse du cordon dans ses rapports avec la grossesse et l'accouchement*. Thèse, Paris.

Leinzinger, E. (1972) Totaler Nabelschnurabriss intra partum bei Hydramnion. *Zentralblatt für Gynäkologie*, **94**, 1233–1238.

Leissner, P. (1967) *Génèse et signification des anomolies d'insertion du cordon ombilical et des artères ombilicals uniques*. Thèse Médicin, Strasbourg, No. 71.

Leissner, P., Dellenbach, P. and Muller, P. (1968) II. Signification clinique et génèse des anomalies d'insertion du cordon ombilical (insertion velamenteuse du cordon) *Revue Francaise de Gynécologie et d'Obstétrique*, **63**, 613–624.

le Marec, R., Kerisit, J., de Villartay, A., Ferrand, B., Toulouse, R. and Senecal, J. (1972) L'artère ombilicale unique: etude de 31 cas. *Journal de Gynécologie, Obstétrique et Biologie de la Reproduction*, **1**, 825–841.

Lenoski, E.F. and Medovy, H. (1962) Single umbilical artery: incidence, clinical significance, and relation to autosomal trisomy. *Canadian Medical Association Journal*, **87**, 1229–1231.

Lerat, M.F., Macre, J. and Lebret, M. (1969) Lésions du cordon. *Bulletin de la Fédération des Sociétés de Gynécologie et d'Obstétrique de Langue Francais*, **21**, 567–570.

Leung, A.K.C. and Robson, W.L.M. (1989) Single umbilical artery – a report of 159 cases. *American Journal of Diseases of Children*, **143**, 108–111.

Lewenthal, H., Alexander, D.J. and Ben-Adereth, N. (1967) Single umbilical artery: a report of 50 cases. *Israel Journal of Medical Sciences*, **3**, 899–902.

Lewis, A.J. (1962) Autosomal trisomy. *Lancet*, **i**, 866.

Lilja, M. (1991) Infants with single umbilical artery studied in a national registry: general epidemiological characteristics. *Paediatric and Perinatal Epidemiology*, **5**, 27–36.

Lilja, M. (1992) Infants with single umbilical artery studied in a national registry. 2. Survival and malformations in infants with a single umbilical artery. *Paediatric and Perinatal Epidemiology*, **6**, 416–422.

Little, W.A. (1961) Umbilical artery aplasia. *Obstetrics and Gynecology*, **17**, 695–700.

Lockwood C.J., Scioscia, A.L. and Hobbins, J.C. (1986) Congenital absence of the umbilical cord resulting from maldevelopment of embryonic body folding. *American Journal of Obstetrics and Gynecology*, **155**, 1049–1051.

Lucchetti, A. (1965) Considerazioni clinico-statistiche sulla patologia del funicolo. *Clinica Ostetrice e Ginecologica*, **67**, 1–92.

Lundgren, A.T. and Boice, W.A. (1939) True knotting of the umbilical cord. *Illinois Medical Journal*, **76**, 451–458.

Lupovitch, A. and McInerney, T.S. (1968) Hematoma of the umbilical cord: a dissecting aneurysm of the umbilical vein. *American Journal of Obstetrics and Gynecology*, **102**, 902–904.

Lurie, S., Fenakel, K. and Gorbacz, S. (1990) Antenatal maceration of umbilical cord: a case report. *European Journal of Obstetrics, Gynecology and Reproductive Biology*, **35**, 279–281.

McLennan, H., Price, E., Urbanska, M., Craig, N. and Fraser, M. (1988) Umbilical cord knots and encirclements. *Australian and New Zealand Journal of Obstetrics and Gynaecology*, **28**, 116–119.

McLennan, J.E. (1968) Implications of the eccentricity of the human umbilical cord. *American Journal of Obstetrics and Gynecology*, **101**, 1124–1130.

Malaponte, E., Costa, V., Calabrese, A., Canfora, A. and Massimino, S. (1985) Fibroangioma cavernoso del funicolo associato a pseudo-ematoma del cordone ombelicale. *Minerva Ginecologia*, **37**, 51–55.

Mallard, E.C., Williams, C.E., Johnston, B.M. and Gluckman, P.D. (1994) Increased vulnerability to neuronal damage after umbilical cord occlusion in fetal sheep with advancing gestation. *American Journal of Obstetrics and Gynecology*, **170**, 206–214.

Malpas, P. (1964) Length of the human umbilical cord at term. *British Medical Journal*, **i**, 673–674.

Marchesoni, M. and Helfer, A. (1956) Spunti per una nuova interpretazione eziopatogenetica della torsionimia del funicolo ombelicale. *Annali di Ostetricia e Ginecologia*, **78**, 637–645.

Mateu-Aragones, J.M. (1956) Ruptura del cordon umbilical. *Acta Gynaecologica et Obstetrica Hispano-Lusitana*, **5**, 5–10.

Matheus, M. and Sala, M.A. (1980) The importance of placental examination in newborns with single umbilical artery. *Zeitschrift für Geburtshilfe und Perinatologie*, **184**, 231–232.

Mele, V. (1968) Anomalia del funicolo causa di morte intrauterina del feto. *Quaderni di Clinica Ostetrica e Ginecologia*, **23**, 1122–1130.

Meyer, W.W., Lind, J. and Moinian, M. (1969) An accessory fourth vessel of the umbilical cord: a preliminary study. *American Journal of Obstetrics and Gynecology*, **105**, 1063–1068.

Miller, J.Q., Picard, E.H., Alkan, M.K., Warner, S. and Gerald, P.S. (1963) A specific congenital brain defect (arhinencephaly) in 13–15 trisomy. *New England Journal of Medicine*, **268**, 120–124.

Miller, M.E., Higginbottom, M. and Smith, D.W. (1981) Short umbilical cord: its origin and relevance. *Pediatrics*, **67**, 618–621.

Mishriki, Y.Y., Vanyshelbaum, Y., Epstein, H. and Blanc, W.A. (1987) Hemangioma of the umbilical cord. *Pediatric Pathology*, **7**, 43–49.

Mital, V.K., Garg, B.K. and Gupta, U. (1969) Single umbilical artery: its association with congenital malformation. *Journal of Obstetrics and Gynaecology of India*, **19**, 583–587.

Moessinger, A.C., Mills, J.L., Harley, E.E., Ramakrishnan, R., Berendes, H.W. and Blanc, W.A. (1986) Umbilical cord length in Down's syndrome. *American Journal of Diseases of Children*, **140**, 1276–1277.

Molz, G. (1965) Aplasie einer Nabelarterie und angeborene Fehlbildungen. *Helvetica Paediatrica Acta*, **20**, 403–414.

Molz, G., Tondury, G. and Manestar M. (1980) Eventration associated with attachment of fetus to placenta: a combination of malformations with female preponderance. *Zeitschrift für Kinderchirurgie*, **31**, 70–81.

Monie, I.W. (1965) Velamentous insertion of the cord in early pregnancy. *American Journal of Obstetrics and Gynecology*, **93**, 276–281.

Monie, I.W. (1970) Genesis of single umbilical artery. *American Journal of Obstetrics and Gynecology*, **108**, 400–405.

Monie, I.W. and Khemmani, M. (1973) Absent and abnormal umbilical arteries. *Teratology*, **7**, 135–142.

Morin, L.R., Bonan, J., Vendrolini, G. and Bourgeois, C. (1987) Sonography of umbilical cord hematoma following genetic amniocentesis. *Acta Obstetricia et Gynecologica Scandinavica*, **66**, 669–670.

Müller, G., Dehalleux, J.M., Trutt, B., Philippe, E., Dreyfus, J. and Gandar, R. (1969) L'artère ombilicale unique – à propos de 54 cas. *Bulletin de la Société Belge de Gynécologie et d'Obstétrique*, **39**, 333.

Nadkarni, B.B. (1969) Congenital anomalies of the human umbilical cord: a light and electron microscope study. *Indian Journal of Medical Research*, **57**, 1018–1027.

Naeye, R.L. (1985) Umbilical cord length: clinical significance. *Journal of Pediatrics*, **107**, 278–281.

Naftolin, F. and Mishell, D.R., Jr (1965) Vasa previa. *Obstetrics and Gynecology*, **26**, 561–565.

Nayak, S.K. (1967) Thrombosis of the umbilical cord vessels. *Australian and New Zealand Journal of Obstetrics and Gynaecology*, **7**, 148–154.

Nelson, L.H., Melone, P.J. and King, M. (1990) Diagnosis of vasa previa with transvaginal and color flow Doppler ultrasound. *Obstetrics and Gynecology*, **76**, 506–509.

Nickell, K.A. and Stocker, J.T. (1987) Placental teratoma: a case report. *Pediatric Pathology*, **7**, 645–650.

Nieder, J. and Link, M. (1970) Ein Beitrag zue Pathologie der Nabelschnurgeschwülste. *Zentralblatt für Gynäkologie*, **92**, 420–428.

Nöldeke, H. (1934) Geburtskomplikationen bei Insertio velamentosa. *Zentralblatt für Gynäkologie*, **58**, 351–356.

Ottolenghi-Preti, G.F. and Bailo, P. (1950) I funicoli lunghi (studio clinico-statistico su quasi 30 000 parti) *Annali di Ostetricia e Ginecologia*, **72**, 293–312.

Ottolenghi-Preti, G.F., Magnani, L. and Paghera, A. (1972) L'ematoma del funicolo: presentazione di due casi e rassegna della litteratura. *Annals di Ostetricia, Ginecologia e Medicina Perinatale*, **93**, 562–578.

Ottow, B. (1922) Interposito velamentosa funiculi umbilicalis, eine bisher übersehene Nabelstranganomalie, ihre Entstehung und klinische Bedeutung. *Archiv für Gynäkologie*, **116**, 176–199.

Ottow, B. (1923) Über die Insertio furcata der Nabelschnur. *Archiv für Gynäkologie*, **118**, 378–382.

Overbeck, L. (1960) Hematome der Nabelschnur. *Zeitschrift für Geburtshilfe und Gynäkologie*, **155**, 381–393.

Pal, A.K., Chopra, S.K., Barua, S.C. and Misuriya, A.K. (1973) Stricture of the umbilical cord. *Indian Journal of Paediatrics*, **40**, 415–416.

Palliez, R., Benoit, M. and Delecour, M. (1956) Tumeur du cordon ombilical: kyste du canal omphalomesenterique. *Bulletin de la Fédération des Sociétés de Gynécologie et d'Obstétrigue de Langue Francais*, **8**, 346–347.

Papadatos, C. and Paschos, S. (1965) Single umbilical artery and congenital malformations. *Obstetrics and Gynecology*, **26**, 367–370.

Paulino, E.H. (1970) Clinical review of vasa praevia in a ten-year period. *Medical Annals of the District of Columbia*, **39**, 251–252.

Peckham, C.H. and Yerushalmy, J. (1965) Aplasia of one umbilical artery: incidence by race and certain obstetric factors. *Obstetrics and Gynecology*, **26**, 359–366.

Perrin, E.V.D.K. and Kahn-Vander Bel, J. (1965) Degeneration and calcification of the umbilical cord. *Obstetrics and Gynecology*, **26**, 371–376.

Petrikovsky, B.M., Nochimson, D.J., Campbell, W.A. and Vintzileos, A.M. (1988) Fetal jejunoileal atresia with persistent omphalomesenteric duct. *American Journal of Obstetrics and Gynecology*, **158**, 173–175.

Philippe, E., Ritter, J., Dehalleux, J.M., Renaud, R. and Gandar, R. (1968) De la pathologie des avortements spontanés. *Gynécologie et Obstétrique*, **67**, 97–118.

Picinelli, G. and Picinelli, M.L. (1968) Considerazioni sulle caratteristiche cliniche di alcuni casi di brevita assoluta del funicolo. *Minerva Ginecologica*, **20**, 1322–1329.

Piraux, P. (1957) Un cas rare d'anomolie du cordon umbilical ayant entraine la mort du foetus par anoxia. *Bulletin de la Société Belge de Gynécologie et Obstétrique*, **27**, 354.

Pollack, M.S. and Bound, L.M. (1989) Hemangioma of the umbilical cord: sonographic appearances. *Journal of Ultrasound in Medicine*, **8**, 163–166.

Purola, E. (1968) The length and insertion of the umbilical cord. *Annales Chirurgia et Gynaecologia Fenniae*, **57**, 621–622.

Quek, S.P. and Tan, K.L. (1972) Vasa praevia. *Australian and New Zealand Journal of Obstetrics and Gynaecology*, **12**, 206–209.

Quinlan, D.K. (1965) Coarctation in cord of twenty-one-week-old fetus, with atresia, fibrosis, secondary torsion. *South African Journal of Obstetrics and Gynaecology*, **3**, 1–2.

Qureshi, F. and Jacques, S.M. (1994) Marked segmental thinning of the umbilical cord vessels. *Archives of Pathology and Laboratory Medicine*, **118**, 826–830.

Raaflaub, W. (1959) Zur Kausalitt der Nabelschnurkomplikationen. *Gynaecologia*, **148**, 145–148.

Ragucci, N. and Morandi, C. (1969) Le distocie del funicolo ombelicale (contributo clinico-statistico) *Minerva Ginecologica*, **21**, 653–655.

Rehn, K. and Kinnunen, O. (1962) Antepartum rupture of the umbilical cord: case report. *Acta Obstetricia et Gynecologica Scandinavica*, **41**, 86–89.

Resta, R.G., Luthy, D.A. and Mahoney, B.S. (1988) Umbilical cord hemangioma associated with extremely high alphaprotein levels. *Obstetrics and Gynecology*, **72**, 488–491.

Richards, D.S., Lutfi, E., Mullins, D., Sandler, D.L. and Raynor, B.D. (1995) Prenatal diagnosis of disseminated intravascular coagulation associated with umbilical cord arteriovenous malformation. *Obstetrics and Gynecology*, **85**, 860–862.

Robertson, R.D., Rubinstein, L.M., Wolfson, W.L., Lebherz, T.B., Blanchard, J.B. and Crandall, B.F. (1981) Constriction of the umbilical cord as a cause of fetal demise following midtrimester amniocentesis. *Journal of Reproductive Medicine*, **26**, 325–327.

Roberts-Thomson, M.E. (1973) The hazards of umbilical cord haematoma. *Medical Journal of Australia*, **1**, 648–650.

Robinson, L.K., Jones, K.L. and Benirschke, K. (1983) The nature of structural defects associated with velamentous and marginal insertion of the umbilical cord. *American Journal of Obstetrics and Gynecology*, **146**, 191–193.

Rosen, R.H. (1955) The short umbilical cord. *American Journal of Obstetrics and Gynecology*, **66**, 1253–1259.

Rucker, M.P. and Tureman, G.R. (1945) Vasa previa. *Virginia Medical Monthly*, **72**, 202–207.

Russell, C.S. and McKichan, M.D. (1962) Thalidomide and congenital abnormalities. *Lancet*, **i**, 429–430.

Rust, W. (1937) Seltsame veranderungen an der Nabelschnurgefassen. *Archiv für Gynäkologie*, **165**, 58–62.

Ruvinski, E.D., Wiley, T.L., Morrison, J.C. and Blake, P.G. (1981) In utero diagnosis of umbilical cord hematoma by ultrasonography. *American Journal of Obstetrics and Gynecology*, **140**, 833–834.

Saller, D.N., Jr and Neiger, R. (1994) Cytogenetic abnormalities among perinatal deaths demonstrating a single umbilical artery. *Prenatal Diagnosis*, **14**, 13–16.

Saller, D.N., Jr, Keene, C.L., Sun, C.C. and Schwartz, S. (1990) The association of single umbilical artery with cytogenetically abnormal pregnancies. *American Journal of Obstetrics and Gynecology*, **163**, 922–925.

Sauramo, H. (1960) Obstetric complications due to secundines. *Annales Chirurgiae et Gynaecologia Fenniae*, **49**, 291–297.

Scheffel, T. and Langanke, D. (1970) Die Nabelschnurkomplikationen an der Universitäts Frauenklinik Leipzig von 1955 bis 1967. *Zentralblatt für Gynäkologie*, **92**, 429–434.

Scheuner, G. (1965) Über die mikroskopische Struktur der Insertio velamentosa. *Zentralblatt für Gynäkologie*, **87**, 38–49.

Schiff, I., Driscoll, S.G. and Naftolin, F. (1976) Calcification of the umbilical cord. *Obstetrics and Gynecology*, **126**, 1046–1048.

Schreier, R. and Brown, S. (1962) Hematoma of the umbilical cord: report of a case. *Obstetrics and Gynecology*, **20**, 798–800.

Schroderus, K.A. (1950) Tumours of the umbilical cord in the light of a rare case. *Acta Obstetricia et Gynaecologica Scandinavica*, **29**, 351–360.

Schultze, K.W. (1969) Intrauteriner Fruchttod durch Nabelschnurtorsion. *Zentralblatt für Gynäkologie*, **91**, 694–696.

Scott, J.S. (1960) Placenta extrachorialis (placenta marginata and placenta circumvallata) *Journal of Obstetrics and Gynaecology of the British Empire*, **67**, 904–918.

Segovia, J.P. (1967) Anomalias vasculares del condon umbilical (con especial consideracion a la arteria umbilical unica) *Revista de Obstetricia y Ginecologia de Venezuela*, **27**, 421–457.

Seifer, D.B., Ferguson, J.E., Behrens, C.M., Zemel, S., Stevenson D.K. and Ross, J.C. (1985) Nonimmune hydrops fetalis in association with hemangioma of the umbilical cord. *Obstetrics and Gynecology*, **66**, 283–286.

Seki, M. and Strauss, L. (1964) Absence of one umbilical artery: analysis of 60 cases with emphasis on associated developmental aberrations. *Archives of Pathology*, **78**, 446–453.

Sepulveda, W.H. (1991) Antenatal sonographic detection of single umbilical artery. *Journal of Perinatal Medicine*, **19**, 391–395.

Shanklin, D.R. (1958) The human placenta: a clinico-pathologic study. *Obstetrics and Gynecology*, **11**, 129–138.

Siddiqi, T.A., Bendon, R., Schultz, D.M. and Miodovnik, M. (1992) Umbilical artery aneurysm: prenatal diagnosis and management. *Obstetrics and Gynecology*, **80**, 530–533.

Sikorski, J. and Legiewski, A. (1974) Guzy naczyniowe pepowiny. (Vascular tumours of the umbilical cord.) *Ginekologia Polska*, **45**, 877–879.

Sirivongs, B. (1974) Vasa previa: report of 3 cases. *Journal of the Medical Association of Thailand*, **57**, 261–268.

Slavov, J. (1966) Haematoma of the umbilical cord. *Akusherstvo i Ginekologiya*, **5**, 171–175.

Slemens, J.L. (1916) The results of a routine study of the placenta. *American Journal of Obstetrics*, **74**, 204–215.

Smith, D. and Majmudar, B. (1985) Teratoma of the umbilical cord. *Human Pathology*, **16**, 190–193.

Soernes, T. and Bakke, T. (1986) The length of the human umbilical cord in vertex and breech presentations. *American Journal of Obstetrics and Gynecology*, **154**, 1086–1087.

Soma, H. (1963) Correlation between umbilical vascular anomaly and fetal abnormalities. *Japanese Journal of Obstetrics and Gynaecology*, **15**, 1056.

Sondergaard, G. (1994) Hemangioma of the umbilical cord. *Acta Obstetricia et Gynecologica Scandinavica*, **73**, 434–436.

Sopracordevole, F. and Perissinotto, M.G. (1991) Il nodo vero di funicolo: implicazioni cliniche. *Minerva Ginecologia*, **43**, 109–113.

Stephan, U. and Thomas, J. (1963) Plazentaanomalien und Fruchtentwicklung. *Archiv für Kinderheilkunde*, **168**, 266–273.

Strong, T.H., Elliot, J.P. and Radin, T.G. (1993) Non-coiled umbilical blood vessels: a new marker for the fetus at risk. *Obstetrics and Gynecology*, **81**, 409–411.

Strong, T.H., Jarles, D.L., Vega, J.S. and Feldman, D.B. (1994) The umbilical coiling index. *American Journal of Obstetrics and Gynecology*, **170**, 29–32.

Summerville, J.W., Powar, J.S. and Ueland, K. (1987) Umbilical cord hematoma resulting in intra-uterine fetal death: a case report. *Journal of Reproductive Medicine*, **32**, 213–216.

Suppi, G. and Maschio, C. (1960) Le formazioni cistiche del cordone ombellicale. *Attualita di Ostetricia e Ginecologia*, **6**, 461–468.

Swanberg, H. and Wiqvist, N. (1951) Rupture of the umbilical cord during pregnancy: report of a case. *Acta Obstetricia et Gynecologica Scandinavica*, **30**, 203–210.

Szabo, L.G. and Esztergaly, S. (1981) Prenatal development of umbilical cord hematoma. *Zentralblatt für Gynäkologie*, **103**, 102–104.

Szecsi, K. (1955) Beitrage zur spontanen Zerreissung der zu kurzen Nabelschnur. *Zentralblatt für Gynäkologie*, **77**, 1024–1028.

Szpakowski, M. (1974) Morphology of arterial anatomoses in the human placenta. *Folia Morphologica* (Warsaw), **33**, 53–60.

Tavares-Fortuna, J.F. and Lourdes-Pratas, M. (1978) Coarctation of the umbilical cord: a cause of intrauterine fetal death. *International Journal of Gynaecology and Obstetrics*, **15**, 469–473.

Thomas, J. (1961) Untersuchungsergebnisse über die Aplasie einer Nabelarterie unter besonderer Berucksichtigung der Zwillingsschwangerschaft. *Geburtshilfe und Frauenheilkunde*, **21**, 984–992.

Thomas, J. (1962) Die Entwicklung von Fetus und Placenta bei Nabelgefssanomalien. *Archiv für Gynäkologie*, **198**, 216–223.

Tollison, S.B. and Huang, P.H. (1988) Vasa previa: a case report. *Journal of Reproductive Medicine*, **33**, 329–330.

Torrey, W.E., Jr (1952) Vasa previa. *American Journal of Obstetrics and Gynecology*, **63**, 146–152.

Tortora, M., Chervanek, F.A., Mayden, K. and Hobbins, J.C. (1984) Antenatal sonographic diagnosis of single umbilical artery. *Obstetrics and Gynecology*, **63**, 693–696.

Uchida, I., Bowman, J.M. and Wang, H.C. (1968) The 18-trisomy syndrome. *New England Journal of Medicine*, **266**, 1198–1201.

Uher, M. (1975) Pretrzeni pupechniku za porodu. (Rupture of the umbilical cord during delivery.) *Ceskoslovensk Gynekologie*, **40**, 727–728.

Uyanwah-Akpom, P.O. and Fox, H. (1977) The clinical significance of marginal or velamentous insertion of the umbilical cord. *British Journal of Obstetrics and Gynaecology*, **84**, 941–943.

VanDrie, D.M. and Kammeraad, L.A. (1981) Vasa previa case report: review and presentation of a new diagnostic method. *Journal of Reproductive Medicine*, **26**, 577–580.

van Leeuwen, G., Behringer, B. and Glenn, L. (1967) Single umbilical artery. *Journal of Pediatrics*, **71**, 103–106.

Vestermark, V., Christensen, I., Kay, L. and Windfeldt, M. (1990) Spontaneous intra-uterine rupture of a velamentous umbilical cord: a case report. *European Journal of Obstetrics, Gynecology and Reproductive Biology*, **35**, 279–281.

Virgilio, L.A. and Spangler, D.B. (1978) Fetal death secondary to constriction and torsion of the umbilical cord. *Archives of Pathology and Laboratory Medicine*, **102**, 32–33.

Virot, S., Mce, J., Virot, J.G. and Blanc, J.M. (1981) L'hématome du cordon rapport de l'echographie. *Revue Francaise de Gynécologie et d'Obstétrique*, **77**, 131–135.

Vlietinck, R.F., Thiery, M., Orye, E., de Clercq, A. and van Vaerenbergh, P. (1972) Significance of the single umbilical artery; a clinical, radiological, chromosomal and dermatologic study. *Archives of Disease in Childhood*, **47**, 639–642.

von Franqué, O. (1900) Zur Pathologie der Nachgeburtsheile. *Zeitschrift für Geburtshilfe und Gynäkologie*, **43**, 463–498.

Vous-Kristiansen, F. and Thue-Nielsen, V. (1985) Intra-uterine fetal death and thrombosis of the umbilical vessels. *Acta Obstetricia et Gynecologica Scandinavica*, **64**, 331–334.

Wagner, H., Baretton, G., Wisser, J., Babic, R. and Lohrs, U. (1993) Teratom der Nabelschnur: Kasuistik mit Literaturubersicht. *Patholge*, **14**, 395–398.

Walker, C.W. and Pye, B.G. (1960) The length of the human umbilical cord: a statistical report. *British Medical Journal*, **i**, 546–548.

Walz, W. (1947) Über das Ödem der Nabelschnur. *Zentralblatt für Gynäkologie*, **69**, 144–148.

Weber, J. (1963) Constriction of the umbilical cord as a cause of foetal death. *Acta Obstetricia et Gynecologica Scandinavica*, **42**, 259–267.

Wessell, J., Gerhold, W., Unger, M., Lichtenegger, W., and Vogel, M. (1992) Nabelschnur-komplikationen als Ursache des intrauterinen Fruchttodes. *Zeitschrift für Geburtshilfe und Perinatologie*, **196**, 173–176.

Weyerts, L.K., Jones, M.C., Grafe, M. and Scioscia, A.L. (1993) Umbilical cord haemangioma associated with an eruptive cutaneous haemangioma in a female infant. *Prenatal Diagnosis*, **13**, 61–64.

Wilson, R.D., Magee, J.F., Sorensen, P.H.B. and Johnson, A. (1994) In utero decompression of umbilical cord angiomyxoma followed by vaginal delivery. *American Journal of Obstetrics and Gynecology*, **171**, 1383–1385.

Yavner, D.L. and Redline R.W. (1989) Angiomyxoma of the umbilical cord with massive cystic degeneration of Wharton's jelly. *Archives of Pathology and Laboratory Medicine*, **113**, 935–937.

Zambelli, A. (1942) Cited by Lucchetti (1965).

Zeman, V. (1972) Aplazie umbilikalni arterie. *Ceskoslovensk Pediatrie*, **27**, 78–80.

Zeman, V. and Rauchenberg, M. (1970) Kavernozni a kapilarni hemangiomy pupecniky. *Ceskoslovensk Pediatrie*, **25**, 663–665.

Zienert, A., Bollmann, R., Chaoui, R. and Bartho, S. (1992) Die singulare Umbilikalarterie – Konsequenzen dieser pranatalen Diagnose. *Zentralblatt für Gynäkologie*, **114**, 131–135.

Zink, P. and Reinhardt, G. (1969) Gerichtsmedizinische untersuchungen zum Verhalten der Nabelschnur bei gewaltsamer Zerreissung. *Deutsche Zeitschrift für die gesampte gerichtliche Medizin*, **66**, 86–96.

16

PATHOLOGY OF
THE MEMBRANES

The pathology of the placental membranes (Fig. 16.1) is a subject that has, until relatively recently, lain in the shadow of a profound neglect, being shunned by both pathologists and obstetricians, who tended to regard the membranes simply as an inert sac. Three events, however, have conspired to change this situation: first, there was the appearance, in 1962, of Bourne's classic monograph *The Human Amnion and Chorion*, which laid the foundations for a logical study of the pathology of these structures and stimulated many workers to regard them with a somewhat greater awareness. Secondly, there has been a growing realization that the membranes are of considerable functional importance, a change of attitude that has led to a new interest in their physiology, biochemistry and immunology, with results that have been summarized by Hoyes (1975), Schmidt (1992) and Sutcliffe (1992). Thirdly, Torpin's (1968) monograph on the role played by the amnion in the production of congenital abnormalities of the fetus has provoked an understanding of the importance of a detailed study of the membranes in both teratologists and pathologists.

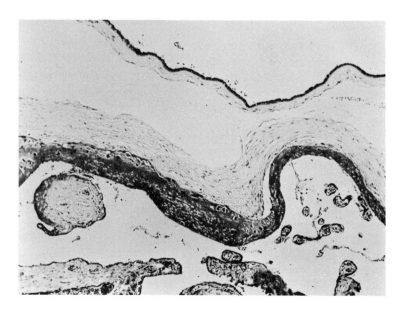

Figure 16.1. The amnion (above) and chorion (below) of a normal placenta. The amniotic epithelium is formed of a single layer of cuboidal cells (H & E ×60).

It must, nevertheless, be admitted that an account of the pathology of the extraplacental membranes will still appear rather skimpy and fragmented, and I feel that the definitive pathological studies of these structures have still to be undertaken.

EPITHELIAL CELL ABNORMALITIES

The amniotic epithelium is generally cuboidal but a small proportion of normal cells may be columnar in shape. Bourne (1962) has also noted that abnormal vacuolated columnar cells may be present, a change that he considers is due to the effects of meconium. He further described a 'club-foot' deformity, in which the cells are tall and irregular and have nuclei situated at their extreme apex, and a 'palisade' deformity, in which the cells are tall but regular, and although joined at their apices by tight adhesions, are separated from each other along their lateral margins by dilated intercellular canals. Pseudostratification, epithelial disorganization, epithelial cell necrosis, and 'basket' deformities may also be seen, the latter consisting of small areas of dead cells with immediately adjacent degenerate cells, which make a concave margin for the necrotic tissue. The significance of some of these changes is uncertain and Hoyes (1975) has counselled against accepting too readily that an abnormality of cellular form is necessarily an indication of pathological damage, pointing out that the shape and vacuolation of the amniotic epithelial cells may be altered very considerably by folds in the membrane, by alterations in amniotic tension, and by variability in the technique of fixation.

An interesting abnormality sometimes seen in the amniotic epithelium is the presence of 'giant goblet cells'. These have been variously considered as fat-containing cells (Bautzmann and Schroder, 1955) or as aggregated vacuolated cells (Petry and Damminger, 1956), but Bourne (1962) has shown quite convincingly that they are not cells at all but are distended or grossly dilated intercellular canals. The pathogenesis and significance of this change is unknown, but Bourne suggests that it may be indicative of an abnormality in the transfer of fluid across the membranes.

Fine vacuolation of the amniotic epithelial cells has been noted in association with fetal gastroschisis (Ariel & Landing, 1985) and electron microscopic examination has shown that the vacuoles contain lipid of unknown origin and nature (Grafe & Benirschke, 1990). This abnormality is present in most cases of gastroschisis and is virtually diagnostic of that condition.

SQUAMOUS METAPLASIA

Bourne (1962) has given a full description of this abnormality; indeed, his lucid account of squamous metaplasia is, to the best of my knowledge, the only detailed study of this lesion in the English-language literature, and I have no hesitation in drawing rather heavily on his writings.

Squamous metaplasia is seen on the fetal surface of the amnion and umbilical cord, though in the latter site it would better be termed squamous hyperplasia. Any number of lesions may be present and they tend to be aggregated most strikingly around the site of cord insertion. The foci of squamous metaplasia are grey or white, range in size up to a few millimetres in diameter, are slightly elevated, are rough and granular to the touch, and can only be separated from the amnion with difficulty; occasionally the foci may coalesce to form large, smooth plaques measuring several centimetres across.

Histologically (Fig. 16.2) the foci consist of stratified squamous epithelial cells, the number of layers varying from six to 20. There is usually a sharp transition at the edge of the lesion from columnar to squamous epithelium, and the cells at the base of the nodule, which are deeply staining, are referred to as 'reserve cells'. Sinha (1971), who examined plaques of amniotic squamous metaplasia electron-optically, showed that the reserve cells are in fact very similar to normal amniotic cells; also, he confirmed the truly squamous nature of the metaplastic epithelium, which in its fine structure is very similar to normal fetal skin.

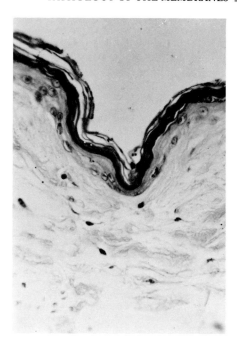

Figure 16.2. Squamous metaplasia of the amnion (H & E ×360).

The incidence of squamous metaplasia is in some doubt because, whilst Benirschke and Kaufmann (1995) maintain that it can be found in 60% of term placentas, Bourne (1962) was able to detect it in only 4% and Paddock (1924) in only 2.5%. Irrespective of its incidence, it is generally agreed that squamous metaplasia is of no clinical or pathological significance. It is not specifically associated with oligohydramnios or fetal malformation, and whilst one example has been reported of its concurrence with congenital ichthyosis (Coston, 1908), a full review of the available data indicates that there is no true association between the two lesions (Bourne, 1962).

AMNION NODOSUM

This condition, in which the fetal surface of the amnion is studded with multiple small nodules, was originally described by Pilgrim in 1889, but it was not until 1950 that Landing introduced the term 'amnion nodosum'. This was not a very striking terminological innovation, as these lesions had been known as 'Amnionknotchen' for many years previously in the German-language literature (von Franqué, 1897; Sitzenfrey, 1912; Bergendal, 1930; Nordenson, 1932). Landing was, however, the first to point out that these nodules were usually associated with oligohydramnios and thus were particularly likely to be found in cases of fetal renal agenesis, congenital obstruction of the fetal urinary tract or extramembranous pregnancy, an observation that has subsequently been amply confirmed (Scott & Bain, 1958; Jeffcoate & Scott, 1959; Thompson, 1960; Blanc, 1961; Blanc et al, 1962; Bryans et al, 1962; Dierickx et al, 1966; Masson et al, 1966; Dellenbach et al, 1967; Porrazzi & Vecchione, 1967; Molinengo et al, 1968; Esquivel & Colo, 1974). There are, however, well-documented examples of amnion nodosum occurring in the membranes of healthy infants (Chades y Suarez, 1967). Although the condition is usually seen in term pregnancies, it has been noted in first-trimester abortions (Bourne, 1962).

On naked-eye inspection, amnion nodosum is seen as small, slightly elevated plaques or nodules on the fetal surface of the amnion (Fig. 16.3); these occur with greatest frequency on that part of the amnion directly overlying the placenta, particularly around the site of insertion of the cord, but they do also develop on the extraplacental amnion and on that covering the umbilical cord. The nodules measure 1–5 mm across, are usually round, often geometrically so, but may be ovoid: they are shiny,

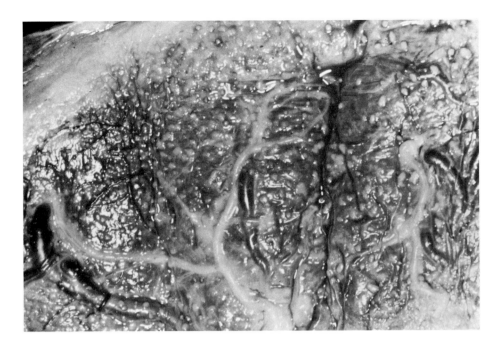

Figure 16.3. Macroscopic appearances of amnion nodosum in the amnion covering the fetal surface of the placenta. The tiny nodules are seen most clearly above and to the right.

greyish-yellow and may be easily detached from the amnion to leave a ragged saucer-like depression. The nodules not infrequently coalesce to form irregular plaques, and if one of these is picked off it is found to be soft, waxy and rather granular to the touch.

On light microscopy (Fig. 16.4) the nodules consist largely of amorphous or granular eosinophilic material which is sometimes arranged in broad fibrillar bands; embedded in this are cells, cell fragments and, occasionally, fragments of hair. The amorphous material is PAS and alcian blue positive, but stains negatively for keratin, amyloid and fibrin. Salazar and Kanhour (1974) and Bourne (1962) are in some disagreement about the relationship between the nodule and the amniotic epithelium: the former maintain that the amniotic basement membrane beneath the nodule is always intact, and that between this and the nodule the amniotic epithelium may be totally preserved, partially persistent or completely absent; the latter is of the opinion that the basement membrane is often breached and the amniotic-epithelium nearly always absent, so that the amniotic connective tissue is in direct contact with the matrix of the nodule. My own experience of this condition is too limited to allow me to enter into this controversy, but there is rather more general agreement that the amnion may grow over the superficial surface of the nodule in an attempt to 'epithelialize' it.

Electron-optical examination of the amnion nodosum has been undertaken by Bartman and Driscoll (1968) and Salazar and Kanhour (1974), the findings of both groups being very similar. The amorphous material noted on light microscopy is seen, at this level, to consist of interlacing bundles of electron-dense fibrillar material, which shows no periodicity and is admixed with cellular fragments and cells of various types which, however, all appear epithelial in nature.

There is now little support for the view that the nodules represent foci of squamous metaplasia which have undergone necrosis, and most would agree with the view, originally proposed by von Franqué (1897) and later espoused by Blanc (1961), that the nodules are probably deposits of vernix caseosa. Salazar and Kanhour (1974) argue that the amorphous material represents bundles of tonofilaments resulting from destruction by maceration of the superficial layers of the fetal epidermis, and suggest that the cellular component of the lesion may come not only from fetal skin but also from the fetal oral cavity or urinary tract or, possibly, from the amnion itself. It is less clear, however,

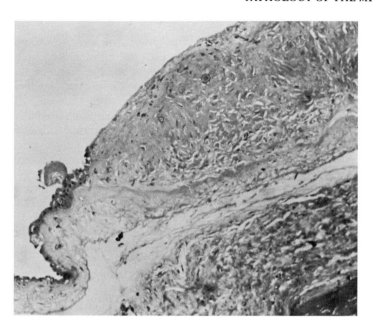

Figure 16.4. Histological appearances of a nodule of amnion nodosum (above and to the right). Cellular fragments are embedded in amorphous eosinophilic material (H & E ×250).

just why this fetal material is deposited on the membranes. Bourne (1962) postulated that there may be a primary abnormality of the membranes, which is implicated in the development of both the oligohydramnios and the amnion nodosum. An alternative stance is that the nodules are a non-specific result of oligohydramnios and that the fetal elements are simply concentrated in the scanty amniotic fluid and thus easily form myriads of small deposits on the amnion.

The only pathological or clinical significance of amnion nodosum is that it is an excellent, though not entirely absolute, hallmark of oligohydramnios, and its presence should alert one to the possibility of a congenital abnormality in the newborn infant.

MECONIUM STAINING

Meconium staining of the membranes is found in nearly 20% of placentas (Nathan et al, 1994; Benirschke & Kaufmann, 1995) but occurs most commonly in placentas from pregnancies prolonged beyond the 42nd week of gestation (Usher et al, 1988; Steer et al, 1989). Meconium staining has traditionally been regarded as evidence of intrauterine fetal hypoxia and distress (Krebs et al, 1980; Starks, 1980) but in recent years this long-held view has been challenged by those who maintain that there is no clear-cut correlation between meconium passage and either the clinical status of the neonate or laboratory measures of fetal hypoxia and acidosis (Meis et al, 1982; Dooley et al, 1985; Dijxhoorn et al, 1986; Steer et al, 1989; Yeomans et al, 1989; Trimmer & Gilstrap, 1991; Baker et al, 1992). Houlihan and Knuppel (1994) reviewed the often conflicting studies on this topic and came to the conclusion that the vast majority of fetuses with meconium staining of the membranes, even those who have acidaemia at delivery, have not been subjected to a chronic hypoxic insult. Nevertheless, Nathan et al (1994) found meconium passage to be associated with a small, but significant, risk of an unfortunate fetal outcome whilst both Mahomed et al (1994) and Berkus et al (1994) have claimed that the passage of 'thick' meconium is, quite independently of any other factor, significantly related to an adverse fetal outcome. The definition of 'thick' as opposed to 'thin' meconium is obviously highly subjective but it is almost certain that any increase in perinatal mortality associated with heavy meconium passage is due principally to an increased incidence of the meconium aspiration syndrome.

In view of the lack of clinical agreement as to the significance of meconium passage, the pathologist should clearly note the presence of meconium staining of the membranes but should refrain from expressing any view about the pathogenesis or importance of this finding.

Benirschke and Kaufmann (1995) divide meconium staining of the membranes into 'acute', characterized by the presence of green, slimy meconium, 'subacute', with dark discoloration of the membranes, and 'chronic', in which the membranes are dull and greenish-brown. They correlate the subacute and chronic, but not acute, staining with fetal complications but this subdivision appears somewhat subjective and non-reproducible. If meconium has been in contact with the amnion for several hours, degenerative changes such as vacuolation, piling up of cells and, later, necrosis may be seen on histological examination of the stained membranes. There may also be meconium-induced damage to the musculature of the fetal vessels on the maternal surface of the placenta (Altshuler & Hyde, 1989), a subject considered more fully in Chapter 15. Meconium-laden macrophages may be seen, first in the amnion and then later in the chorion. It has been demonstrated from *in vitro* studies that meconium-containing macrophages are present within the amnion within 1 hour after exposure of the membranes to meconium and within the chorion within 3 hours (Miller et al, 1985). How far it is possible to extrapolate these findings to the *in vivo* situation is a moot point but from our general knowledge of the rapidity with which macrophages can ingest particulate matter it is probable that meconium-containing macrophages could be found within a very short time of exposure to meconium. It may be necessary to distinguish between meconium and haemosiderin in amniotic macrophages, a distinction easily accomplished with a Prussian blue stain.

AMNIOTIC POLYPS

Numerous polyps on the fibrous surface of the membranes were noted in a triploid conceptus by Schlegel et al (1966); the polyps were derived from the amniotic epithelium, and, whilst some had slender single stalks, others had a stouter arborizing pattern. It was postulated that the polyps were a marker for triploidy, but, to the best of my knowledge, this has been neither confirmed nor refuted, and their significance is, to say the least, uncertain.

Faulk et al (1988) have also described multiple amniotic polyps in association with neonatal epidermolysis bullosa. These polyps appear to consist largely of protrusions of connective tissue through epithelial defects and they are partially covered by degenerating epithelial cells (Benirschke & Kaufmann, 1995).

INFLAMMATION OF THE MEMBRANES

This important topic is discussed in Chapter 11.

PREMATURE RUPTURE OF THE MEMBRANES

In this section I use the term 'premature rupture of the membranes' in its conventional obstetrical sense, i.e. rupture of the membranes during the later months of pregnancy but before the 37th week of gestation with subsequent onset of premature labour and delivery. The membranes may, of course, rupture at a much earlier stage of gestation and this can result in abortion, extramembranous pregnancy or extra-amniotic pregnancy, subjects that will be considered separately.

Premature rupture of the membranes is an important cause of preterm delivery; it is estimated that in approximately one-third of such deliveries the membrane rupture is the initial event, occurring prior to, and presumably being responsible for, the early onset of labour (Lockwood, 1994). This has naturally focused attention on the state and condition of the membranes in premature rupture, and it has been variously proposed that under such circumstances there may be an inherent weakness, a mechanical deficiency or a degenerative change. There is now no doubt that infection, in the form of a chorioamnionitis, is an important factor in the aetiology of premature rupture, accounting for up to 55% of cases (Romero et al, 1988), and this relationship is discussed in Chapter 11. Nevertheless, premature membrane rupture can occur in the complete absence of any clinical or pathological evidence of infection and it is in these cases that the possibility of a mechanical defect in the membranes has been raised (Polzin & Brady, 1991). It is worth noting that epidemiological studies of premature membrane rupture (Evaldson et al, 1980; Harger et al, 1990) often do not distinguish between those related to infection and those in which non-infective factors appear more important, a deficiency that dilutes markedly the value of such studies.

Several studies of the mechanical properties of the membranes have consistently shown that the tensile strength (as measured by the load necessary per unit width of membrane to cause rupture) is approximately the same in those membranes which rupture prematurely as in those which remain intact until term (Danforth et al, 1953; Embrey, 1954; Polishuk et al, 1962, 1964, 1965; Meudt & Meudt, 1967). Artal et al (1976) have measured a variety of stress–strain characteristics of the membranes and have found that the modulus of elasticity (which is an indication of the stiffness of a material and which is measured by the slope of a load–deformation curve) is lower in prematurely ruptured than in non-prematurely ruptured membranes. They point out that in physiological terms this suggests that, for the same stress, those membranes that rupture prematurely demonstrate more strain than do those which persist unruptured to term, or, alternatively, that they develop the same strain at a lower stress.

A reduced content of either total collagen or, more specifically, collagen type III in membranes that have ruptured prematurely has been noted in several studies (Skinner et al, 1981; Kanayama et al, 1985; Andreucci et al, 1986; Andreucci & Rosolia, 1989; Ghoneim et al, 1993); and has been variously attributed to increased amniotic fluid levels of trypsin or collagenase or to decreased levels of amniotic fluid alpha-1-antitrypsin, collagenase inhibitor or tissue inhibitor of metalloproteinases (Ruiz & Lama, 1990; Polzin & Brady, 1991; Kelly, 1995). Teodoro et al (1990) made the remarkable observation, which clearly requires confirmation, that the low collagen content found by them in prematurely ruptured membranes was associated with a decreased content of collagen both in the placenta and in the umbilical cord vessels, suggesting that the membrane abnormality was simply one facet of a more widespread collagen deficiency. Opinion on this matter has not been unanimous, however, and others have been unable to demonstrate any deficiency of collagen in prematurely ruptured membranes (Al-Zaid et al, 1980; Evaldson et al, 1987).

An alternative approach to this problem has been to suggest that premature rupture of the membranes is related to a decreased production of surfactant by the amnion (Hills & Cotton, 1984; Hills, 1994), it being argued that the consequently diminished lubrication may lead to high local stress at any point in the membranes that is prevented from moving relative to adjacent tissues.

Whether there is or is not a subtle change in membrane collagen content or metabolism or in membrane surfactant synthesis is not, of course, a matter of great moment for the pathologist looking at conventionally stained sections of ruptured membranes. Artal et al (1976) did, however, claim that the thickness of the membranes was reduced near the rupture site in prematurely ruptured membranes, their results in this respect being in conflict with those of earlier workers (Polishuk et al, 1962) but in accord with the histological studies of Bourne (1962), Malak and Bell (1994) and Lai (1994). Bourne noted degenerative changes in prematurely ruptured membranes that were confined to the cervical and dependent membranes; in essence, he found that the amniotic epithelium in this area was largely necrotic and was reduced to a thin, narrow band of amorphous eosinophilic material in which only a very few viable cells were present, whilst the chorionic cells were bloated and isolated in fibrin. These changes are of uncertain origin and are a little difficult to evaluate, because Bourne noted that similar appearances could be found in a proportion of membranes that had remained unruptured until term. Meudt and Meudt (1967) have suggested that the necrosis is due to meconium, but, as Bourne (1962) has pointed out, the lesions produced by meconium differ from those seen in premature rupture and, furthermore, do not affect just the cervical membranes. The dependent membranes are, however, probably particularly vulnerable to ischaemia and it is possible that vascular factors are involved in the pathogenesis of these lesions. Arias et al (1993) have, in fact, identified a group of patients in whom a maternal placental vasculopathy appeared to be associated with premature rupture of the membranes: the vasculopathy identied by them was of the type seen in pregnancy-induced hypertension and in many cases of intrauterine fetal growth retardation, i.e. due to inadequate placentation. It is difficult to accept, however, that there is a clear-cut relationship between a vascular lesion of this type and premature membrane rupture if only because multivariate analysis excludes hypertension as a risk factor for premature membrane rupture (Harger et al, 1990). Arias et al (1993) did note that their results should be interpreted with caution and admitted that it is difficult to identify the link between premature membrane rupture and a failure to establish adequate haemochorial placentation; nevertheless, this is an interesting approach which merits further study.

EXTRAMEMBRANOUS PREGNANCY

In this condition, gestation continues after rupture of both amnion and chorion during early or mid-pregnancy so that the fetus develops, either partly or fully, outside the membranes. Torpin (1966) has reviewed the earlier reports of this unusual event, pointing out that whilst most of the first accounts came from Germany and France, the condition appears subsequently to have exerted an unusual fascination for South American workers, who have reported a considerable number of cases, this being in contrast to the extreme paucity of such reports in the English-language literature. This latter deficiency appears to have been partially rectified because, in addition to Torpin's own account of two cases in 1966, further instances have, in recent years, been described in English by Carpenter (1965), Kohler et al (1970), Gregersen (1976), Perlman et al (1980) and Davies and Lomeli (1983). Examples have also been recorded in the non-English literature by Nold (1957), Rosset (1957), Dellenbach et al (1967), Ringe (1967), Weise and Link (1970), van Drooge and Okken (1982) and Hoekstra and de Boer (1990).

In most cases the membranes have ruptured between the 11th and 23rd weeks of pregnancy, and delivery has occurred between the 27th and 35th weeks, with there being, in the intervening period, a continuous or intermittent loss of liquor. A very high proportion of the infants have died during the neonatal period, either from prematurity alone or from this combined with infection.

The placenta from an extramembranous pregnancy is invariably circumvallate, whilst the membranous sac is unduly small and clearly of too limited a capacity to have contained the fetus. Characteristically, the sac wall is rather firm and usually has, at the margins of the rupture site, a thick, rolled edge (Fig. 16.5), though this is not invariably the case (Perlman et al, 1980). Nodules of amnion nodosum may be present and there may be extensive deposition of haemosiderin in the membranes (Benirschke & Kaufmann, 1995).

It is a moot point whether the placenta is circumvallate because the pregnancy has been extramembranous or whether the pregnancy is extramembranous because of the vallate form of the placenta. Torpin (1966) has argued forcibly for the latter view, maintaining that in circumvallate placentation, which he believes to be due to excessively deep implantation of the fertilized ovum (see Chapter 3), the membranes are unduly restricted in area and will, with the subsequent stretching attendant upon the growth of the fetus, be unusually liable to rupture. It is equally possible, however, that the rupture is traumatic in origin (Vago & Chavkin, 1980) and that the subsequent loss of fluid predisposes to the development of a circumvallate placenta.

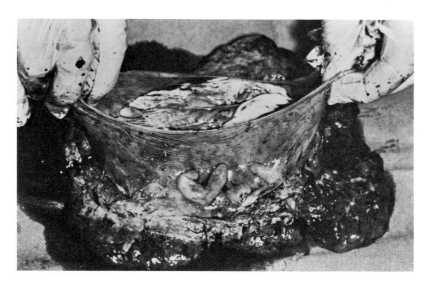

Figure 16.5. Placenta and membranes from an extramembranous pregnancy. The placenta is circumvallate, whilst the membranes are short and thick with a rolled edge. The membranous sac was far too small to have contained the fetus.

EXTRA-AMNIOTIC PREGNANCY

In this form of gestation, rupture of the amnion occurs in early pregnancy but the fetus continues to survive in the intact chorion. This appears, at first sight, to be an extremely infrequent phenomenon, because only a handful of cases have been reported in which this diagnosis was based on examination of the placenta and fetal membranes (Kovacs, 1933; Hückel, 1936; Meyer-Rüegg, 1939; Torpin, 1968; Kohler & Jenkins, 1976; Yang et al, 1984; Yang, 1990; Sherer et al, 1991). Whilst, however, it is certainly the case that an uncomplicated extra-amniotic term pregnancy is distinctly rare, there are good reasons for believing that the frequency of this form of gestation is underestimated because amniotic band formation, now widely though not universally held to be a complication of early amniotic rupture, is much less uncommon. Indeed, the amniotic band syndrome (discussed below) is often used as a surrogate for early amniotic rupture and this syndrome was found in 18 of 1010 pre-viable fetuses examined by Kalousek and Bamforth (1988).

Following amniotic rupture there is no external loss of liquor, although there may be oligohydramnios and the pregnancy, though probably often aborted, may well proceed to term; the placenta is of normal form and the infant may be completely normal. The diagnosis can be made by recognizing that the amnion is represented only by a small apron-like 'cuff' or 'collar' around the insertion of the cord (Fig. 16.6) or by noting the presence of amniotic strings. Amnion nodosum may be present in some cases (Yang et al, 1984).

The aetiology of amniotic rupture in the early months of gestation is a matter of conjecture. Torpin (1968) thought that abdominal trauma may be an aetiological factor though Ossipoff and Hall (1977) found only very slender evidence for this belief. Some cases of amniotic band syndrome have followed diagnostic amniocentesis or chorionic villus sampling in early pregnancy (Rehder, 1978; Moessinger et al, 1981; Ashkenazy et al, 1982; Kohn, 1987; Christiaens et al, 1989; Kanayama et al, 1995) but Lage et al (1988) have, with some justice, cast a sceptical eye on these selective reports. There has been one case which was associated, almost certainly coincidentally, with the presence of an intrauterine contraceptive device (Csecsei et al, 1987). Deformities caused by amniotic bands have been described in infants born to mothers who had taken LSD during pregnancy (Blanc et al, 1971) and have occurred in fetuses with the Ehlers-Danlos syndrome or osteogenesis imperfecta (Young et al, 1985) whilst there

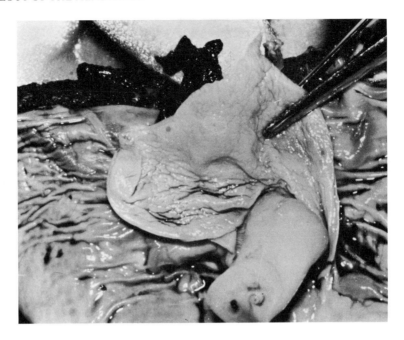

Figure 16.6. An extra-amniotic pregnancy. The amnion is represented only by a small, shrunken, but grossly thickened, remnant which forms a 'collar' around the insertion of the cord.

have been a few instances of familial amniotic band syndrome (Etches et al, 1982; Lubinsky et al, 1983). In the vast majority of cases, however, no aetiological factor can be identified.

AMNIOTIC BANDS AND STRINGS

It has been recognized almost since antiquity that a wide, but characteristic, range of fetal abnormalities (including constriction rings, intrauterine amputations, syndactyly, fusion defects of the cranium and face, and club-feet) are often found in association with amniotic bands, strings and adhesions. These combinations have evoked several explanatory hypotheses, only two of which merit serious attention.

Streeter (1930) maintained that the fetal abnormalities were due to a defect of development dating back to the formation of the amniotic cavity and the laying down of the germ disc, and he thus regarded the constriction rings as being due to a primary abnormality of the limb buds and the 'amniotic' bands as sloughed off, abnormal, redundant tissue. This concept was subsequently supported by Keith (1940) and Patterson (1962). The alternative view is that of Torpin who, in a series of papers (Torpin et al, 1964a,b; Torpin, 1965) that culminated in a monograph devoted to the subject (Torpin, 1968), proposed that amniotic bands and strings were a consequence of amniotic rupture during early pregnancy. He showed that following this event the amnion tends to become partially or totally detached from the chorion and may then fragment, shred and shrink down to form a collar around the insertion of the cord, or roll up to form a rope-like structure, the distal end of which may be free or still attached to the chorion. Following amniotic detachment, the mesoblastic tissue on the maternal surface of the separated amnion and that on the fetal surface of the denuded chorion tends to be drawn out into thin fibrous strings. The stage is then set for the possible entanglement of fetal limbs or digits within these bands or strings, with the subsequent development of constriction rings which, in extreme cases, lead to intrauterine amputations. Furthermore, the raw chorion rapidly absorbs liquor, and in the resulting oligohydramniotic state, which is probably responsible for the development of club-feet, the fetus may rub against the rough chorion and sustain abrasions to which the mesoblastic strings may become attached, producing fusion deformities, particularly of the head and face. Finally, the fetus may actually swallow a mesoblastic string, and this will result eventually in an adhesion between membranes and face, with a further risk of fusion deformities at this site.

Torpin's views were based on careful examination and study of many placentas; it is not surprising, therefore, that his theories have won many adherents (Baker & Rudolph, 1971; Chemke et al, 1973; Krag, 1974; Ornoy et al, 1974; Mahmood & Altshuler, 1975; Isacsohn et al, 1976; Seidman et al, 1989), and that constriction rings in the digits and limbs and intrauterine amputations are now generally thought to be caused by amniotic bands or strings, though these bands are now known to consist of both amnion and mesoderm (Moerman et al, 1992). Such bands can also cause syndactyly, by encircling the developing digits, or abdominal constriction rings (Imber et al, 1974), and can, even more alarmingly, encircle the neck and cause intrauterine decapitation (Ehrhardt, 1956; Swinburne, 1967). Even if the fetus escapes malformation by amniotic bands or strings, it still faces a threat to its continued existence, because a band may encircle the umbilical cord and constrict it sufficiently to cause fetal compromise and, usually, death (Fig. 16.7). Reports of such a catastrophe include those of James et al (1969), Hinze (1970), Linz (1970), Kohler and Collins (1972), Hamann and Rohde (1974), Duchesne et al (1975), Burrows and Phillips (1976), Ashkenazy et al (1982), Heifetz (1984b), Reles et al (1991), Rolon and Acosta (1991), Pommerenke and Sadenwasser (1992) and Kanayama et al (1995). It is indeed the effects of constriction of the umbilical cord by an amniotic band that is the strongest evidence for Torpin's theory, as this cannot be explained by Streeter's hypothesis.

As long as the consideration of amniotic bands is limited to easily explained mechanical effects, the situation is straightforward. The relatively simple concept of fetal deformities that are clearly caused by a mechanical constriction has, however, been widened to include visceral and body wall abnormalities which, together with the limb deformities, are collectively grouped together as 'amniotic band syndrome', 'amniotic band sequence', 'amnion rupture sequence', 'amniotic band disruption complex' or 'amniotic deformity, adhesions and mutilations (ADAM) complex'. Quite apart from whatever one wishes to call this complex, some have attributed it in its entirety to early

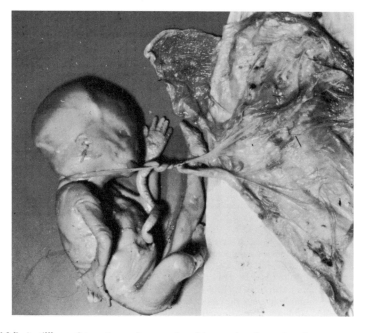

Figure 16.7. A stillborn fetus. A membranous band is running from the placenta to the fetal occipital region and is constricting the umbilical cord.

amniotic rupture and the mechanical effects of band formation (Higginbottom et al, 1979; Miller et al, 1981; Lin et al, 1989; Scheijgrond et al, 1989; Seidman et al, 1989; Bokmand et al, 1991) whilst others have considered that it is due to other factors such as vascular compromise, genetic disruption or germ disc disruption and regard the amniotic bands as being of no pathogenetic significance (Stock & Stock, 1979; Herva & Karkinen-Jaaskelainen, 1984; Hunter & Carpenter, 1986; Van Allen et al, 1987; Donnai & Winter, 1989; Lockwood et al, 1989; Bamforth, 1992). This is, of course, simply a resurgence of the Streeter *versus* Torpin argument, but now applied to a wider spectrum of abnormalities. The resolution of this argument lies outside both the scope of this book and my own embryological knowledge, but the views of Moerman et al (1992) seem to me to be highly persuasive and provide for a synthesis between the conflicting viewpoints. These workers point out that constrictive tissue bands clearly result from primary amnion rupture, that most craniofacial abnormalities in this syndrome are the result not of amnion rupture but of a vascular disruption sequence with or without cephalo-amniotic adhesions and that the body wall and visceral abnormalities (the 'limb–body wall complex') result from a vascular disruption occurring in the presence of an intact amniotic sac which may, however, secondarily rupture with ensuing formation of constrictive bands

If called upon to examine a placenta from a child with presumed amniotic band deformities, the pathologist would be well advised to immerse the organ in water, a technique that allows for the delicate amniotic strings to be more easily seen and recognized; subsequent histological examination will show that the amnion is absent from the placental surface.

TUMOURS

Some placental teratomas, themselves a debated entity, may lie within the membranes but the only genuine primary tumours to be described in the membranes have been single instances of a leiomyoma (Misselevich et al, 1989) and a haemangioma (Heifetz, 1984a).

REFERENCES

Altshuler, G. and Hyde, S. (1989) Meconium induced vasoconstriction: a potential cause of cerebral and other fetal hypoperfusion and of poor pregnancy outcome. *Journal of Child Neurology*, **4**, 137–142.

Al-Zaid, N.S., Bou-Resli, M.N. and Goldspink, G. (1980) Bursting pressure and collagen content of fetal membranes and their relation to premature rupture of the membranes. *British Journal of Obstetrics and Gynaecology*, **87**, 227–229.

Andreucci, D., Cossermelli, W., Rosolia, W.P. and Pinto, M.N. (1986) The low hydroxyproline content of prematurely ruptured human fetal membranes. *Brazilian Journal of Medical and Biological Research*, **19**, 351–354.

Andreucci, D. and Rosolia, W.P. (1989) Reduction of hydroxyproline content in the vessels of the human umbilical cord in premature rupture. *Gynecologic and Obstetric Investigation*, **28**, 138–140.

Arias, F., Rodriquez, L., Rayne, S.C. and Kraus, F.T. (1993) Maternal placental vasculopathy and infection: two distinct subgroups among patients with preterm labor and preterm ruptured membranes. *American Journal of Obstetrics and Gynecology*, **168**, 585–591.

Ariel, I.B. and Landing, B.H. (1985) A possible distinctive vacuolar change of the amniotic epithelium associated with gastroschisis. *Pediatric Pathology*, **2**, 283–289.

Artal, R., Sokol, R.J., Neuman, M., Burstein, A.H. and Stojkov, J. (1976) The mechanical properties of prematurely and non-prematurely ruptured membranes: methods and preliminary results. *American Journal of Obstetrics and Gynecology*, **125**, 655–659.

Ashkenazy, M., Borenstein, R., Katz, Z. and Segal, M. (1982) Constriction of the umbilical cord by an amniotic band after midtrimester amniocentesis. *Acta Obstetricia et Gynecologica Scandinavica*, **61**, 89–91.

Baker, C.J. and Rudolph, A.J. (1971) Congenital ring constrictions and intrauterine amputations. *American Journal of Diseases of Children*, **121**, 393–400.

Baker, P.N., Kilby, M.D. and Murray, H. (1992) An assessment of the use of meconium alone as an indication for fetal blood sampling. *Obstetrics and Gynecology*, **80**, 792–796.

Bamforth, J.S. (1992) Amniotic band sequence: Streeter's hypothesis revisited. *American Journal of Medical Genetics*, **44**, 280–287.

Bartman, J. and Driscoll, S.G. (1968) Amnion nodosum and hypoplastic cystic kidneys: an electron microscopic and microdissection study. *Obstetrics and Gynecology*, **32**, 700–705.

Bautzmann, H. and Schroder, R. (1955) Vergleichende Studien über Bau und Funktion des Amnions: neue Befunde an menschlichen Amnion miet Einschluss seiner freien Bindgewebs- oder sog. Hofbauerzellen. *Zeitschrift für Anatomie und Entwicklungsgeschichte*, **119**, 7–22.

Benirschke, K. and Kaufmann, P. (1995) *Pathology of the Human Placenta*, 3rd edn. New York: Springer-Verlag.

Bergendal, S. (1930) Ueber Amnionknotchen. *Acta Obstetricia et Gynecologica Scandinavica* **9**, 41–57.

Berkus, M.D., Langer, O., Samueloff, A., Xenakis, E.M.J., Field, N.T. and Ridgway, L.E. (1994) Meconium-stained amniotic fluid: increased risk for adverse neonatal outcome. *Obstetrics and Gynecology*, **84**, 115–120.

Blanc, W.A. (1961) Vernix granulomatosis of amnion (amnion nodosum) in oligohydramnios: lesion associated with urinary anomalies, retention of dead fetuses and prolonged leakage of amniotic fluid. *New York State Journal of Medicine*, **61**, 1492–1495.

Blanc, W.A., Aperson, J.W. and McNally, J. (1962) Pathology of the newborn and of the placenta in oligohydramnios. *Bulletin of the Sloane Hospital for Women in the Columbia Presbyterian Medical Center*, **8**, 51–64.

Blanc, W.A., Mattison, D.R., Kane, R. and Chauhan, P. (1971) LSD, intrauterine amputations and amniotic band syndrome. *Lancet*, **ii**, 158–159.

Bokmand, S., Bangsboll, S. and Ornvold, K. (1991) Tidlig amnionruptursekvens eller amnionbandsyndromet. *Ugeskrift for Laeger* (Copenhagen), **153**, 1846–1848.

Bourne, G. (1962) *The Human Amnion and Chorion*. London: Lloyd-Luke (Medical Books).

Bryans, A.M., Bails, J.V. and Haust, M.D. (1962) Amnion nodosum: report of a case. *American Journal of Obstetrics and Gynecology*, **84**, 582–585.

Burrows, S. and Phillips, N. (1976) Strangulation of umbilical cord by amniotic band. *American Journal of Obstetrics and Gynecology*, **124**, 697–698.

Carpenter, C.W. (1965) Extramembranous pregnancy with hydrorrhea gravidarum: report of a case. *Obstetrics and Gynecology*, **25**, 405–408.

Chades y Suarez, A. (1967) Amnios nodoso: presentacion de 17 casos. *Revista Peruana de Patologia* **10**, 279–285.

Chemke, J., Graff, G., Hurwitz, N. and Liban, E. (1973) The amniotic band syndrome. *Obstetrics and Gynecology*, **41**, 332–336.

Christiaens, G.C.M.L., van Baarlen, J., Huber, J. and Leschot, N.J. (1989) Fetal limb constriction: a possible complication of CVS. *Prenatal Diagnosis*, **9**, 67–71.

Coston, H.R. (1908) Report of a case of ichthyosis fetalis: placenta and membranes involved. *American Journal of Obstetrics*, **58**, 650–654.

Csecsei, K., Szeifert, G.T. and Papp, Z. (1987) Amniotic bands associated with early rupture of amnion due to an intrauterine device. *Zentralblatt für Gynäkologie*, **109**, 738–741.

Danforth, D.N., McElin, T.W. and States, M.N. (1953) Studies on fetal membranes. i. Bursting tension. *American Journal of Obstetrics and Gynecology*, **65**, 480–487.

Davies, B.R. and Lomeli, R.M. (1983) Pressure malformations from a chronic leakage of amniotic fluid: possible iatrogenic origin of extramembranous pregnancy and the extrachorial placenta. *American Journal of Obstetrics and Gynecology*, **147**, 838–839.

Dellenbach, P., Szwarcberg, R., Philippe, E. and Gillet, J.Y. (1967) Grossesse extramembraneuse avec amnion nodosum: considérations cliniques et anatomiques. *Revue Francaise de Gynécologie et d'Obstétrique*, **62**, 157–162.

Dierickx, J., Parmentier, R. and Wilkin, P. (1966) L'amnion nodosum. *Bulletin de la Société Belge de Gynécologie et d'Obstétrique*, **36**, 403–417.

Dijxhoorn, M.J., Visser, G.H., Fidler, V.J., Touwen, B.C. and Huisjes, H.J. (1986) Apgar scores, meconium and acidaemia at birth in relation to neonatal neurological morbidity in term infants. *British Journal of Obstetrics and Gynaecology*, **93**, 217–222.

Donnai, D. and Winter, R.M. (1989) Disorganisation: a model for 'early amnion rupture'? *Journal of Medical Genetics*, **26**, 421–425.

Dooley, S.L., Pesavento, D.J., Depp, R., Socol, M.L., Tamara, R.K. and Wiringa, K.S. (1985) Meconium below the vocal cords at delivery: correlation with intrapartum events. *American Journal of Obstetrics and Gynecology*, **153**, 767–771.

Duchesne, C., Verschelden, G. and Lemay, M. (1975) Syndrome des bandelettes amniotiques. *Union Médicale du Canada*, **104**, 1793–1796.

Ehrhardt, L. (1956) Seltene Spontanamputation durch Amnionstrang: Akephalus. *Zentralblatt für Gynäkologie*, **78**, 1509–1513.

Embrey, M.P. (1954) On the strength of the foetal membranes. *Journal of Obstetrics and Gynaecology of the British Empire*, **61**, 793–796.

Esquivel, A.C. and Colo, J.A.S. (1974) Amnion nodosum: estudio histopatologico de un case. *Ginecologia y Obstetricia de México*, **35**, 135–140.

Etches, P.C., Stewart, A.R. and Ives, E.J. (1982) Familial congenital amputations. *Journal of Pediatrics*, **101**, 448–449.

Evaldson, G., Lagrelius, A. and Winiarski, J. (1980) Premature rupture of the membranes. *Acta Obstetricia et Gynecologica Scandinavica*, **59**, 385–393.

Evaldson, G., Larsson, B. and Jiborn, H. (1987) Is the collagen content reduced when the fetal membranes rupture? A clinical study of term and prematurely ruptured membranes. *Gynecologic and Obstetric Investigation*, **29**, 92–94.

Faulk, W.P., Hsi, B.L., Yeh, C.J.G., McIntyre, J.A. and Stevens, P.J. (1988) Epidermolysis bullosa fetalis: an immunogenetic disease of extraembryonic exoderm? *American Journal of Obstetrics and Gynecology*, **158**, 150–157.

Ghoneim, F.A., Fateen, B.A., Rashad, M. et al (1993) Collagen type III in normal and prematurely ruptured amniotic membranes. *Journal of The Egyptian Public Health Association*, **68**, 49–62.

Grafe, M.J. and Benirschke, K. (1990) Ultrastructural study of the amniotic epithelium in a case of gastroschisis. *Pediatric Pathology*, **10**, 95–101.

Gregersen, E. (1976) Extramembranous pregnancy with amniorrhoea. *Acta Obstetricia et Gynecologica Scandinavica*, **55**, 69–71.

Hamann, H. and Rohde, E. (1974) Eine seltene amniogene Missbildung. *Zentralblatt für Gynäkologie*, **96**, 1403–1406.

Harger, J.H., Hsing, A.W., Tuomala, R.E. et al (1990) Risk factors for preterm premature rupture of fetal membranes: a multicenter case-control study. *American Journal of Obstetrics and Gynecology*, **163**, 130–137.

Heifetz, S.A. (1984a) Chorangioma of the placental membranes. *Military Medicine*, **149**, 621.

Heifetz S.A. (1984b) Strangulation of the umbilical cord by amniotic bands: report of 6 cases. *Pediatric Pathology*, **2**, 285–304.

Herva, R. and Karkinen-Jaaskelainen, M. (1984) Amniotic adhesion malformation syndrome: fetal and placental pathology. *Teratology*, **29**, 11–19.

Higginbottom, M.C., Jones, K.L., Hall, B.D. and Smith, D.W. (1979) The amniotic band disruption complex: timing of amniotic rupture and variable spectra of consequent defects. *Journal of Pediatrics*, **95**, 544–549.

Hills, B.A. (1994) Further studies of the role of surfactant in premature rupture of the membranes. *American Journal of Obstetrics and Gynecology*, **170**, 195–201.

Hills, B.A. and Cotton, D.C. (1984) Premature rupture of membranes and surface energy: possible role of surfactant. *American Journal of Obstetrics and Gynecology*, **149**, 896–902.

Hinze, E. (1970) Intrauteriner Fruchttod durch Amnionstrange. *Zentralblatt für Gynäkologie*, **92**, 74–75.

Hoekstra, J.H. and de Boer, R. (1990) Very early prolonged premature rupture of membranes and survival. *European Journal of Pediatrics*, **150**, 859.

Houlihan, C.M. and Knuppel, R.A. (1994) Meconium-stained amniotic fluid: current controversies. *Journal of Reproductive Medicine*, **39**, 888–898.

Hoyes, A.D. (1975) Structure and function of the amnion. In *Obstetrics and Gynecology Annual*, Vol. 4, Wynn, R.M. (Ed.), pp. 1–38. New York: Appleton-Century-Crofts.

Hückel, H. (1936) Uber extraamniale Schwangerschaft. *Zentralblatt für Gynäkologie*, **60**, 1276–1282.

Hunter, A.G.W. and Carpenter, B.F. (1986) Implications of malformations not due to amniotic bands in the amniotic band sequence. *American Journal of Medical Genetics*, **24**, 691–700.

Imber, G., Guthrie, R.H., Jr and Goulian, D., Jr (1974) Congenital band of the abdomen and the amniotic etiology of bands. *American Journal of Surgery*, **127**, 753–754.

Isacsohn, M., Aboulafia, Y., Horowitz, B. and Ben-Hur, N. (1976) Congenital annular constrictions due to amniotic bands. *Acta Obstetricia et Gynecologica Scandinavica*, **55**, 179–182.

James, P.D., Beilby, J.O.W. and Steele, S.J. (1969) An unusual cause of intrauterine death. *Journal of Obstetrics and Gynaecology of the British Commonwealth*, **76**, 752–754.

Jeffcoate, T.N.A. and Scott, J.S. (1959) Polyhydramnios and oligohydramnios. *Canadian Medical Association Journal*, **80**, 77–86.

Kalousek, D.K. and Bamforth S. (1988) Amnion rupture in previable fetuses. *American Journal of Medical Genetics*, **31**, 63–73.

Kanayama, M.D., Gaffey, T.A. and Ogburn, P.L., Jr (1995) Constriction of the umbilical cord by an amniotic band, with fetal compromise illustrated by reverse diastolic flow in the umbilical artery: a case report. *Journal of Reproductive Medicine*, **40**, 71–73.

Kanayama, N., Terao, T., Kawashima, Y., Huriuchi, K. and Fujimoto, D. (1985) Collagen types in normal and prematurely ruptured amniotic membranes. *American Journal of Obstetrics and Gynecology*, **153**, 899–903.

Keith, A. (1940) Concerning the origin and nature of certain malformations of the face, head and foot. *British Journal of Surgery*, **28**, 173–192.

Kelly, T. (1995) The pathophysiology of premature rupture of the membranes. *Current Opinion in Obstetrics and Gynecology*, **7**, 140–145.

Kohler, H.G. and Collins, M.L. (1972) Ligation of the umbilical cord by torn amniotic membranes. *Journal of Obstetrics and Gynaecology of the British Commonwealth*, **79**, 183–184.

Kohler, H.G. and Jenkins, D.M. (1976) Extra-amniotic pregnancy: a case report. *British Journal of Obstetrics and Gynaecology*, **83**, 251–253.

Kohler, H.G., Peel, K.R. and Hoar, R.A. (1970) Extra-membranous pregnancy and amniorrhoea. *Journal of Obstetrics and Gynaecology of the British Commonwealth*, **77**, 809–812.

Kohn, G. (1987) The amniotic band syndrome: a possible complication of amniocentesis. *Prenatal Diagnosis*, **7**, 303–305.

Kovacs, F. (1933) Uber die extraamniale Schwangerschaft. *Zentralblatt für Gynäkologie*, **57**, 415–425.

Krag, D. (1974) Amnionic rupture and birth defects of the extremities. *Human Pathology*, **5**, 69–77.

Krebs, H.B., Peters, R.E., Dunn, L.J., Jordan, H.V.F. and Segreti, A. (1980) Intrapartum fetal heart rate monitoring. III. Association of meconium with abnormal fetal heart rate patterns. *American Journal of Obsetrics and Gynecology*, **137**, 936–940.

Lage, J.M., VanMarter, L.J. and Bieber, F.R. (1988) Questionable role of amniocentesis in the etiology of amniotic band formation: a case report. *Journal of Reproductive Medicine*, **33**, 71–73.

Lai, R.S. (1994) Evaluation of the mechanism of decreased tensile strength of fetal membrane in premature rupture of the membranes. *Chinese Journal of Obstetrics and Gynecology*, **28**, 567–568.

Landing, B.H. (1950) Amnion nodosum: a lesion of the placenta apparently associated with deficient secretion of fetal urine. *American Journal of Obstetrics and Gynecology*, **60**, 1339–1342.

Lin, H.H., Wu, C.C., Hsieh, C.Y. and Lee, T.Y. (1989) Amniotic rupture sequence: report of five cases. *Asia and Oceania Journal of Obstetrics and Gynaecology*, **15**, 343–350.

Linz, O. (1970) Intrauteriner Fruchttod infolge Strangulation der Nabelschnur durch einen amnion Faden. *Zentralblatt für Gynäkologie*, **92**, 684–687.

Lockwood, C.J. (1994) Recent advances in elucidating the pathogenesis of preterm delivery, the detection of patients at risk, and preventative therapies. *Current Opinion in Obstetrics and Gynecology*, **6**, 7–18.

Lockwood, C., Ghidini, A., Romero, R. and Hobbins, J.C. (1989) Amniotic band syndrome: reevaluation of its pathogenesis. *American Journal of Obstetrics and Gynecology*, **160**, 1030–1033.

Lubinsky, M., Sujansky, E., Sanger, W., Salyards, P. and Severn, C. (1983) Familial amniotic bands. *American Journal of Medical Genetics*, **14**, 81–87.

Mahmood, K. and Altshuler, G. (1975) Amniotic band syndrome in an immature fetus. *Obstetrics and Gynecology*, **45**, 349–351.

Mahomed, K., Nyoni, R. and Masona, D. (1994) Meconium staining of the liquor in a low risk population. *Paediatric and Perinatal Epidemiology*, **8**, 292–300.

Malak, T.M. and Bell, S.C. (1994) Structural characteristics of term human fetal membranes: a novel zone of extreme morphological alteration within the rupture site. *British Journal of Obstetrics and Gynaecology*, **101**, 375–386.

Masson, J.C., Philippe, E., Korn, R., Irrmann, M., Dehalleux, J.M. and Gandar, R. (1966) Amnion nodosum. *Revue Francaise de Gynécologie et d'Obstétrique*, **61**, 701–707.

Meis, P.J., Hobel, C.J. and Ureda, J.R. (1982) Late meconium passage in labor – a sign of fetal distress? *Obstetrics and Gynecology*, **59**, 332–336.

Meudt, R. and Meudt, E. (1967) Rupture of the fetal membranes: an experimental, clinical and histological study. *American Journal of Obstetrics and Gynecology*, **99**, 562–568.

Meyer-Rüegg, H. (1939) Zur Pathogenese der Graviditas extra-amniales. *Zentralblatt für Gynäkologie*, **63**, 594–597.

Miller, M.E., Graham, J.M., Higginbottom, M.C. and Smith, D.W. (1981) Compression related defects from early amniotic rupture: evidence for mechanical teratogenesis. *Journal of Pediatrics*, **98**, 292–297.

Miller, P.W., Coen, R.W. and Benirschke, K. (1985) Dating the time interval from meconium passage to birth. *Obstetrics and Gynecology*, **66**, 459–462.

Misselevich, I., Abramovici, D., Reiter, A. and Boss, J.H. (1989) Leiomyoma of the fetal membranes: report of a case. *Gynecologic Oncology*, **33**, 108–111.

Moerman, P., Fryns, J.P., Vandenberghe, K. and Lauweryns, J.M. (1992) Constrictive amniotic bands, amniotic adhesions, and limb body wall complex: discrete disruption sequences with pathogenetic overlap. *American Journal of Medical Genetics*, **42**, 470–479.

Moessinger, A.C., Blanc, W.A., Byrne, J., Andrews, D., Warburton, D. and Bloom, A. (1981) Amniotic band syndrome associated with amniocentesis. *American Journal of Obstetrics and Gynecology*, **141**, 588–591.

Molinengo, L., Biressi, P.C. and Scorta, A. (1968) 'Amnion rodosum'. *Minerva Ginecologica*, **20**, 1340–1344.

Nathan, L., Leveno, K.J., Carmody, T.J., Kelly, M.A. and Sherman, M.I. (1994) Meconium: a 1990's perspective on an old obstetric hazard. *Obstetrics and Gynecology*, **83**, 329–332.

Nold, B. (1957) Ein weiterer Fall von Graviditas Exochorialis. *Zentralblatt für Gynäkologie*, **79**, 860–863.

Nordenson, N.G. (1932) Beitrag zur Kenntnis von den 'Amnionkn otchen'. *Acta Obstetricia et Gynecologica Scandinavica*, **12**, 267–281.

Ornoy, A., Sekeles, E. and Sadovsky, E. (1974) Amniogenic bands as a cause of syndactyly in a young human fetus. *Teratology*, **9**, 129–134.

Ossipoff, V. and Hall, B.D. (1977) Etiologic factors in the amniotic band syndrome: a study of 24 patients. *Birth Defects*, **13**, 117–132.

Paddock, R. (1924) Recent observations of certain pathological conditions of the amnion. *American Journal of Obstetrics and Gynecology*, **8**, 546–554.

Patterson, T.J.S. (1962) Amniotic bands. In *The Human Amnion and Chorion*, Bourne, G.L. (Ed.), pp. 250–264. London: Lloyd-Luke (Medical Books).

Perlman, M., Tennenbaum, A., Menash, M. and Ornoy, A. (1980) Extramembranous pregnancy: maternal, placental, and perinatal implications. *Obstetrics and Gynecology* **55**, 34s–37s.

Petry, G. and Damminger, K. (1956) Untersuchungen über den Bau des menschlichen Amnions. *Zeitschrift für Zellforschung und mikroskopische Anatomie*, **44**, 225–262.

Pilgrim, H. (1889) *Die Zotten und Karunkeln des menschlichen Amnion*. Marburg: Pfiel.

Polishuk, W.Z., Kohane, S. and Peranio, A. (1962) The physical properties of fetal membranes. *Obstetrics and Gynecology*, **20**, 204–210.

Polishuk, W.Z., Kohane, S. and Hadar, A. (1964) Fetal weight and membrane tensile strength. *American Journal of Obstetrics and Gynecology*, **88**, 247–250.

Polishuk, W.Z., Ben-Sira, M.Y. and Kohane, S. (1965) Variations in foetal membrane tensile strength. *Journal of Obstetrics and Gynaecology of the British Commonwealth*, **72**, 422–425.

Polzin, W.J. and Brady, K. (1991) Mechanical factors in the etiology of premature rupture of the membranes. *Clinical Obstetrics and Gynecology*, **34**, 702–714.

Pommerenke, F. and Sadenwasser, W. (1992) Nabelschnurkompression durch Amnionstrang. *Zentralblatt für Gynäkologie*, **114**, 557–559.

Porrazzi, L.C. and Vecchione, R. (1967) 'L'amnion nodosum' (studio di due casi) *Rivista di Anatomia Patologica e di Oncologia*, **31**, 281–295.

Rehder, H. (1978) Fetal limb deformities due to amniotic constrictions (a possible consequence of preceding amniocentesis) *Pathology Research and Practice*, **162**, 316–326.

Reles, A., Friedmann, W., Vogel, M. and Dudenhausen, J.W. (1991) Intrauteriner Fruchttod nach Strangulation der Nabelschnur durch Amnionbander. *Geburtshilfe und Frauenheilkunde*, **51**, 1006–1008.

Ringe, A.D. (1967) Graviditas extramembranacea (extrachorialis) *Zentralblatt für Gynäkologie*, **89**, 284–288.

Rolon, P.A. and Acosta, A. (1991) Bride foeticide du cordon ombilical. *Journal de Gynécologie, Obstétrique et Biologie de la Reproduction*, **20**, 589–590.

Romero, R., Quintero, R., Oyarzun, E. et al (1988) Intraamniotic infection and thoriale Schwangerschaft. *Zentralblatt für Gynäkologie*, **79**, 863–865.

Rosset, W. (1957) Über eine exochoriale Schwangerschaft. *Zentralblatt für Gynäkologie*, **79**, 863–865.

Ruiz, A. and Lama, M.S. (1990) Collagen metabolism in premature rupture of amniotic membranes. *Obstetrics and Gynecology*, **75**, 84–88.

Salazar, H. and Kanhour, A.I. (1974) Amnion nodosum: ultrastructure and histopathogenesis. *Archives of Pathology*, **98**, 39–46.

Scheijgrond, W.J., Rodrigues-Pereira, R., Roorda, R.J. and Jansen, F.H. (1989) Vroege amnioruptur als oorzak van multiple congenitale afwijkingen bij de pasgeborene. *Nederlands Tijdschrift voor Kindergeneeskunde*, **57**, 58–60.

Schlegel, R.J., Beu, R., Lead, J.C., Fariase, E., Lewczak, P. and Gardner, L. (1966) Arborizing amniotic polyps in triploid conceptus: a diagnostic anatomic lesion? *American Journal of Obstetrics and Gynecology*, **96**, 357–361.

Schmidt, W. (1992) The amniotic fluid compartment: the fetal habitat. *Advances in Anatomy, Embryology and Cell Biology*, **127**, 1–100.

Scott, J.S. and Bain, A.D. (1958) Amnion nodosum. *Proceedings of the Royal Society of Medicine*, **51**, 512–513.

Seidman, J.D., Abbondanzo, S.L., Watkin, W.G., Ragsdale, B. and Manz, H.J. (1989) Amniotic band syndrome: report of two cases and review of the literature. *Archives of Pathology and Laboratory Medicine*, **113**, 891–897.

Sherer, D.M., Smith, S.S., Metlay, L.A. and Woods, J.R., Jr (1991) Sonographic and pathologic features of circumvallate placenta associated with early amnion rupture. *Journal of Clinical Ultrasound*, **19**, 241–243.

Sinha, A.A. (1971) Ultrastructure of human amnion and amniotic plaques of normal pregnancy. *Zeitschrift für Zellforschung und mikroskopische Anatomie*, **122**, 1–14.

Sitzenfrey, A. (1912) Ueber Amnionanomalien. *Beitrage zur Geburtshilfe und Gynäkologie*, **17**, 1–10.

Skinner, S.J.M., Campos, G.A. and Liggins, G.C. (1981) Collagen content of human amniotic membranes: effect of gestation length and premature rupture. *Obstetrics and Gynecology*, **57**, 487–489.

Starks, G.C. (1980) Correlation of meconium-stained amniotic fluid, early intrapartum fetal pH and Apgar scores as predictors of perinatal outcome. *Obstetrics and Gynecology*, **56**, 604–608.

Steer, P.J., Eigbe, F., Lissauer, T.J. and Beard, R.W. (1989) Interrelationships among abnormal cardiotocograms in labor, meconium staining of the amniotic fluid, arterial cord blood pH, and Apgar scores. *Obstetrics and Gynecology*, **74**, 715–721.

Stock, R.J. and Stock, M.E. (1979) Congenital annular constrictions and intrauterine amputations revisited. *Obstetrics and Gynecology*, **53**, 592–598.

Streeter, G.L. (1930) Focal deficiencies in fetal tissues and their relation to intrauterine amputation. *Contributions to Embryology. Carnegie Institution of Washington*, **22**, 1–44.

Sutcliffe, R.G. (1992) Amnion: physiological roles and clinical significance. In *Immunological Obstetrics*, Coulam, C.B., Faulk, W.P. and McIntyre, J.A. (Eds), pp. 189–201. New York: Norton.

Swinburne, L.M. (1967) Spontaneous intrauterine decapitation. *Archives of Disease in Childhood*, **42**, 636–641.

Teodoro, W.R., Andreucci, D. and Palma, J.A. (1990) Placental collagen and premature rupture of fetal membranes. *Placenta*, **11**, 549–551.

Thompson, V.M. (1960) Amnion nodosum. *Journal of Obstetrics and Gynaecology of the British Empire*, **67**, 611–614.

Torpin, R. (1965) Amniochorionic mesoblastic fibrous strings and amnionic bands: associated constricting fetal malformations or fetal death. *American Journal of Obstetrics and Gynecology*, **91**, 65–75.

Torpin, R. (1966) Extramembranous pregnancy. *Journal of the Medical Association of Georgia*, **55**, 174–179.

Torpin, R. (1968) *Fetal Malformation Caused by Amnion Rupture During Gestation*. Springfield, Illinois: Charles C. Thomas.

Torpin, R., Goodman, L. and Gramling, Z.W. (1964a) Amnion string swallowed by the fetus. *American Journal of Obstetrics and Gynecology*, **90**, 829–831.

Torpin, R., Miller, G.T. and Culpepper, B.W. (1964b) Amniogenic fetal digital amputations associated with clubfoot. *Obstetrics and Gynecology*, **24**, 379–384.

Trimmer, K.J. and Gilstrap, L.C. (1991) 'Meconiumcrit' and birth asphyxia. *American Journal of Obstetrics and Gynecology*, **165**, 1010–1013.

Usher, R.H., Boyd, M.E., McLean, F.H. and Kramer, M.S. (1988) Assessment of fetal risk in postdate pregnancies. *American Journal of Obstetrics and Gynecology*, **158**, 259–264.

Vago, T. and Chavkin, J. (1980) Extramembranous pregnancy: an unusual complication of amniocentesis. *American Journal of Obstetrics and Gynecology*, **137**, 511–512.

Van Allen, M.I., Curry, C. and Gallagher, L. (1987) Limb body wall complex. I. Pathogenesis. *American Journal of Medical Genetics*, **28**, 529–548.

Van Drooge, P.H. and Okken, A. (1982) Extramembraneuze zwangerchap. *Nederlands Tijdschrift voor Geneeskunde*, **126**, 1819–1823.

von Franqué, O. (1897) Zur Kenntnis der Amnionanomalieen. *Monatsschrift für Geburtshilfe und Gynäkologie*, **6**, 36–41.

Weise, W. and Link, M. (1970) Beitrag zur Hydrorrhoea uteri gravidi bei extrachorialer Schwangerschaft. *Zentralblatt für Gynäkologie*, **92**, 674–679.

Yang, S.S. (1990) ADAM sequence and innocent amniotic band: manifestations of early amnion rupture. *American Journal of Medical Genetics*, **37**, 562–568.

Yang, S.S., Levine, A.J., Sanborn, J.R. and Delp, R.A. (1984) Amniotic rupture, extra-amniotic pregnancy, and vernix granulomata. *American Journal of Surgical Pathology*, **8**, 117–122.

Yeomans, E.R., Gilstrap, L.C., Leveno, K.J. and Burris, J.S. (1989) Meconium in the amniotic fuid and fetal acid-base status. *Obstetrics and Gynecology*, **73**, 175–179.

Young, I.D., Lindenbaum, R.H., Thompson, E.M. and Pembrey, M.E. (1985) Amniotic bands in connective tissue disorders. *Archives of Disease in Childhood*, **60**, 1061–1063.

PATHOLOGICAL EXAMINATION OF THE PLACENTA

There are many who feel that the placenta should be examined in its fresh state as soon as possible after delivery. However, unless an urgent pathological opinion on a placenta is required (a situation that does not arise with any great frequency), I prefer to delay examination of the organ for several days and allow it to fix whole in 10% formalin; this permits easier handling, facilitates cutting of the organ, and allows for better recognition of gross lesions. It is perhaps only fair to point out that Benirschke and Kaufmann (1995) disagree quite strongly with me about the merits of formalin fixation, maintaining that this makes critical examination of the placenta more difficult: they recommend simple storage and refrigeration. I find, however, that the unfixed placenta is difficult to handle and even more difficult to cut, but this may be no more than a tribute to my lack of manual dexterity.

On initial examination, any gross abnormality of shape, such as accessory lobe or bilobate placenta, will usually be obvious; note should also be taken as to whether the placenta is of the extrachorial type or not. The site of cord insertion is recorded, and if there is a velamentous insertion the vessels running from the cord to the placenta are scrutinized with care for evidence of traumatic damage or bleeding. The colour, glossiness and translucency of the membranes covering the cord are noted, and the cord is examined for oedema and for focal lesions such as torsion, haematoma, true knot or stricture. If the cord appears to be unusually thick, its diameter can be measured, but I can seen little point in routinely measuring the length of the cord, reserving this procedure for those cords which are overtly either excessively long or unduly short. The cord is then cut off from the placenta at a point about 2–4 cm above its insertion into the fetal surface; the cut surface of the cord is examined and the number of vessels recorded. A transverse section for histological examination is then taken from the cut end of the cord and a further transverse section from about the middle of the cord; sections will also be taken from any macroscopically abnormal area of the cord.

The extraplacental membranes are then examined; their degree of glossiness and translucency is noted and a search is made for amnion nodosum and for meconium staining. The point of membrane rupture is established and it is often of value, particularly in cases of suspected placenta praevia, to measure the distance from the margin of the rupture site to the placental edge. It is my usual practice to take a section of the membranes from the edge of the rupture site and from the membranes at the placental margin. Benirschke's (1961) technique of taking a membrane roll for histological examination has, however, much to recommend it, particularly in cases of suspected chorioamnionitis. This is done by cutting a segment of the membranes from the point of rupture to the placental margin and then rolling this segment into a 'jam-roll' like structure, which can be tied with a thin thread and then subsequently sectioned transversely.

Attention is next paid to the fetal surface of the placenta, and again the translucency and colour of the membranes in this site are noted and a search made for amnion nodosum. A subamniotic haematoma, if present, will usually be obvious, whilst note should be taken of any tuberous projections that could signal the presence of a massive subchorial thrombosis. The large vessels on the fetal surface of the placenta are examined and palpated for thrombi, aneurysms or traumatic damage. The maternal surface of the placenta is then examined and an attempt should be made to lift off any adherent blood clot; if this can be removed, particular attention should be paid to whether or not this has caused an indentation of the surface. The only other lesion that may be apparent on inspection of the maternal surface is heavy calcification.

I do not usually measure the diameter or thickness of the placenta as I think that the results obtained are of little value, finding it sufficient simply to indicate if the placenta appears to be unusually small or unduly bulky. For reasons which are discussed in Appendix 2, I do not weigh the placenta.

Further examination of the placenta requires that it be cut up, and the common practice of making a few random slicing cuts with a knife is quite inadequate. The entire placenta should be cut into vertical strips, each of about 0.5 cm thickness; I find a bacon slicer admirable for this purpose though a sharp knife will suffice if this invaluable aid is not available. The placental strips are then laid out in order and all visible abnormalities and lesions noted. In theory, all visible lesions should be examined histologically, but I see little point in subjecting to microscopic study those lesions that can be readily and specifically identified on naked-eye examination, e.g., septal cysts, intervillous thrombi and subchorionic fibrin plaques. It should be emphasized, however, that it is often extremely difficult to distinguish plaques of perivillous fibrin from old infarcts unless histological examination is performed, and that only if all areas of undue pallor are studied histologically will the diagnosis of fetal artery thrombosis be made with any degree of certainty.

In addition to taking sections from those lesions whose nature is not obvious on naked-eye examination, it is of importance to choose blocks of macroscopically normal placental tissue for microscopic examination. These require considerable care in their selection because the villous appearances in different areas of the placenta are not constant but vary from the centre to the periphery of the organ and from the fetal to the maternal surface (Fox, 1964): the potential hazards introduced by this morphological variability can only be overcome by taking blocks from standard areas of the placenta. I recommend taking four placental slices from the area between the lines CD and EF in Fig. A1.1 and then cutting a full-thickness block of tissue, from fetal to maternal surface, from the central area of each slice, i.e. from the area 'A' in Fig. A1.2. Sections from each of these blocks are cut and stained, and for general purposes I use a haematoxylin and eosin stain, a PAS stain and a trichrome stain for each section, these being, in my opinion, the most useful for routine practice. A haematoxylin and eosin stain is clearly desirable and will, in itself, suffice for the study of most histological abnormalities of the placental tissue, but a PAS stain is useful for the study of trophoblastic basement membrane changes, whilst a trichrome stain is necessary for the evaluation of stromal fibrosis.

In each block attention should be paid to the villi, the fetal arteries, the chorionic plate and the basal plate. When examining the villi, the variability of their appearance in the vertical plane from fetal to maternal surface must be borne in mind, and I assess villous changes and abnormalities by studying only those villi in the maternal zone of each block (Fig A1.3). This zone is not chosen in a purely arbitrary fashion but is selected because it is probably the area in the placenta where maximal gas transfer between mother and fetus takes place, where villous density is greatest and where the villi appear optimally adapted for transfer purposes. As a first step in examining the villi it is necessary to estimate their maturity and note their vascularity. Attention should then be paid to the number of syncytial knots, vasculo-syncytial membranes and

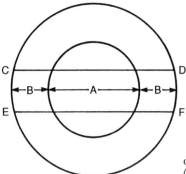

Figure A1.1. Diagrammatic representation of the surface of the placenta; this is divided into central (A) and peripheral (B) zones.

Figure A1.2. Diagrammatic representation of a vertical strip of placenta taken from the area lying between the lines CD and EF in Fig. A1.1. The strip is divided into central (A) and peripheral (B) zones which correspond to those shown in Fig. A1.1.

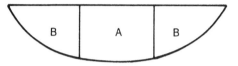

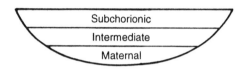

Figure A1.3. Diagrammatic representation of a vertical strip of placenta taken from the area lying between the lines CD and EF in Fig. A1.1. The strip is divided in the vertical plane into subchorionic, intermediate and maternal (or basal) zones.

villous cytotrophoblastic cells, and the thickness of the trophoblastic basement membrane should be noted. In many instances it may be possible to assess these villous changes quite subjectively, insofar as a scan of the tissue will show, for example, that there is clearly no excess of syncytial knots. In some cases, however, it may be felt that a more objective and quantitative result is required, and under these circumstances I count 100 villi in the maternal zone of each of the four blocks and express the final result as a percentage, e.g., syncytial knots on 9% of the villi. The villous stroma is then examined for fibrosis or oedema and any excess of Hofbauer cells noted; evidence of villous inflammation should also be sought. The proportion of villi showing partial or complete fibrinoid necrosis is noted, and any excess of nucleated red blood cells in the fetal villous vessels is recorded.

The fetal stem arteries in each section are examined, and note is taken of any abnormality such as thrombosis or 'obliterative endarteritis'. The basal plate is studied for evidence of necrosis; if any maternal vessels are present in scraps of decidua attached to the plate, careful note should be taken of their structure and condition. The chorionic plate is examined and the presence or otherwise of polymorphonuclear leucocytes in the plate itself or in the subchorionic layer of fibrin is recorded; the condition of the fetal vessels in the chorionic plate is assessed and the condition of the overlying amnion noted.

Included in the histological study of the placenta will also be, of course, the sections taken from the cord and from the extraplacental membranes.

Twin placentas require a special technique of examination and this is outlined in Chapter 4.

REFERENCES

Benirschke, K. (1961) Examination of the placenta. *Obstetrics and Gynecology*, **18,** 309–332.
Benirschke, K. and Kaufmann, P. (1995) *Pathology of the Human Placenta*, 3rd edn. New York: Springer-Verlag.
Fox, H. (1964) The pattern of villous variability in the normal placenta. *Journal of Obstetrics and Gynaecology of the British Commonwealth*, **71,** 749–758.

PLACENTAL WEIGHT

The weighing of the placenta in the delivery room is part of the time-honoured ritual of childbirth and is also considered to be an integral and important aspect of the pathological examination of the placenta. However, it would not be unfair to say that most who make these genuflections towards the altar of supposed scientific measurement rarely pause to consider either the accuracy or the value of this procedure.

Simply weighing the placenta is obviously not a very demanding task, but it is a matter of the greatest difficulty to obtain a true estimate of placental tissue mass. There is, first, no standard technique for weighing the placenta, either in the delivery room or in the laboratory; some weigh the organ with membranes and cord attached and without removing any adherent maternal clot, others remove either the membranes and cord or adherent clot but not both, whilst yet others trim off the membranes, cut off the cord and remove any clot. However, even if a standard technique of weighing the placenta is used, the amount of blood trapped within the placenta represents an often unconsidered variable. Some maternal blood usually remains in the intervillous space, and in a placenta with a weight of 500 g the entrapped maternal blood can account for between 50 and 100 g (Rosa & de Blieck, 1957). Even more importantly, fetal blood is also trapped within the placenta, and the amount of this is dependent, to some extent, upon the technique used for clamping the cord after delivery; if the cord is clamped immediately after the child is born, almost one-third of the infant's blood volume will be trapped in the placenta, but if clamping is delayed for 3 minutes and the placenta allowed to drain by gravity, the proportion of the fetal blood volume remaining in the placenta falls to less than 15% (Yao et al, 1969). However, even if maximal drainage of fetal blood from the placenta is allowed, the residual fetal blood content of the placenta is extremely variable and ranges from 25 to 270 g (Garrow & Hawes, 1971). This factor cannot be controlled or corrected for, and it can only be overcome by embarking on the rather tedious procedure of estimating the blood-free placental weight.

These particular difficulties apply to estimating the weight in both the delivery room and the laboratory, but the pathologist has to face still further complications, because he or she rarely receives the placenta until some, or many, hours after the child is delivered. It has been shown by Lemtis and Hadrich (1974) that the stored placenta loses 4% of its weight in 12 hours, 6% in 24 hours, and 10% in 48 hours. It might be thought that this particular factor could be overcome by fixing the placenta soon after delivery, but my own observations have shown that fixation of this organ produces weight changes of an unpredictable type and degree and makes invalid any attempt to obtain a reasonably accurate estimate of placental weight.

All these uncontrolled factors make weighing the placenta an exercise fraught with hazards, and it is perhaps not surprising that, in 10 large series published in relatively recent years, the suggested figure of the 'normal' placental weight at term has ranged from 430 to 650 g (Garrow, 1970). It is often thought that figures obtained within any individual institution or centre can be compared with each other because the factor, or factors, altering the true placental mass will be the same in each case and will remain constant; however, this is not true, because there is no simple way in which the quantity of fetal blood remaining within the placenta after drainage can either be estimated or controlled, and this represents neither a fixed amount nor a standard proportion of the placental mass, but varies widely for no obvious reason.

Even if a true estimate of placental mass could be obtained, would this information be of any real value? In general terms the placental weight is related to the birth weight of the fetus and simply to know the placental weight is of no importance, it having been long recognized that only the placental/fetal weight ratio is likely to provide any useful information. The rather voluminous literature on this topic has been reviewed by, amongst others, Little (1960), Gruenwald and Minh (1961), Thomson et al (1969) and Nummi (1972), and their general conclusion has been that it is exceedingly difficult to draw useful conclusions from placental/fetal weight ratios and that these correlate poorly with maternal or fetal complications. Little (1960) commented that 'to consider the placental coefficient, per se, as a measure of placental sufficiency or reserve would be a naive view', whilst Thomson et al (1969) concluded that 'weight is a poor indicator of placental adequacy'.

Such conclusions will only appear unjustified to those who fail to consider placental weight in a clear and logical fashion, and who tend to argue that, as small babies usually have small placentas, the baby is small *because* the placenta is small. This, as Gruenwald (1975) has commented, implies that fetal weight is narrowly limited by placental size and that the placenta is therefore functioning at the full stretch of its functional capacity during a normal pregnancy, an assumption that is demonstrably untrue. Indeed, the reverse is almost certainly the case, and when the fetus is small the placenta, being a fetal organ, shares in the generally diminished growth of the fetus; the small placenta, just as the small fetal liver, is a manifestation rather than a cause of poor fetal growth.

In many complicated pregnancies the placental/fetal weight ratio is actually increased and this indicates that in the face of an unfavourable maternal environment, such as in pre-eclampsia, heavy maternal cigarette smoking, severe maternal anaemia, high altitude pregnancy or maternal heart disease, the placenta undergoes some degree of compensatory hypertrophy in an attempt to overcome the baleful influence of the unhealthy maternal milieu. This being the case, it is not surprising that Nummi (1972) found a high placental/fetal weight ratio to be associated with an increased perinatal mortality because the cause of this increased fetal and neonatal demise is the factor, or factors, which also induces placental compensatory hypertrophy. The increased weight ratio is irrelevant except as an indication of the efforts of the placenta to overcome the ill-effects of the unfavourable situation in which both the placenta and the fetus are placed.

It will be seen, therefore, that the techniques for estimating placental weight are riddled with inaccuracies and that the results obtained are of little value; this being the case, I see no reason why the practice of routinely weighing the placenta should be continued.

REFERENCES

Garrow, J.S. (1970) The relationship of fetal growth to size and composition of the placenta. *Proceedings of the Royal Society of Medicine*, **63**, 498–500.

Garrow, J.S. and Hawes, S.F. (1971) The relationship of the size and composition of the human placenta to its functional capacity. *Journal of Obstetrics and Gynaecology of the British Commonwealth*, **78**, 22–28.

Gruenwald, P. (1975) The supply line of the fetus: definitions relating to fetal growth. In *The Placenta and its Maternal Supply Line*, Gruenwald, P. (Ed.), pp. 1–17. Lancaster: Medical and Technical Publishing.

Gruenwald, P. and Minh, H.N. (1961) Evaluation of body and organ weights in perinatal pathology. II. Weight of body and placenta of surviving and of autopsied infants. *American Journal of Obstetrics and Gynecology*, **82**, 312.

Lemtis, H. and Hadrich, G. (1974) Uber die Gewichtsabnahme des Mutterkuchens nach der Geburt und die Bedeutung für den Quotienten aus Plazenta- und Kindsgewicht. *Geburtshilfe und Frauenheilkunde*, **34**, 618–622.

Little, W.A. (1960) The significance of placental/fetal weight ratios. *American Journal of Obstetrics and Gynecology*, **79**, 134–137.

Nummi, S. (1972) Relative weight of the placenta and perinatal mortality: a retrospective clinical and statistical analysis. *Acta Obstetrica et Gynecologica Scandinavica*, Supplement **17**, 1–69.

Rosa, P. and de Blieck, J. (1957) Mesure de la quantité de sang foetal et maternal dans le placenta expulsé. *Bulletin de la Société Belge de Gynécologie et d'Obstétrique*, **27**, 386–392.

Thomson, A.M., Billewicz, W.Z. and Hytten, F.E. (1969) The weight of the placenta in relation to birthweight. *Journal of Obstetrics and Gynaecology of the British Commonwealth*, **76**, 865–872.

Yao, A.C., Moinian, M. and Lind, J. (1969) Distribution of blood between infant and placenta after birth. *Lancet*, **ii**, 871–873.

ADDENDUM

The above was written for the first edition of this book and nothing that has occurred or has been written in the intervening 18 years has caused me to change my views about the value of weighing the placenta. I am quite happy to describe placentas as being of 'average size' or as 'small' whilst I would describe those placentas that probably weigh over 600 g as 'large': I would reserve the term 'unduly bulky' for hydropic placentas. These are, of course, imprecise terms but they nevertheless convey a general impression of placental size just as much as terms such as 'average height', 'short' and 'tall' convey a widely understood impression of height when describing human beings. Certainly any imprecision in the terms I use to describe placentas is more than matched by the imprecision of weighing the placenta.

PLACENTAL BIOPSY

The technique of villous sampling of the early placenta to obtain information about fetal genetic or metabolic abnormalities is, of course, now well established. A much more contentious topic is biopsy of the third-trimester placenta in order to obtain placental tissue for the diagnosis of placental abnormalities. A technique of transabdominal needle biopsy of the placenta was described by Alvarez (1966, 1968) and Aladjem (1969); the villi thus obtained were examined in the fresh state by phase contrast microscopy. This technique was used, to some extent, by workers in Germany (Werner, 1971; Gerl et al, 1973) and Japan (Yoshida et al, 1974) and although Coles (1971) considered placental biopsy to be potentially dangerous, Aladjem (1969) performed 215 placental biopsies without any apparent maternal or fetal complications and obtained villous tissue in 40% of the patients biopsied.

It appears, therefore, that placental biopsy may, in experienced hands, be a reasonably safe procedure; however, it is difficult to accept that the tissue obtained is representative of the organ as a whole, because, as pointed out in Chapter 1, the villi vary morphologically not only within the placenta as a whole, from maternal to fetal surface and from the central to peripheral areas, but also within individual lobules. Coles (1971) and Carceller Blay and Palacin Forgue (1972) have investigated the sampling error in placentas from both normal and complicated pregnancies with particular reference to the potential use of placental biopsy. They concluded that arbitrarily chosen fragments of tissue fail to give a representative picture of villous morphology in the placenta as a whole.

Despite the above findings, a plea for the value of placental biopsy has recently re-emerged after a gap of nearly a quarter of a century during which interest in this topic has been dormant and was indeed thought to be extinct (Kliman et al, 1995). In a study of needle biopsies of delivered placentas it was found that two diagnoses were seen commonly enough and had enough positive predictive value to be potentially useful clinically, these being villous oedema and an increased number of syncytial knots. As discussed in the main text of this volume, the diagnosis of villous oedema is highly subjective whilst the clinical significance of finding villous oedema is uncertain: the significance of an excess number of syncytial knots is also a matter for some debate. I would therefore hesitate to subscribe to the view that placental biopsy is a reasonably sensitive technique for diagnosing villous abnormalities that reflect acute and chronic stresses in the placenta and I find it difficult to envisage a role for placental biopsy.

REFERENCES

Aladjem, S. (1969) Fetal assessment through biopsy of the human placenta. In *The Foeto-Placental Unit*, Pecile, A. and Finzi, C. (Eds), pp. 392–402. Amsterdam: Excerpta Medica.
Alvarez, H. (1966) Diagnosis of hydatidiform mole by transabdominal placental biopsy. *American Journal of Obstetrics and Gynecology*, **95**, 538–541.

Alvarez, H. (1968) Placental biopsy: results, limitations and topographic differences. In *Diagnosis and Treatment of Fetal Disorders*, Adamsons, K. (Ed.), pp. 50–71. New York: Springer-Verlag.

Carceller Blay, C. and Palacin Forgue, A. (1972) Morfologia placentaria en il parto prematuro y en il crecimento fetal retardo. *Revista Espagnola de Obstetricia y Ginecologica*, **31**, 394–402.

Coles, R.A. (1971) Phase contrast microscopy of the placenta. *American Journal of Obstetrics and Gynecology*, **111**, 369–373.

Gerl, D., Kadner, J., Ehrhardt, G., Estel, C. and Kreuziger, K.P. (1973) Ein Beitrag zur Plazentabiopsie. *Zentralblatt für Gynäkologie*, **95**, 259–262.

Kliman, H.J., Perrotta, P.L. and Jones, D.C. (1995) The efficacy of placental biopsy. *American Journal of Obstetrics and Gynecology*, **173**, 1084–1088.

Werner, C. (1971) Methodik und Wert der Phasenkontrastmikroskopie für die Plazentadiagnostik. *Geburtshilfe und Frauenheilkunde*, **31**, 575–581.

Yoshida, K., Soma, H., Hiraoka, M. and Kiyokawa, T. (1974) Evaluation of placental dysfunction through phase contrast microscopy. In *Proceedings of the 6th Asian Congress of Obstetrics and Gynaecology, Kuala Lumpur, Malaysia*, pp. 241–243.

MEDICO-LEGAL ASPECTS OF PLACENTAL PATHOLOGY

A few decades ago the placenta was rarely, if ever, a subject for discussion in the courts, but today it occupies an almost pivotal position in obstetric litigation.

The principal scenario in which the placenta plays such a star role is commonly a case of either perinatal death or cerebral palsy in which it is maintained that the adverse fetal outcome was the result of negligence on the part of the attending obstetrician, usually during labour and delivery. The defence will then attempt to counter this claim by making one, or more, of the following counterclaims:

1. That examination of the placenta yields evidence of chronic or acute 'stress' which not only antedated the onset of labour but was possibly responsible for the unfortunate outcome of the pregnancy.
2. That there are lesions present in the placenta which, in themselves, could have been responsible for the adverse fetal outcome.
3. That placental examination yields evidence of fetal hypoxia of sufficient duration to have predated the onset of labour.

The pathologist called upon to examine a placenta in such circumstances should proceed with the utmost prudence and should bear in mind that very often the cause of fetal hypoxia or intrapartum death is completely unknown and that our understanding of the pathogenesis of cerebral palsy is, at best, fragmentary.

Quite clearly in some cases a lesion of the placenta or cord will be present that is of considerable importance, such as placental floor infarction, a large chorangioma, a stricture of the cord or very extensive thrombosis of fetal intraplacental vessels. Such a finding is, however, the exception rather than the rule and in the absence of such a lesion the pathologist should be extremely cautious in the assessment of the significance of such findings as villitis, villous oedema or chorioamnionitis; the evidence that any of these findings either cause or reflect fetal stress is unconvincing.

The most important cause of chronic fetal hypoxia is chronic uteroplacental ischaemia and the principal morphological hallmark of such ischaemia is an undue number and prominence of villous cytotrophoblastic cells. A secondary result of uteroplacental ischaemia is vasoconstriction of the fetal vessels with resultant 'endarteritis obliterans' of the fetal stem arteries, diminished villous perfusion and increased syncytial knot formation. Such findings allow the pathologist to infer that there has been chronic uteroplacental ischaemia, the most probable cause of which is inadequate conversion of spiral arteries into uteroplacental vessels during the process of placentation. However, it is very important to note that the vast majority of infants whose placentas show these changes are fully healthy and there is certainly no clear association between these changes and cerebral palsy.

The pathologist is often pressed to say if there is evidence of fetal hypoxia and, if so, how long such hypoxia has been present, the aim being, of course, to establish that the duration of fetal hypoxia is such as to antedate labour and delivery. In this respect emphasis is often placed upon the presence of meconium and of nucleated fetal red blood cells. In the past the passage of meconium was usually thought to be indicative of fetal hypoxia but, as discussed in the main body of this text, the validity of this view has been progressively questioned and it would now be unwise to maintain that the presence of meconium in the placental tissues is indicative of there having been fetal hypoxia. The reality of the situation is that, in our present state of knowledge, no inference as to the well-being or otherwise of the fetus can be drawn from the mere presence of meconium in the placental tissues.

The presence of nucleated red blood cells in the fetal vessels of the placenta is, however, of greater import. In 1967 I published a paper showing that an excess of nucleated erythrocytes in the fetal blood in the placental vessels (defined as being more than one nucleated cell per 1000 red cells) was indicative of fetal hypoxia (Fox, 1967). I received no reprint requests for this paper and during the next 20 years it was never cited (not even by myself). In the mid-1980s this paper was, however, rescued from its total obscurity by those interested in diagnosing fetal hypoxia by placental examination and it has now become widely accepted, not just on the basis of my own paper but also of many other studies, that in the absence of factors such as haemolytic anemia, feto-maternal haemorrhage or fetal infection, the presence of easily detectable nucleated fetal red cells is a good indication that the fetus has been subjected to hypoxia. Within the medico-legal context the problem then arises, however, as to whether one can tell from the presence of nucleated red blood cells if the hypoxia is of long-standing duration, i.e. antedates labour, or is of recent onset. In very general terms the increase in nucleated erythrocytes is due to increased fetal production of erythropoietin and it is probable that it takes several days for erythropoietin levels to rise and exert their effect on fetal erythropoiesis. I have, however, seen an excess of intraplacental fetal nucleated red cells in cases in which it was known that an episode of fetal hypoxia occurred 1–2 hours before delivery and Benirschke (1994) has recorded a case in which nucleated erythrocytes were found in neonatal blood within 1 hour of an acute fetal blood loss. It is possible, therefore, that there is a population of nucleated red cells sequestrated in the liver and spleen which can be almost immediately released into the circulation if the fetus is subjected to acute hypoxia. In my opinion the finding of nucleated fetal red cells does not, therefore, permit the pathologist to give any view as to the duration of the fetal hypoxia or about the temporal relationship between an episode of fetal hypoxia and birth.

I am certain that many of the opinions expressed here will be regarded as unduly negative in some circles: my own view would be that they are cautious but realistic.

REFERENCES

Benirschke, K. (1994) Placenta pathology questions to the perinatologist. *Journal of Perinatology*, **14,** 371–375.

Fox H. (1967) The incidence and significance of nucleated erythrocytes in the foetal vessels of the mature human placenta. *Journal of Obstetrics and Gynaecology of the British Commonwealth*, **74,** 40–43.

INDEX

Page references in **bold** denote main entries